Illustrated Tips and Tricks in

Hip and Knee Reconstructive and Replacement Surgery

Illustrated Tips and Tricks in

Hip and Knee Reconstructive and Replacement Surgery

Daniel J. Berry

L.Z. Gund Professor of Orthopedic Surgery
Chairman, Emeritus
Department of Orthopedic Surgery
Mayo Clinic
Rochester, Minnesota

Mark W. Pagnano

Professor and Chairman
Department of Orthopedic Surgery
Mayo Clinic
Rochester, Minnesota

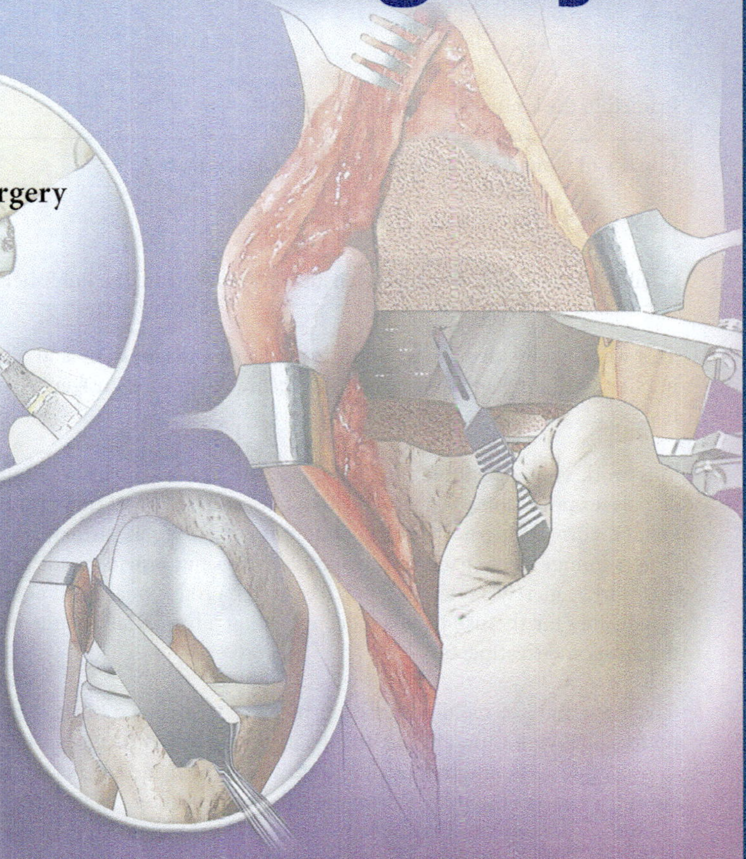

Wolters Kluwer

Philadelphia • Baltimore • New York • London
Buenos Aires • Hong Kong • Sydney • Tokyo

Acquisitions Editor: Brian Brown
Development Editor: Sean McGuire
Editorial Coordinator: Jeremiah Kiely
Marketing Manager: Julie Sikora
Production Project Manager: Barton Dudlick
Design Coordinator: Holly McLaughlin
Artist/Illustrator: Jen Clements
Manufacturing Coordinator: Beth Welsh
Prepress Vendor: TNQ Technologies

9 8 7 6 5 4 3

Printed in the United States of America

Library of Congress Cataloging-in-Publication Data

ISBN-13: 978-1-4963-9206-0

Cataloging-in-Publication data available on request from the Publisher.

---

shop.lww.com

MPP0625

This book is dedicated to our colleagues and mentors at Mayo Clinic with whom we have shared the opportunity to deliver outstanding patient care, conduct research that improves patient's lives, and educate residents, fellows, and practicing orthopedic surgeons acrcss the world. We hope that the accumulated insights from this book prove valuable to hip and knee surgeons and make a difference in the surgical care of patients.

Foreword

The field of hip and knee arthroplasty has undergone remarkable growth and maturation over the last five decades. Hip and knee replacements are now among the most successful major operations ever devised. For the surgeon performing these operations there are 4 pillars of success: appropriate patient selection, good clinical judgment and compassionate perioperative care, choice of successful implants, and finally—and very importantly—optimal choice and application of surgical techniques. This book focuses primarily on the last pillar—surgical technique.

The senior authors of the chapters in this book are all members of the Mayo Clinic Department of Orthopedic Surgery. The "tips and tricks" described in this book represent our collective, accumulated knowledge about how to most successfully execute each procedure. Our approaches come from many sources: our mentors during training (some from the Mayo Clinic, some from other institutions), our North American and international arthroplasty colleagues, and the personal experience (usually positive, occasionally negative) gained collectively from performing tens of thousands of primary and revision hip and knee replacements. The experience of surgeons in our department was developed not only by a large volume of joint replacement surgery but also by a high level of case complexity. Equally important, our department members pride themselves on evolving operative techniques collaboratively, exchanging ideas and information about what works and what does not. And we try to tether our subjective beliefs to rigorous, objective evaluation of short- and long-term results, documented in our unique resource, the Mayo Clinic Joint Registry, and reported in the peer reviewed literature. Because the book comes from one orthopedic department, it provides a coherent approach to many challenges, but the reader should recognize there are many ways "to skin the cat" and this book does not attempt to describe every technique ever devised.

As this book was envisioned, written, and edited, we tried to focus on essential aspects of each operation and on the practical, and sometimes subtle, technical points of hip and knee arthroplasty. We hope this book will allow the user to perform these operations more successfully, more easily, more efficiently, and with fewer complications.

Acknowledgments

We offer our sincere gratitude to the outstanding knee and hip surgeons who have shared their wisdom, technical tips, and decision-making insight in this volume.

We recognize the strong work of the publisher and staff, including Brian Brown, Jeremiah Kiely, and Sean McGuire. Furthermore, we would like to thank Ms. Karen Fasbender for her outstanding work and administrative support as this book was developed.

Finally, we offer our sincere appreciation to each of our families for the incredible support they have provided throughout our careers as we recognize that we could not have accomplished what we have without them.

Contributors

Matthew P. Abdel, MD
Professor
Department of Orthopedic Surgery
Mayo Clinic
Rochester, Minnesota

Timothy B. Alton, MD
Previous Adult Reconstruction Fellow
Department of Orthopedic Surgery
Mayo Clinic
Rochester, Minnesota;
Currently Proliance Orthopedic Associates
Renton, Washington

Nicholas A. Bedard, MD
Adult Reconstruction Fellow
Department of Orthopedic Surgery
Mayo Clinic
Rochester, Minnesota

Daniel J. Berry, MD
L.Z. Gund Professor of Orthopedic Surgery
Chairman, Emeritus
Department of Orthopedic Surgery
Mayo Clinic
Rochester, Minnesota

Joshua S. Bingham, MD
Assistant Professor
Department of Orthopedic Surgery
Mayo Clinic
Scottsdale, Arizona

Timothy S. Brown, MD
Previous Adult Reconstruction Fellow
Department of Orthopedic Surgery
Mayo Clinic
Rochester, Minnesota;
Currently Assistant Professor
Department of Orthopedics and Rehabilitation
University of Iowa Hospitals and Clinics
Iowa City, Iowa

Brian P. Chalmers, MD
Orthopedic Surgery Resident
Department of Orthopedic Surgery
Mayo Clinic
Rochester, Minnesota

Cory G. Couch, MD
Adult Reconstruction Fellow
Department of Orthopedic Surgery
Mayo Clinic
Rochester, Minnesota

Diane L. Dahm, MD
Professor
Department of Orthopedic Surgery
Mayo Clinic
Rochester, Minnesota

Ashton H. Goldman, MD, LCDR, MC, USN
Previous Adult Reconstruction Fellow
Department of Orthopedic Surgery
Mayo Clinic
Rochester, Minnesota;
Currently Assistant Professor in Orthopaedic Surgery
Department of Surgery
Uniformed Services University of Health Sciences
Portsmouth, Virginia

Arlen D. Hanssen, MD
Professor, Emeritus
Department of Orthopedic Surgery
Mayo Clinic
Rochester, Minnesota

Adam Hart, MD
Previous Adult Reconstruction Fellow
Department of Orthopedic Surgery
Mayo Clinic
Rochester, Minnesota;
Currently Assistant Professor
McGill University
Montreal, Quebec, Canada

Nicholas M. Hernandez, MD
Orthopedic Surgery Resident
Department of Orthopedic Surgery
Mayo Clinic
Rochester, Minnesota

David G. Lewallen, MD
Professor
Department of Orthopedic Surgery
Mayo Clinic
Rochester, Minnesota

Tad M. Mabry, MD
Associate Professor
Department of Orthopedic Surgery
Mayo Clinic
Rochester, Minnesota

R. Kyle Martin, MD, FRCSC
Adult Reconstruction Fellow
Department of Orthopedic Surgery
Mayo Clinic
Rochester, Minnesota

Kapil Mehrotra, MD
Previous Orthopedic Surgery Resident
Department of Orthopedic Surgery
Mayo Clinic
Rochester, Minnesota;
Currently Fellow
Hospital for Special Surgery
New York, New York

Heath P. Melugin, MD
Orthopedic Surgery Resident
Department of Orthopedic Surgery
Mayo Clinic
Rochester, Minnesota

Mark W. Pagnano, MD
Professor and Chairman
Department of Orthopedic Surgery
Mayo Clinic
Rochester, Minnesota

Graham D. Pallante, MD
Orthopedic Surgery Resident
Department of Orthopedic Surgery
Mayo Clinic
Rochester, Minnesota

Kevin I. Perry, MD
Assistant Professor
Department of Orthopedic Surgery
Mayo Clinic
Rochester, Minnesota

Stephen M. Petis, MD, MSc, FRCSC
Previous Adult Reconstruction Fellow
Department of Orthopedic Surgery
Mayo Clinic
Rochester, Minnesota;
Currently Department of Orthopaedic Surgery
Woodstock General Hospital
Woodstock, Ontario, Canada

Rafael J. Sierra, MD
Professor
Department of Orthopedic Surgery
Mayo Clinic
Rochester, Minnesota

Joseph M. Statz, MD
Orthopedic Surgery Resident
Department of Orthopedic Surgery
Mayo Clinic
Rochester, Minnesota

Alan K. Sutak, MD
Previous Orthopedic Surgery Resident
Department of Orthopedic Surgery
Mayo Clinic
Rochester, Minnesota;
Currently Fellow
Duke University Medical Center
Department of Orthopedic Surgery
Durham, North Carolina

Michael J. Taunton, MD
Associate Professor
Department of Orthopedic Surgery
Mayo Clinic
Rochester, Minnesota

Matthew W. Tetreault, MD
Adult Reconstruction Fellow
Department of Orthopedic Surgery
Mayo Clinic
Rochester, Minnesota

Robert T. Trousdale, MD
Professor
Department of Orthopedic Surgery
Mayo Clinic
Rochester, Minnesota

Brandon J. Yuan, MD
Assistant Professor
Department of Orthopedic Surgery
Mayo Clinic
Rochester, Minnesota

Table of Contents

Part II Revision Total Hip Arthroplasty

Section A Preoperative Planning/Templating for Revision THA

Section B Exposures and Implant Removal in Revision THA

Section C Revision THA Implants

Section D Revision THA Implants

Part III Primary Knee

Section A Preoperative Planning/Templating for Primary THA

Part I
Primary Total Hip Arthroplasty

Chapter 1
Preoperative Planning and Templating for Primary Total Hip Arthroplasty

TIMOTHY B. ALTON
DANIEL J. BERRY

Introduction

- Preoperative planning allows the surgeon to predict intraoperative needs and challenges and to work out an operative plan and to prepare for contingencies in advance of surgery. This, in turn, helps the surgeon execute the operation accurately and efficiently.
- Preoperative planning helps ensure the optimal instruments and implants will be available at surgery.
- Successful total hip arthroplasty (THA) requires precise positioning of femoral and acetabular components, appropriately sized for the patient's femoral and pelvic anatomy, to minimize complications and optimize biomechanical function and implant longevity. Preoperative planning and careful templating helps the surgeon accomplish optimal restoration of hip biomechanics.
- Digital templating allows fast, precise, calibrated measurements and digital storage in the electronic medical record for access and review at the time of surgery.

History

- Careful documentation of symptoms
  - Pain location, duration, alleviating and aggravating interventions, etc
- Prior non-operative treatment
  - Injections, physical therapy, weight loss, nonsteroidal anti-inflammatory drugs (NSAIDs), etc
- Detailed medical history to identify modifiable and nonmodifiable risk factors
  - Lumbar spine issues, hernias, diabetes, myocardial infarction, blood clots, patient or family clotting disorders, dental problems, etc
  - Send for preoperative medical clearance as indicated
- Detailed surgical history focused on the operative hip and limb
  - Prior arthroscopy, infections, osteotomies, trauma, etc

Physical Examination

- Observe patient standing and walking
  - Identify/document gait abnormalities, coronal plane deformities, foot drop, etc
- Examination of the operative hip
  - Leg length evaluation with detailed preoperative documentation of differences
    - Note scoliosis and pelvic tilt issues that can contribute to actual and perceived leg length discrepancies.

- Different methods exist to measure true and apparent leg length. The authors usually use apparent leg length measured in the supine position. However, when major deformities or contractures exist, true leg length measurement may be used. Blocks to test the leg length that levels the patient's pelvis and feels comfortable to the patient are helpful.
- Evaluate range of motion
  - Flexion, extension (can flex contralateral hip to isolate operative hip), internal and external rotation
- Careful examination and documentation of distal motor/sensory function
- Palpate for dorsalis pedis and posterior tibial pulses
- Careful examination of the skin for open sores and prior scars, plan accordingly.

Radiographs

- Three views
  - Standing AP pelvis, AP hip, and true lateral hip radiographs
    - When previous femoral trauma or deformity is present, make sure radiographs are available showing the entire femur that will be instrumented.
    - True lateral hip radiographs can be valuable in identifying predominantly anterior or posterior hip arthritis.
    - Note prior lumbar fusion and pelvic obliquity and plan accordingly.

Templating

Goals

- Restoration of "normal" biomechanics
  - Equalizing limb lengths and recognizing pre-operative discrepancies
  - Normalizing femoral offset to optimize abductor muscle function and hip joint stability
- Correct implant sizing
  - Decreases intraoperative fracture risk, streamlines implant inventory, and lessens risk of implant undersizing and component loosening
- Assess bone
  - Femur: assess morphology and bone quality and determine implant type and design and implant fixation type that will provide best fixation and restoration of hip biomechanics.
  - Femur: identify proximal femoral deformity.
  - Acetabulum: anticipate need for bone grafting (large cysts, protrusio deformity, acetabular dysplasia), and identify defects that may require special management.
  - Identify retained acetabular or femoral hardware that may require removal.

Steps

- Magnification (Figure 1.1)
  - Determine magnification of radiograph based on radiographic marker (Figure 1.2) or known dimension of retained implant (for example, the diameter of the femoral head from contralateral THA).
- Leg length (Figure 1.3)
  - Recognize pelvic orientation using fixed anatomic landmarks (teardrop, ischial tuberosity).
  - Draw a line from the inferior border of right teardrop to the inferior border of the left teardrop. Measure the vertical distance from this line to the superior border of the lesser trochanter of each femur and correct for magnification (Figure 1.3). The difference between the measurements from side to side represents the leg length discrepancy at the hip. Remember, notable hip flexion contracture on one side will alter this measurement and also this measurement does not take into account leg length discrepancy contributions from further down the femur or the leg nor does it take into account functional leg length discrepancies related to pelvic obliquity or other contractures or deformities.
- Acetabular component position (Figure 1.4)
  - Place digital template at an abduction angle of 40 to 45° relative to pelvic axis centered within the osseous confines of the acetabulum. Medial reference relative to Kohler's line; cranial and caudal position determined by teardrop and superior-lateral acetabular bone.
  - This will set the center of rotation (COR) of the acetabular component.

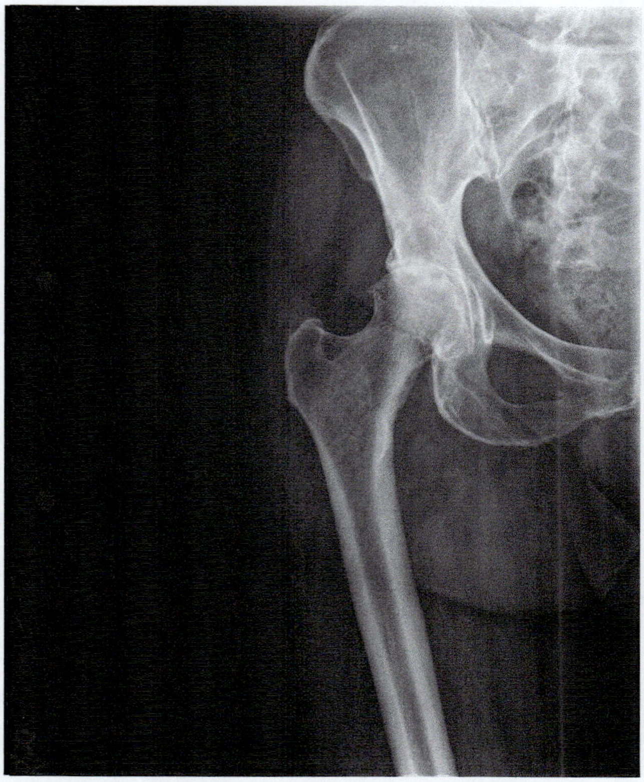

Figure 1.1 | Preoperative anteroposterior (AP) radiograph of the right hip shows advanced arthritis. Magnification standardization software shows multiple options for magnification correction.

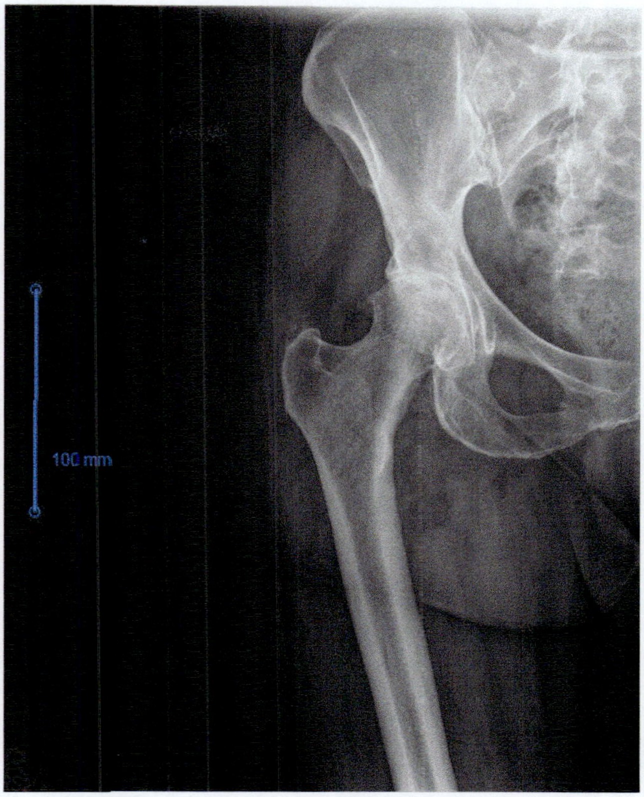

Figure 1.2 | Preoperative anteroposterior (AP) radiograph of the right hip showing magnification correction using radiographic markers of a known standard distance.

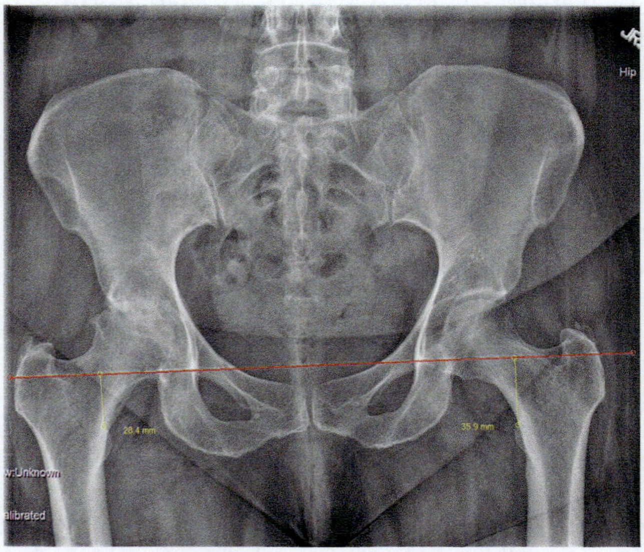

Figure 1.3 | Preoperative anteroposterior (AP) pelvis radiograph showing leg length evaluation with line drawn from the inferior teardrop on the right hemipelvis to the inferior teardrop on the left hemipelvis. The difference in vertical distance from this line to the superior border of the lesser trochanter between the left and right hips is calculated to determine leg length difference (35.9–28.4 = 7.5 mm).

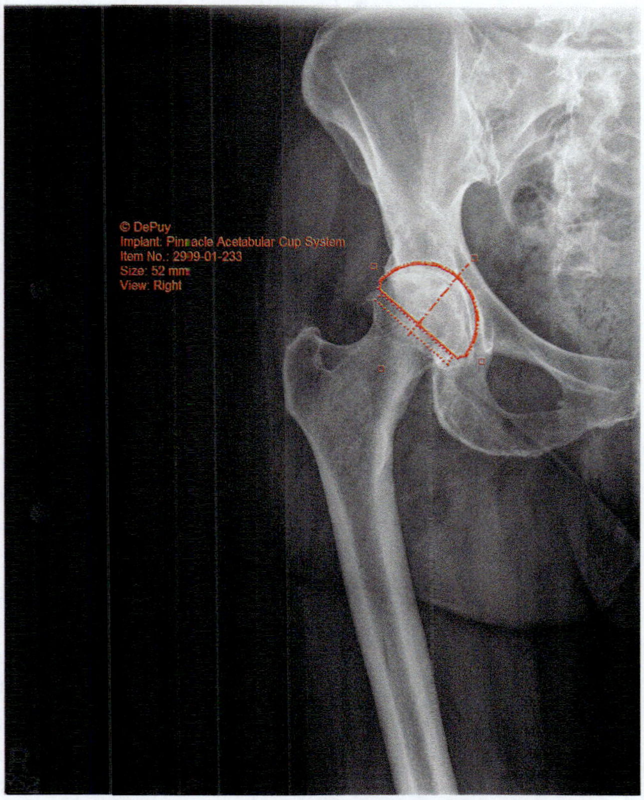

Figure 1.4 | Preoperative anteroposterior (AP) radiograph of the right hip shows templated position of the acetabular component after magnification correction.

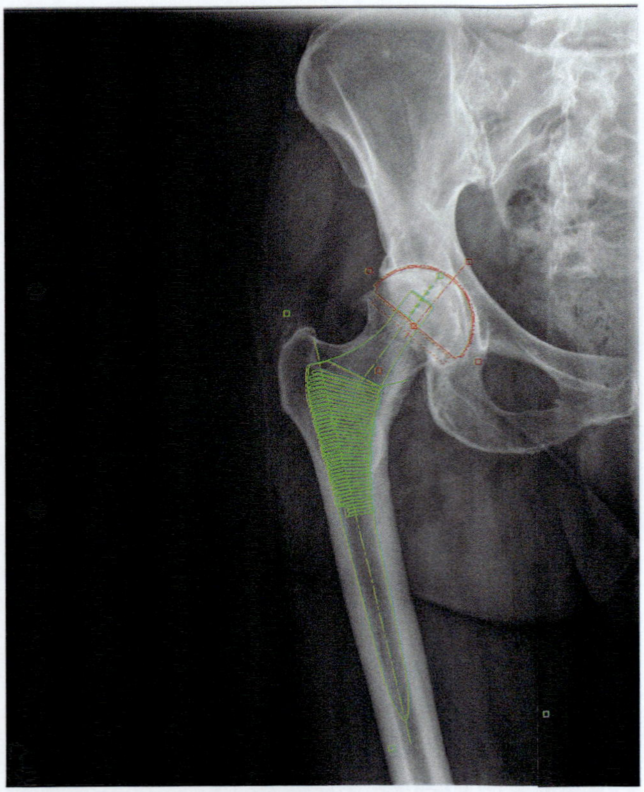

Figure 1.5 | Preoperative anteroposterior (AP) radiograph of the right hip shows templated position of the femoral component after magnification correction.

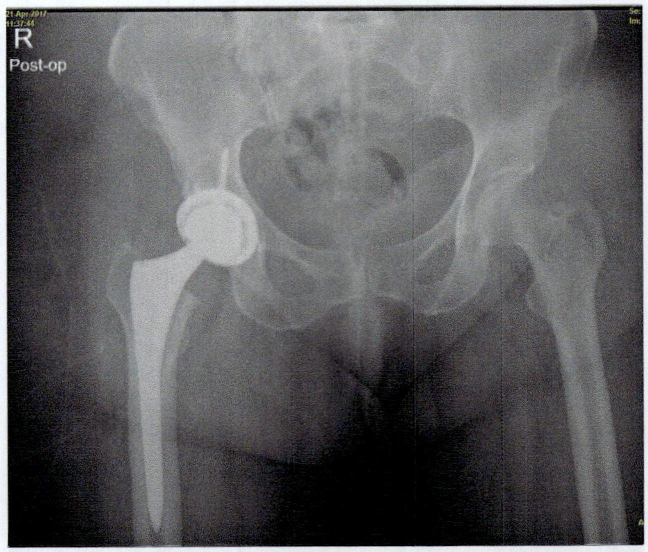

Figure 1.6 | Postoperative anteroposterior (AP) pelvis radiograph shows final position of femoral and acetabular components.

- Femoral component size (Figure 1.5)
  - Implant size is based on inner diameter of diaphyseal and metaphyseal bone; implant selection is based on fit of implant to confines of femoral anatomy.
    - Femoral deformity (trauma, prior surgery, dysplasia) may dictate implant selection.
    - Remember many arthritic hips have an external rotation contracture which can make the femoral metaphysis appear less broad from medial to lateral than it is in reality. Implant sizing may need to be adjusted accordingly. In extreme cases, templating the femoral component size based on the opposite undiseased hip may be helpful.
  - Implant offset selected to restore "normal" hip offset.
- Femoral component position (Figure 1.5)
  - Place template to optimize fit within proximal femur (as outlined above) and to restore leg length and offset.
    - The COR of the femoral component can now be compared with the COR of the acetabular component to determine the postreconstruction leg length and offset. For example, if the templated femoral COR is proximal to the acetabular COR, the leg length will be increased, and if the femoral COR is inferior to the acetabular COR, the leg length will be decreased. Likewise if the femoral COR is medial to the acetabular COR, the lateral offset of the hip will be increased, whereas if the femoral COR is lateral to the acetabular COR, the lateral offset of the hip will be decreased. Lateral offset of the hip is essentially equivalent to femoral offset of the hip, unless the hip COR changed by acetabular component placement.
    - Templating is an iterative process optimizing the femoral neck resection level, femoral implant size and offset, and planned modular femoral neck length to optimally reproduce hip biomechanics.
    - Remember that many arthritic hips have an external rotation contracture that will make the femoral offset appear less than it is in reality. One may compensate for this by measuring the femoral offset of the opposite hip if it is not diseased.
  - At this point, the appropriate-sized acetabular and femoral components are known as are the anticipated modular femoral head neck length, femoral head diameter, and femoral neck resection level needed to restore leg length and femoral offset. Radiographs after surgery ideally will closely match the preoperative plan (Figure 1.6).

Chapter 2
Posterior Approach

TIMOTHY S. BROWN
ROBERT T. TROUSDALE

Key Concepts

- Lateral positioning with patient rigidly immobilized at the pelvis is critical to prevent the pelvis from tilting which can lead to malposition of the acetabular component.
- Incision placement lateral over the trochanter, with approximately 2/3 distal and 1/3 proximal to the tip of the trochanter.
- Clean dissection of piriformis, short external rotators with capsule imperative for proper closure.
- Circumferential exposure of the acetabulum is obtained with several straight Hohmann retractors and the femur retracted anteriorly.
- Exposure of the femur is obtained with a wide Hohmann and a Mueller neck retractor.
- Good posterior capsular and muscular repair is a must to prevent problems with postoperative dislocation.

Sterile Instruments and Implants

- Two self-retaining cerebellar retractors
- Charnley retractor
- Five straight Hohmann retractors
- One wide Hohmann retractor
- One Mueller femoral neck retractor
- 6.0 mm round burr

Preoperative Planning

- Preoperative planning includes
  - Low anteroposterior (AP) pelvis radiograph for leg-length measurements and assessment of contralateral disease
  - AP hip and cross-table lateral of the hip for templating

Bone, Implant, and Soft Tissue Techniques

Introduction

The posterior approach to the hip has long been a standard surgical approach for primary and revision hip arthroplasty. With evolution of the miniposterior approach and the addition of a robust capsular repair, functional and clinical outcomes of the posterior approach for primary hip arthroplasty make it the most commonly used approach for total hip arthroplasty (THA) today.

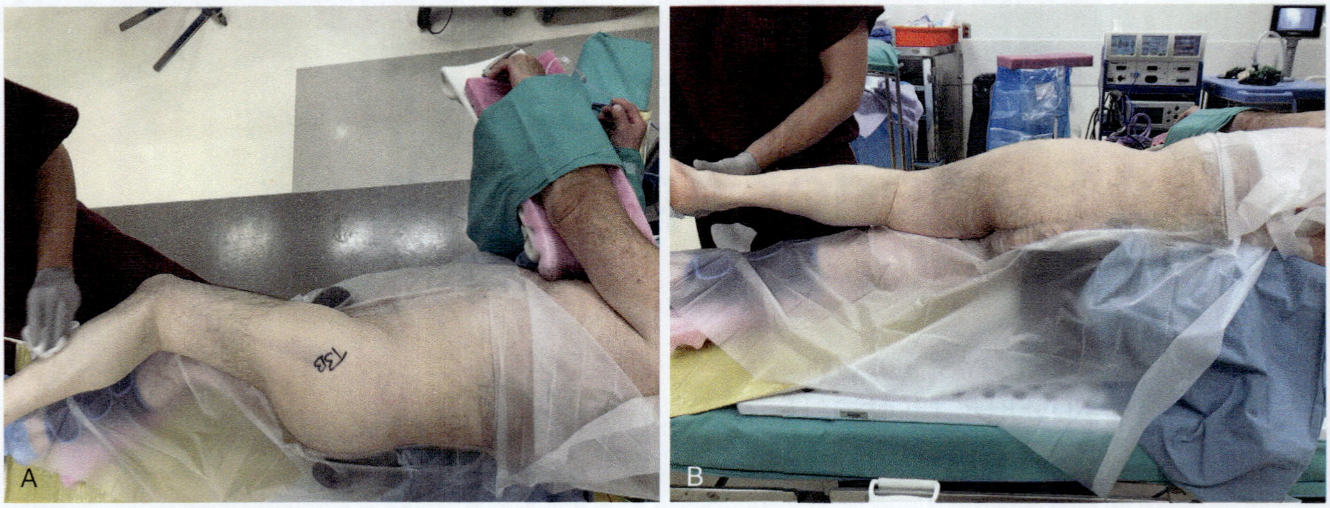

Figure 2.1 | A, B. Patient positioning in lateral decubitus position for the posterior approach.

Technique

Patient positioning (Figure 2.1A and B). Patient positioning in lateral decubitus position for the posterior approach.

- Feel leg-lengths before incision in the lateral position lining up the knees and lower leg.
- Skin incision (Figure 2.2).
  - Greater trochanter palpated with the hip in abduction and neutral rotation. The anterior superior iliac spine (ASIS) can be a reliable landmark in large patients. If the tip of the surgeon's long finger is placed on the ASIS and the hand placed orthogonal to the patient, the extended thumb will land close to the tip of the greater trochanter.
  - Incision directly lateral, centered on the greater trochanter.
  - Approximately 5 cm distal, 3 cm proximal angled 15° posterior-proximal to anterior-distal. Increase as needed for exposure.
- Fascial incision (Figure 2.3A and B). Incision through the fascia in line with the skin incision, curved posteriorly in line with the fibers of the gluteus maximus proximal.
  - Feel anterior soft spot in fascia at gluteus maximus insertion.
  - Start fascial incision there and follow skin incision.
  - Take care not to dive deep with the knife or cautery and injure the vastus lateralis or the gluteus medius.
  - Tag or mark fascia for accurate post-op repair.

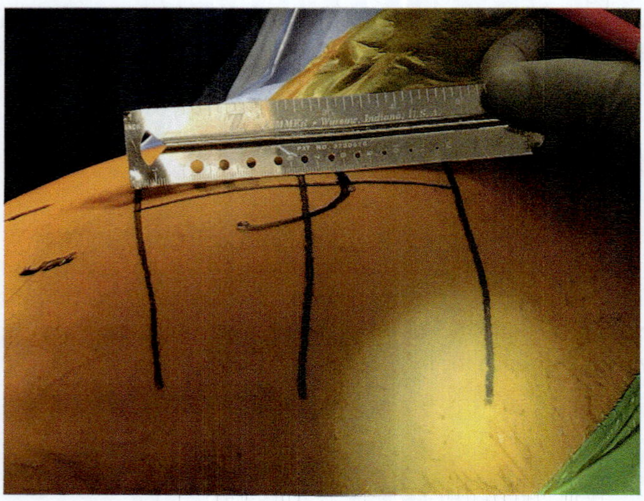

Figure 2.2 | Marking out the skin incision on the patient.

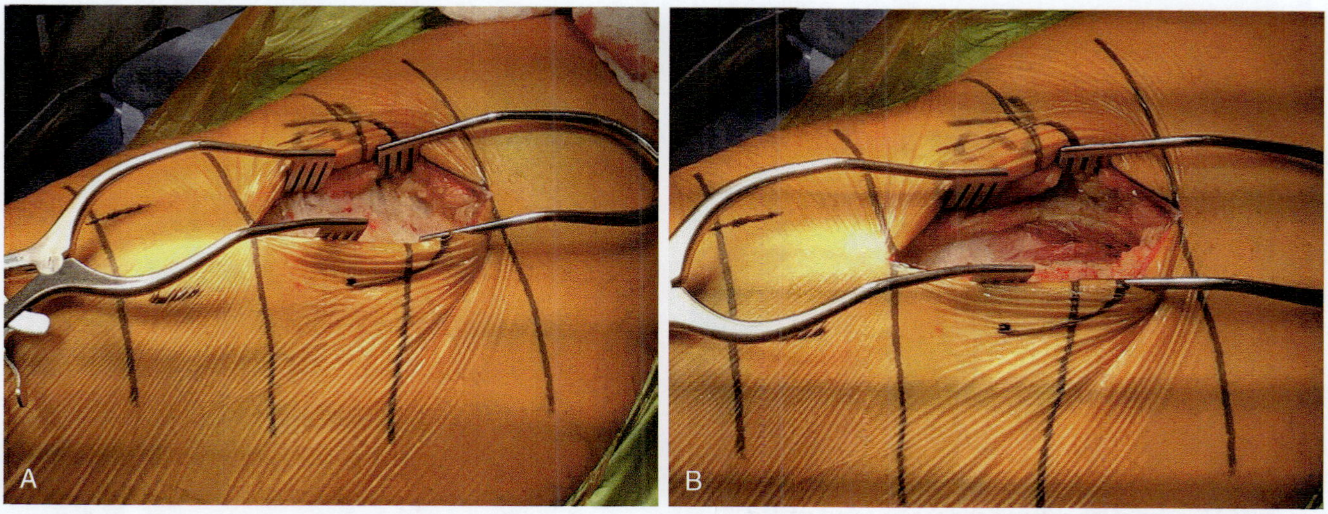

Figure 2.3 | A, B. Incision through the fascia in line with the skin incision, curved posteriorly in line with the fibers of the gluteus maximus proximally.

- Abduct hip and bluntly split gluteus maximus proximally.
- Place Charnley retractor with bend cephalad.
- Identification of piriformis.
  - Retractor under anterior gluteus maximus.
  - Use electrocautery longitudinally through first layer of bursa taking care to cauterize vessels. Use sponge to bluntly clear bursa from piriformis and short external rotators.
  - Develop the plane between gluteus medius and minimus with a Cobb elevator and place a narrow Dever retractor in this interval.
  - Identify gluteus minimus and piriformis proximally (Figure 2.4).
- Takedown of rotators and hip capsule.
  - Place Ava retractor between external rotators and quadratus femoris distally
  - External rotators and capsule can be taken together or as separate anatomic layers. We take them as one layer, providing a sturdy repair at the conclusion of the case.
  - Take down piriformis and conjoint tendon of short external rotators directly off back of femur.
  - Tag piriformis and short external rotators with separate sutures (Figure 2.5).
  - Make capsulotomy from proximal to distal, taking care to remove directly from the femur (Figure 2.6). If capsule is left on the femur, it will leave less capsule for a good repair at closure.
  - Ensure labrum is divided superiorly.
  - Stop dissection distally at level of quadratus femoris or lesser trochanter.
  - Dislocate the hip slowly with flexion, adduction, and internal rotation. A bone hook under the femoral neck can facilitate dislocation especially in large patients with an intact round ligament.

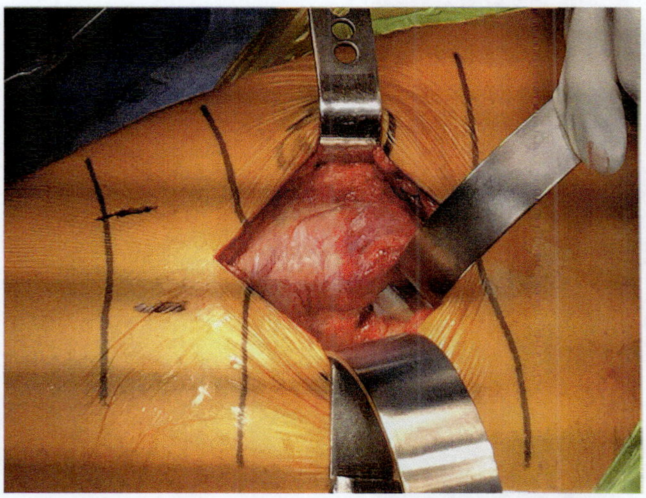

Figure 2.4 | Identification of the piriformis and gluteus minimus.

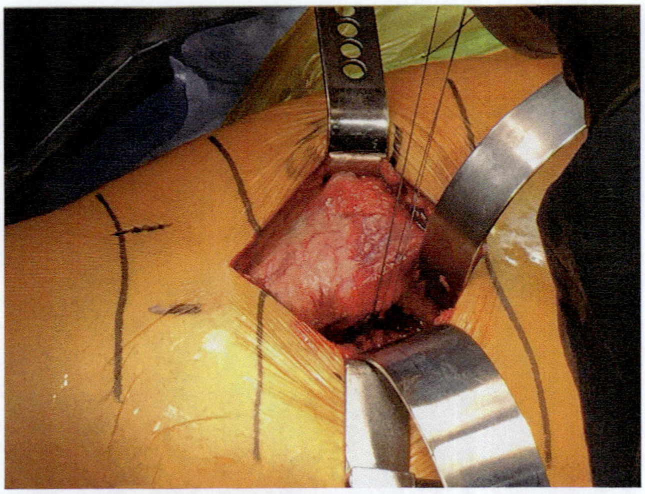

Figure 2.5 | Tagging of the piriformis and short external rotators.

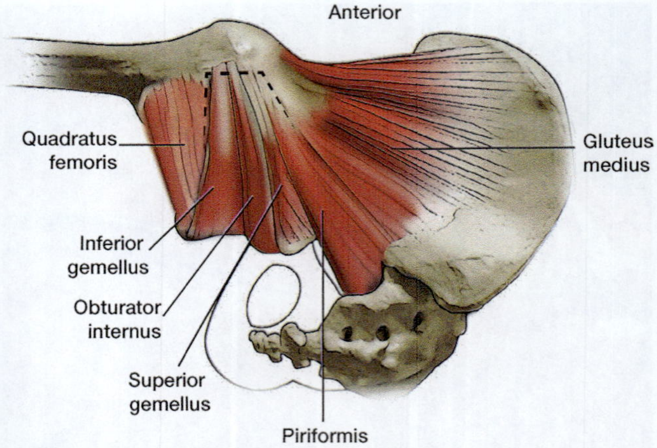

Figure 2.6 | Illustration of the capsulotomy.

- Femoral osteotomy.
  - With the hip dislocated, place wide Hohmann around the lesser trochanter for exposure (Figure 2.7).
  - Measure neck length for osteotomy using exposed lesser trochanter as reference point.
  - Use implant template for angle of femoral neck osteotomy.
  - Use large sagittal blade for neck osteotomy, taking care not to lever against greater trochanter during removal. Take care not to damage greater trochanter with saw.
  - Incise the anterior synovium and capsule as needed for exposure.
  - Place retractor over anterior column, retracting the femur carefully.
- Acetabular exposure.
  - Use a large bone hook to retract the femur anteriorly. While retracting, resect anterior synovium and excess anterosuperior capsule to prevent impingement during hip flexion and internal rotation. Place a straight Hohmann anteriorly between the capsule and the labrum. Aim to lodge the retractor into the ilium, and retract the femur out of the way with this retractor. Place the operative leg in a flexed and internally rotated position off the bed to facilitate exposure. The foot may be placed on a padded Mayo stand.
  - Place an additional straight Hohmann posteriorly between the capsule and labrum into the ischium. Use a mallet to firmly lodge this retractor in place.

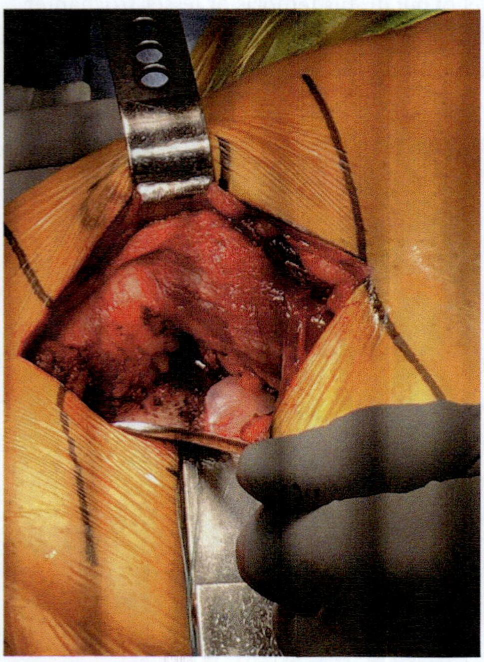

Figure 2.7 | Exposure of the proximal femur for neck osteotomy.

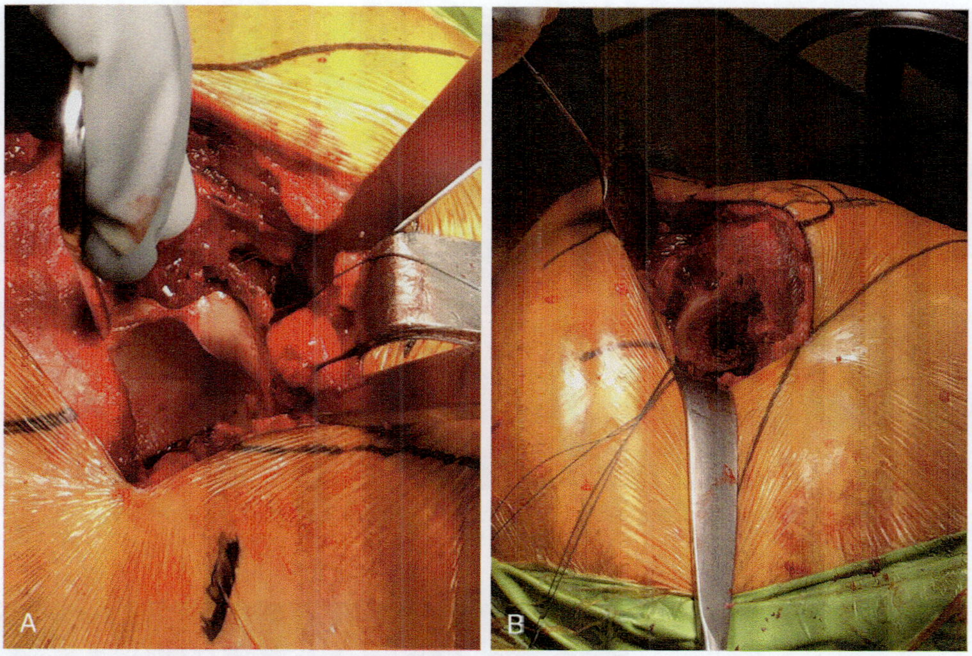

Figure 2.8 | A, Acetabular exposure with Hohmann retractors. B, Femoral exposure with wide Hohmann and Mueller retractors.

- Additional straight Hohmann retractors can be used for circumferential exposure of the acetabulum. Anterior superior and posterior superior placement can be helpful (Figure 2.8).
- Femoral exposure.
  - With the leg internally rotated and the hip at neutral, a wide Hohmann is placed under the lesser trochanter. The hip is then flexed and adducted.
  - A Mueller retractor is placed under the anterior and medial femoral neck, exposing the proximal femur for preparation (Figure 2.8).
  - Electrocautery and heavy forceps are used to remove soft tissue from the piriformis fossa.
  - A 6-mm round burr can be used to remove posterior and lateral bone of the femoral neck to create a starting point for femoral preparation in the posterolateral quadrant of the proximal femur.
- Closure.
  - Closure begins with repair of the capsulotomy. A heavy braided suture is used to repair the piriformis, rotators, and capsule to the posterior trochanter. In our technique, we use a tapered needle and heavy wire driver, as we find this will work in most cases and eliminates the risk of placing several drill holes into the trochanter (Figures 2.9 and 2.10).

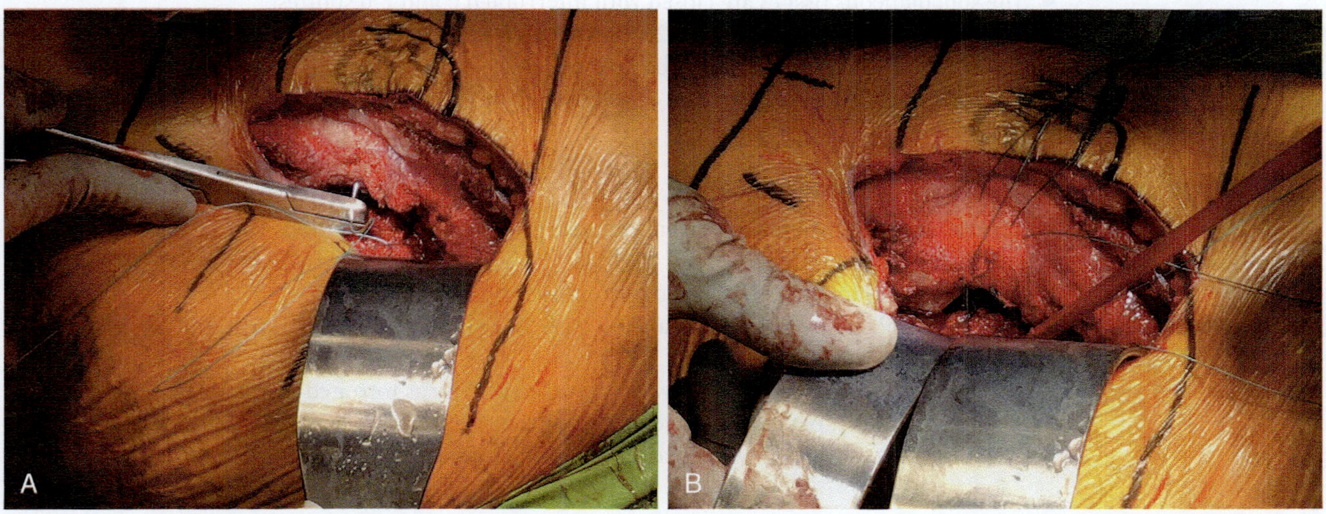

Figure 2.9 | A, Placement of suture through the posterior greater trochanter with a heavy needle driver. B, Sutures through posterior trochanter.

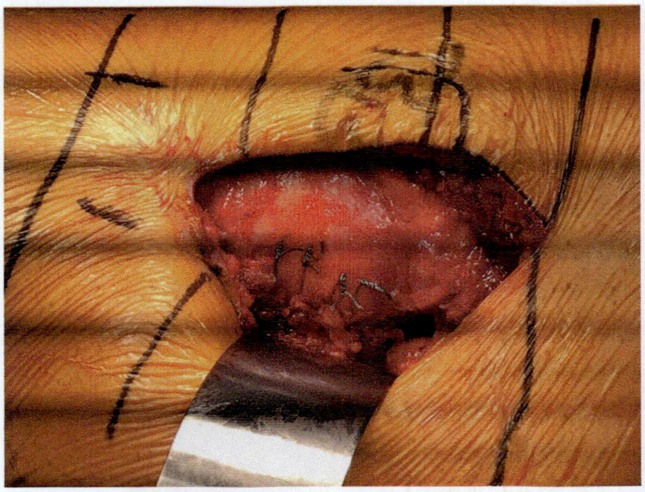

Figure 2.10 I Posterior repair of capsule and short external rotators.

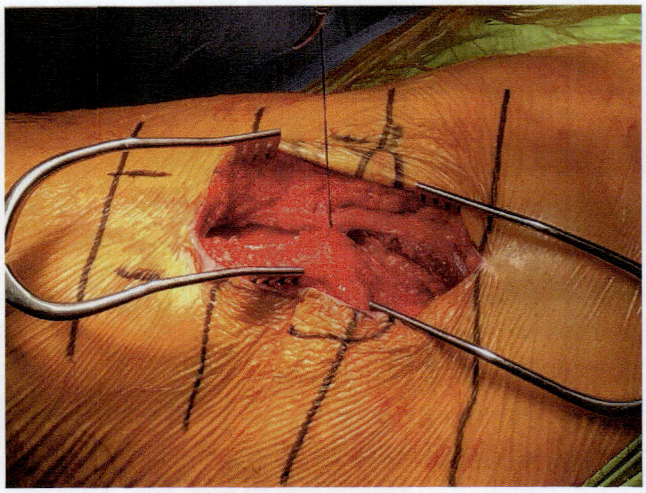

Figure 2.11 I Closure of the fascia.

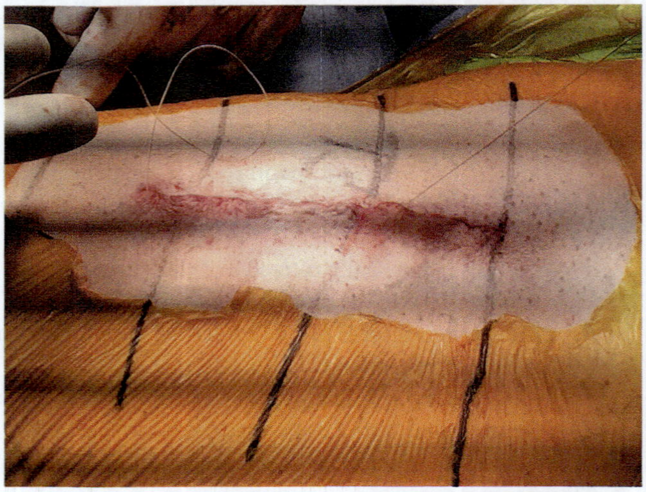

Figure 2.12 I Closure of the skin with a running monofilament.

- Closure of the fascia begins with a single braided suture, the tails of which are not cut. This stitch is used as a retractor to keep the fascial closure from diving too deep (Figure 2.11).
- The fascial repair is then completed with a running barbed suture or large monofilament suture.
- The subcutaneous tissues are closed with interrupted 0 and 2-0 sutures.
- The skin is closed with a running 2-0 barbed monofilament (Figure 2.12).
- The authors prefer the incision to be dressed with 2-octyl cyanoacrylate and a silver-impregnated barrier dressing.

Postoperative care

- Postoperatively, the patients are given minimal posterior hip precautions (if flex hip past 90° have legs abducted) for 3 months.
- Weight-bearing as tolerated is allowed for routine primary THA.
- Crutches or walker are used for balance with weaning as tolerated starting at about 2 weeks postoperatively.
- Return to gym at 2 weeks is allowed with increased activity as tolerated for routine primary THA.
- At the 3-month visit, patients are released from these precautions but advised to always bend forward with the legs abducted when reaching for the ground.

Chapter 3
Anterolateral Approaches

STEPHEN M. PETIS
KEVIN I. PERRY

Key Concepts

- The anterolateral approach to the hip, also known as the modified Hardinge approach, is a well-established surgical approach to the hip for performing total hip arthroplasty.
- This approach provides excellent exposure of the acetabulum and proximal femur for reconstructive purposes.
- Preoperative gait and abductor muscle assessment should be performed before surgery to anticipate abductor insufficiency that may require repair using this approach.
- Careful takedown and repair of the abductor musculature is critical to optimize postoperative function and hip biomechanics and mitigate the risk of hip instability.
- The senior author favors a course of protected weight bearing postoperatively to facilitate healing of the abductor repair.

Sterile Instruments and Implants

Instruments

- Routine hip retractors, including a Charnley retractor, and assortment of blunt and sharp Hohmann retractors
- A 2.5- or 3.2-mm drill
- Blunt or sharp bone hook

Implants

- Cementless or cemented total hip system

Positioning

- Lateral decubitus or supine—surgeon preference
- Two hip bolsters for lateral decubitus position
- Operative leg draped free for ease of acetabular and femoral exposure

Surgical Approach (for Lateral Decubitus Position; Modify as Needed for Supine Position)

- The patient is positioned in the lateral decubitus position with the operative hip up (Figure 3.1). A hip bolster is applied posteriorly just proximal to the gluteal cleft and anteriorly on the pubic symphysis to immobilize the pelvis during surgery. Additional bolsters can be applied to the upper back and sternum for additional immobilization.
- It is critical to ensure the operative leg can be moved through a full range of motion before draping to permit optimal acetabular and femoral exposure.

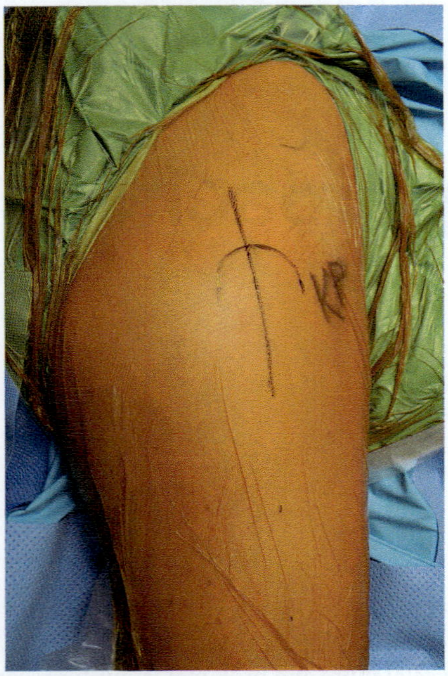

Figure 3.1 | Preoperative photo with the skin incision marked out.

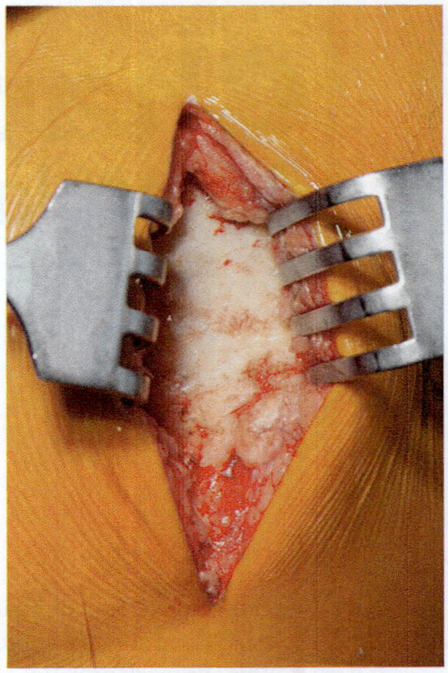

Figure 3.2 | Visualization of the fascia after superficial dissection.

- A 10- to 15-cm incision is made centered over the tip of the greater trochanter. Angling the incision posterior-proximal to anterior-distal can assist in accessing the femoral canal during femoral reconstruction (Figure 3.1). Typically, extending the incision proximally assists with femoral exposure, and extending distally assists with acetabular access.
- Identify the fascia latae (Figure 3.2). A small split is made distally in the fascia in-line with the femoral diaphysis. Abduct the leg and sweep deep under the fascia to break up bursa adherent to the fascia. Identify the interval between tensor fascia latae and gluteus maximus and split the remaining fascia along this interval.
- A Charnley retractor is often placed under the anterior and posterior fascia latae flaps to assist with exposure.
- Identify and assess the gluteus medius muscle (Figure 3.3). The muscle is split proximally along its fibers as it inserts onto the greater trochanter. There is often a raphe that will split naturally with blunt dissection, and this represents an approximately 35% anterior, 65% posterior split in the muscle (Figure 3.4). Scissors can then be placed through the raphe (Figure 3.5) and replaced with retractors (Figure 3.6) to expose the gluteus minimus and capsule overlying the femoral neck.
- Identify the tendon of the gluteus medius. Occasionally, overlying bursal tissue may have to be excised to improve exposure. A cuff of tendon is dissected off the greater trochanter and ends at the vastus ridge distally (Figures 3.7 and 3.8). Carrying the tenotomy too far distally into the vastus lateralis can lead to increased bleeding.
- A leash of vessels often is present over the gluteus minimus and capsular layer that should be cauterized. A full-thickness split of the gluteus minimus and capsule is made along the superior aspect of the femoral neck, leaving an anterior and posterior cuff of tissue for later repair (Figures 3.9 and 3.10). Alternatively, the gluteus minimus and capsule can be dissected as separate layers and split in a similar fashion.
- The gluteus minimus, medius, and capsular tissue are elevated off the anterior aspect of the femur to the level of the lesser trochanter. A blunt Hohmann retractor placed along the inferolateral aspect of the femoral neck, as well as hip flexion and external rotation, can help with exposure during deep dissection.
- With a blunt or sharp bone hook placed along the femoral neck, an assistant provides traction and external rotation to dislocate the hip. If this is difficult, ensure that the joint capsule has been split proximally to the level of the superolateral acetabulum and distally to the lesser trochanter.

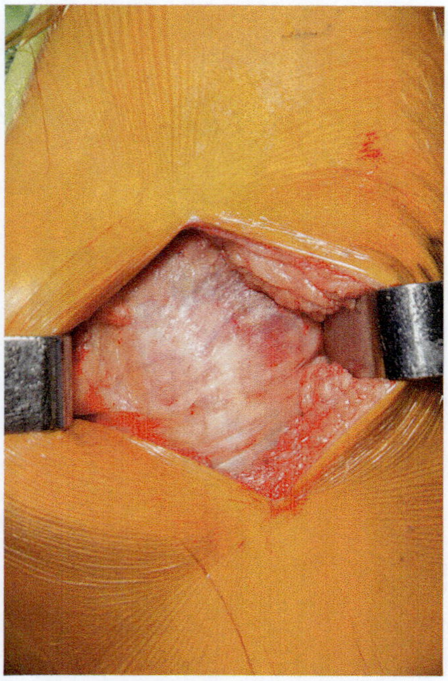

Figure 3.3 | Exposure of the trochanter, gluteus medius, and vastus lateralis.

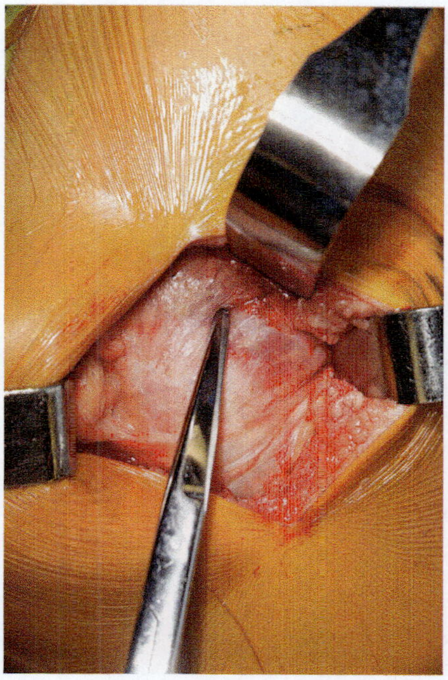

Figure 3.4 | The tip of the scissors shows where the anterior portion of the gluteus medius will be taken down.

- Place blunt Hohmann retractors around the femoral neck and perform a femoral neck osteotomy based on preoperative templating (Figures 3.11-3.13). Ensure that the limb is orientated in the neutral position so the inclination and version of the osteotomy can be performed accurately.
- For acetabular exposure, position the limb in the neutral position with slight hip flexion. Make a small split in the anterior capsulolabral junction at the 3-o'clock position for a right hip. A sharp Hohmann retractor is carefully placed anteriorly to avoid neurovascular injury.
- A sharp, bent Hohmann retractor is placed posteriorly at the 8-o'clock position in the same fashion. If positioned appropriately, this retractor may rest on the femoral calcar to aid in retracting the

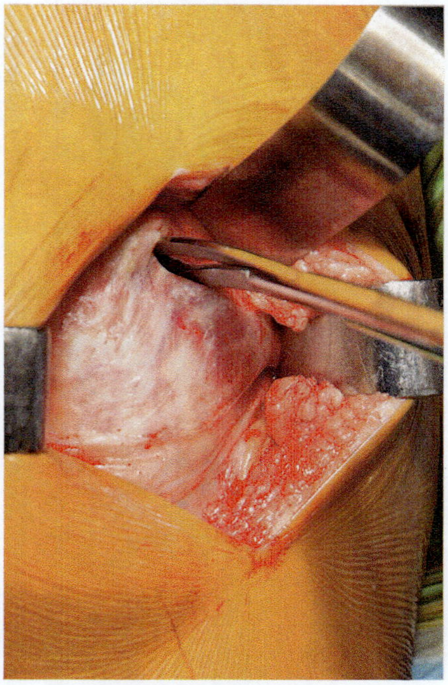

Figure 3.5 | The tip of the scissors penetrates the gluteus medius.

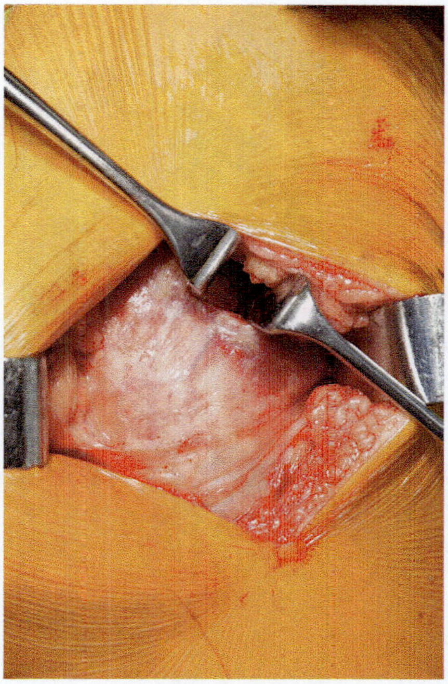

Figure 3.6 | Two knee retractors are placed through the gluteus medius.

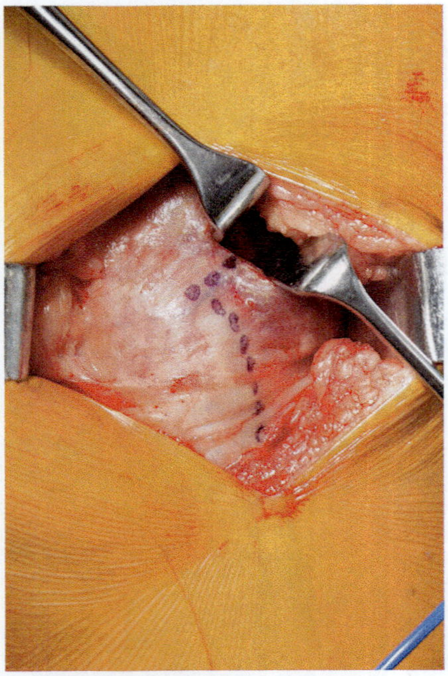

Figure 3.7 | The dissection of the gluteus medius through the tendinous insertion onto the greater trochanter is marked out with a marking pen before being carried out.

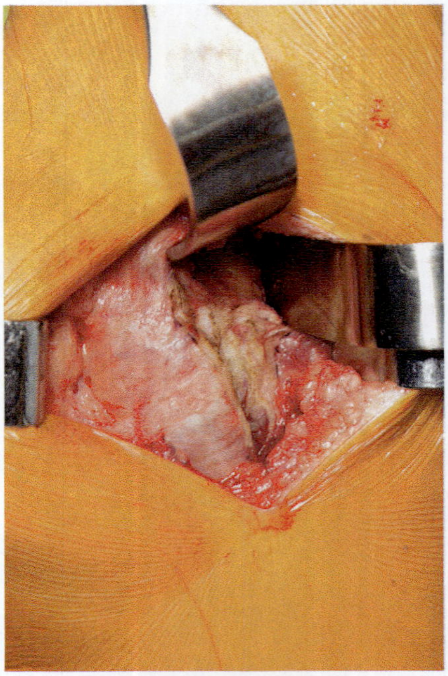

Figure 3.8 | Intraoperative photo demonstrating the gluteus minimus after the gluteus medius has been reflected.

proximal femur posteriorly. Typically, this provides adequate acetabular exposure (Figure 3.14). If this exposure is inadequate, a blunt or sharp bone hook can aid in displacing the femur posteriorly. Additionally, rotating the femur internally or externally can improve exposure.

- Release the capsule inferiorly to the level of the transverse acetabular ligament at the 6-o'clock position. Take care not to dissect into the iliopsoas muscle and tendon or beyond the inferior acetabular margin as this can lead to bleeding. A blunt Hohmann retractor is placed along the inferior margin of the acetabulum. A sponge can be tied to this retractor and secured to the Charnley retractor.
- If additional exposure is required, a sharp Hohmann can be impacted into the anterosuperior quadrant of the pelvis. Perform the acetabular reconstruction.

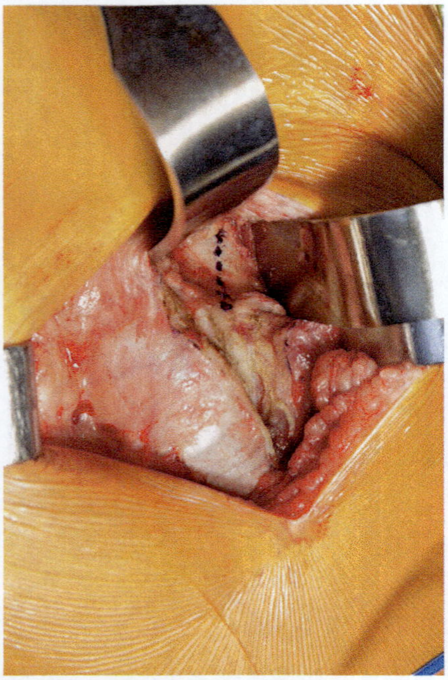

Figure 3.9 | Intraoperative photo showing the planned incision through the gluteus minimus and capsule.

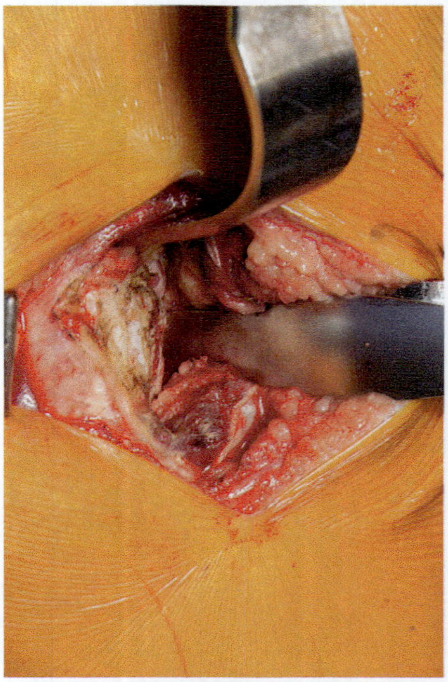

Figure 3.10 | Exposure of the femoral head and neck after dissection through the gluteus minimus and capsule.

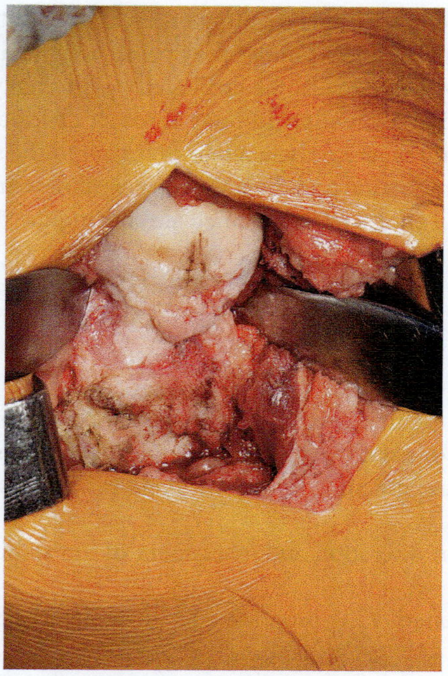

Figure 3.11 | Intraoperative photo after the femoral head has been dislocated anteriorly.

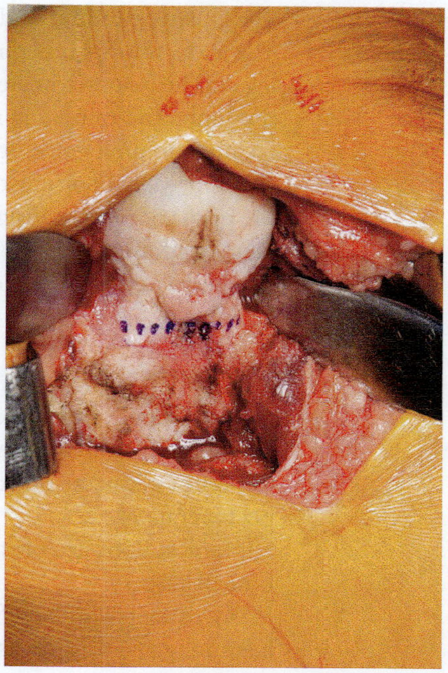

Figure 3.12 | Planned femoral neck osteotomy marked out.

- For femoral exposure and reconstruction, place a blunt retractor along the posterolateral aspect of the greater trochanter. This retractor will help displace the femur anteriorly to access the femoral canal. Position the limb in a hip bag in the figure 4 position. Ensure the lower leg and knee are orientated vertically to assist with femoral version assessment.
- Two additional Hohmann retractors assist with femoral exposure. One is placed along the medial femoral neck and the other posterior to rest along the calcar. This second retractor will assist in retracting the abductor muscles and skin during femoral preparation. Before inserting this retractor, additional posterior capsule may need to be resected along the posterior femoral cortex to optimize entry into the femoral canal. Femoral entry should be posterior to avoid thinning of the anterior femoral cortex during reconstruction. Complete the femoral reconstruction.

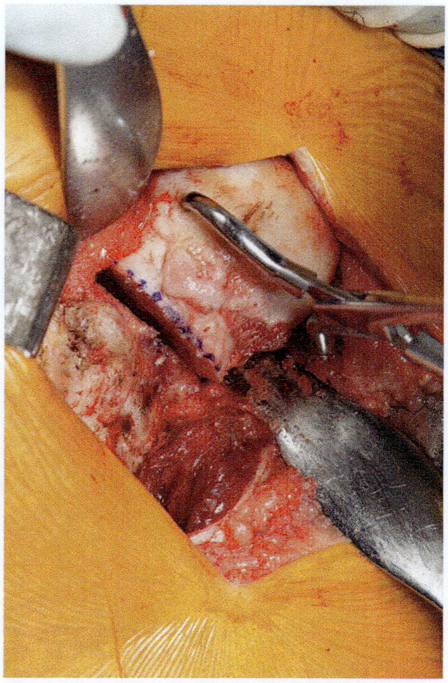

Figure 3.13 | After the femoral neck osteotomy.

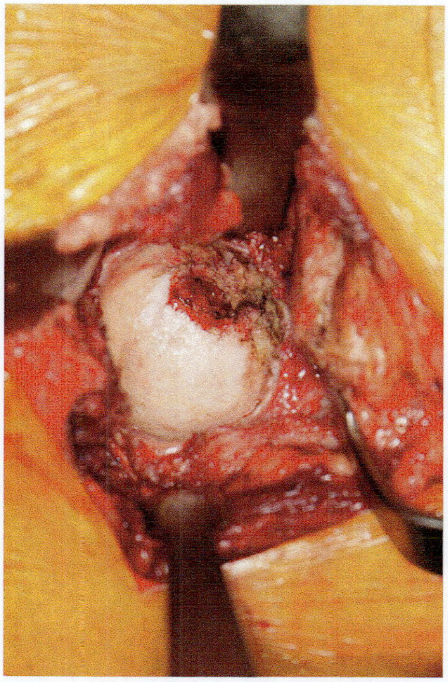

Figure 3.14 | Exposure of the acetabulum.

- The gluteus minimus and capsule are approximated with either running or interrupted suture.
- The abductor repair begins by placing sterile drapes or towels under the operative leg to abduct the leg and help approximate the abductor tenotomy. This can also be facilitated by internally rotating the limb. The muscle is repaired tendon-to-tendon, or tendon-to-bone through drill holes based on surgeon preference. An excellent, anatomic, and secure muscle repair is critical to the success of this approach. Poor muscle healing with muscle retraction and then abductor weakness and limp is the primary complication of this approach, and all efforts must be aimed at reducing the risk of this complication.
- The fascia and skin are closed in routine fashion.

Postoperative Care

- Patients should be protected weight bearing for the first several weeks after surgery to protect the abductor repair. Assistive devices, such as a cane or a walker, are recommended for the first 6 weeks to permit abductor muscle healing. Abductor strengthening is also withheld for the first 6 weeks postoperatively.
- Hip precautions are prescribed based on surgeon discretion and assessment of hip stability at the time of surgery.
- Many patients will benefit from an abductor strengthening program after this operative approach, beginning at 6 to 8 weeks postoperatively.

Chapter 4
Direct Anterior Approach

MICHAEL J. TAUNTON
TIMOTHY B. ALTON

Key Concepts

- The direct anterior approach (DAA) provides access to the hip joint through an intramuscular, internervous interval without abductor disruption.
- Originally described by Smith-Peterson in the 1940s and later modified by Heuter in the 1950s, this approach has gained popularity recently by arthroplasty surgeons and may lead to earlier restoration of gait kinematics and have a lower dislocation rate.
- Fluoroscopy is easily used in conjunction with this approach, and it can be performed with the patient supine with the leg free on a standard operating room table or on a specialty table.
- Supine positioning places the pelvis in a neutral position, facilitates correct acetabular cup placement, and allows more accurate intraoperative assessment of leg length and stability.
- Femoral exposure and access is more limited than for other anterolateral and posterior approaches. This limits the type of femoral components that can be used easily with this approach. Some studies have reported higher rates of femoral component loosening and femoral fracture with the DAA.
- The lateral femoral cutaneous nerve may be injured in this approach, and this can bother patients.

Indications

- All patients who meet classic indications for total hip arthroplasty are candidates for DAA.
- For new adopters of the approach, patients who are thin and flexible, with low muscle bulk, good bone quality, and normal femoral offset (lack of coxa breva) are the best patients to operate on.
- Contraindications:
  - Skin infection or irritation at surgical site, excessive pannus.
  - Depends on surgeon expertise; excessive femoral or acetabular deformity may require more extensile exposures or osteotomies.

Technical Considerations

- Obese patient
  - Abdominal girth can be problematic; retract and hold with tape
    - May lead to wound healing problems
    - Consider suture closure in morbid obesity
  - Positioning on specialized table
    - Supine, arms on arm boards at 90°
    - Ensure excellent padding of feet in boots attached to table
    - Peroneal post between legs, source of countertraction, well padded

Sterile Instruments and Implants

Instruments

- 2 Ava retractors, 2 Mueller-type retractors, 2 Meyerding retractors, 1 sharp Hohmann retractor, 2 curved cobra-type retractors
- A 3.5-mm burr
- Femoral elevator hook

Implants

- Cementless or cemented total hip system
- Broach-only femoral stem with trochanteric relief is preferred for standard cases

Positioning

- Supine
- Traction table
  - Well-padded perineal post, well-padded traction boots, support under nonoperative leg
  - Prep out from 5 cm proximal to the anterior superior iliac spine (ASIS), distally to above the knee, anteriorly to 5 cm medial to the ASIS, and posteriorly to the posterior thigh
- Standard table
  - Prep both legs free with stockinettes to allow for "figure 4" position

Surgical Approach

- The patient is positioned in the supine position either on a specialized traction table (Figure 4.1A and B) or on a standard operating table. It is important to ensure proper padding on the perineal post and around the traction boots if utilized. A 10- to 12-cm incision is made 2 cm distal and 2 cm lateral to the ASIS, centered over tensor fascia latae (TFL) muscle belly (Figure 4.2). This is usually about 15° off of a line subtended from the ASIS to the patella. The incision may be extended at either end for additional exposure. Extending the incision proximally and releasing the anterior 1 cm of TFL may aid in femoral exposure.
- Superficial dissection is continued through the subcutaneous adipose tissue. If the lateral femoral cutaneous nerve or branches are encountered, protect and retract them medially. The fascia overlying the TFL is encountered. The purple hue of the TFL muscle belly should be noted (Figure 4.3). If this is not appreciated, it is likely that the approach has been made too medially. Once the TFL is properly identified, incise the fascia over TFL and develop the medial plane inside of fascia, over the TFL muscle belly (Figure 4.4).
- A finger can then drop superior to the femoral neck, medial to the TFL muscle belly. An Ava-type retractor is then placed superior to the neck. A Meyerding retractor then retracts the TFL laterally (Figure 4.5). A sharp Hohmann retractor retracts the rectus muscle off of the inferior neck. The lateral femoral circumflex vessel branches are identified and coagulated. The deep layer of the TFL fascia and investing fat over the anterior femoral neck may be excised. An Ava retractor can then be placed inferior to the neck. The capsulotomy is then made in line with the anterior superior femoral neck. It is then continued in line with the intertrochanteric line, with the surgeon paying attention not to leave a cuff of capsule that would otherwise need to be removed for proper releases (Figure 4.6). This inferior limb of the capsulotomy may then be tagged with a #5 Ethibond suture to allow for identification and retraction during acetabular preparation. The Ava retractors may then be placed inside of the capsule superior and inferior to the femoral neck.
- The preoperatively planned femoral neck cut level may then be checked with a radiodense marker such as a long cautery tip with the use of C-arm. Otherwise, the surgeon may use the lesser trochanter as a reference point if C-arm is not utilized. The femoral neck cut is made utilizing a standard stiff saw blade. The actual neck cut is begun in the anterior cortex, a cut approximately 6 to 9 mm superior to that level is made completely across the superior femoral neck, and then the definitive femoral neck cut is completed. This creates a "napkin ring" that may be removed for aid in femoral head removal. Applying light traction to the leg may aid in completion of the neck cut.

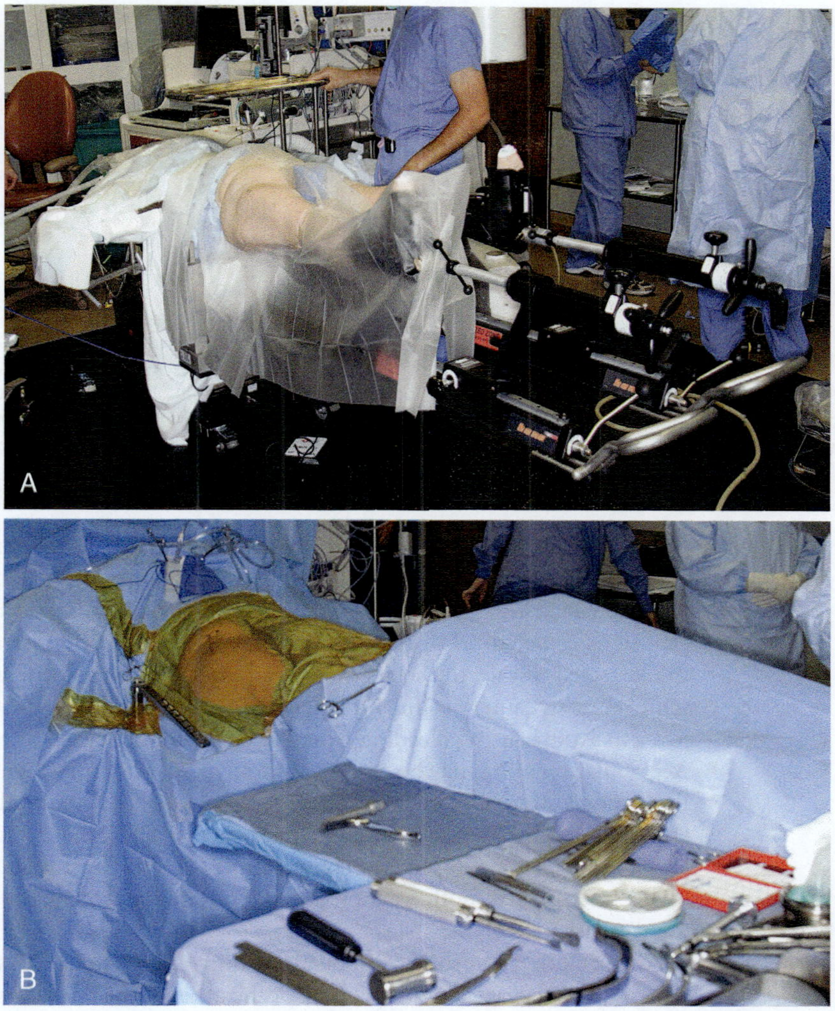

Figure 4.1 | A, B. Intraoperative photograph demonstrating supine patient positioning on a specialized table.

- At this point, a wound protector/retractor may be placed to protect the skin edges and the TFL. This is placed deep to the deep layer of the TFL fascia laterally and deep to the sartorius medially.
- The leg is then externally rotated to 40° to 80°; the anterior capsule may be further released to allow for further posterior translation of the femur to aid in acetabular exposure if needed. The leg is then left in the 40° externally rotated position, and a cork screw is placed in the anterior aspect of the femoral head, and it is removed (Figure 4.7).

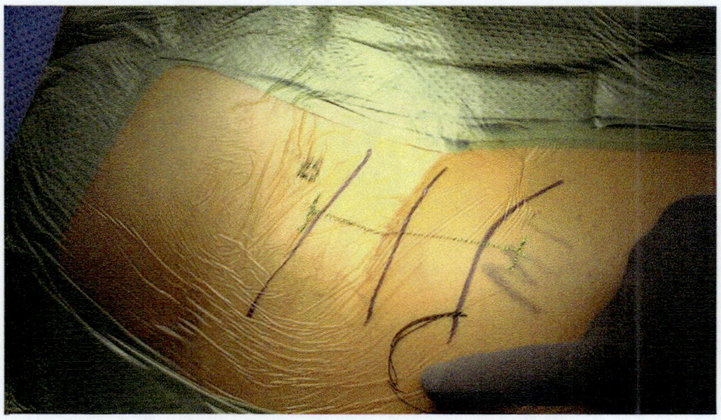

Figure 4.2 | Intraoperative photograph demonstrating incision placement. The incision is placed 1 finger breadth lateral and distal to the ASIS and usually is 10 to 12 cm in length.

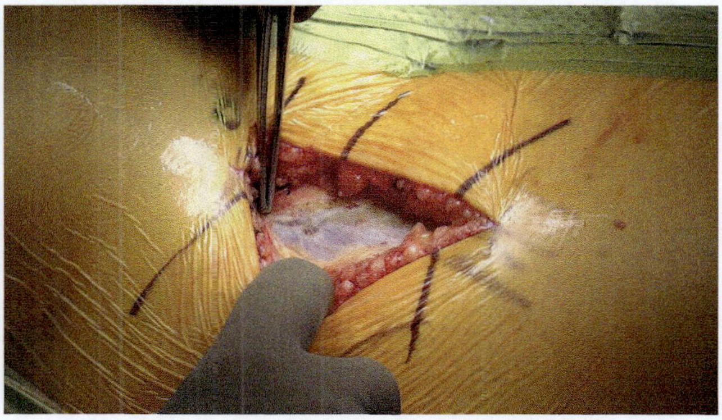

Figure 4.3 | Intraoperative photograph demonstrating the fascia over the TFL.

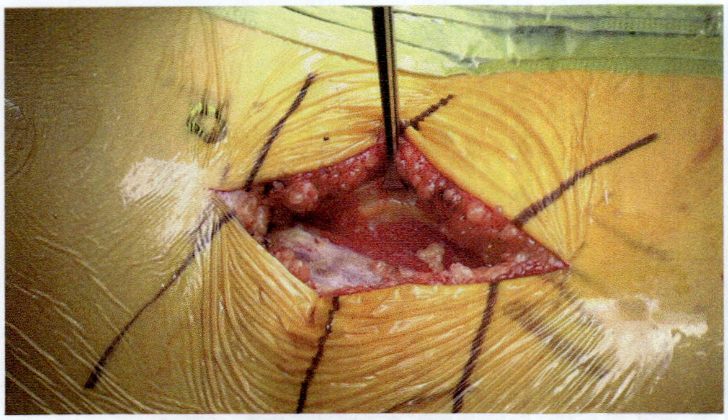

Figure 4.4 | Intraoperative photograph demonstrating elevation of the medial aspect of the TFL fascia after split, and elevation of the facia to facilitate dissection inside of the fascia on the medial aspect of the TFL.

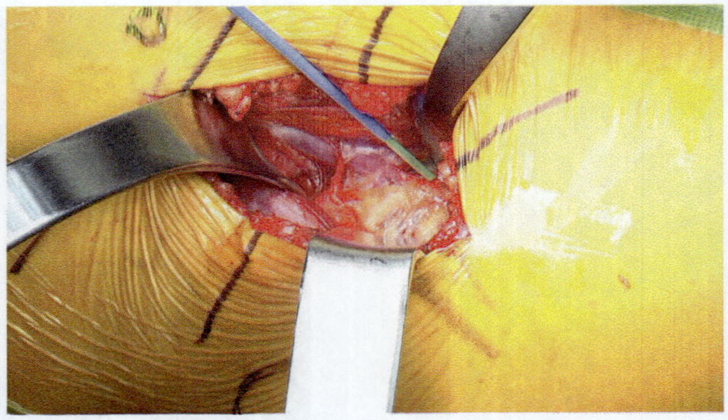

Figure 4.5 | Intraoperative photograph demonstrating Ava retractors superior and inferior to the femoral neck, and identification and cauterization of the medial circumflex vessels.

- Once the femoral head is removed, the leg is positioned in neutral extension and externally rotated 40°. An anterior retractor is placed inside the capsule inferior to the psoas tendon crossing of the anterior rim. This allows the psoas tendon to protect the neurovascular bundle. A cuff of posterior capsule is elevated off of the ilium to allow for a posterior retractor to be placed inside the capsule directed toward the sciatic notch (Figure 4.8). The labrum and pulvinar tissues should then be removed with cautery to fully delineate the borders of the acetabulum. Care should be taken in the fovea to avoid causing bleeding from the obturator artery.
- Acetabular reaming may be carried out in a regular fashion (Figure 4.9).
- If utilizing a straight reamer handle, care should be taken to avoid having the femur push the reamer anteriorly, as it may cause the surgeon to excessively ream the anterior wall. Reaming with fluoroscopic guidance may optimize component position. If using fluoroscopy, correct the angle of the image intensifier in both rotation and inlet/outlet to provide proper anteroposterior (AP) image of the patient's pelvis.
    - The projected ellipse of component opening indicates anteversion.
    - It may be necessary to remove one or the other of the retractors to facilitate reamer and cup placement in a less invasive exposure.
- Femoral exposure—specialized orthopedic table technique:
    - Ensure that there is no traction on the operative leg before femoral exposure.
    - The leg is externally rotated to a goal of 120°; this may be limited in the case of contractures.
    - A Mueller-type retractor is placed on the posterior-medial calcar to translate the femur laterally during broaching.
    - A specialized femoral elevator is inserted around the posterior proximal femur just proximal to the gluteus maximus insertion to allow for femoral elevation during broaching.
    - The leg is then hyperextended and adducted. The arm of the specialized table is usually on the floor. The nonoperative leg should be resting in a neutral position.

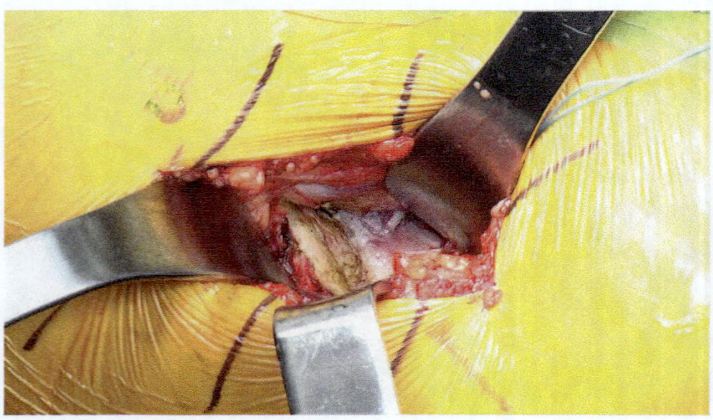

Figure 4.6 | Intraoperative photograph demonstrating anterior-superior capsular split, which is then continued in line with the intertrochanteric line.

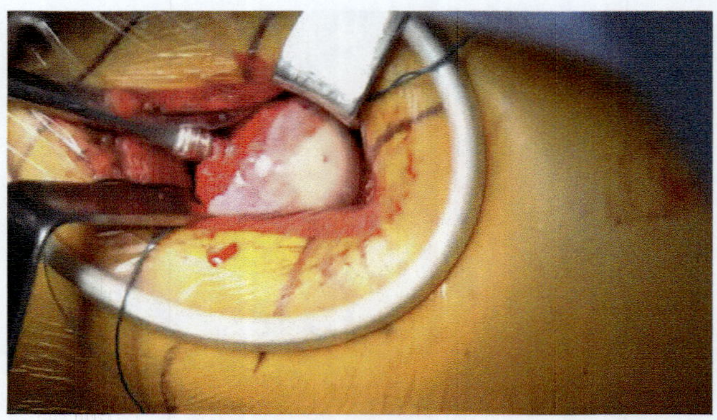

Figure 4.7 | Intraoperative photograph demonstrating femoral head removal.

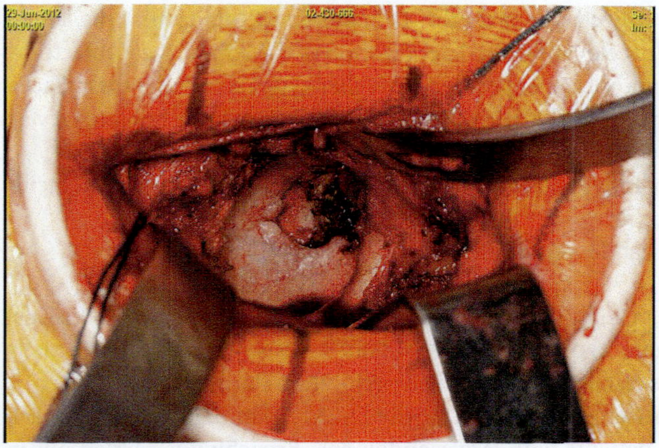

Figure 4.8 | Intraoperative photograph demonstrating acetabular exposure with anterior retractor and medial capsular release.

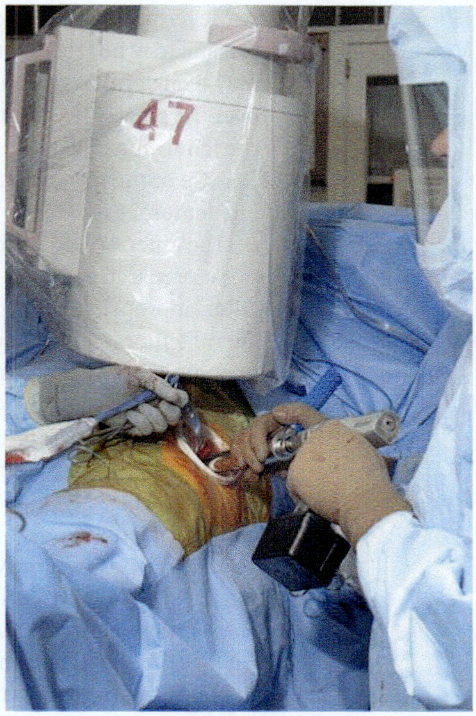

Figure 4.9 | Intraoperative photograph demonstrating reaming with fluoroscopic guidance.

- A Meyerding-type retractor is then utilized to retract the TFL and abductors so that the lateral capsule may be released to further allow elevation and lateralization of the femur. After the capsule is released, the Meyerding retractor is removed and another Mueller-type retractor is placed over the greater trochanter to further expose the calcar.
- The femoral elevator hook is then raised to allow for full femoral exposure.
- Release of the piriformis and subsequently the conjoined tendon is rarely required but can facilitate femoral exposure in select cases.
  - Trendelenburg positioning can facilitate femoral exposure.
  - Even more rarely, the anterior 1 to 2 cm of the TFL can be released (Figure 4.10).

- Femoral exposure—standard table technique:
  - If utilizing a standard table, a sand bag may be placed under the hemipelvis on the operated side. The patient is positioned so that the break in the bed is at the level that allows for leg extension relative to the pelvis. The leg portion of the bed is dropped 30° to 45°. The nonoperative extremity is supported in neutral position on a Mayo stand. The operative extremity can then be placed in a "figure 4" position, adducted, externally rotated, and extended posterior to the nonoperative limb.

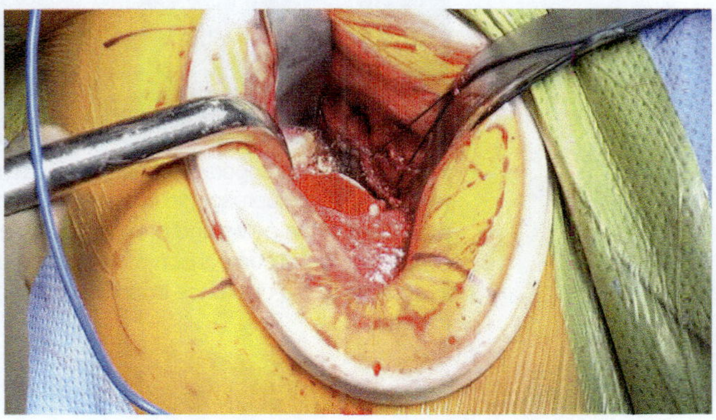

Figure 4.10 | Intraoperative photograph demonstrating elevation of the femur with the femoral elevator hook, with the leg positioned in extension, adduction, and external rotation.

- A Meyerding-type retractor is then utilized to retract the TFL and abductors so that the lateral capsule may be released to further allow elevation and lateralization of the femur. A capsulectomy may be helpful in tight patients for appropriate exposure. A Mueller-type retractor is then placed over the greater trochanter to further expose the calcar. Assistants may use a bone hook to elevate the femur if needed.
- Release of the piriformis and subsequently the conjoined tendon is rarely required but can facilitate femoral exposure in select cases.
  - The anterior 1 to 2 cm of the TFL can be released.

- Femoral preparation:
  - After appropriate femoral exposure, a high-speed burr safely and effectively removes residual lateral femoral neck before further femoral preparation. A "rat tail" rasp is very helpful to initially open up the femur and sound for the canal to avoid cortical perforation during broaching.
    Broach-only–type stems are the most efficient for use in the DAA. Additionally, offset broach handles can be helpful especially in patients with larger abdomens. Broaching is carried out in a standard fashion. The broach is typically biased against varus, flexion, and overanteversion (Figure 4.11).
- Checking leg length, offset, and stability:
  - The supine position provides a distinct advantage by facilitating the ready use of fluoroscopy. An intraoperative preresection fluoroscopic image of the operative hip should be saved. This should be performed after adjusting the fluoroscopy to provide a normalized AP pelvis projection. After trials are inserted and the hip is reduced, another image can be obtained at the same magnification. These images can be printed and compared by an overlay technique. Alternatively, several proprietary software programs can perform a similar task. Assess leg length, offset and femoral component position, and component fill of proximal femur (Figure 4.12).
  - In the case of femoral neck fracture, or proximal femoral deformity, a "flipped" view of the contralateral hip can help ensure more anatomic reconstruction.
  - After real implants are inserted, the capsulotomy may be closed with braided resorbable suture. The fascia is closed with a running barbed suture.
  - Skin closure is most usually done with running suture in the subcuticular layer. An occlusive dressing is placed to protect the wound in the first 2 weeks.

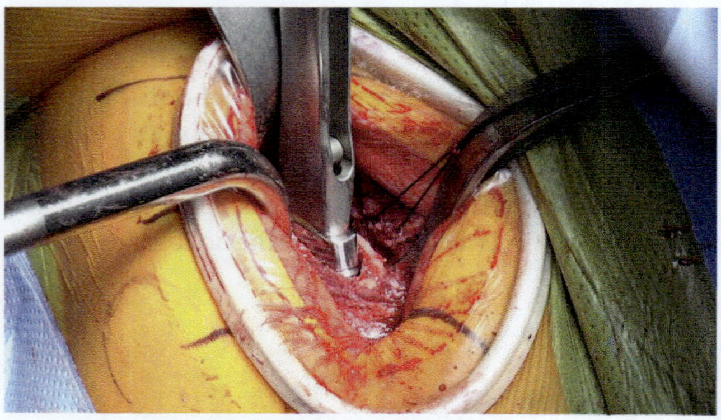

Figure 4.11 | Intraoperative photograph demonstrating offset broach handle for femoral broaching.

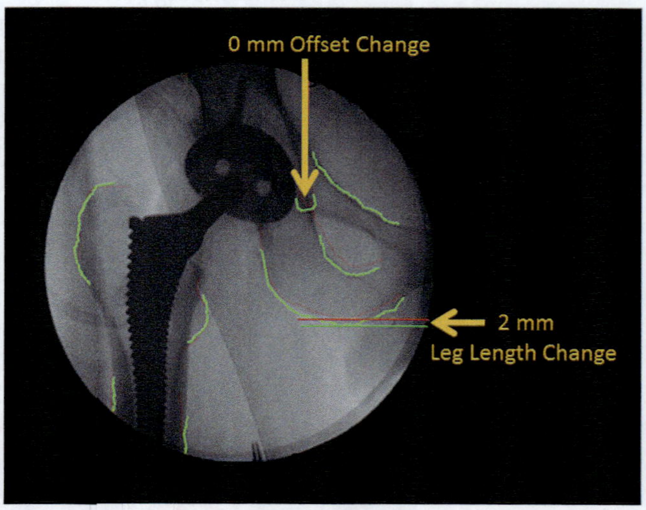

Figure 4.12 | Intraoperative photograph demonstrating the overlay technique. Two fluoroscopic images are printed out. The anatomic structures of the pelvis and proximal femur are outlined. The films are overlaid, and the comparison of the teardrops demonstrates change in offset, and the difference in ischial height demonstrates leg length change.

Suggested Reading

1. Taunton MJ, Trousdale RT, Sierra RJ, Kaufman K, Pagnano MW. Randomized clinical trial of direct anterior and miniposterior approach THA: which provides better functional recovery? *Clin Orthop Relat Res*. 2018;476(2):216-229.
2. Anterior Total Hip Arthroplasty Collaborative Investigators, Bhandari M, Matta JM, Dodgin D, et al. Outcomes following the single-incision anterior approach to total hip arthroplasty: a multicenter observational study. *Orthop Clin North Am*. 2009;40(3):329-342. doi:10.1016/j.ocl.2009.03.001.
3. Taunton MJ, Mason JB, Odum SM, Springer BD. Direct anterior total hip arthroplasty yields more rapid voluntary cessation of all walking aids: a prospective, randomized clinical trial. *J Arthroplasty*. 2014. doi:10.1016/j.arth.2014.03.051. pii:S0883-5403(14)00340-4.
4. Poehling-Monaghan KL, Kamath AF, Taunton MJ, Pagnano MW. Direct anterior versus miniposterior THA with the same advanced perioperative protocols: surprising early clinical results. *Clin Orthop Relat Res*. 2014;473(2):623-631.

Chapter 5
Transtrochanteric Approaches

DANIEL J. BERRY

Key Concepts

- Transtrochanteric approaches to the hip joint are not needed for most primary total hip arthroplasties (THA) but when used can provide wide exposure to the hip joint, for both the acetabulum and femur.
- A number of variations of transtrochanteric approaches exist, and each has its pros and cons. Different techniques are indicated in different circumstances. All provide the benefit of enhanced exposure to the hip compared with routine anterior, posterior, or anterolateral/direct lateral exposures to the hip, but they also carry the risk of trochanteric nonunion.
- The main techniques are conventional trochanteric osteotomy with reflection of the trochanter and abductors proximally (Figure 5.1); trochanteric slide in which the abductors, greater trochanter (GT), and vastus lateralis are maintained in continuity (Figure 5.2); and extended greater trochanteric osteotomy (Figure 5.3). Detailed techniques of extended trochanteric osteotomy are described in Chapter 23.
- Conventional GT osteotomies allow the GT and abductors to be reflected proximally: this protects the superior gluteal nerve and can be helpful when wide exposure to the lateral ileum is needed (Figure 5.4). The trochanteric slide keeps the abductors, GT, and vastus lateralis in continuity, which may maintain better abductor function should healing of the osteotomy fail to occur.
- Conventional trochanteric osteotomies or trochanteric slide is most frequently used for the following indications: severe hip stiffness that precludes safe access to the hip with a conventional exposure or with in situ femoral neck osteotomy (Figure 5.5); proximal femoral deformity in which the GT overhangs the femoral canal precluding safe access to the canal for femoral preparation without abductor damage (Figure 5.6); selected revision hip arthroplasties, particularly when the femoral component will be retained and is bulky and wide access to the acetabulum is needed.

Sterile Instruments and Implants

- Routine instrumentation for THA
- Oscillating saw
- Trochanteric fixation of choice: 18-gauge wires, double Luque wires, trochanteric claw/cables, trochanteric hook plate and instrumentation
- Wire and/or cable tighteners
- Wire/cable cutters

Positioning

- Lateral decubitus or supine depending on surgeon preference for THA.
- If lateral decubitus is chosen, a leg bag on the ventral side of the patient is used when the hip is dislocated anteriorly.

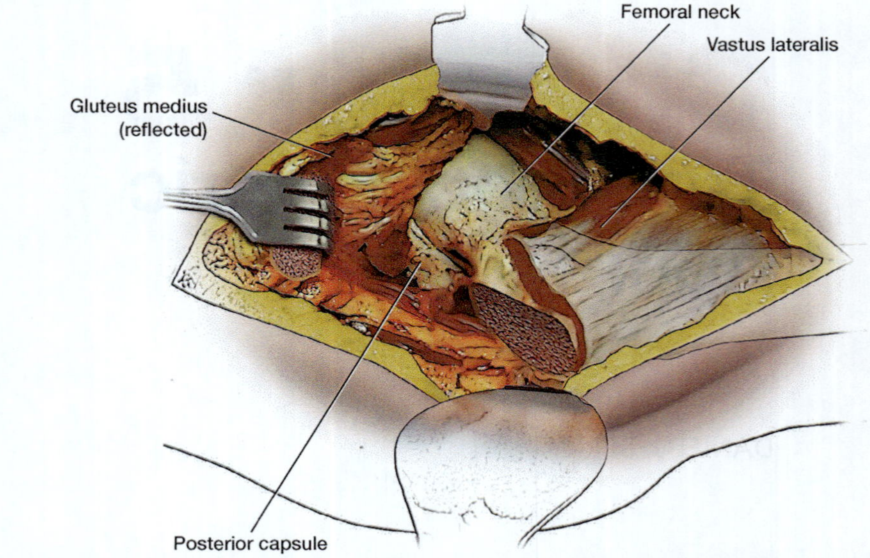

Figure 5.1 | Conventional greater trochanteric osteotomy with reflection of the greater trochanter and abductors proximally.

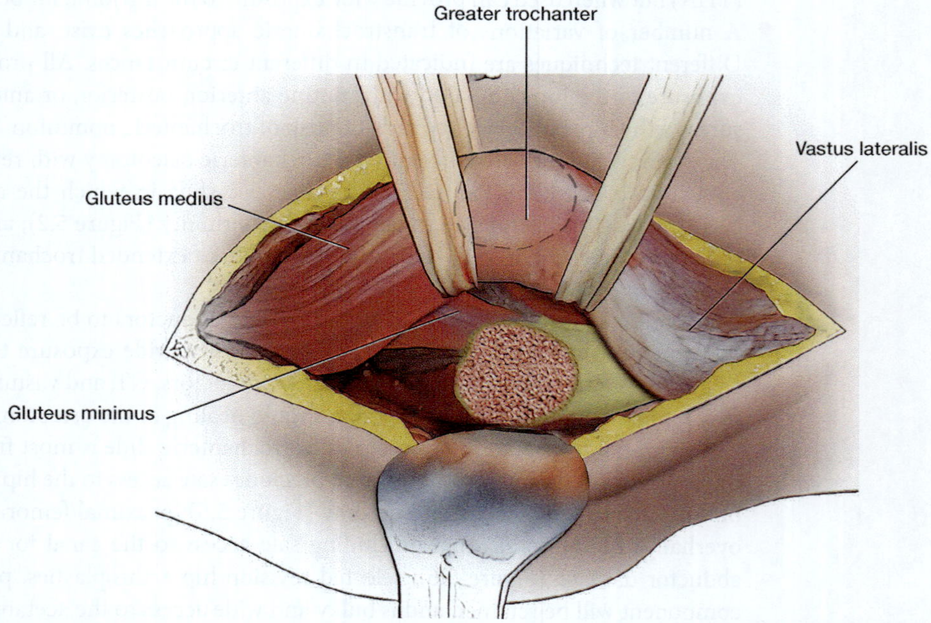

Figure 5.2 | Greater trochanteric slide: the abductors, greater trochanter, and vastus lateralis are kept in continuity.

Surgical Approaches

- The transtrochanteric approach can be used in combination with anterior or posterior dislocation of the hip. However, in general, it is preferable to avoid taking down the abductors (such as in an anterolateral or direct lateral approach to the hip) when a transtrochanteric approach subsequently will be used because this devascularizes the GT and muscle reattachment also is more difficult.

Preoperative Planning

- Identify the patient in whom a transtrochanteric approach may be needed (see notes concerning indications in the Key Concepts section).
- Determine what style of GT osteotomy will be most effective for the specific operative challenge.
- Perform routing templating and preoperative planning for the planned primary or revision THA procedure.

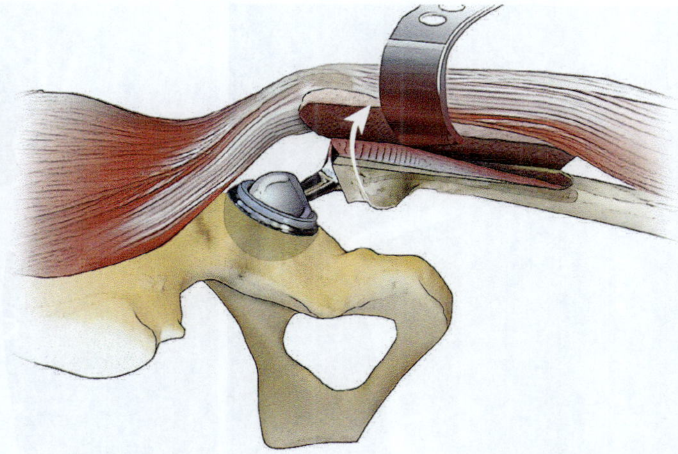

Figure 5.3 | Extended greater trochanteric osteotomy.

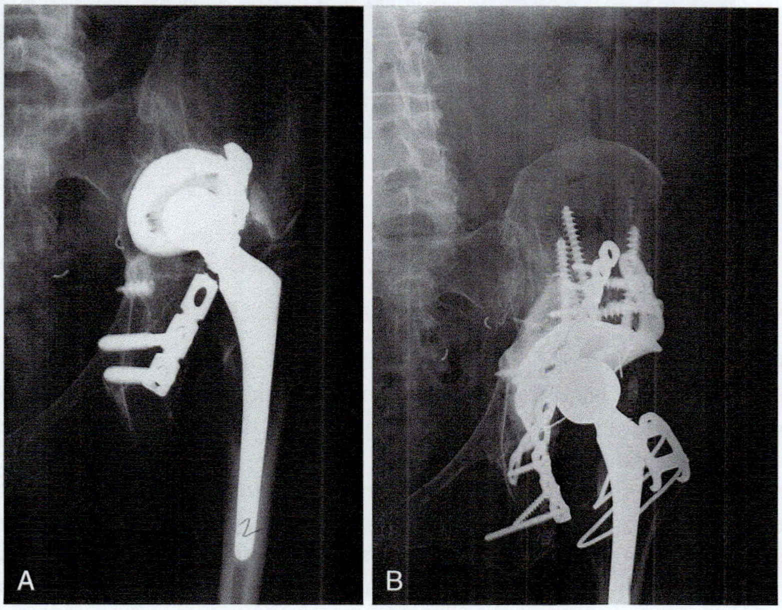

Figure 5.4 | A, Radiograph of failed THA with massive acetabular bone loss requiring wide acetabular exposure and exposure of the lateral ilium for reconstruction. B, Postoperative radiograph after THA using conventional greater trochanteric osteotomy.

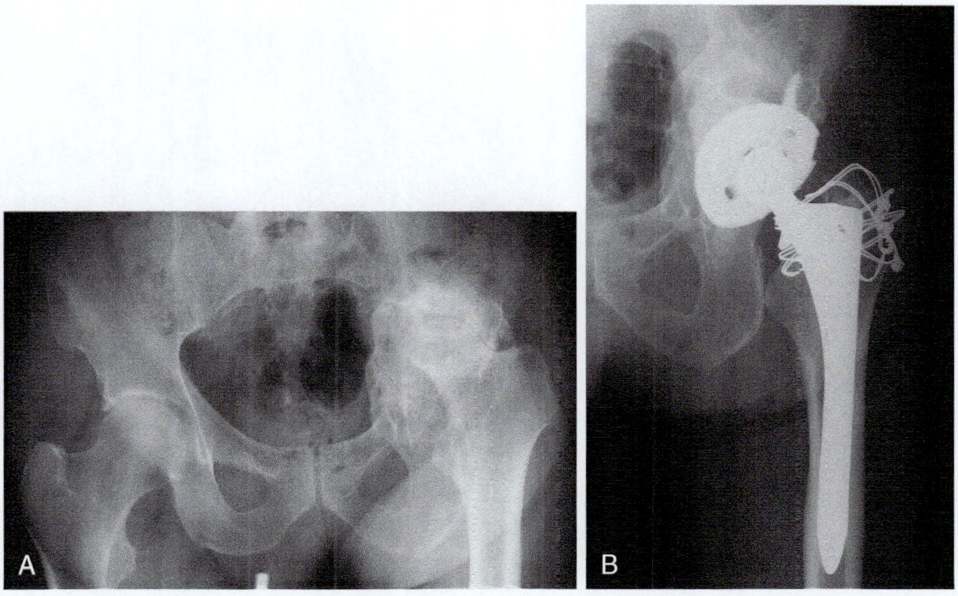

Figure 5.5 | A, Radiograph of hip with severe medial migration of the femoral head. B, Postoperative radiograph after THA using greater trochanteric osteotomy.

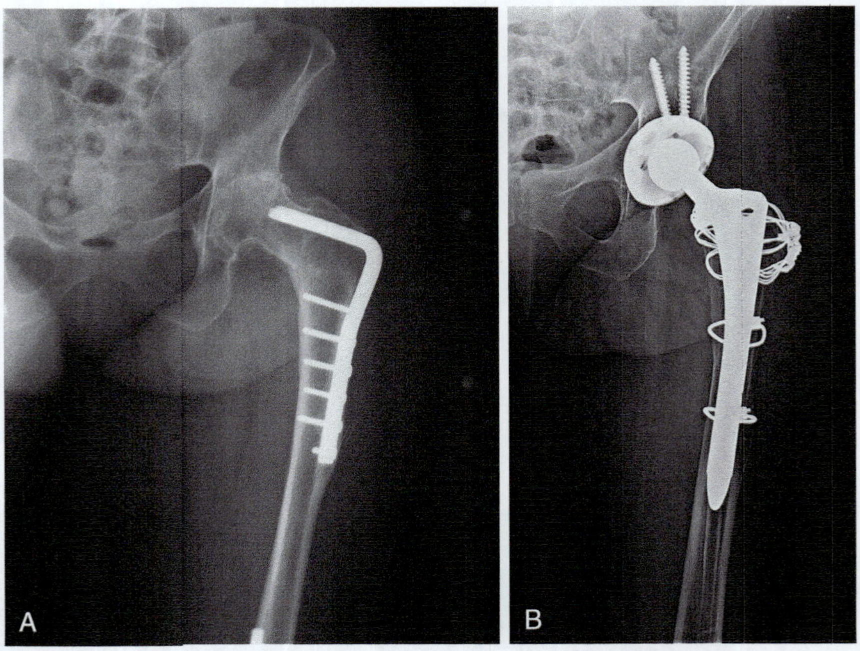

Figure 5.6 | A, Radiograph of hip with varus proximal femoral deformity after intertrochanteric osteotomy with greater trochanter overhanging the femoral canal. B, Postoperative radiograph after THA using greater trochanteric osteotomy.

Bone, Implant, and Soft Tissue Techniques

Conventional Greater Trochanteric Osteotomy

- Make a straight lateral or Kocher-style incision over the hip centered roughly over the GT.
- Incise the iliotibial band longitudinally and carry the incision proximally by splitting the gluteus maximus in the direction of its fibers or by splitting the interval between the gluteus maximus and the tensor fascia lata muscle.
- Identify the vastus tubercle, and reflect several centimeters of proximal vastus lateralis to provide access to the vastus tubercle. This will serve as the entry point for the osteotomy (Figure 5.7).
- Use an instrument such as a curved hemostat to identify the depth of the abductor attachments on the GT. The exit point for the osteotomy should be just deep to the muscle attachments (Figure 5.8).

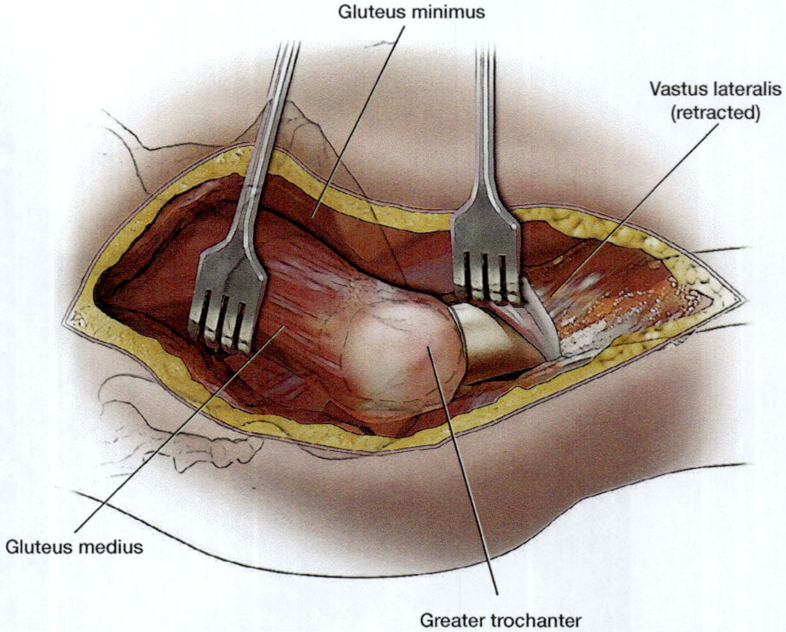

Figure 5.7 | The entry point for the conventional greater trochanteric osteotomy is provided by reflecting a small amount of vastus lateralis.

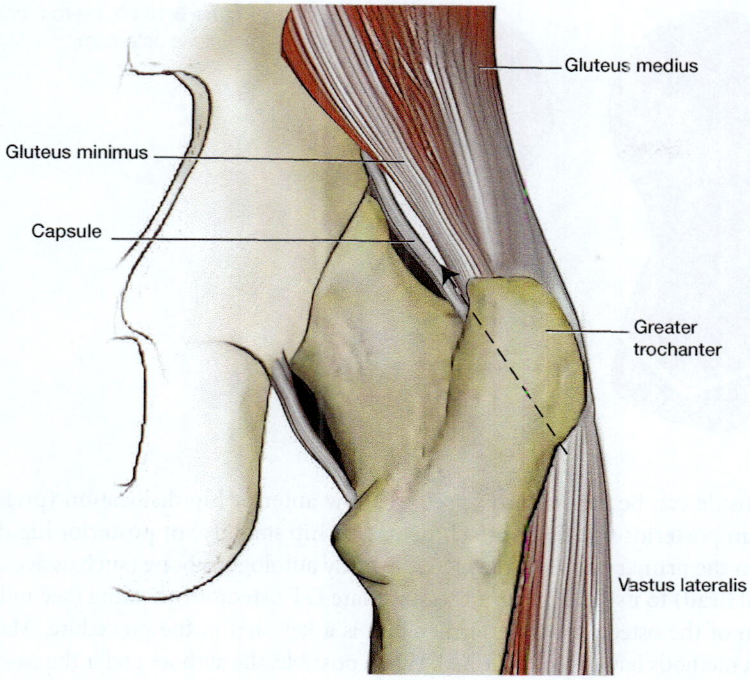

Figure 5.8 | The exit point for the conventional greater trochanteric osteotomy is just deep to the gluteus minimus insertion.

- Use an oscillating saw to perform the osteotomy. This is the critical step, and care should be taken to make the osteotomy in the proper orientation and to make the osteotomy fragment the proper thickness. Ideally the fragment should be thick enough to provide a strong fragment for reattachment but not so thick that the bed of the GT osteotomy will be severely depleted during femoral preparation. Usually the osteotomy fragment will be about 1 cm thick.
- Different osteotomy configurations may be used. A flat osteotomy (Figure 5.9) is the easiest to perform and allows leeway for adjustment of the GT position during reattachment. A "Chevron" osteotomy (Figure 5.10) provides more inherent rotational stability of the osteotomy, but care must be taken to avoid splitting the fragment vertically. When performing a Chevron osteotomy, the osteotomy should be oriented apex-lateral. Placing one saw blade in the osteotomy after the first pass with a saw for the first limb of the osteotomy provides a guide for the second pass with the saw for the second limb of the osteotomy (Figure 5.11).
- After the osteotomy is completed, the GT and abductors are reflected proximally by dissecting the abductors away from the underlying capsule and lateral ilium.

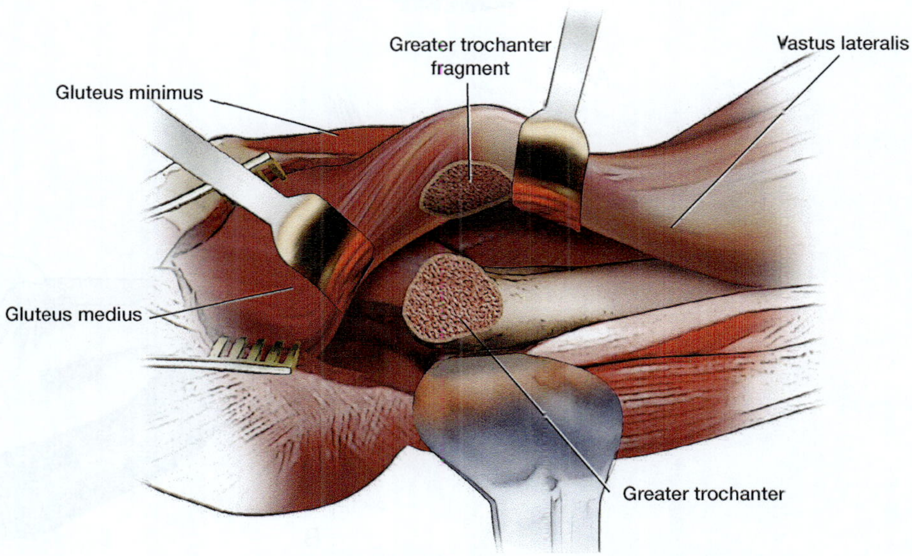

Figure 5.9 | Flat greater trochanteric osteotomy.

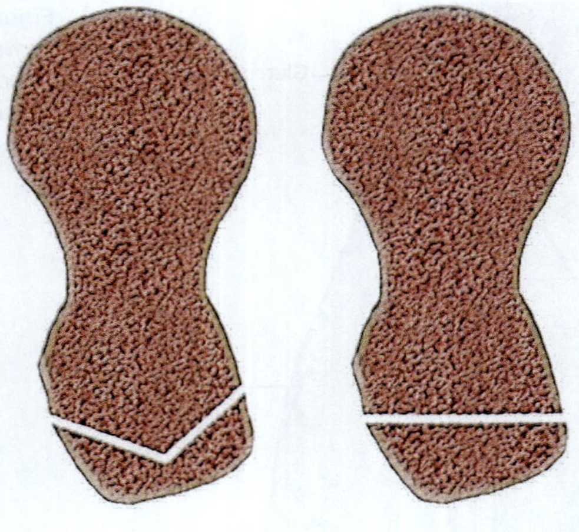

Figure 5.10 I "Chevron" configuration greater trochanteric osteotomy.

- The capsule can be incised or excised to allow anterior hip dislocation (preferred in most cases to maintain posterior soft tissue attachments and hip stability) or posterior hip dislocation.
- Perform the primary or revision THA. Save any autologous bone (such as acetabular reamings or the femoral head) to use as bone graft to stimulate GT osteotomy healing (see following text).
- Fixation of the osteotomy is performed and is a key step in the procedure. Many different osteotomy fixation methods have been described. When possible, the authors prefer the so-called 4-wire technique. Trochanteric claw and cable fixation is strong but creates risk of cable fretting and debris and trochanteric irritation from the claw. Claw plates are bulky and may devascularize the bone and are used rarely.
- Fixation with the 4-wire technique uses 2 vertical and 2 horizontal wires (either 18-gauge or double Luque wires) (Figure 5.12). Drill 2 holes through the lateral cortex of the femur about 1 cm distal to the osteotomy and pass the vertical wires. For the horizontal wires, often the proximal wire is passed through a drill hole in the proximal lesser trochanter and the distal wire is passed inferior to the lesser trochanter. The wires may be passed over the GT or through drill holes in the GT. In most cases passing wires over the GT works well. Abduct the hip, hold the osteotomy fragment in the desired position with a sharp rake, and tighten the wires sequentially and firmly and then secure the wires with twists or wire knots.
- Fixation with a GT claw can be performed with several different cable configurations (Figure 5.13). Do not pass cables vertically over the top of the GT. These can fray and create cable debris in the

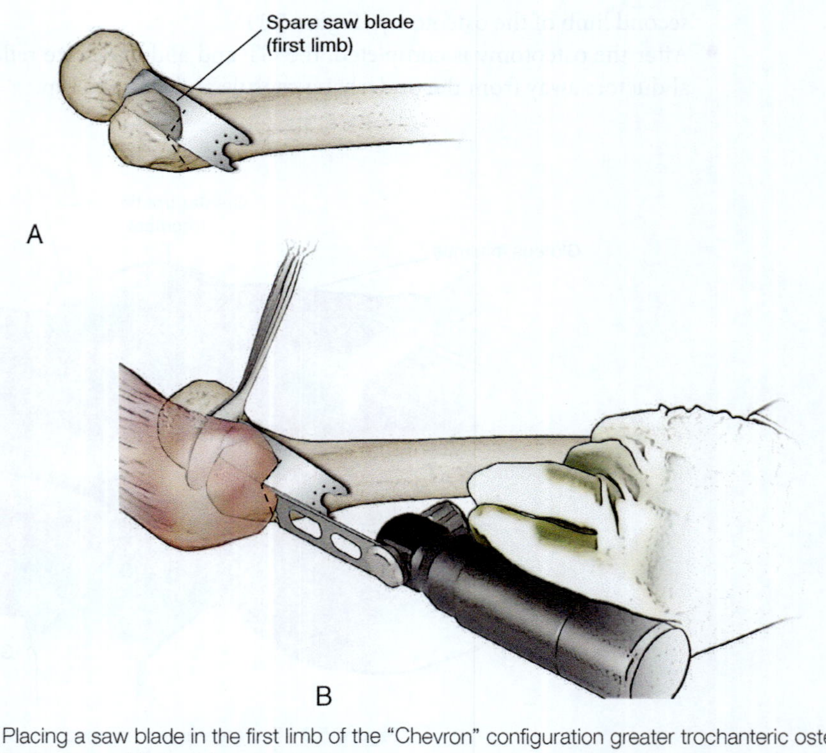

Figure 5.11 I Placing a saw blade in the first limb of the "Chevron" configuration greater trochanteric osteotomy provides a guide for the second limb of the osteotomy.

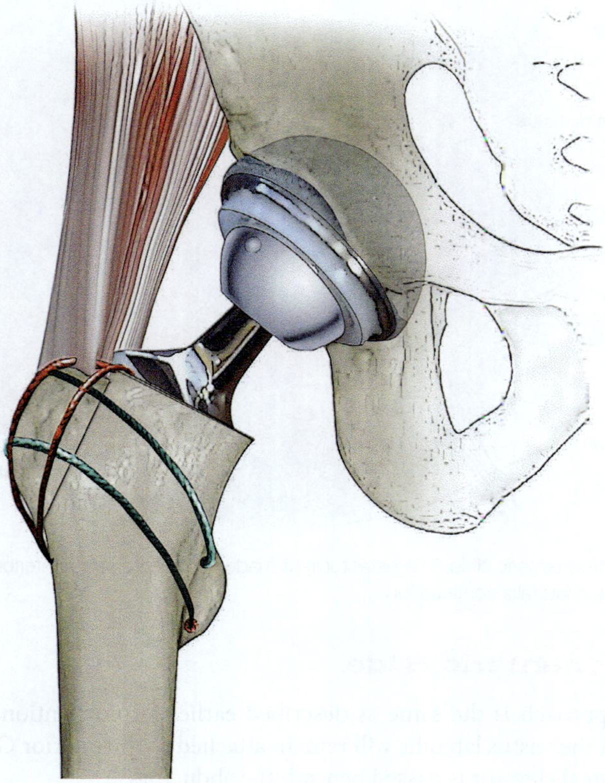

Figure 5.12 | Four-wire configuration fixation of conventional greater trochanteric osteotomy.

joint. Abduct the hip, hold the osteotomy carefully in correct orientation with a sharp rake, and sequentially tighten, then fasten, the cables.

- If desired the GT may be advanced moderately on its bed to improve abductor tension. Make sure good contact between the GT and the bed of the GT is maintained. A saw may be used to lengthen the bed distally if need (maintain the bed as a flat surface, which will match the underside of the osteotomized GT).
- If autogenous bone graft from the THA is available, pack this around the GT osteotomy.
- Close the vastus lateralis with strong suture to the soft tissues remaining on the inferior GT.

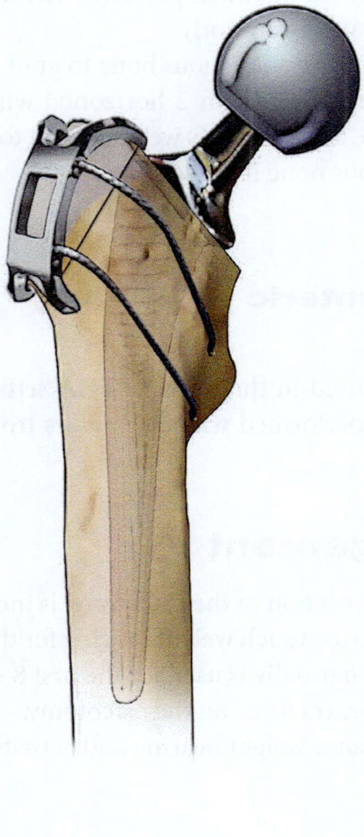

Figure 5.13 | Greater trochanteric osteotomy fixation with claw and cables.

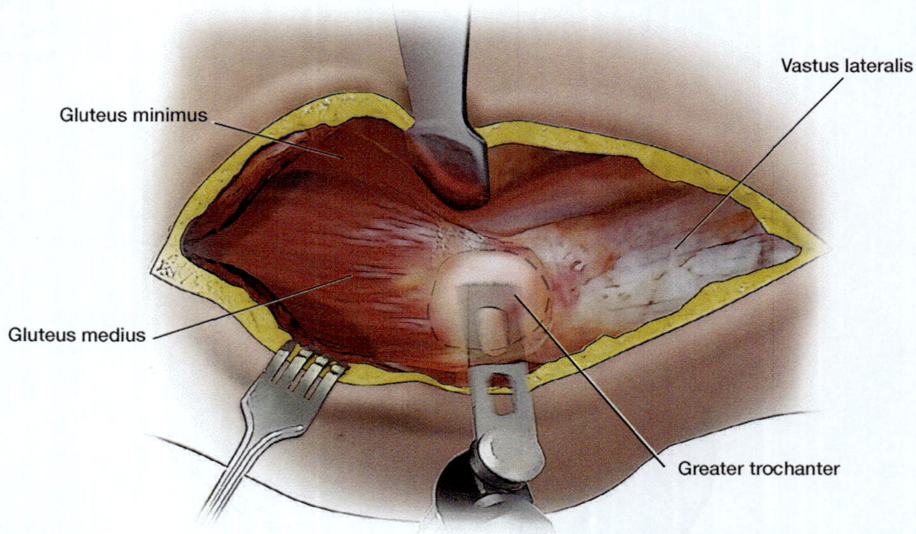

Figure 5.14 | Greater trochanteric slide. The osteotomy is made from posterior to anterior and maintains abductor–greater trochanter–vastus lateralis continuation.

Greater Trochanteric Slide

- The operative approach is the same as described earlier for conventional GT osteotomy. The key difference is that the vastus lateralis will remain attached to the inferior GT.
- A snap or periosteal elevator is passed beneath the abductors.
- A snap or periosteal elevator is passed from posterior to anterior deep to the origin of the vastus lateralis just distal to the vastus ridge.
- The osteotomy is made with an oscillating saw from posterior to anterior (Figure 5.14). The depth of the osteotomy should be as described earlier for a conventional osteotomy: thick enough to provide a strong osteotomy fragment and to maintain abductor and vastus lateralis attachments to the fragment but not so thick that the bed of the GT will be ruined during femoral preparation for the THA. Usually the osteotomy fragment will be about 1 cm thick.
- The adductors, GT, and vastus lateralis are reflected anteriorly by dissecting the abductors away from the underlying capsule and (if needed) the lateral ilium and the vastus lateralis away from the proximal lateral femur (see Figure 5.2).
- The hip usually is dislocated anteriorly (to maintain posterior soft tissue attachments for posterior hip stability), but it also may be dislocated posteriorly.
- Perform the primary or revision THA. Save autologous bone to graft the osteotomy site.
- Fixation of the osteotomy most commonly is with 2 horizontal wires or a trochanteric claw and cables. Make sure the fixation is secure and the GT is well opposed to its bed.
- Graft the osteotomy site with autologous bone if available.
- Close the wound in layers.

Extended Greater Trochanteric Osteotomy

- See Chapter 23 for details.
- When an extended GT osteotomy is used in the primary THA setting, the anterior and posterior osteotomy longitudinal limbs can be performed with saw passes from posterior to anterior before hip dislocation if desired.

Postoperative Management

- Osteotomy healing is important, so protection of the osteotomy is indicated until healing occurs.
- Weight bearing typically is restricted to toe touch weight bearing for the first 8 weeks postoperatively.
- A hip guide brace with 15° of abduction usually is used for the first 8 weeks to protect the osteotomy from adduction of the leg, which puts extra force on the osteotomy.
- Follow serial hip radiographs and advance weight bearing and activity based on osteotomy healing.

Chapter 6
Uncemented Acetabular Components

JOSEPH M. STATZ
RAFAEL J. SIERRA

Key Concepts

- Choosing an uncemented acetabular component over a cemented acetabular component for total hip arthroplasty (THA) is largely surgeon preference in the majority of patients.
- The vast majority of acetabular components (cups) implanted in the United States are uncemented owing to excellent clinical outcomes, decreased operating time, ability to add adjuvant screw fixation for primary stability, and versatility of use with the availability of differing head diameter and bearing surface liner options.
- Advantages of uncemented acetabular components:
  - Survivorship: Excellent long-term survivorship in clinical series and registries
  - Versatility: Can be used in nearly any case
  - Decreased operating time
  - Acetabular version or hip center of rotation can be altered after cup insertion by changing the cup position or by using different liner options
  - Ease of modular liner exchange if that should be needed for hip stability or other reasons
- Disadvantages of uncemented acetabular components:
  - Risk of acetabular fracture when impacting component with a press-fit.
  - Bone needs to grow into the cup for long-term stability.
  - Conventional uncemented cups are contraindicated in irradiated, necrotic, and allograft bone. This problem has been mostly solved with highly porous uncemented cups.
- The goal of implanting an uncemented acetabular component is to obtain adequate component stability against adequate bone that will support the component and to obtain long-term fixation by bone ingrowth.
  - To aid in initial stability, underreaming the acetabular bone by 1 to 2 mm smaller than the acetabular component will create hoop stresses between the component and bone, stabilizing the component with this press-fit.
  - Adding acetabular screws can also increase initial fixation to the acetabular bone and should be used when adequate press-fit is not achieved.
  - Almost all uncemented cups have external surfaces that are coated with 3-dimensional matrices that lead to bone ingrowth and/or roughened surfaces that lead to bone ongrowth. Three-dimensional porous surfaces have a strong track record of resisting loosening even if osteolysis occurs.
- Two main types of uncemented acetabular components exist for primary and revision THA (Figure 6.1).
  - Hemispherical acetabular components have a constant radius of curvature throughout the entire component. Obtaining a press-fit with a hemispherical cup will create relatively uniform hoop stresses at all contact points between the cup and bone.

- Elliptical acetabular components have an increasing radius of curvature of the outer surface of the cup when comparing the center of the component to the edges of the component. Obtaining a press-fit with an elliptical cup will create stronger hoop stresses at the periphery of the cup and weaker hoop stresses at the center of the cup. These cups are usually reamed line to line as the periphery of the cup is usually thicker than the last reamer used.

Sterile Instruments and Implants

- Routine hip retractors
- Uncemented acetabular component (with instrumentation)

Positioning

- Surgeon preference for primary THA; the author utilizes a posterolateral approach with the patient in the lateral decubitus for primary and revision THA.

Surgical Approaches

- Uncemented acetabular components can be inserted through any THA approach. Please refer to Chapters 2-5.

Preoperative Planning

- Template acetabular component size and acetabular version. It can be useful to template cup diameter on a cross-table lateral view in addition to an anteroposterior (AP) view (Figures 6.2 and 6.3). An uncemented cup gets most of its press-fit from the anterior and posterior walls, which are best seen on the cross-table lateral view. This is especially helpful in cases in which superolateral defects exist, whereby templating from the AP radiographs might lead to overestimation of cup diameter. Placing

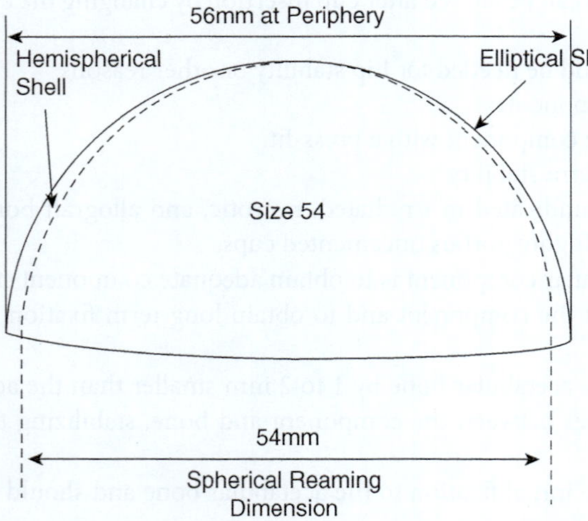

Figure 6.1 | Hemispherical cups (shells) have a constant radius of curvature from the center of the cup toward the periphery (dotted line), whereas elliptical cups have a radius of curvature that increases from the center of the cup toward the periphery. In this example, if the acetabulum was reamed with a 54-mm reamer, a 54-mm hemispherical cup would have no press-fit, whereas a 54-mm elliptical cup would have 2 mm of press-fit at the periphery where the diameter is 56 mm and no press-fit at the center of the cup where the diameter is 54 mm. (With permission from Haidukewych GJ, Jacofsky DJ, Hanssen AD, Lewallen DJ. Intraoperative fractures of the acetabulum during primary total hip arthroplasty. *J Bone Joint Surg Am*. 2006;88(9):1952-1956.)

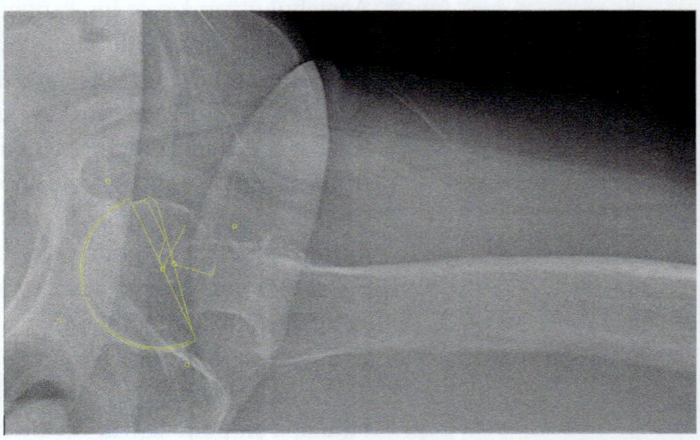

Figure 6.2 | Preoperative templating on a cross-table lateral reproduces an accurate cup size as this shows the anterior and posterior walls, which provide most of the stability when obtaining a press-fit.

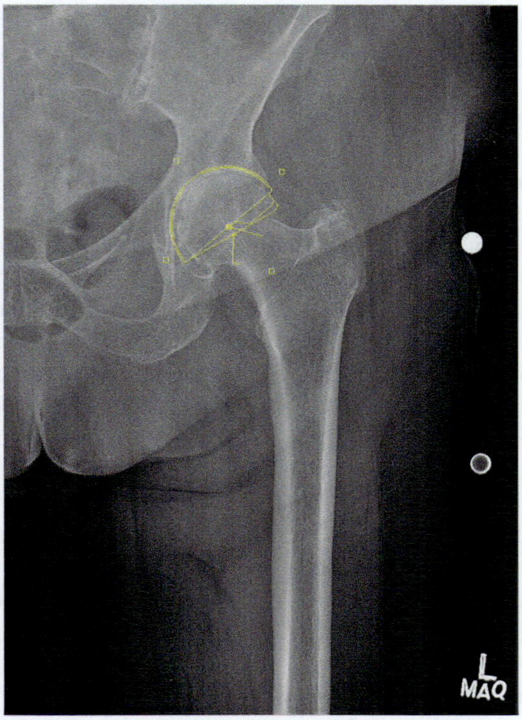

Figure 6.3 | Templating should also be performed on an AP radiograph of the hip with the cup sitting on or near the medial wall and contacting the superior rim of the acetabulum.

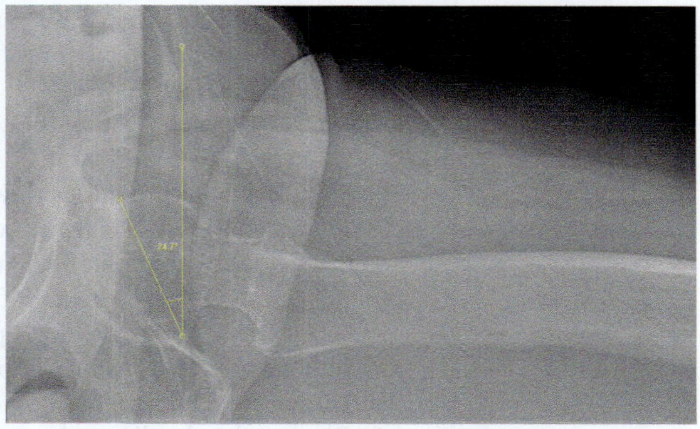

Figure 6.4 | The cross-table lateral can also be useful for judging the native anteversion of the acetabulum. In this case, the patient's native anteversion is 24.7°.

the templated acetabular component from the lateral radiograph on the AP radiograph should give the surgeon an idea as to whether appropriate coverage laterally will be achieved without bone grafting or superior placement of the acetabular component. Getting an idea of the patient's preoperative acetabular version on this lateral view will also allow the surgeon to judge acetabular component version intraoperatively (Figure 6.4).

- Template and clinically examine preoperative leg length discrepancy.
- Choose and template an appropriate femoral component. Please refer to Chapter 1.

Bone, Implant, and Soft Tissue Techniques

- Perform the desired approach to the hip joint.
- Perform the femoral neck osteotomy using templates as a guide.
- Prepare the femur for an appropriately sized and positioned femoral component. This can also be done after acetabular preparation and is the author's preference.
- Expose the acetabulum with appropriate retractors, making sure to place all retractors peripherally enough that they will not interfere with or get caught on the acetabular reamers. A posterior cobra retractor into the ischium or above it in the lesser sciatic notch and an anterior curved retractor to translate the femur anteriorly are the workhorse for acetabular exposure. A third straight retractor into the iliac bone to retract the gluteus minimus is added if needed.
- Remove the acetabular labrum circumferentially. This is usually most easily removed by using an outside-in technique with sharp dissection to peel the labrum off of the outer acetabular rim into the acetabulum.
- Clear the cotyloid fossa of the ligamentum teres and synovium to expose the floor of the fovea. Review preoperative radiographs, noting the position of the femoral head and center of rotation and medial and anterior and posterior acetabular osteophytes.
- Examine the native acetabulum, noting the native version, the center of the acetabulum, any asymmetric wear, the presence of osteophytes in the cotyloid fossa, the presence of dysplasia, and any

other abnormalities. The native version can be judged with preoperative templating as well as by examining the transacetabular ligament (TAL) intraoperatively, which normally closely parallels the desired acetabular version.

- Determine asymmetry within the acetabular fossa. Avoid reaming too anterior or posterior with the first reamers.
- There are several techniques with which to ream an acetabulum, but they all have the same goal of creating a good press-fit against bone that is strong enough to support an acetabular component and that also has circumferential punctate bleeding that will allow for bone ingrowth/ongrowth. In general, elevating the hip center of rotation, overreaming the anterior or posterior wall, and over-medialization should be avoided. Specific anatomic landmarks should help avoid these conditions.
- The author's preferred method of preparing an acetabulum is to start with a reamer 6 mm smaller than the templated size and ream medially to the floor of the cotyloid fossa of the acetabulum (Figure 6.5). The templated radiographs and restoration of offset should dictate how medially the cup will be placed, but in general the author reams just medial to Kohler's line. It is important to ream straight down to the fossa without deviating anterior, posterior, or superior. Deviating will lead to insufficient support of the cup and nonanatomic cup placement.
    - When reaming medially, the surgeon should make sure that the reamer is not off center; the most common error is to ream too posteriorly. If the surgeon does not take into account the position of the first reamer, then subsequent reamers will differentially ream posteriorly, leading to problems with the integrity of the posterior wall. Hugging the anterior wall with the reamer will avoid this complication (Figure 6.6).
    - Reaming should then be carried out in 2-mm increases; the surgeon should be aware of the location of the reamer as it pertains to the transverse ligament. In general, a reamer that sits over the TAL requires either medialization or increase in depth of reaming superiorly. A reamer that sits just inside the TAL is generally in correct position. In most cases the goal is for reaming to the depth of the floor of the fovea, which provides restoration or slight medialization of the hip center. The true medial wall is a few millimeters deeper than the floor of the fovea. Reaming all the way to the true medial wall usually is needed only in special cases such as developmental hip dysplasia in which deep medialization is required for adequate cup coverage.

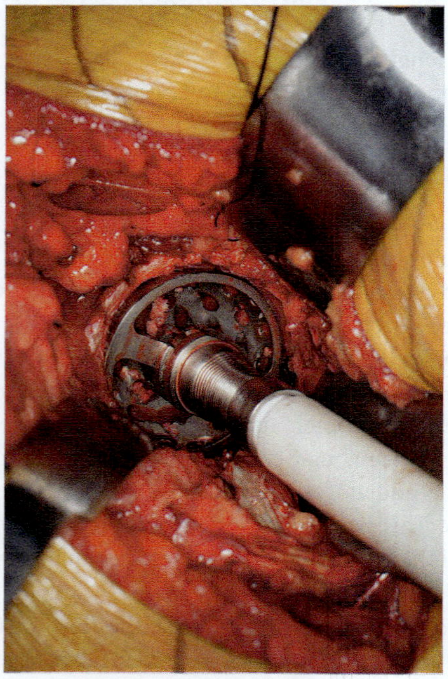

Figure 6.5 | The first reamer should be 6 mm smaller than the templated cup size and used to ream to the bottom of the cotyloid fossa (medial wall) of the acetabulum.

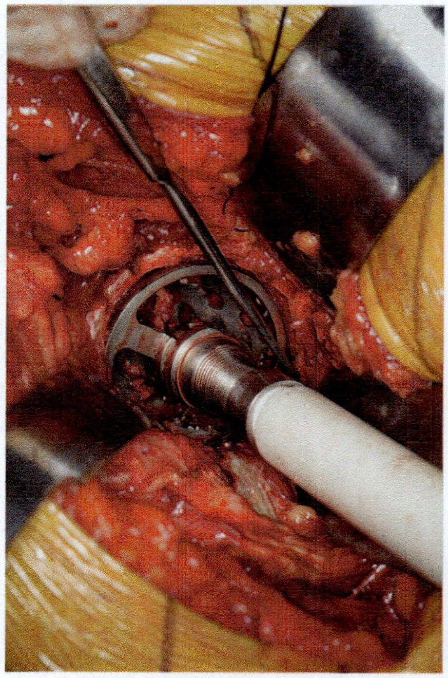

Figure 6.6 | Ensure that the reamer is centered in the acetabulum. Reaming the posterior wall more than the anterior wall, or vice versa, should be avoided.

- With each sequential reamer, equal contact should be made anteriorly, posteriorly, and superiorly, and usually an equal amount of bone should be removed from each of these areas. Reaming should stop when appropriate peripheral contact is achieved with circumferential punctate bleeding bone, which is usually with a reamer that is 2 mm smaller than the templated cup diameter. The surgeon should then decide whether 1 or 2 mm of press-fit is desired based on bone quality. Most of the time, if not always, a 1-mm press-fit is appropriate.
- The final reamer is used to ream medially and peripherally to the same diameter to avoid creating an "hourglass deformity" whereby the center of the acetabulum is reamed to a smaller diameter than the periphery, which can interfere with the press-fit of the cup. Going further than the medial wall will create a defect into the pelvis. Judging how medial to go depends on the templated radiograph and can be determined intraoperatively based on the stepoff created by the reamed bone surface, the floor of the fovea, and, in some cases, the medial wall. Care should be taken when coxa profunda is noted radiographically. In such situations, reaming should not be carried out into the depth of the medial acetabular wall but should be left lateralized as compared with the medial wall. The depth of the current reamer can be judged by visualizing bone through the inside of the reamer.
- If desired, a trial cup can be placed to ensure that a true hemisphere was reamed and that appropriate version and position can be obtained during insertion of the real cup. If using a trial cup, a nerve hook can be used to ensure that good contact is being made in all quadrants of the hemisphere. A trial cup 1 mm smaller than the last reamer usually works well for this. The surgeon may elect to use the trial cup and trial femoral component to optimize cup version based on the stability of the hip before definitive component implantation.
- Once acetabular preparation is complete, the acetabulum is cleaned with saline and a sponge. It is important that there is no fibrous tissue obstructing full seating of the cup as this will interfere with bone ingrowth (Figure 6.7).
- A real uncemented acetabular component 1 to 2 mm larger than the last reamer is then opened and inserted into the acetabulum. Getting the cup into the acetabulum sometimes involves maneuvering, twisting, and tilting the cup. The surface of the cup is rough and disposed to adhering to tissue on the way in. Once the component is positioned in the desired version and abduction at the rim of the acetabulum, a mallet is used to impact the component (Figure 6.8A). The component should be

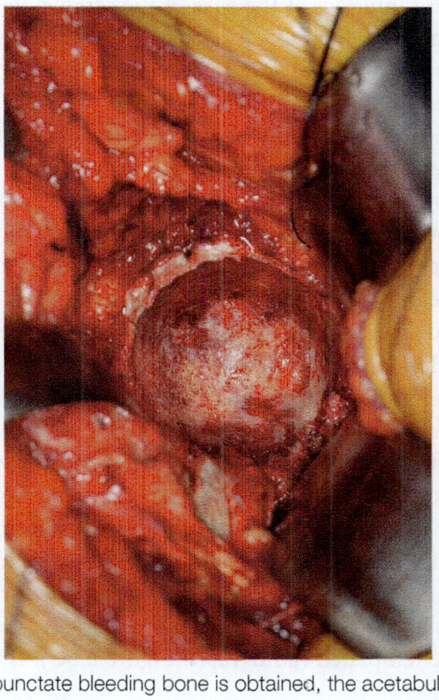

Figure 6.7 | Once circumferential, punctate bleeding bone is obtained, the acetabulum should be thoroughly irrigated and all fibrous tissue be removed with a sponge so that the cup can seat fully against bone without any interposed fibrous tissue.

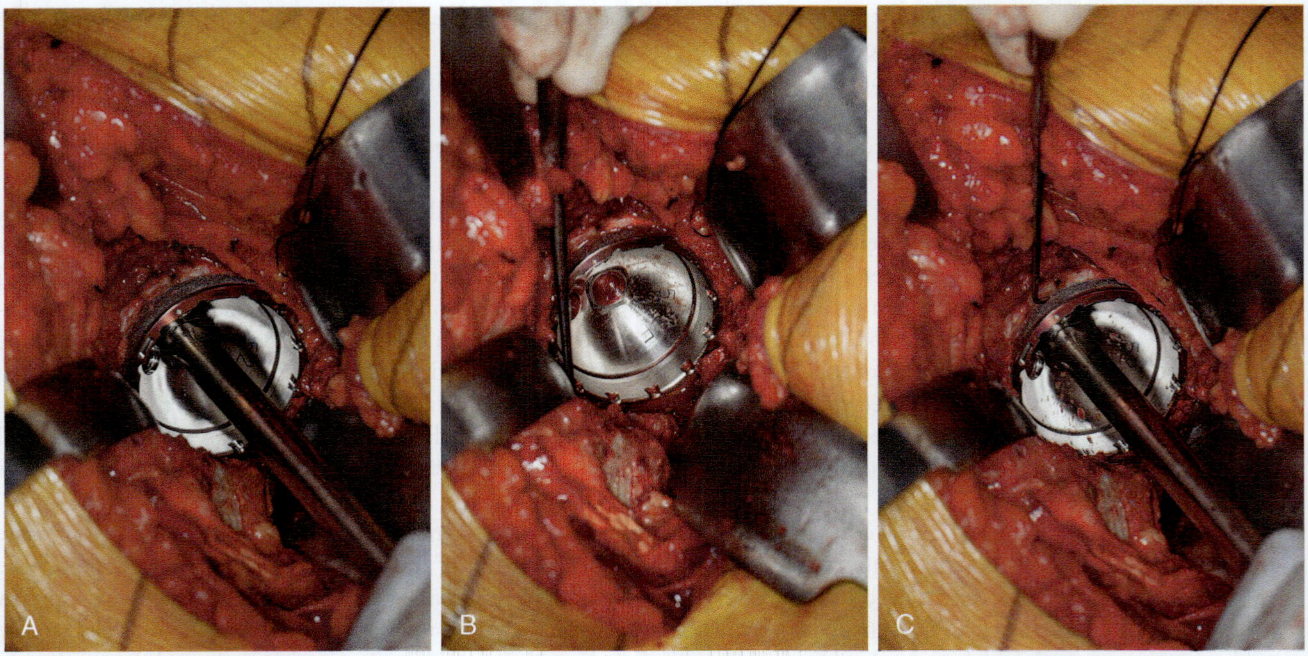

Figure 6.8 | A, The cup should be inserted in the desired version and abduction and impacted with a mallet. The cup should generally be placed in 5 to 25° of anteversion and 30 to 50° of abduction. The anteversion should generally parallel the TAL, and the inferior portion of the cup should be just deep to the TAL. B, The anterior wall should be palpated with a nerve hook and been felt to be flush with the anterior rim of the cup. C, The superior uncoverage of the cup should be examined, which is indicated in this figure with a nerve hook. This should be compared with the preoperative templating. If there is more uncoverage intraoperatively, the cup is more horizontal than templated. If there is less uncoverage, the cup is more vertical than templated.

seated all the way down to bone centrally and peripherally. This can be judged by a change in pitch of the mallet strikes, the lack of advancement of the component, and by directly examining the bone-implant interface at the base of the screw holes in the cup with a nerve hook. Peripheral impaction with a face-type impactor can assure that the implant is seated into the depth of the reamed bone.

- The position of the acetabular component should be verified using anatomic landmarks. In general terms:
  - The inferior rim of the cup should not sit lateral to the TAL. If it does, then the acetabulum is not reamed medially and/or superiorly enough or cup position is too vertical.
  - The anterior wall should be palpated with a nerve hook (Figure 6.8B). The anterior wall and the anterior acetabular cup rim should be flush with one another or the cup should be inset relative to the rim. Cup prominence anteriorly can lead to iliopsoas impingement. Alternatively, if the native acetabular wall is markedly overhanging the cup anteriorly, then the cup probably has either too much anteversion or the acetabulum has been reamed superiorly. Noting posterior wall coverage will help determine whether it is the former or latter situation. If the posterior wall is also prominent, then the cup may have been reamed to a superiorly positioned hip center. This situation should be avoided.
  - After removing anterior and posterior osteophytes, note the position of the TAL and its corresponding trajectory with regards to the acetabular opening. It should sit parallel to it in the majority of cases. Exceptions include patients with overanteverted native acetabulums, such as those with hip dysplasia or patients with severe acetabular retroversion. It is important for the surgeon to note the femoral version as well to determine the best position of the acetabular component.
  - The superolateral uncoverage of the acetabular component should be noted and compared with the templated radiograph (Figure 6.8C). If the cup uncoverage is more than templated, then the

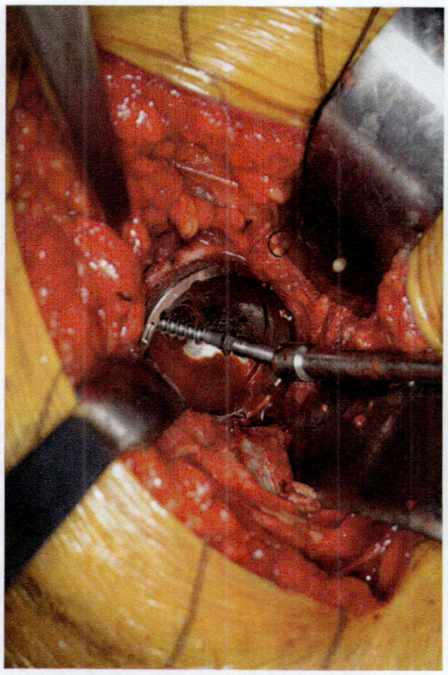

Figure 6.9 | Acetabular screws can be used to enhance fixation but are not always necessary if excellent press-fit is obtained.

acetabular component is horizontal. On the other hand, if there is no uncoverage then the cup may have been placed too vertical. A moderate amount of cup uncoverage is acceptable if the implant is inherently captured by the socket and stable.
- A final check of acetabular anteversion can be made by placing a finger into the sciatic notch to determine the orientation of the acetabular opening in reference to that anatomic landmark. A line that connects the posterior acetabular ridge to the greater sciatic notch is perpendicular to a line connecting the anterior and posterior acetabular walls.

- If desired, acetabular screws can be placed to aid in securing the cup (Figure 6.9). Usually 1 to 2 screws are placed into the ilium in between the inner and outer surfaces of the ilium between the anterior superior iliac spine and sciatic notch. These are usually unicortical screws that gain purchase when the threads make contact with the inner cortex of the ilium. If needed to obtain fixation, additional screws can be placed into the ischial bone and pubic bone. Care should be taken to not plunge with the drill in these locations, as injury to neurovascular structures is more likely with these trajectories. A "safe zone" for screw placement has been defined and should be familiar to the surgeon.
- A trial head and liner can be placed to determine appropriate tension, range of motion, stability, and leg lengths. Obtain an intraoperative radiograph if desired to confirm appropriate component positioning.
- Impact the real acetabular liner into the cup and real femoral head onto the femoral trunnion. Check to make sure the liner is properly and securely locked into the metal shell.
- Irrigate the wound thoroughly.
- Close the hip capsule and perform a routine closure specific to the chosen approach.
- Apply a sterile dressing.
- Postoperative radiographs can be obtained as a baseline for future follow-up (Figure 6.10A-C) and to document proper implant position and hip reduction.

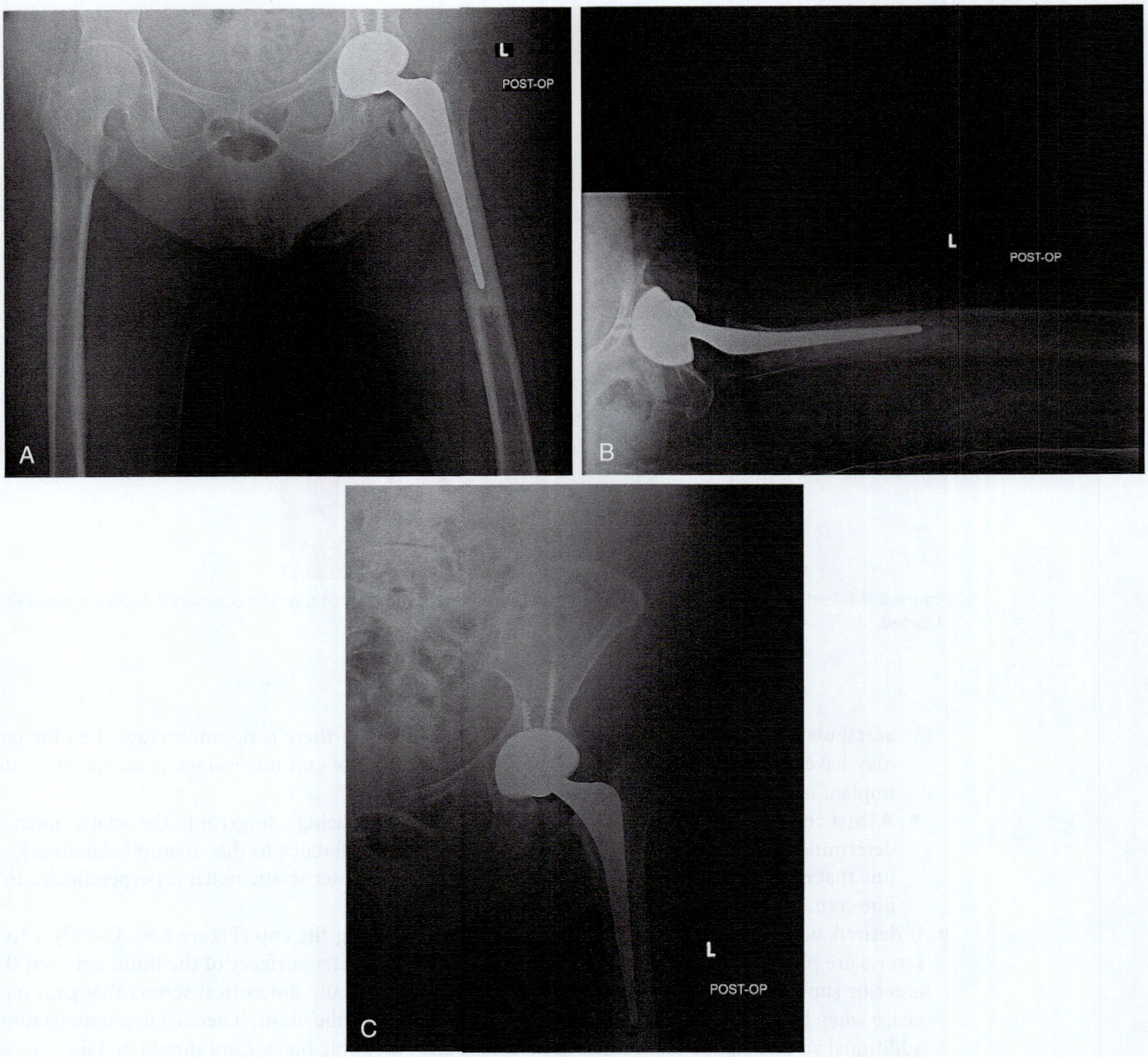

Figure 6.10 | A-C. Postoperative x-rays can be obtained as a baseline for future examinations.

Postoperative Care

The patient may weight bear as tolerated with standard THA precautions.

Chapter 7
Uncemented Tapered Stems

TIMOTHY S. BROWN
MICHAEL J. TAUNTON

Key Concepts

- The starting point for preparation of the femur is key and can differ by implant
- Special attention must be paid to lateralize during the preparation process to keep the final component from being placed in a varus position.
- Stable initial fixation with scratch-fit and appropriate stem sizing is critical for long-term ingrowth and implant fixation.

Sterile Instruments and Implants

- Retractors specific for the surgeon's preferred approach (Figure 7.1)
- Round high-speed burr
- Reamers, broaches, trials specific to the selected cementless tapered implant (Figures 7.2 and 7.3)

Surgical Approaches

- Posterolateral: Care must be taken when reaming to avoid extending the femoral component.
- Anterolateral: Care must be taken when reaming to avoid flexing the femoral component.
- Direct anterior: Adequate exposure of the femur is necessary for safe preparation. The abdomen may push the reamer into varus and flexion.

Preoperative Planning

- Preoperative evaluation of the femoral bone quality and any deformity can help the surgeon decide which type of stem will fit best. A tight canal with a wide metaphysis may be more amenable to a ream and broach system that allows expansion of the diaphysis to allow for a sufficiently large stem to provide good fit in the metaphysis.
- Preoperative templating for femoral stem sizing and position is useful for planning stem insertion relative to the greater trochanter (Figure 7.4).

Bone, Implant, and Soft Tissue Techniques

- After initial exposure of the proximal femur, a sharp Hohmann retractor is placed on the anterior border of the greater trochanter to move the gluteus medius and minimus away from the path of reaming and broaching.
- An entry point posterolaterally near the piriformis fossa is made with the high-speed burr (Figure 7.5).
- A T-handled starting reamer is used to define the femoral canal.

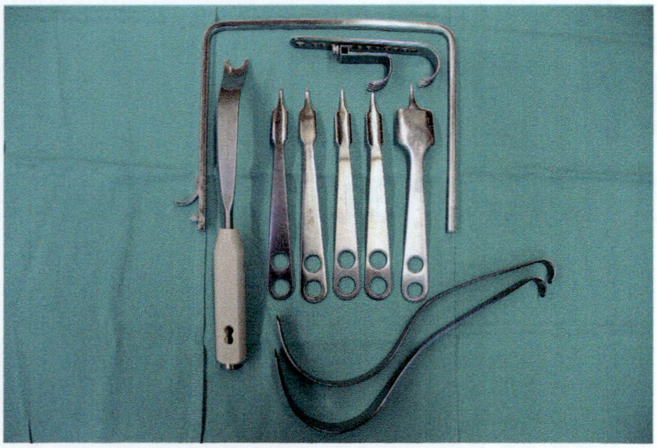

Figure 7.1 | Retractors utilized by authors for a primary posterior approach.

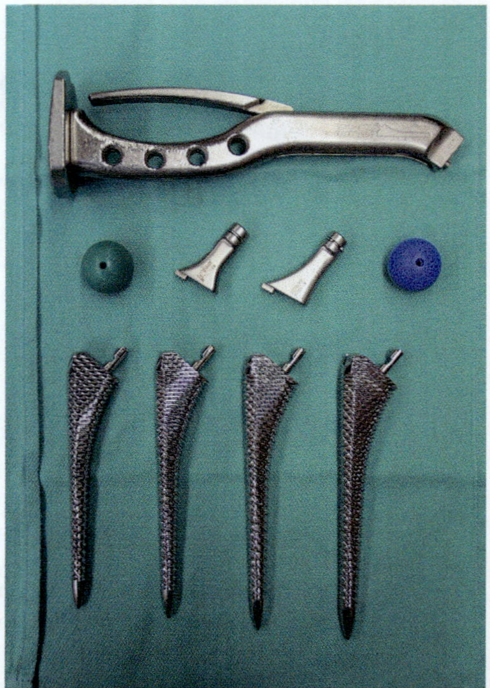

Figure 7.2 | Reamers, broaches, and trials for a ream and broach cementless tapered femoral stem.

Ream and Broach

- For a ream and broach system, the reamers are used sequentially up to the templated size. Care should be taken not to ream past the distal extent of where the stem will sit. Care should also be taken to keep the reamer out of varus alignment. Often, this will mean lateralization of the reamer partially into the greater trochanter.
- After completion of the femoral reaming, the femoral broaches are used sequentially up to the size templated. In general, the version of the native femoral neck is followed to maximize the size of the stem that can be used.

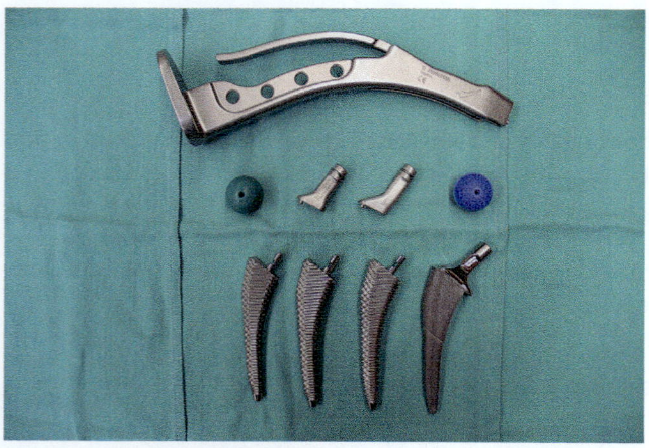

Figure 7.3 | Broaches and trials for a broach-only cementless tapered femoral stem.

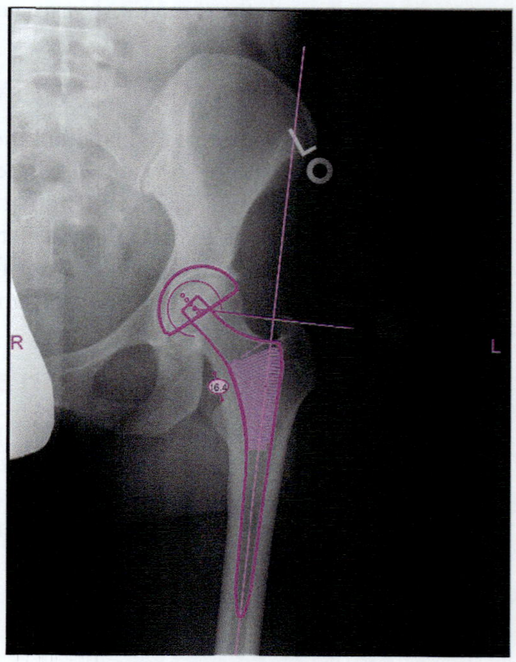

Figure 7.4 | Anteroposterior radiograph of hip with planned stem size and position.

- For patients with retroverted anatomy, we will aim to provide 10 to 15° anteversion with the femoral stem. In such circumstances the broach envelope will be created in a somewhat more anteverted orientation than the patient's femoral neck. Working the posterolateral aspect of the broach posteriorly into the femoral neck allows greater anteversion to be obtained because this creates more space anteriorly for the medial flare of the broach, even in the retroverted femoral neck.
- One may impact on the broach handle in a direction that biases the broach laterally to prevent the broach from heading into a varus position.
- Once a broach size is found that is axially and rotationally stable within the proximal femur, a trial neck and trial femoral head are placed. The hip is reduced and checked for leg length, stability, and impingement.
- An intraoperative anteroposterior radiograph with the broach in place is helpful to determining stem sizing and positioning.
- Before removing the broach, attention must be paid to the depth at which the broach has seated.
- While the broach is in place and after the broach is removed, the calcar should be inspected for fracture. If a fracture is present, or the surgeon feels there is a likelihood of postoperative fracture, a cerclage wire or cable should be placed above the lesser trochanter.
- The definitive femoral component is then inserted and impacted into position. Care should be taken to ensure the implant follows the exact anteversion of the previously prepared broach envelope. Impaction with multiple blows of modest magnitude is the safest way to ensure full seating with low risk of femoral fracture. Pushing the stem laterally during insertion can facilitate full seating. Pay attention to the implant insertion handle during impaction to make sure it is not being forced against the greater trochanter, which can lead to fracture.
- The final implant should seat at approximately the same level as the broach. If the implant is proud, the version should be checked. If the implant sinks below this level, the proximal femur should be carefully evaluated for fracture (Figure 7.6). If the implant does not seat deeply enough, it best to withdraw the implant and reprepare the femur to a slightly deeper level with reamers and broaches, rather than impact the implant so forcefully that a fracture is caused.
- After final seating of the implant, inspect the femoral neck area to make sure a fracture is not present. If even a small crack is present, treat it with a cerclage wire or cable and make sure the implant remains perfectly stable axially and rotationally.

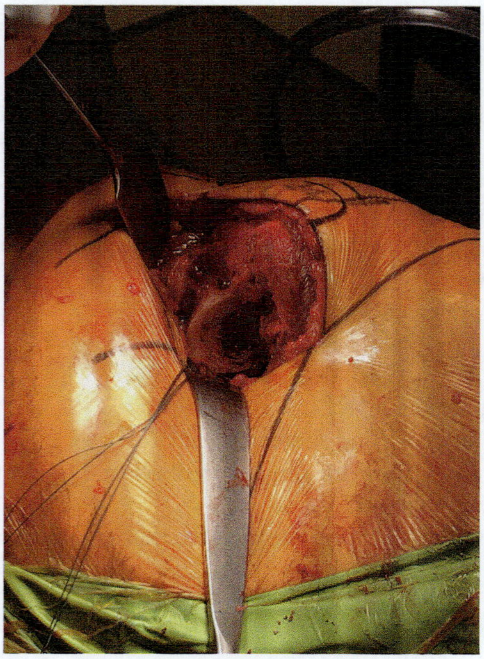

Figure 7.5 | Proximal femoral exposure for preparation of the femur.

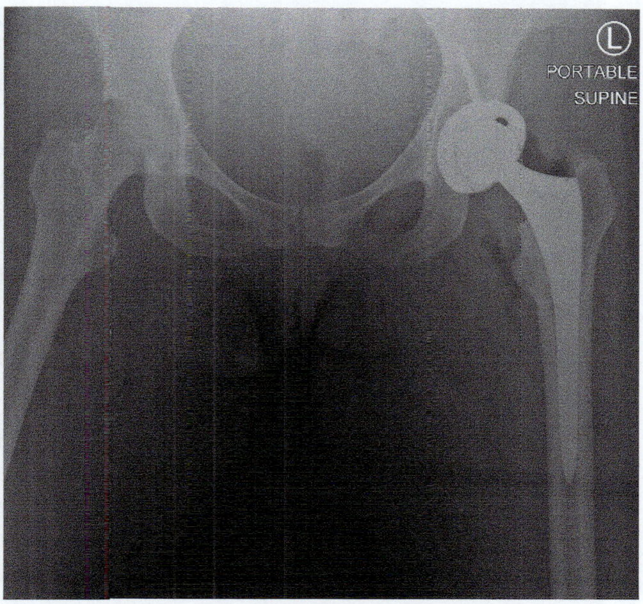

Figure 7.6 | Anteroposterior radiograph of a ream and broach cementless tapered stem.

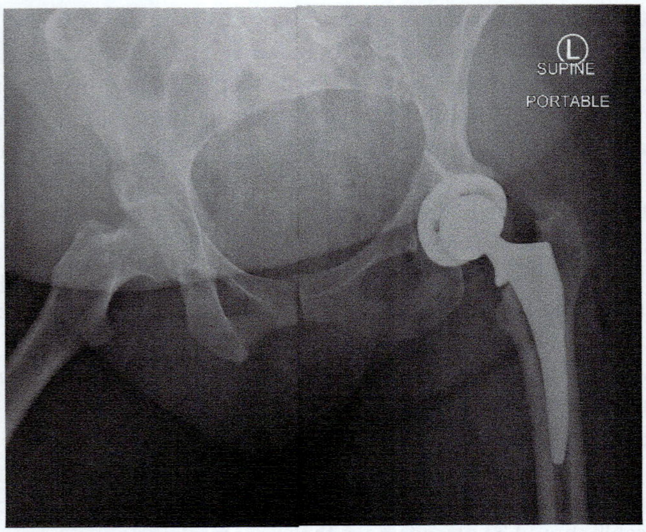

Figure 7.7 | Anteroposterior radiograph of a broach-only cementless tapered stem.

Broach Only

- A box osteotome is utilized to open the canal laterally.
- A starter femoral broach that is significantly smaller than the rest of the broaches is then utilized to direct initial direction for broaching.
- Femoral broaches are then used sequentially up to the size templated. In general, the version of the native femoral neck is followed to maximize the size of the stem that can be used. For patients with retroverted anatomy, we will aim to provide 10 to 15° anteversion with the femoral stem (see earlier comments related to ream and broach implants).
- It is our preference to impact on the broach handle in a direction that biases the broach laterally, to prevent the broach from heading into a varus position.
- Once a broach size is found that is axially and rotationally stable within the proximal femur, a trial neck and trial femoral head are placed and the hip is tested for length and stability.
- If the implant has a collar, attention is paid to where the broach sits while trialing. A calcar reamer is utilized so that a fixed level can be identified for final implant seating.
- While the broach is in place and after the broach is removed, the calcar should be inspected for fracture. If a fracture is present, or the surgeon feels there is a likelihood of postoperative fracture, a cerclage wire or cable should be placed above the lesser trochanter.
- Before removing the broach, look at the depth to which the broach has seated. The final implant should seat at this same level. If the implant is proud, the version should be checked. If the implant sinks below this level, the proximal femur should be carefully evaluated for fracture (Figure 7.7).
- After final seating of the implant, inspect the femoral neck area to make sure a fracture is not present. If even a small crack is present, treat it with a cerclage wire or cable and make sure the implant remains perfectly stable axially and rotationally.

Postoperative Care

- Weight bearing as tolerated is usually allowed postoperatively.
- Hip precautions are dependent on the surgical approach and surgeon preference.
- Postoperative radiographs on the day of surgery are helpful for surgeon feedback and to identify any component malposition or fracture that was not noted intraoperatively.
- Radiographs are taken at early follow-up (6-12 weeks) to ensure adequate fixation and stable position of the femoral stem.

Chapter 8
Uncemented Cylindrical Stems

TAD M. MABRY

Key Concepts

- The surgeon must take great care to obtain excellent femoral exposure, as cylindrical stems require both preparation and implantation in line with the femoral canal.
- Initial axial and rotational stability is achieved by way of a diaphyseal "scratch fit" over a distance of 5 to 7 cm.
- Although these stems have been used successfully across a very wide spectrum of femoral morphologies, the surgeon should consider alternative means of stem fixation at the extremes of femoral canal dimensions, and in the setting of coxa vara with significant trochanteric overhang (Figure 8.1).

Sterile Instruments and Implants

- Surgical approach-specific hip retractors
- Large-diameter high-speed burr and/or lateralizing reamer
- Instruments specific to the selected cementless, cylindrical component

Surgical Approaches

- Cylindrical stems may be implanted via any of the hip arthroplasty approaches.
- However, these straight, rigid stems are not forgiving of suboptimal femoral exposure. To gain appropriate fixation, the femur must be prepared and the implant inserted in line with the diaphysis.
  - Given the excellent femoral exposure offered, the posterolateral approach and the direct lateral approach are typically favored when using this style of femoral component.

Preoperative Planning

- Before detailed planning for a cylindrical stem, the surgeon should assess for any femoral deformity that might lend itself better to alternative methods of reconstruction.
  - Angular deformity
  - Rotational deformity
  - Compromised bone quality (significant osteoporosis, thin cortices, excessively narrow or wide femoral canal dimensions)
- The intended hip center is first determined from templating the acetabular side of the hip reconstruction.
- The femoral reconstruction is then planned in such a way as to effect the necessary change (or maintenance) in leg length. The following 3 key features of the intended stem are then determined (Figure 8.2):
  - Stem diameter—the goal is diaphyseal contact over 5 to 7 cm.

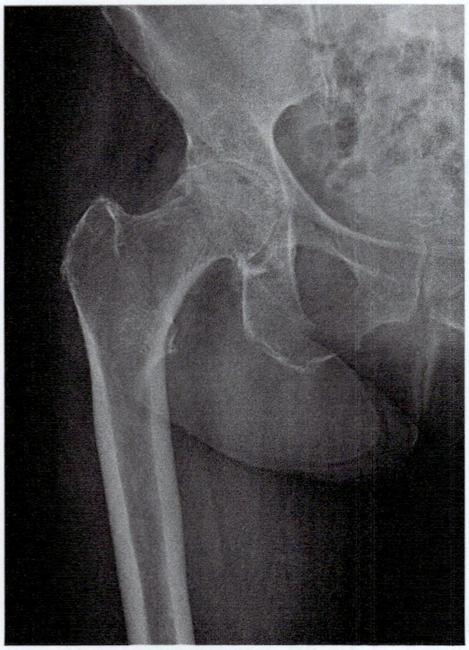

Figure 8.1 | Attempting to use a cylindrical stem in the setting of coxa vara with significant trochanteric overhang risks trochanteric fracture and/or stem malposition. In a case such as this, one should consider alternative stem designs.

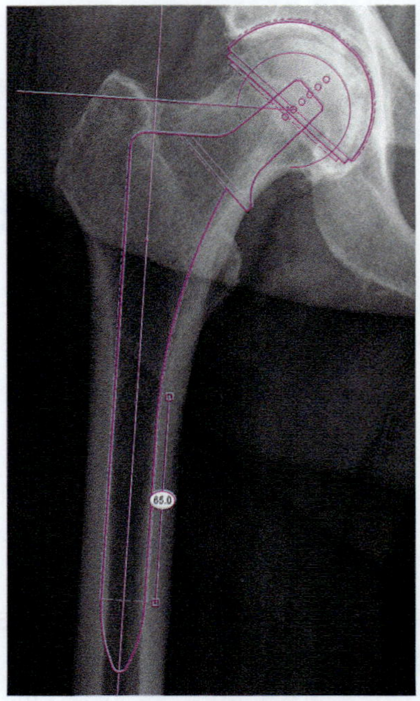

Figure 8.2 | Templated cylindrical stem noting ideal stem diameter (6.5 cm of cortical contact), metaphyseal fill, and restoration of offset.

- Metaphyseal fill—most cylindrical stems have a roughly triangular metaphyseal segment of varying sizes. The goal is to maximize metaphyseal fill without excess bone removal and without impeding rigid diaphyseal fixation.
- Stem offset—the goal is to maintain, or slightly increase, femoral offset, given the beneficial effects on hip stability and wear mechanics.
  - Note, the options for stem offset may relate to the size of the metaphyseal segment in some systems.

Bone, Implant, and Soft Tissue Techniques

Femoral Neck Osteotomy

- Create the femoral neck osteotomy at the desired site based on preoperative templating.
  - An over-long neck cut will inhibit acetabular exposure.
  - A too-short neck cut removes valuable bone for final seating of the collared portion of the stem and reduces stability of the metaphyseal segment.

Exposure

- Ensure circumferential visualization of the proximal femur, including the entire femoral calcar and the junction of the lateral femoral neck and trochanter.

Starting Point

- Open the proximal canal in the vicinity of the piriformis fossa, taking great care to avoid impingement of either the greater trochanter or the abductors on the intramedullary instruments, which would tend to push the implant into varus ± flexion.
  - It is very difficult to "lateralize" the femoral starting point with cylindrical reamers. It is therefore necessary to establish this starting point using a high-speed burr or lateralizing reamer to ensure femoral preparation in line with the diaphysis.
  - The degree of anticipated impingement from the trochanter should be assessed at the time of preoperative templating.

Reaming

- A T-handle starting reamer is often useful to initiate the process.
- Begin reaming with cylindrical reamers of the smallest diameter, increasing by 1-mm increments until cortical contact is first achieved.
  - Further expand the starting point as needed if the reamer seems to be deflected away from the central axis of the femoral canal.
  - Control the depth of reaming by reconciling measurements on the reamers with local bony landmarks.
    - The surgeon must prepare for the full length of the stem to avoid underseating of the final implant or femoral fracture, while avoiding unnecessary removal of bone from reaming to an excessive depth.
- Thereafter, increase the cylindrical reamer diameter by 0.5-mm increments until cortical reaming is achieved over a length of 5 to 7 cm to the desired depth.
  - This can be estimated by inserting the reamer as far as possible with gentle pressure. The surgeon can then measure the amount of reamer still exposed, which would correspond to the length of anticipated femoral canal contact.
  - Typically, the flutes of the final 2 to 3 reamers should be filled with cortical bone when removed from the canal. "Cortical chatter" during reaming does not always correspond to the actual reaming of cortical bone.
- The final reamer should be 0.5 mm less than the diameter of the anticipated real component to obtain the appropriate "scratch fit" in the femoral canal.

Broaching

- Begin broaching with the smallest metaphyseal segment 2 to 3 sizes below the stem for which you have prepared the canal.
  - Special attention must be paid to the appropriate stem anteversion beginning with the initial broach, to maximize bony contact with the final stem.
- Once the broach corresponding to the planned femoral stem diameter has been fully seated, the amount of bone remaining in the metaphysis is assessed. If there remains adequate space, the broach corresponding to the next larger metaphyseal segment is then fully seated.
  - The size of the metaphyseal segment is most often known from preoperative templating.
  - In some cases, a high-speed burr may be necessary to open the cortex of the femoral calcar if it would appear to be impinging upon final seating of the broach, which may help to avoid a proximal fracture.

Trialing and Radiographs

- Using the final broach as a trial, the surgeon should assess leg length, soft tissue tension, and hip stability in the standard fashion.
- Consideration should be made to obtain plain radiographs in 2 planes with the final broach in place to assess size, alignment, and appropriate depth of reaming (Figure 8.3A-C). This is especially important if the surgeon is early in her or his experience with the use of these devices.

Final Implantation

- The diameter of the real stem can be measured very accurately with a hole gauge (Figure 8.4). If the stem size varies slightly from the stated size, reamed sized may be adjusted by 0.05 mm if needed.
- The real femoral stem is first inserted by hand as far as possible, and in the appropriate amount of anteversion, corresponding to the preparation with the final broach.
  - If the stem seems to be excessively proud, the surgeon should consider removing the stem and slightly deeper line-to-line reaming as needed, until the real stem can be inserted by hand with only 5 to 7 cm remaining for further insertion. The surgeon is attempting to balance the appropriate scratch fit without excessive force required for implantation.
- The stem is then carefully impacted with repetitive mallet blows. It is critical that the surgeon uses an assistant as needed to control the stem anteversion during final seating of the implant. Without

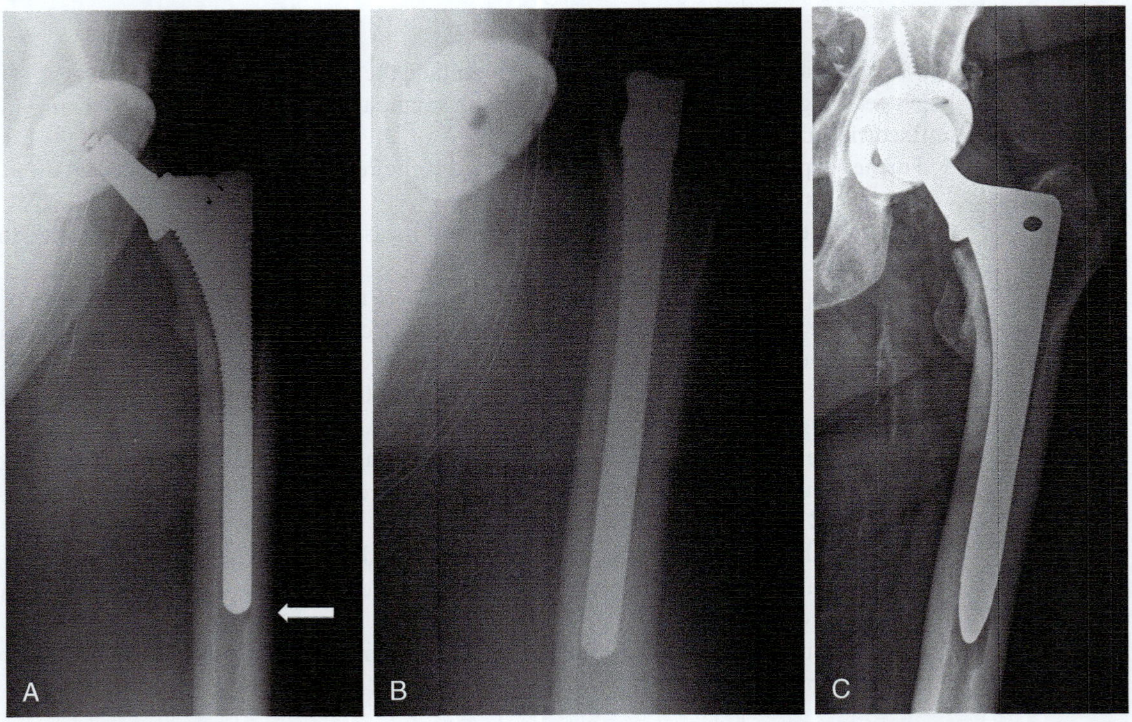

Figure 8.3 | A-C. Intraoperative trial radiographs obtained in 2 planes (A, B) with the final broach. Note that the stem is slightly undersized, with notching of the lateral femoral cortex (see arrow) secondary to varus reaming. Before placing the final stem, the starting point was lateralized and additional reaming was performed in line with the femoral canal to go up 1 stem size. AP radiograph at 10-year follow-up (C) with excellent clinical and radiographic result.

this control, the stem can rotate into a suboptimal position that cannot be corrected intraoperatively. Some components have a hole in the proximal implant through which a rigid instrument can be inserted to provide powerful rotational forces to optimize implant version as the implant is driven into the diaphysis.

- During final insertion, one should visualize slow and steady progress of the stem. Especially over the last 1 to 2 cm, if it appears that the stem advances an unexpectedly great distance with a single mallet blow, one should assess for a distal fracture with intraoperative radiographs.

Postoperative Care

- The vast majority of patients may bear weight as tolerated immediately following the procedure; however, the surgeon may wish to restrict the patient to more limited weight bearing for the first 4 to 6 weeks in 2 situations:
  - When the stem seats more easily than anticipated.
  - If the postoperative radiograph demonstrates significant stem malalignment and/or suboptimal canal fill.

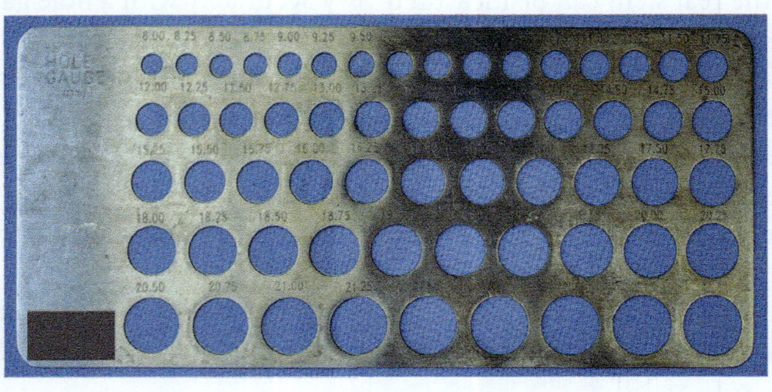

Figure 8.4 | Hole gauge used to accurately measure the diameter of extensively porous coated stems.

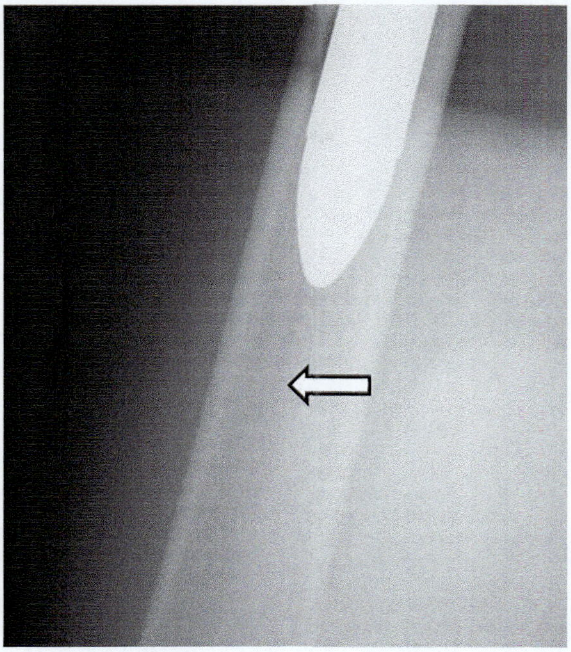

Figure 8.5 | Distal expansion fracture (see arrow) as seen on a postoperative radiograph that does not exit the cortex. This fracture was treated successfully with protected weight bearing.

- Immediate postoperative radiographs must include 2 views that capture the entire construct, including the tip of the femoral stem.
  - Distal short longitudinally oriented expansion cracks that do not exit the cortex on either view may be treated with protected weight bearing (Figure 8.5).
  - Distal expansion cracks that exit the cortex should be considered less stable and are typically treated with cable cerclage.

Chapter 9
Uncemented Modular Stems

BRIAN P. CHALMERS
KEVIN I. PERRY

Key Concepts

- Patients may have proximal femoral anatomic abnormalities that make it difficult to fit a conventional off-the-shelf uncemented femoral component, for a number of reasons. These include developmental dysplasia of the hip (DDH) (Figure 9.1), Perthes disease (Figure 9.2), other developmental anomalies, and trauma.
- Patients with DDH often have complex proximal femoral anatomy, including excessive femoral neck anteversion, a valgus neck shaft angle, metaphyseal-diaphyseal mismatch with a stenotic diaphyseal canal, and proximal femoral hypoplasia, rendering femoral component placement during primary total hip arthroplasty (THA) challenging; furthermore, these patients often have prior proximal femoral hardware from prior surgery compromising metaphyseal fixation.
- Although cemented femoral fixation allows for appropriate compensation of these complex deformities, uncemented femoral fixation allows for biologic ingrowth and potentially superior long-term component durability in this relatively young patient population.
- Uncemented combined metaphyseal and diaphyseal fixation allows improved component fixation in patients with metaphyseal-diaphyseal mismatch and prior proximal femoral hardware.
- The modularity of an uncemented, modular femoral stem is technically easier and allows surgeons to appropriately restore femoral version and offset to optimize hip stability in patients with complex proximal femoral deformities.
- Because these implants use ream-only techniques for femoral preparation they are well suited to situations in which proximal sclerotic bone makes bone preparation with a broach difficult (Figure 9.3).

Sterile Instruments and Implants

Instruments

- Routine hip retractors
- Implant-specific instrumentation

Implants

- Uncemented primary acetabular component of surgeon's choice (with instrumentation)
- Uncemented primary uncemented modular stem (with instrumentation)

Positioning

- Lateral decubitus position

Surgical Approaches

- The surgical approach should allow good femoral exposure and be extensile if needed. Milling of the proximal femur for the modular sleeve requires more exposure than routine roach-only or ream and broach femoral preparation.

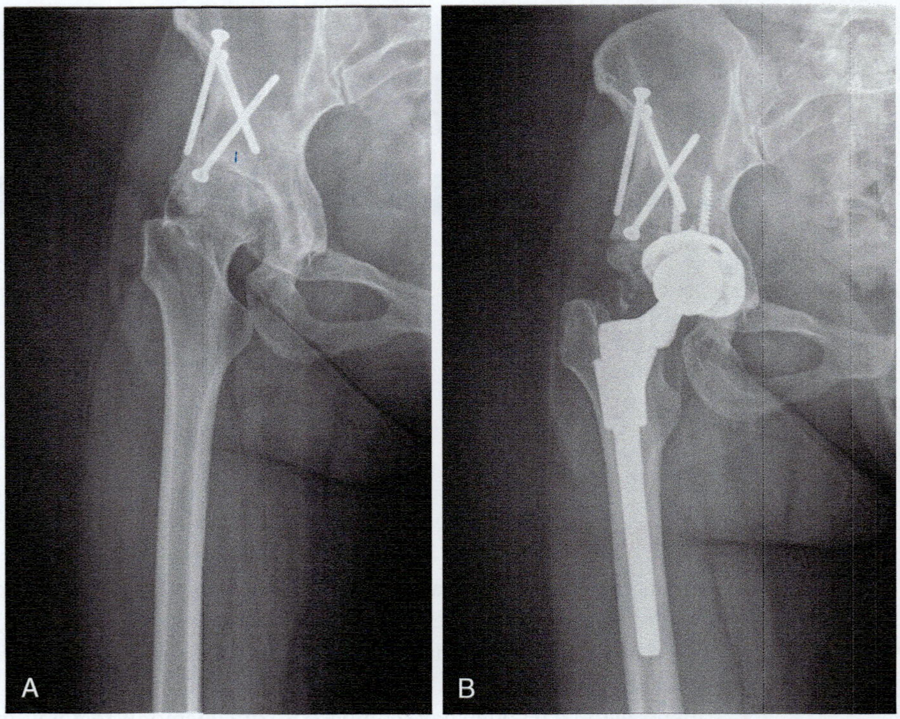

Figure 9.1 | A, Radiograph of patient with developmental dysplasia of the hip and proximal femoral bone deformity including anteversion abnormality. B, Radiograph after reconstruction with uncemented modular stem that allowed management of proximal bone deformity including the abnormal anteversion. (Courtesy of Daniel J. Berry, MD.)

- It may be wise to avoid the direct anterior approach in this patient population because of complex and altered anatomy on both the femoral and acetabular sides that need to be addressed and because making the approach very extensile is challenging.

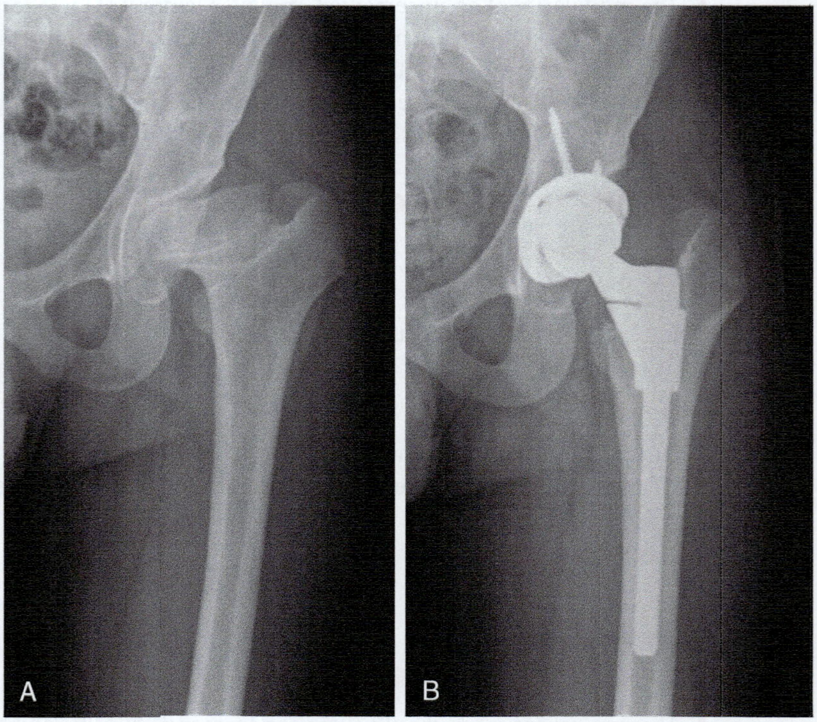

Figure 9.2 | A, Radiograph of patient with history of Perthes disease and abnormally shaped proximal femoral metaphysis. B, Radiograph after THA using modular femoral stem to management bone deformity. (Courtesy of Daniel J. Berry, MD.)

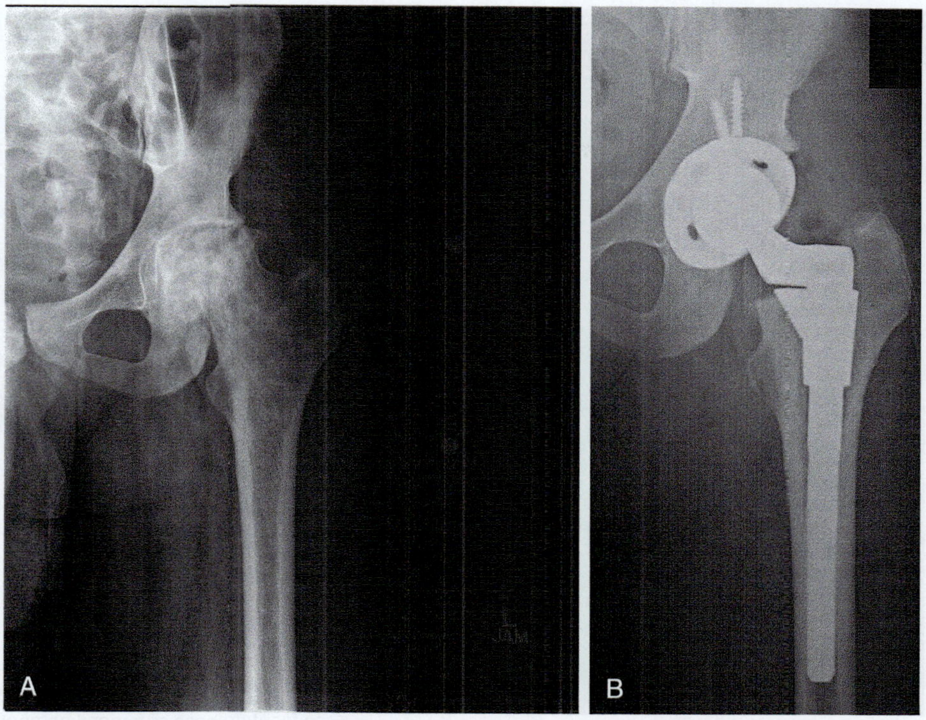

Figure 9.3 | A, Radiograph of patient with osteonecrosis of both femoral heads due to sick cell disease. There are bone infarcts in the metaphyses that make broaching very difficult. B Radiograph after bilateral THA using uncemented modular implant that allowed bone preparation with reaming rather than with broaching. (Courtesy of Daniel J. Berry, MD.)

Preoperative Planning

- The recognition of potential proximal femoral deformities in patients with DDH undergoing primary THA is paramount to preoperative planning (Figure 9.4).
- Be prepared to perform a subtrochanteric shortening osteotomy in patients with Crowe IV DDH undergoing primary THA, as discussed extensively in Chapter 16.
- If a patient has had prior surgery, knowledge of existing hardware and a plan for implant removal is needed.
- It is important to assess leg length and rotational profile of the lower extremities on prone physical examination.
- Preoperative templating for potentially complex acetabular and femoral anatomy is paramount; surgeons should template multiple femoral stem options including an uncemented, modular femoral stem and have multiple femoral reconstruction options readily available.

Bone, Implant, and Soft Tissue Techniques

- The hip is exposed per the surgeon's routine and dislocated.
- The femoral neck is osteotomized in an L-shaped fashion to allow proper femoral component preparation (Figure 9.5).
- The acetabulum is prepared, addressing any bony deficiency or high hip dysplasia, if present, as discussed in previous chapters.
- Attention is then turned to the femur. A high-speed burr is utilized to access the femoral canal and burr the lateral shoulder of the proximal femur to provide direct access to the canal recognizing any anatomic abnormalities. An AO starter reamer is then utilized to ensure that the surgeon has found the femoral canal and begins reaming in the proper trajectory.
- Cylindrical reamers are then utilized to ream the diaphysis (Figure 9.6), starting with an 8- or 9-mm reamer and reaming by 0.5-cm increments until good cortical contact is achieved; preoperative templating of component size is especially helpful; cylindrically ream 0.5 mm above the minor diameter of the planned stem (which is typically 0.5-0.75 mm less than the major diameter [the outside of the splines] of the stem).

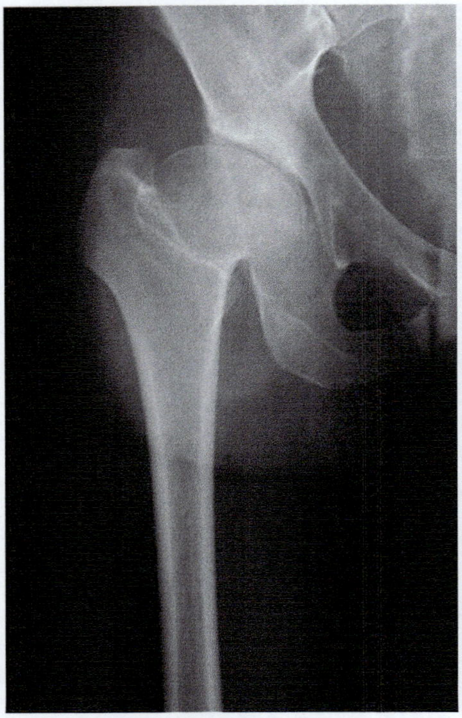

Figure 9.4 | A patient with severe developmental hip dysplasia and proximal femoral deformity undergoing primary total hip arthroplasty. A modular uncemented femoral stem was utilized to easily address this deformity and ensure adequate component fixation.

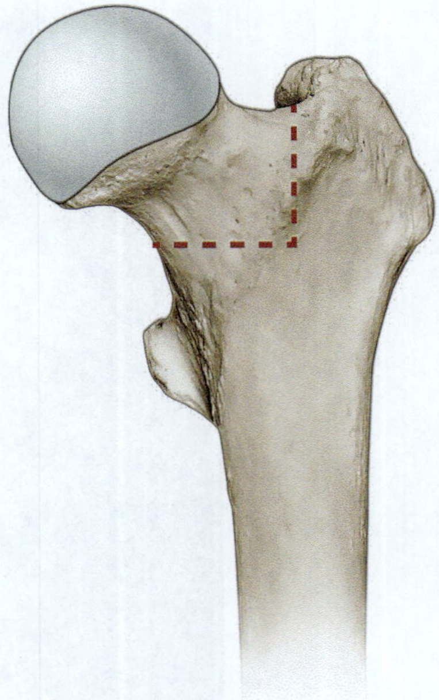

Figure 9.5 | The femoral osteotomy is made in an L-shaped fashion to facilitate ease of femoral component preparation and insertion. (Redrawn with permission of Mayo Foundation for Medical Education and Research. All rights reserved.)

- Place the appropriately sized proximal metaphyseal reaming guide into the femoral canal to ream for the proximal metaphyseal fixation; in the senior authors' preferred implant system, these are color coded based on the size of diaphysis and metaphyseal sleeve to be inserted; sequentially ream the proximal metaphysis with the stem extension in place until the metaphysis is appropriately filled (Figure 9.7). This usually involves cortical contact with the anterior femoral metaphysis and can be seen by looking into the metaphysis at intervals during reaming. Be careful to avoid anterior perforation.
- The senior authors' preferred implant system has a separate reamer and guide to prepare the femur for the triangular sleeve "spout" that fills the medial metaphysis. Make sure that the reaming guide is flush with the anterior cortex and appropriately seated into the metaphysis; orient the reamer in line with the native version of the femoral neck; bury this reamer to the appropriate depth based on what the patient's anatomy will accept (Figure 9.8).
- Insert the appropriate metaphyseal sleeve trial based on what was obtained from final reaming.
- Impact the trial stem; the real stem typically engages with the metaphyseal sleeve as a taper fit; place the femoral stem in the appropriate anteversion to achieve a combined anteversion of 30 to 40° with the acetabular component.
- Reduce the hip and test the trial of range of motion, assessing for hip stability and impingement; excessive anteversion of the femoral stem will cause impingement in extension and external rotation, whereas too little femoral anteversion will cause impingement in flexion and internal rotation.
- Adjust the modular neck to the appropriate femoral anteversion and retrial until satisfied with the stability of the hip in all positions.

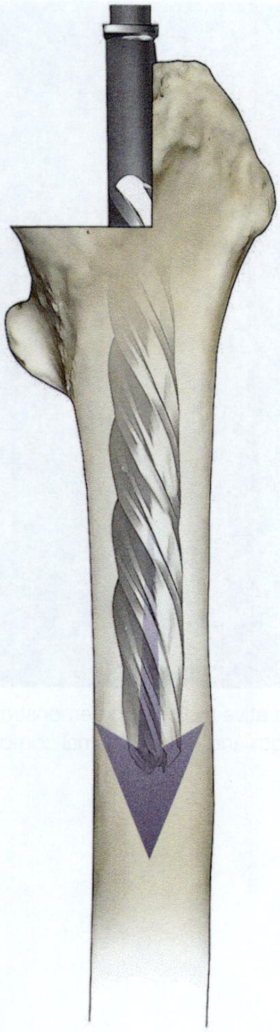

Figure 9.6 | Cylindrical reaming of the diaphysis for the uncemented modular femoral stem. (Redrawn with permission of Mayo Foundation for Medical Education and Research. All rights reserved.)

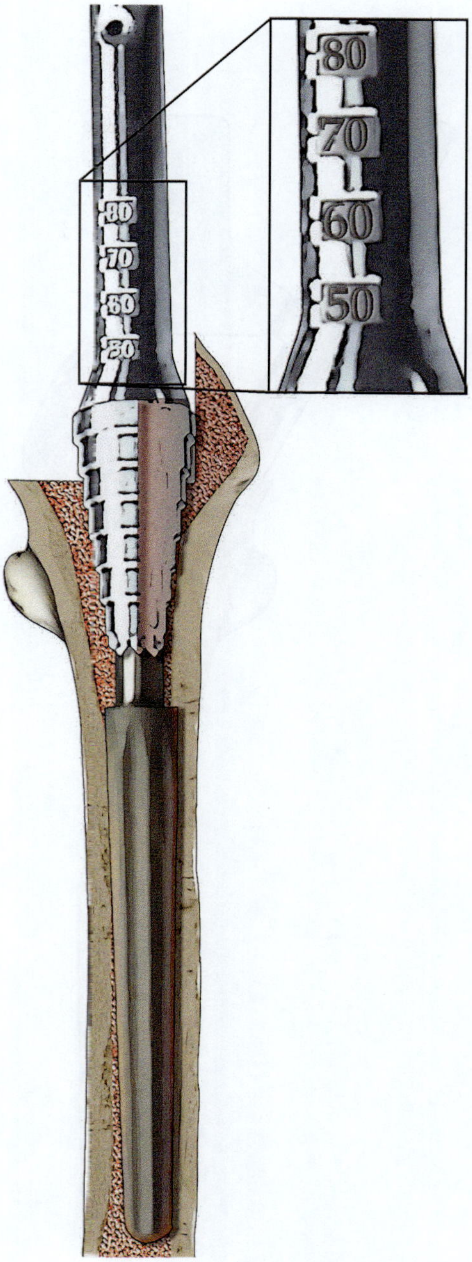

Figure 9.7 | Proximal metaphyseal conical reaming for uncemented modular femoral stem. (Redrawn with permission of Mayo Foundation for Medical Education and Research. All rights reserved.)

- Mark the desired anteversion on the patient's femoral neck with electrocautery before removal of the trials for future reference.
- Obtain an intraoperative radiograph to assure appropriate femoral component fit and restoration of leg length and offset (Figure 9.9).
- Implant the real metaphyseal sleeve in the native femoral anteversion as previously reamed with the instrumented inserter.
- Impact the real femoral stem at the premarked appropriate anteversion, which is often markedly different from the patient's native anteversion (Figure 9.10).

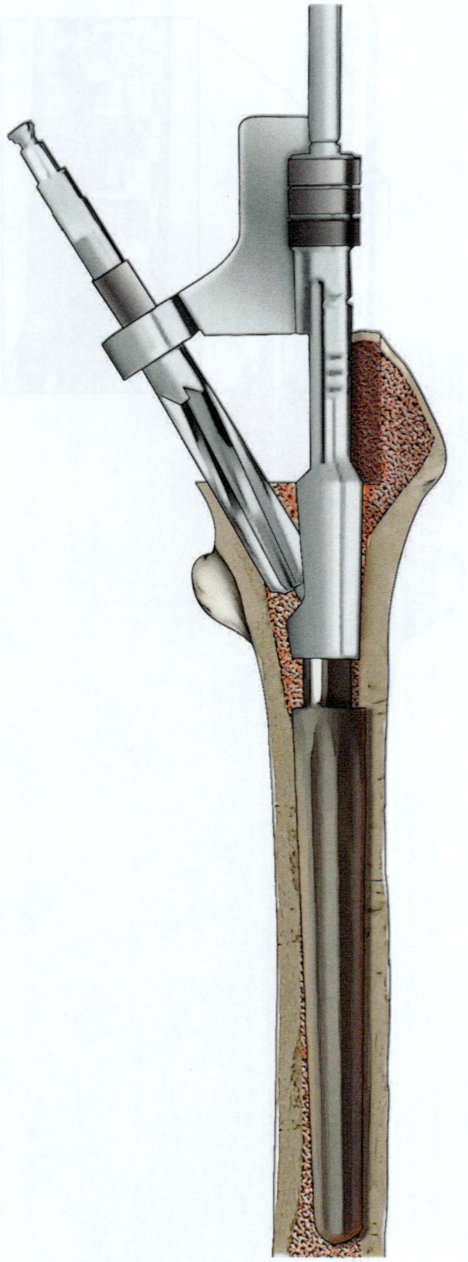

Figure 9.8 | Reaming for the triangular portion of the metaphyseal sleeve of the uncemented modular femoral stem. (Redrawn with permission of Mayo Foundation for Medical Education and Research. All rights reserved.)

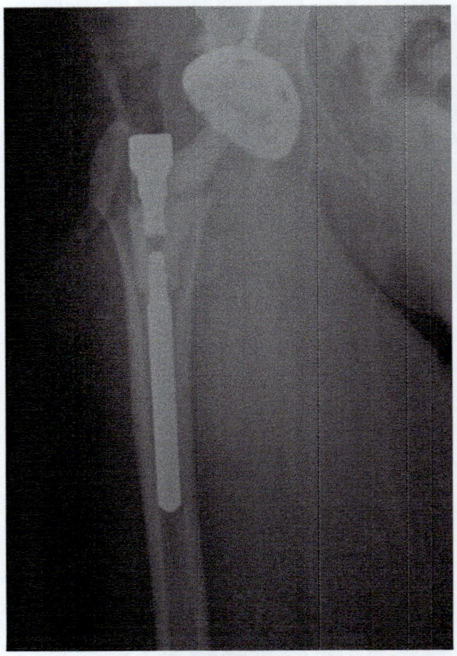

Figure 9.9 | Intraoperative radiograph demonstrating appropriate restoration of leg length and offset with trial components in place.

- Place the trial femoral head and retrial the hip in all positions until satisfied with the hip stability; increase or decrease the neck length as needed to optimize length and offset.
- Impact the final femoral head on the trunnion.
- Reduce the hip; take the hip through range of motion to ensure hip stability.
- Perform a layered closure per the surgeon's preferred technique.
- Postoperative radiographs should be obtained to ensure appropriate implant positioning (Figure 9.11).

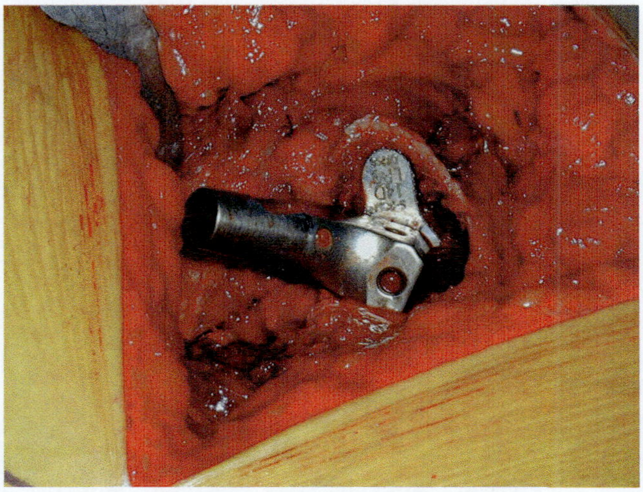

Figure 9.10 | Intraoperative photograph showing the final component in place in the appropriate version to optimize hip stability; there is significant mismatch between appropriate final femoral component version and the patient's native femoral version. Note the metaphyseal sleeve follows the patient's anatomy to provide maximal implant stability. (Courtesy of Daniel J. Berry, MD.)

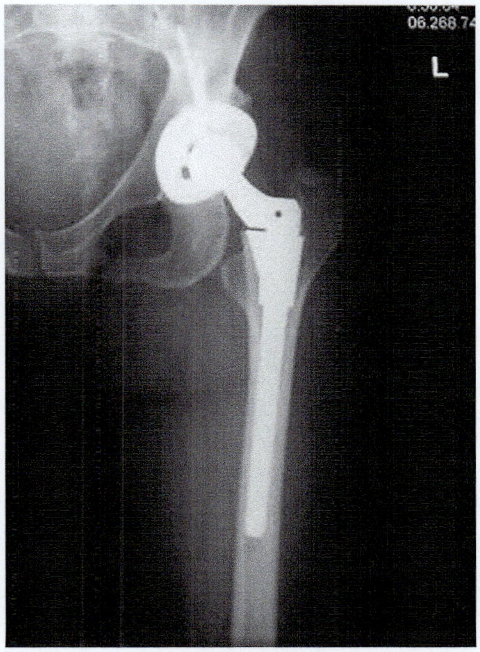

Figure 9.11 | A Postoperative radiograph of patient with severe developmental hip dysplasia and proximal femoral deformity treated with primary total hip arthroplasty. A modular uncemented femoral stem was utilized to easily address this deformity and ensure adequate component fixation. Note good implant fit in the metaphysis and diaphysis. (Courtesy of Daniel J. Berry, MD.)

Postoperative Care

- Weight-bearing protocol postoperatively is based on details of the reconstruction and operative approach. When the reconstruction was performed in the presence of bone deficiency (such as some causes of DDH) or through an anterolateral approach, patients usually are made partial weight bearing for 6 to 8 weeks.
- Hip precautions are prescribed based on surgeon discretion and assessment of hip stability at the time of surgery.

Chapter 10
Uncemented Tapered Fluted Stems

ROBERT T. TROUSDALE

Key Concepts

- Uncemented tapered fluted stems can provide durable fixation during primary total hip arthroplasty.
- These stems are relatively simple to use as they require only reaming the canal until one achieves axial and rotational stability.
- These stems are especially helpful in the face of excessive femoral version, coxa valga, and small femurs and in posttraumatic deformity (Figure 10.1).

Sterile Instruments and Implants

- Routine hip retractors.
- System specific tapered reamers to prepare canal.
- System specific tapered trial implants.
- Trial heads including 28 and 22 mm, as some of these patients will have very small acetabular components.

Surgical Approaches

- Surgical approach may be according to surgeon preference. This implant may be placed easily by various anterior, lateral, or posterior approaches.
- Drape the whole or a majority of femur.
- Position such that it is easy to get an intraoperative radiograph if desired.

Preoperative Planning

- Know patient's preoperative leg length discrepancy.
- Template cup size and position.
- Template femoral component size on anteroposterior and lateral radiographs of the femur. Template the desired neck resection level.
- Using the tip of trochanter as a secondary check for anticipated neck resection is helpful. In general, the tip of greater trochanter should be at the level of the center of the femoral head.

Bone/Implant/Soft Tissue Techniques

- Perform desired approach to hip joint.
- Perform femoral neck osteotomy according to the preoperative plan.
- Prepare acetabulum, place cup with trial liner.

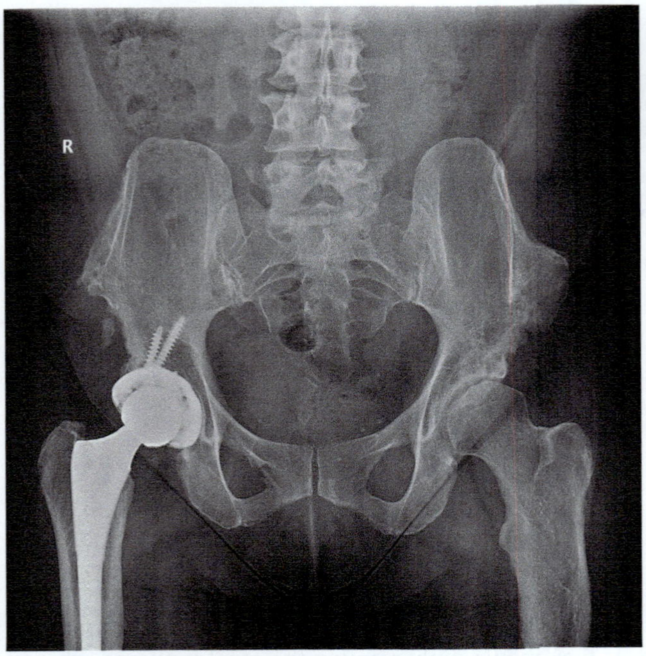

Figure 10.1 | Anteroposterior radiograph of patient with left hip arthritis with proximal femoral deformity. Femur is in varus as well as has torsional malunion deformity.

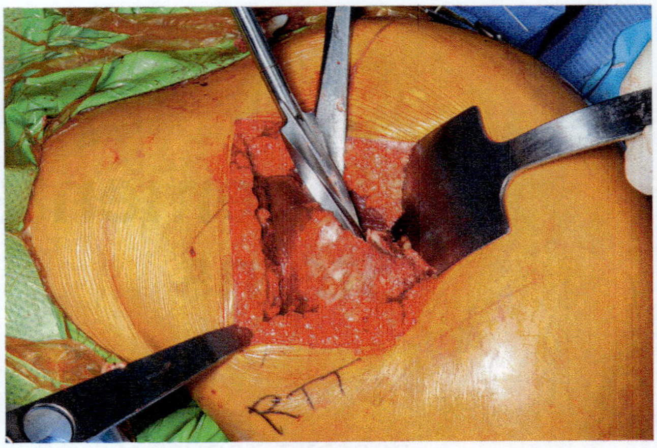

Figure 10.2 | Reaming a cone into left femur.

- Prepare the femur with tapered reamers, either by hand or with power according to system-specific recommendations and surgeon preference. Increase reamer diameter until there is a "cone" of prepared bony where the reamer is tight and obtaining good contact with supportive cortical bone. Goal is to ream to a size where implant will be both rotationally and axially stable. The author prefers to ream by hand initially. When one is close to the size of desired implant, reaming on power is helpful as the reamer gets tight (Figure 10.2).
- Take care to ream a smooth cone that the implant will fit into.
- Obtain an intraoperative radiograph with a trial femoral component in place (Figure 10.3). In most cases, anteroposterior and lateral radiographs of the femur are obtained by rotating the femur 90°.
- Perform trial hip reduction. If satisfied with leg length and hip stability, place the real acetabular liner.
- Ideally the trial finishes with a head length that is in the middle range of length options. That allows one to use a shorter or longer head length depending on exactly where the real implant seats.
- If bone is soft or the surgeon is concerned about the risk of a calcar crack, a prophylactic wire can be placed above the lesser trochanter.
- Insert the real stem. This is done maintaining the desired version, which is determined as soon as the flutes engage the bone. Multiple moderately hard impactions should be utilized for insertion. Continue hitting the implant until it no longer advances. It is critical to have the implant stable in all planes (Figure 10.4).
- Perform one last trial if desired, and impact the chosen real femoral head onto stem.
- Routine closure in layers is performed.
- Obtain a postoperative radiograph in the operating room or recovery area (Figure 10.5).

Postoperative Management

- Weight bearing as tolerated is allowed if the implant went in with excellent fixation.
- Ambulatory aids are used until balance is restored.
- Return to regular activities as tolerated (Figure 10.6A-D).

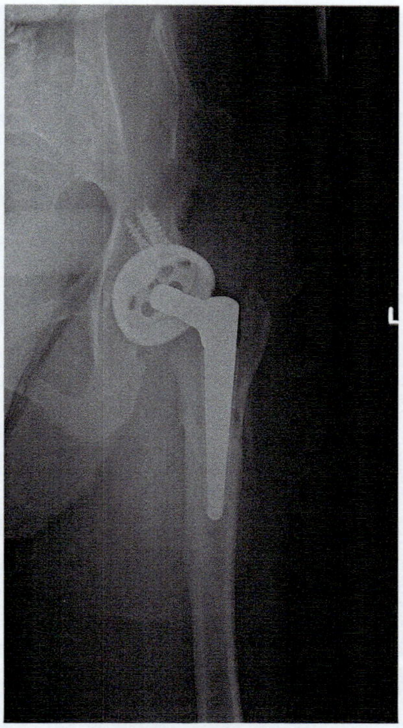

Figure 10.3 | Intraoperative radiograph with trial in place.

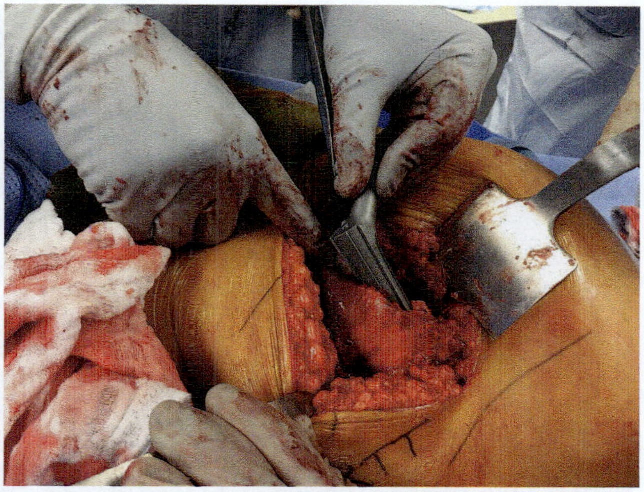

Figure 10.4 | Intraoperative photograph showing insertion of real stem.

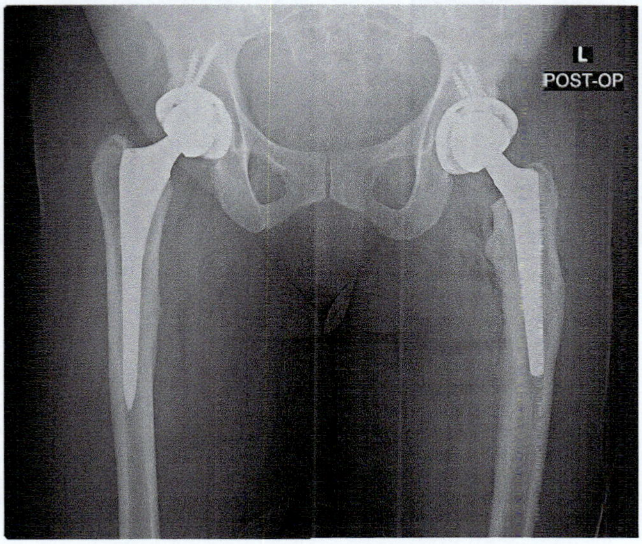

Figure 10.5 | Postoperative radiograph with final implant in place. Note varus deformity has been accommodated with stem.

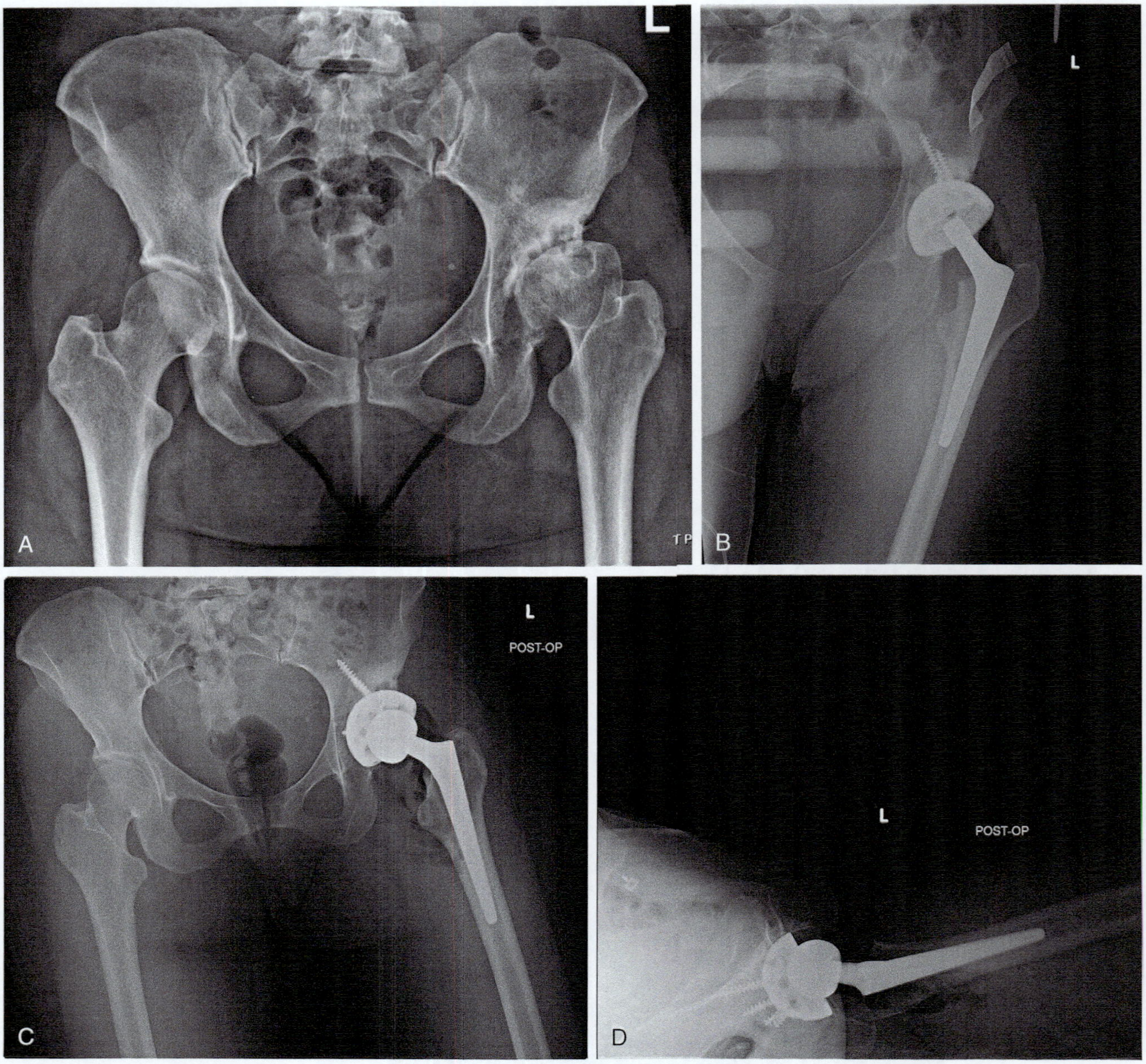

Figure 10.6 | A-D, Preoperative, intraoperative, postoperative anteroposterior, and postoperative lateral radiographs of a dysplastic hip with coxa valga and excess host bone femoral anteversion.

Chapter 11
Cemented Stems

JOSEPH M. STATZ
RAFAEL J. SIERRA

Key Concepts

- Choosing a cemented stem over an uncemented stem is largely surgeon preference in the majority of patients.
- There are 2 main different design principles by which cemented stems work. Both design principles are based on obtaining fixation at the cement-bone interface through cement interdigitation with cancellous bone. However, fixation at the cement-stem interface differs.
  - The composite beam concept utilizes a stem with a roughened or textured surface that allows cement interdigitation with the stem, creating a solid beam composed of bone, cement, and stem.
  - The taper-slip concept utilizes a highly polished, tapered stem with a smooth surface that allows fixation without cement interdigitation but obtains axial stability with its tapered shape and rotational stability with its cross-sectional shape.
- Advantages of cemented stems:
  - Survivorship: Excellent long-term survivorship in clinical series and registries
  - Versatility: Can be used in any case
  - Decreased perioperative fracture risk
  - Fixation with antibiotic cement may decrease infection rates
  - Polished stems may be easily removed from cement mantle, simplifying some revisions
  - Forgiving technique: Basic principles should be followed regardless of stem type; the goal is to implant the stem in appropriate alignment with a solid 2-mm cement mantle surrounding the entire stem
- Disadvantages of cemented stems:
  - Increased operating room time compared with uncemented stem
  - Cement in the femoral canal can be difficult to remove at revision
  - "Cement implantation syndrome" caused by the pressurization of the femoral canal and fat emboli

Sterile Instruments and Implants

- Routine hip retractors
- Pulse lavage irrigator with femoral stem attachment
- Epinephrine-soaked sponges
- Cement plug
- Vacuum cement mixer
- Cement gun with long nozzle and pressurizing attachment
- Cemented femoral component (with instrumentation)

Positioning

Positioning depends on surgeon preference for primary total hip; the author utilizes a posterolateral approach for primary and revision total hip arthroplasty (THA).

Surgical Approaches

Cemented components can be inserted through any THA approach, although this is more difficult through a direct anterior approach. Please refer to Chapters 2-5.

Preoperative Planning

- Template femoral component size. For cemented stems, 2 mm of cement mantle surrounding the implant is preferred, but certain cement philosophies ("French paradox") have shown good results with less than that.
- Template and clinically examine preoperative leg length discrepancy.
- Choose and template an appropriate acetabular component.

Bone, Implant, and Soft Tissue Techniques

- Perform the desired approach to the hip joint.
- The technique described here is for the preparation and placement of a taper-slip design but can be used as a guide for placement of all cemented stems.
- Perform the femoral neck osteotomy using templated preoperative plan as a guide. For a polished tapered designing a precise neck cut is less important; however, too short of a neck cut should be avoided.
- Prepare and implant an appropriately sized and positioned acetabular component. This can also be done before or after femoral preparation (per surgeon preference).
- Establish a femoral entry point (surgeon preference is the use of a round 6.5-mm burr), usually over the posterolateral aspect of the neck (Figure 11.1).
- An AO canal finder is used as a starter to find the trajectory of the femoral canal (Figure 11.2).
- Subsequent hand reaming is performed orienting the femoral stem away from varus and flexion in line with the center of the femoral canal (Figure 11.3).
- Hand ream to open the canal and lateralize the starting point as needed. This helps avoid varus stem alignment, which is associated with a higher rate of loosening.
- Broach the canal to the templated size, making sure to *leave sufficient circumferential cancellous bone (at least 2 mm) around the canal for cement interdigitation* (Figure 11.4). Work broaches against the lateral bone to avoid varus alignment. The final broach should be in line with the native femur with

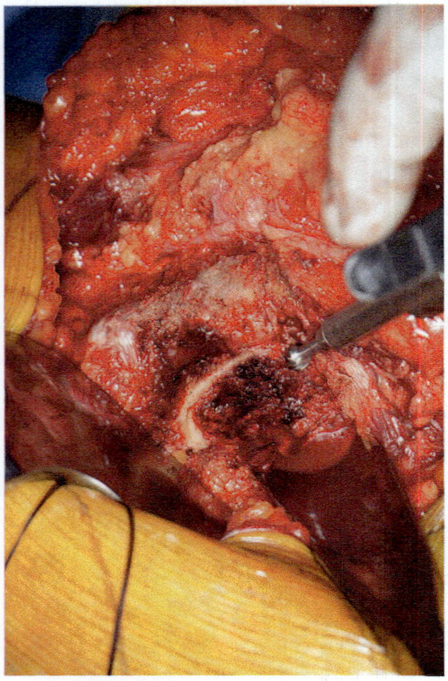

Figure 11.1 | A starting point for femoral stem entry can be established with a burr or box osteotome. This should generally be in the posterolateral quadrant of the cut surface of the femoral neck.

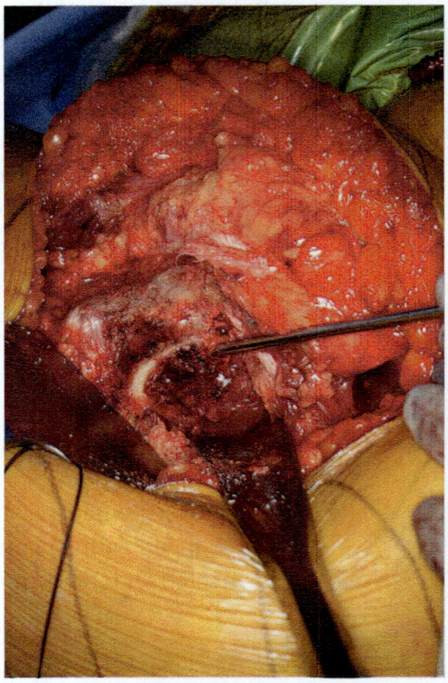

Figure 11.2 | An AO starter reamer is used to palpate the canal and establish a trajectory straight down the femoral canal for subsequent reaming and broaching.

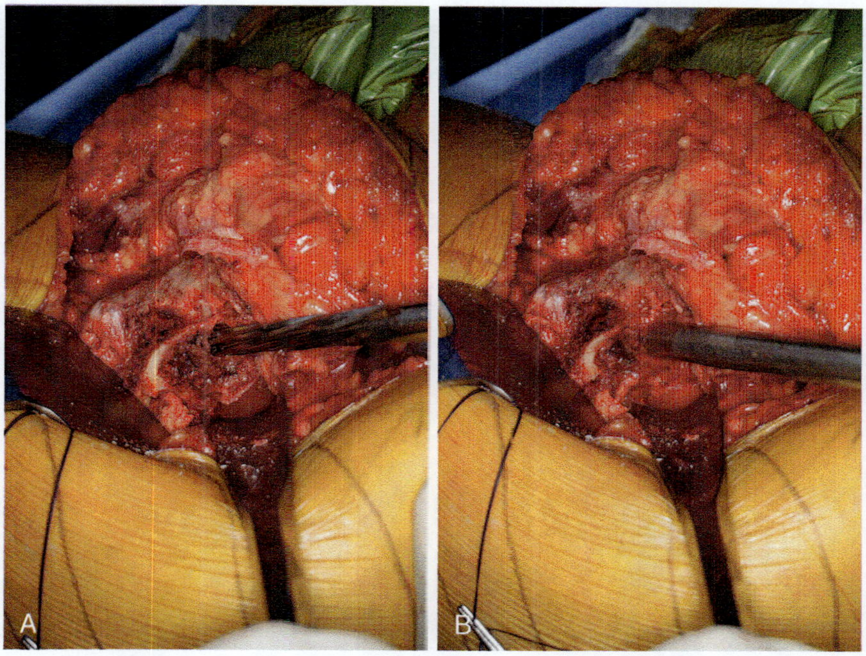

Figure 11.3 | The femoral canal is reamed to an appropriate size, ensuring that 2 to 3 mm of circumferential cancellous bone is preserved in the canal. Note that the reamer is directed away from varus and flexion (A) and the canal will redirect the reamer down the canal as it is advanced (B). A posterior approach was utilized.

respect to varus/valgus and flexion/extension with about 15° to 20° of anteversion, but optimal alignment will also depend on the patient's native femoral version and hip stability achieved at the time of trialing the hip. The final broach should be sized to be against strong cancellous bone, which is typically near the cortex, but not so large as to have removed all the cancellous bone and be directly against the cortical bone.

- Place a cement restrictor down the canal. The depth of insertion can be determined by comparison with the real stem and marking the cement restrictor inserter with a marking pen at the level of the calcar. The cement restrictor should be placed about 1 cm distal to the tip of the stem (Figure 11.5).
- Clean the femoral canal with the pulse lavage irrigator with the femoral stem attachment to clear out any loose bone marrow contents or blood filling the interstices between trabeculae (Figure 11.6).

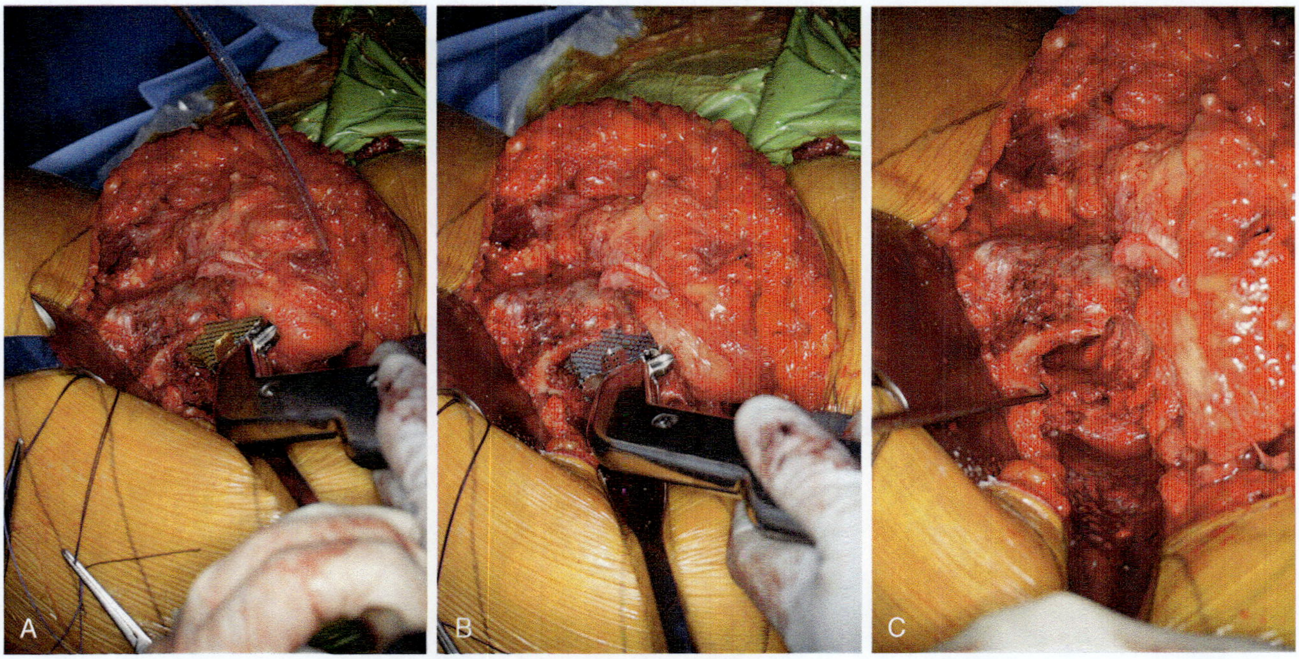

Figure 11.4 | The femur is broached to an appropriate size with appropriate anteversion (A and B). Ensure that 2 to 3 mm of circumferential cancellous bone is left in the canal for cement interdigitation as noted with the nerve hook (C). Appropriate anteversion is generally 15° to 20°.

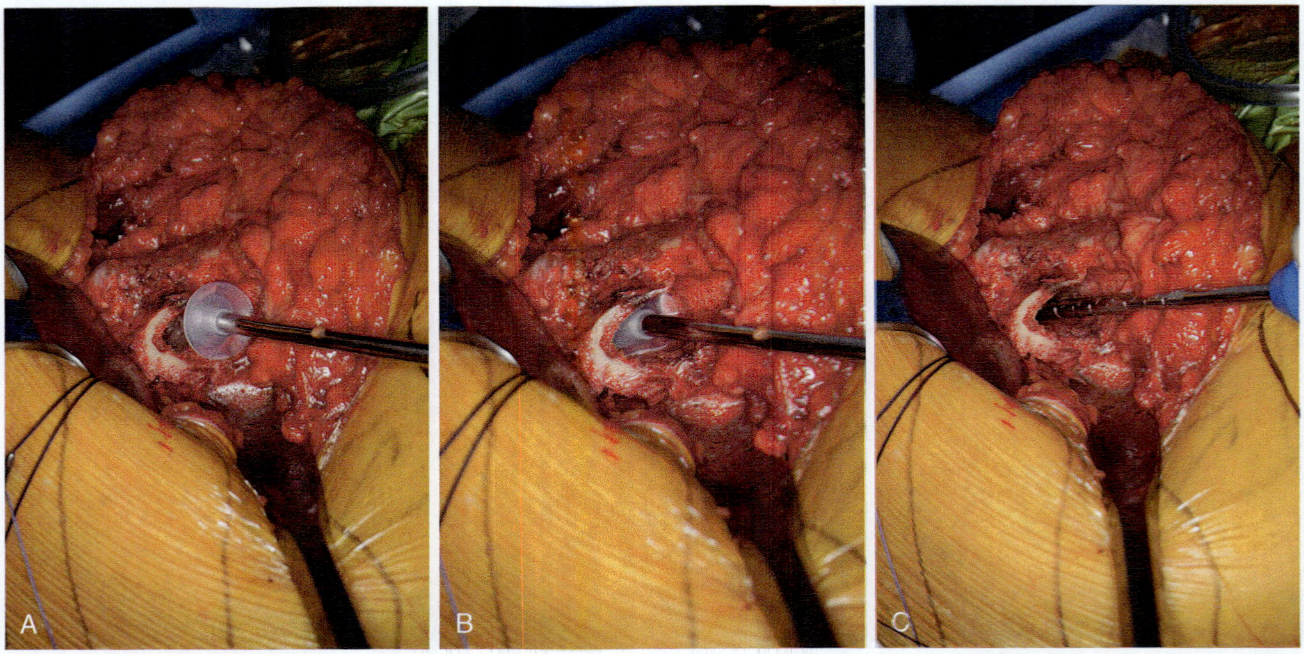

Figure 11.5 | An appropriately sized cement restrictor should be placed down the femur to a depth 1 cm past where the tip of the stem will seat. This should be inserted with gentle taps of the mallet (A, B, and C).

This is an important step to gain good cement fixation. Some surgeons elect to pulse lavage while reaming and broaching for this same purpose in hopes of preventing embolization of marrow contents as the cement restrictor or broaches are inserted down the canal.

- Prepare the femoral canal for cementing. Perform trial reductions to assess for appropriate tension, range of motion, and leg lengths. Obtain an intraoperative radiograph if desired to confirm appropriate component positioning. Suction the canal thoroughly. Fill the canal with epinephrine-soaked sponges (1:100,000 epinephrine: normal saline). It is best to keep a "tail" of each sponge hanging out of the canal and to count the sponges rigorously to avoid leaving a sponge in the canal. The sponges will slow any bleeding into the canal to ensure the canal is as dry as possible. These sponges are removed and replaced with dry sponges—once again count the sponges and leave a tail of each sponge hanging out of the canal to avoid leaving a sponge in the canal. Also place one sponge in the acetabulum to catch any cement that may fall into the cup (Figure 11.7).

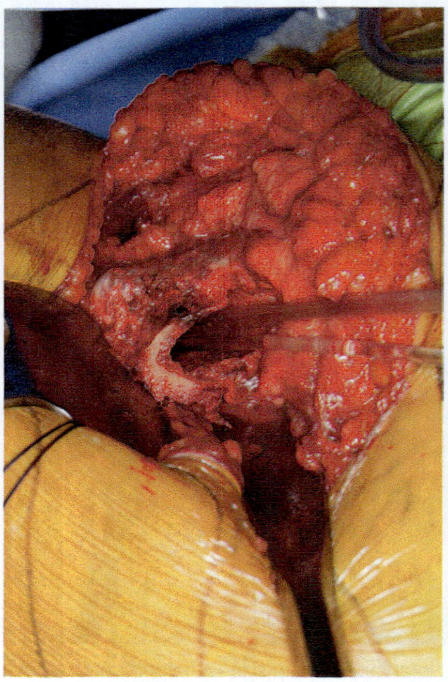

Figure 11.6 | The femoral canal should be thoroughly irrigated and suctioned to remove all marrow elements from the remaining cancellous bone. This will allow for better cement interdigitation as well as decrease the chance of pulmonary emboli during pressurization.

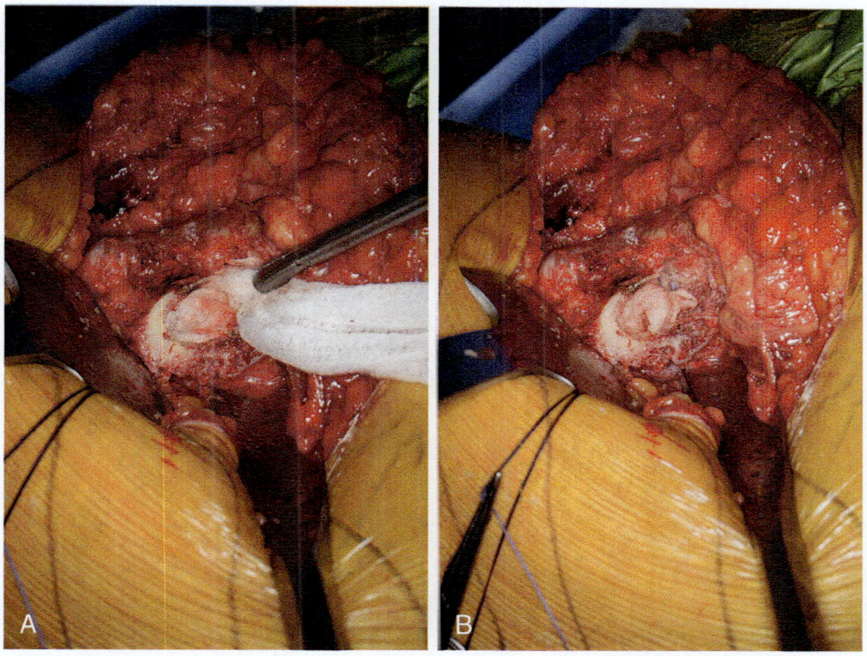

Figure 11.7 | Dilute epinephrine-soaked sponges are inserted into the canal (A) to help with hemostasis, leading to a dry canal amenable to cementation. The sponges are packed tightly into the canal (B).

- Mix cement with a vacuum mixer that loads the cement into a cement gun canister. Mixing cement by hand results in undesirable porosity within the cement mantle.
- Once the cement is slightly doughy, remove the sponges from within the canal and ensure all the sponges have been removed. Insert a small suction catheter into the canal. The suction is placed through the tip of the suction device (Figure 11.8).
- Insert the cement gun nozzle down the canal until the tip hits the cement restrictor (Figure 11.9).
- Squeeze the gun trigger hard and fast to fill the canal with cement. When the nozzle is in the distal canal, you will feel the pressure of the cement push the gun out of the canal. Once cement plugs the suction catheter it can be removed (this usually occurs early once cement is in the depth of the canal,

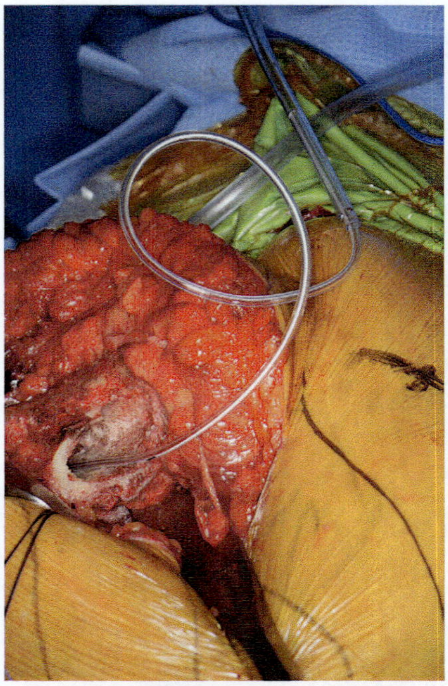

Figure 11.8 | Sponges are removed, and a suction catheter is placed down to the bottom of the femoral canal to thoroughly dry the canal.

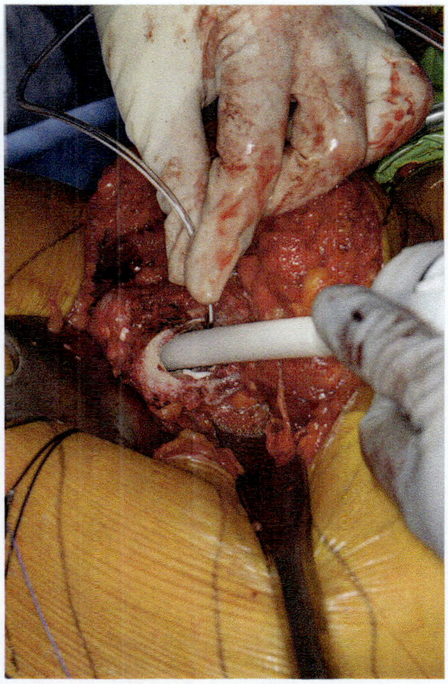

Figure 11.9 | Cement is vacuum mixed into a cement gun with antibiotics. Once the cement is doughy, the gun is inserted into the femoral canal until the tip hits the cement restrictor.

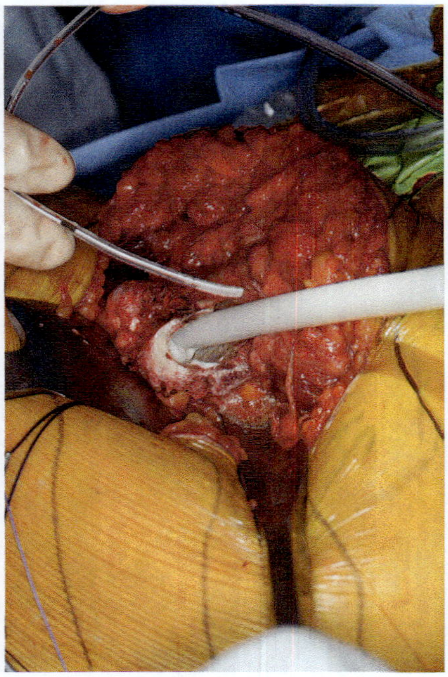

Figure 11.10 I The cement gun is squeezed to forcefully fill the canal with cement and pressurize the cement into the cancellous bone distally, and this will push the cement gun out of the canal. This will also plug the suction catheter with cement, at which time the suction catheter is removed.

Figure 11.10). As the tip of the gun gets pushed more proximally, the cement gun will be pushed out less owing to the increased size of the canal resulting in less pressure pushing on the nozzle. Continue to squeeze the trigger as you remove the nozzle, filling the canal completely up to the level of the femoral neck cut (Figure 11.11) and preventing voids in the cement.

- Unlock the cement gun and insert the cement plunger into the tip to conserve cement and break the long tip off the nozzle. Place a pressurizing attachment over the remaining cement gun tip, choosing the size that obtains a good seal around the femoral neck cut. Place this onto the top of the canal, create a good seal around the metaphysis, and pressurize the canal by squeezing the trigger for a few seconds with good resistance from the pressure (Figures 11.12 and 11.13). Increasing the pressure within the femoral canal will improve cement interdigitation into the bone and improve fixation of the stem.

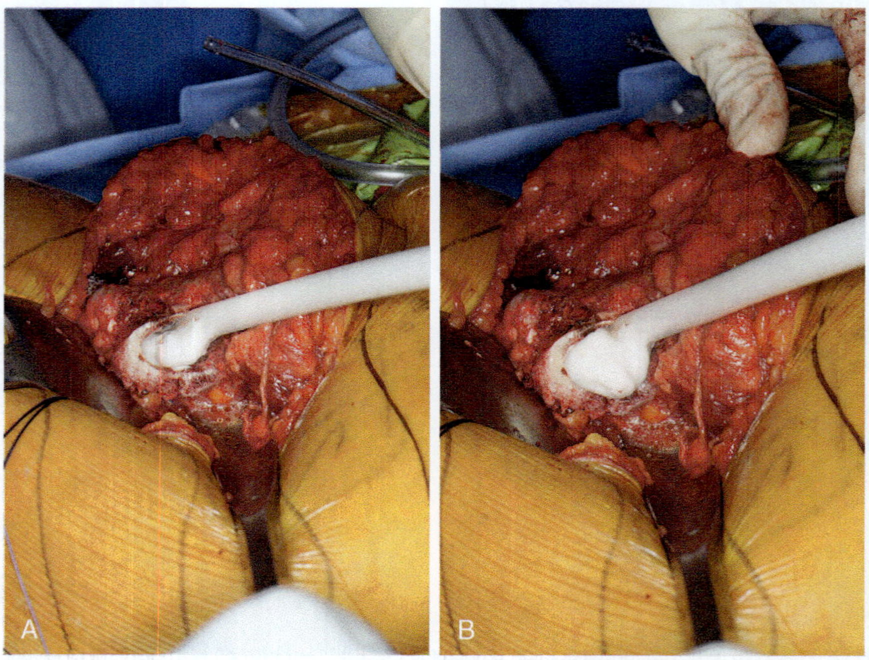

Figure 11.11 I The gun is repeatedly squeezed until the entire femoral canal is filled with cement. The gun is withdrawn and cement is inserted simultaneously (A and B).

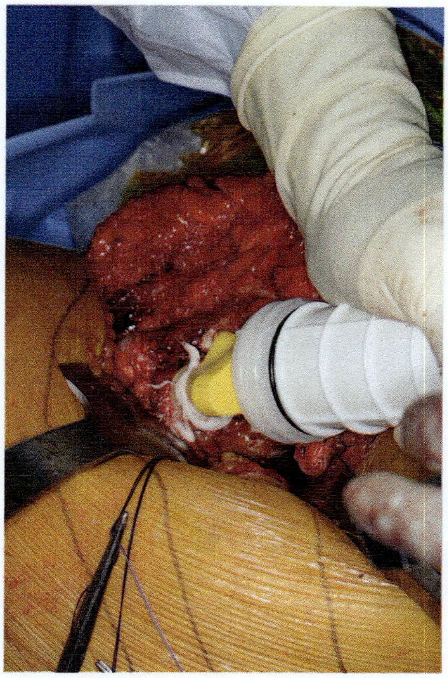

Figure 11.12 I The tip of the cement gun is broken off, and a collar is placed on the end of the gun. This is placed over the cut femoral neck, creating as much of an air-tight seal as possible.

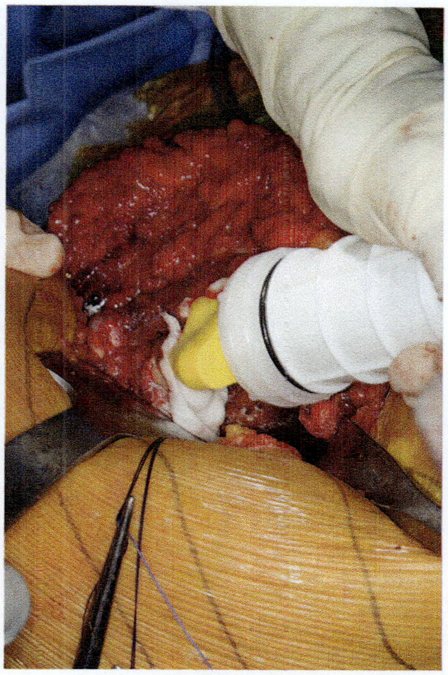

Figure 11.13 I The gun is squeezed again to further pressurize cement.

- Stem insertion and pressurization has been shown to carry a small risk of embolism as shown by transesophageal echo studies. The risk of death in a well-ventilated and hydrated patient is approximately 1/10,000. Communication with the anesthesia team in advance of cementing will ensure that they are aware of the process and will prepare the patient for that step. One may consider skipping this last pressurization step and use only manual pressurization in a patient with compromised cardiopulmonary status such as a high-risk patient undergoing THA or hemiarthroplasty for fracture or for a tumor-related condition.
- The author prefers to heat the polished stem in normal saline, which is heated and placed in a kidney basin. This process in addition to heating 1 of the 2 batches of cement used for cementing allows for the cement to cure faster and decreases the porosity in between the cement and implant interface, improving its bond. There is, however, less working time of the cement, and the surgeon should be aware of this.
- Insert the real stem in appropriate alignment. Most stems have a centralizer attached to the distal tip of the stem to help with distal stem alignment. For the polished taper-slip design stems, the centralizer also allows safe subsidence of the stem as should be expected. The proximal part of the stem is controlled manually, so great care needs to be taken to ensure correct varus/valgus, flexion/extension, and anteversion are placed on the stem during insertion. The position of the stem should be predetermined, and large changes in the stem position should be avoided after the stem is already inserted. This can be estimated by pointing the stem toward the center of the knee and by examining the thickness of the cement mantle around the stem at the level of the femoral neck cut during insertion. While inserting the stem, one hand should hold the stem in appropriate alignment while the other hand has a finger or thumb placed over the calcar region to create increased pressure within the canal at the time of insertion (Figures 11.14 and 11.15). The surgeon's thumb should be removed as the metaphyseal flare of the implant reaches the cement to prevent altering stem alignment (Figure 11.16).
- The mantle around the stem should be equally thick on all sides of the stem. In general, the stem should match the position of the final broach; however, one of the advantages of cement fixation is that the position of the final component does not need to match patient native version.
- Cement extruding from around the stem should be removed during the process of insertion, ensuring the cement does not fall into the cup or extrude into the soft tissues around the femur (Figure 11.17).
- Once the desired stem depth is obtained, hold the stem in place until the cement cures.

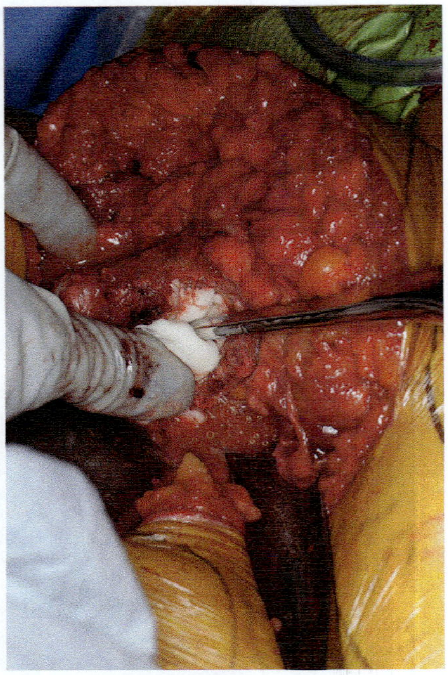

Figure 11.14 | The stem is inserted into the canal directly in line with the femoral canal. In general, the tip of the stem should be inserted toward the posterolateral side of the canal as this is directly over the center of the canal. A thumb is placed over the cement in the area of the calcar.

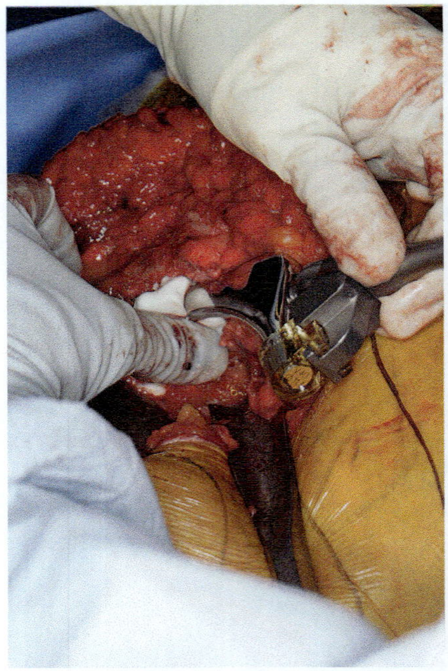

Figure 11.15 | The stem is advanced into the canal in appropriate version and flexion, keeping a thumb over the calcar to increase canal pressure and cement interdigitation.

- For taper-slip stems, a small amount of cement should be placed over the shoulder to prevent it from backing out in the case of a closed reduction attempt with traction for a postoperative dislocation (Figure 11.18).
- Remove the sponge from the acetabulum and inspect the wound for any loose cement.
- Perform trial hip reductions to optimize the femoral neck length of the modular femoral head and the acetabular liner configuration and position (Figure 11.19).
- Impact the real acetabular liner into the cup and real femoral head onto the femoral trunion.
- Irrigate the wound thoroughly.

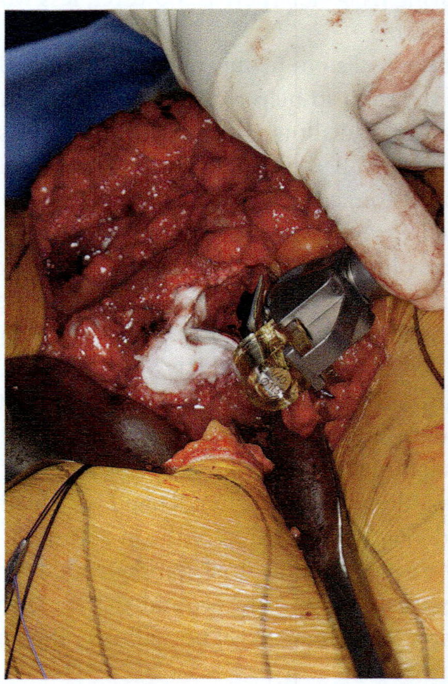

Figure 11.16 | Once the metaphyseal flare of the implant reaches the cement, the thumb is withdrawn to prevent contacting the stem and altering its alignment.

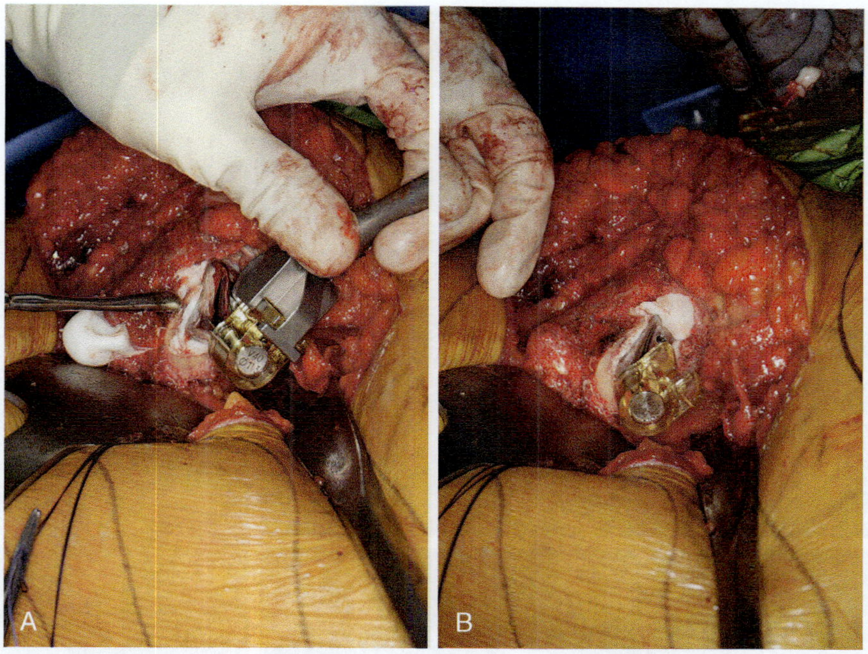

Figure 11.17 | The rest of the stem is inserted in proper alignment, ensuring no large changes in flexion/extension or version are made. An inserter can be used to control stem position during insertion (A) which can then be removed once the cement has hardened (B).

- Close the hip capsule and perform a routine closure specific to the chosen approach.
- Apply a sterile dressing.
- Postoperative radiographs may be obtained as a baseline for future follow-up (Figure 11.20).

Postoperative Care

The patient may weight bear as tolerated with standard THA precautions.

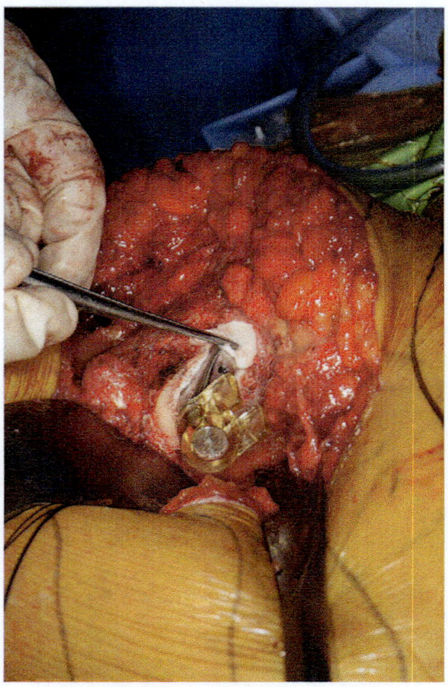

Figure 11.18 | Excess cement is removed from around the stem as it is being inserted, and cement is placed over the shoulder of the implant to prevent it from being pulled out of the canal if a postoperative dislocation requiring reduction should occur.

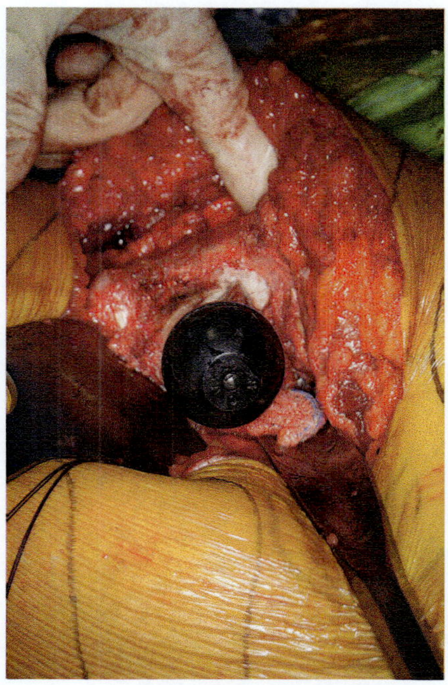

Figure 11.19 | Final trialing takes place once the cement has completely hardened.

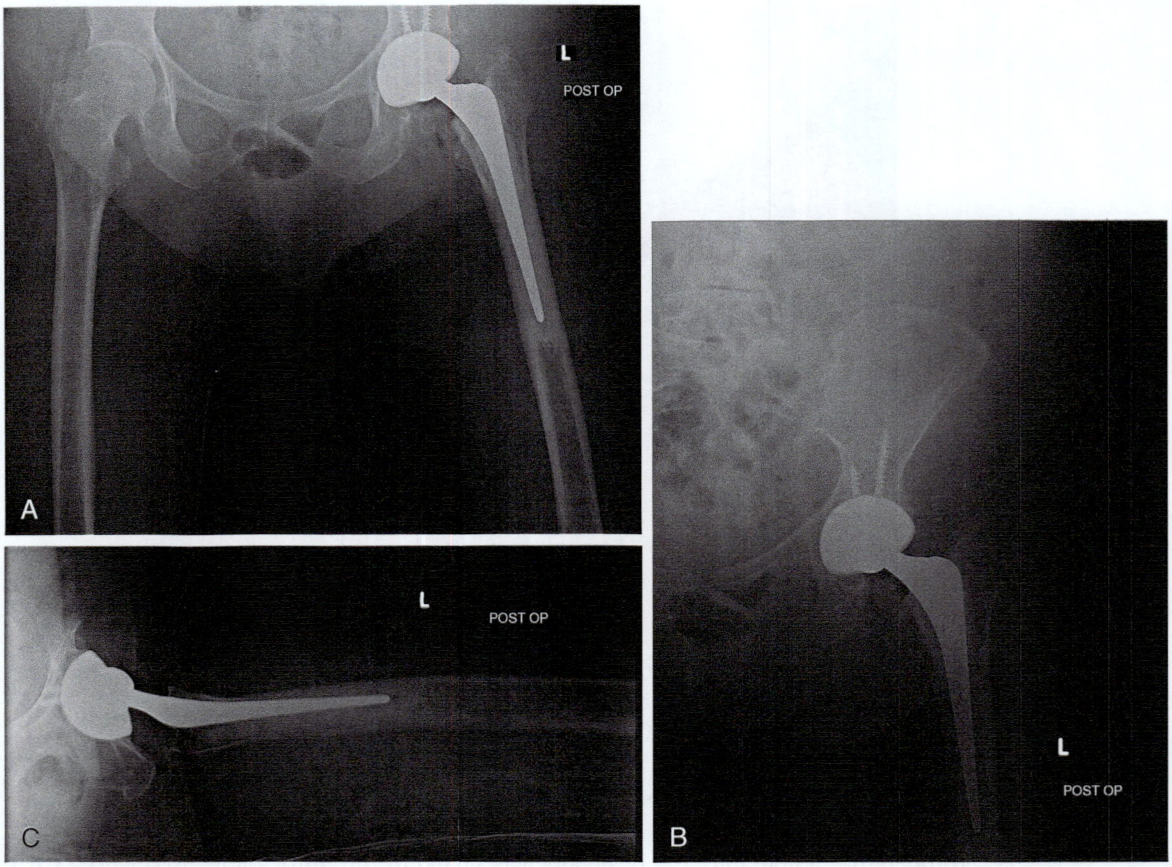

Figure 11.20 | Postoperative x-rays can be obtained as a baseline for future follow-up. The stem position and cement mantle can be seen on anteroposterior pelvis (A), anteroposterior hip (B), and cross table lateral (C) x-rays.

Chapter 12
Acute Hip Fracture

ADAM HART
DANIEL J. BERRY

Key Concepts

- The first decision to make when treating a patient with an acute femoral neck fracture is to consider internal fixation versus replacement. Optimal treatment aims to quickly restore function, minimize complications, and provide a durable result. Furthermore, the patient's age, health, and functional context must also be considered. Although the decision is multifactorial, the following points may help guide treatment (Figure 12.1):
  - Location: Subcapital and mid cervical femoral neck fractures are at higher risk of nonunion because of their intracapsular location. Potential damage to the tenuous retinacular vessels that course along the neck also predisposes the femoral head to avascular necrosis. Conversely, basicervical, intertrochanteric, and subtrochanteric fractures are extracapsular and therefore have a better chance of healing with internal fixation.
  - Displacement: Femoral neck fractures with significant displacement (Garden 3-4) are less stable, more prone to failed internal fixation, and have a higher risk of osteonecrosis of the femoral head. On the other hand, nondisplaced and valgus impacted femoral neck fractures (Garden 1-2) are inherently more stable, have a higher likelihood of healing and a lower likelihood of osteonecrosis of the femoral head, and thus are amenable to internal fixation.
  - Fracture morphology: Fractures with comminution and/or an elevated Pauwels angle (vertically oriented fracture resulting in high shear forces) are less stable and more prone to nonunion or malunion with internal fixation.
  - Patient's age, health, and function: Elderly patients with poor preoperative baseline status and a displaced femoral neck fracture should favor hip replacement to allow for immediate weight bearing and pain relief and to minimize the possibility of additional surgery. On the other hand, younger patients (generally under the age of 65 years) with reasonable health often are better treated with preservation of their native hip by closed (or open if necessary) reduction and internal fixation.
- Once hip replacement has been selected for treatment, the surgeon must consider what type of prosthesis is most appropriate.
  - Hemiarthroplasty: This has the advantage of being a fast and simple surgery while implanting a large diameter head that helps obviate postoperative dislocation. Unfortunately, the metal head that articulates with the patient's native acetabulum may lead to articular cartilage wear and arthritis over time depending on the patient's activity level. Hemiarthroplasty is therefore most appropriate for low-demand, elderly patients and those with predisposing risk factors for dislocation.
  - Total hip arthroplasty: Younger patients who are functionally independent and mobile should be considered for total hip replacement. The advantages of durable pain relief and function outweigh the risk of dislocation in this population. Similarly, patients with preexisting hip arthritis should be considered for total hip replacement over hemiarthroplasty.
- A hip fracture in the geriatric patient should be considered a major, life-threatening injury. Treatment via a multidisciplinary team throughout the perioperative course can improve outcomes.
  - Timely preoperative medical optimization with the goal of surgery within 48 hours of the injury.
  - Minimization of opioid consumption via multimodal pain management and local and regional anesthesia.

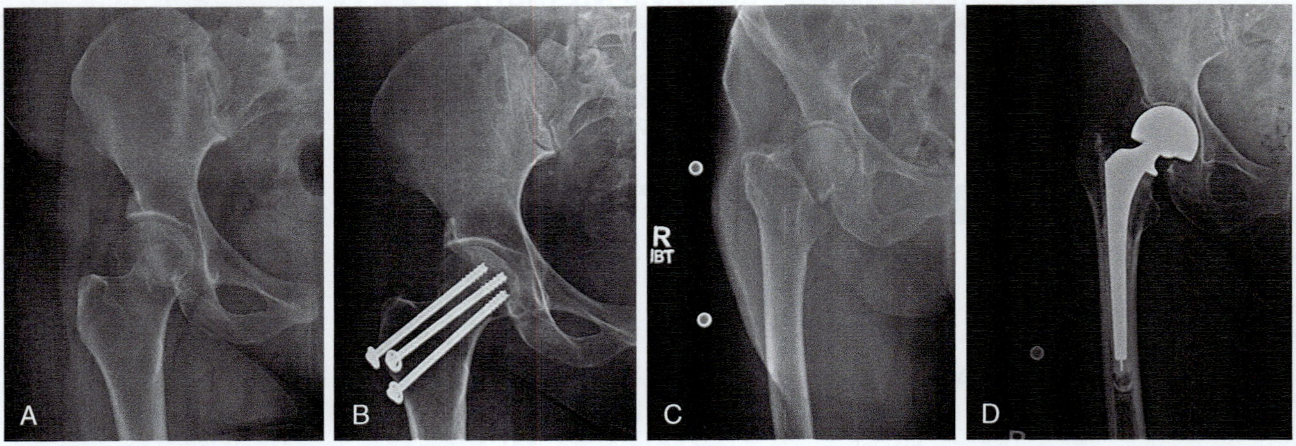

Figure 12.1 I Example of treatment decisions for displaced femoral neck fractures in 2 patients: radiographs of a 35-year-old woman with a valgus-impacted fracture after a fall from 10 feet (A) and 1 year following closed reduction and internal fixation with healed fracture and an intact femoral head (B); radiographs of an 83-year-old woman with a displaced unstable fracture after a fall from own height (C) and 1 year following bipolar hemiarthroplasty (D).

- Immediate postoperative mobilization and rehabilitation.
- Screening and appropriate treatment for osteoporosis, malnutrition, elder abuse, and fall prevention.

Sterile Instruments and Implants

- Perioperative: Consider the use of tranexamic acid, Foley catheterization (for a limited duration), local and regional anesthesia.
- Implants
  - Cemented femoral stem: Despite the widespread popularity of cementless stems, the pathologic/osteopenic bone in the geriatric hip fracture population strongly favors the use of a cemented stem (Figure 12.2). Either a taper-slip or composite beam cemented stem design can be used depending on the surgeon's preference. A cemented stem has the advantage of requiring minimal femoral broaching, solid fixation in osteopenic bone, flexibility in positioning the stem's version and height, and local antibiotic delivery. Most importantly, cemented stems in this population are associated with lower rates of early periprosthetic femur fracture and early femoral component loosening.
  - Hemiarthroplasty: Either a unipolar or bipolar prosthesis may be used depending on surgeon preference. Although a bipolar prosthesis is more expensive, it has the theoretical advantage of decreasing wear of the host acetabular cartilage.
  - Total hip arthroplasty: A cemented or hybrid total hip replacement may be used per the surgeon's preference. The use of a large diameter head (36 or 40 mm) or dual mobility articulation should be considered, especially for patients at increased risk of dislocation (e.g., cognitive impairment, rigidity, fused spine, parkinsonism).

Surgical Approaches

- Anterolateral, direct anterior, or posterolateral operative approaches may be used according to surgeon preference. These patients are at particularly high risk owing to hip dislocation; therefore, the authors prefer to use an anterolateral approach to mitigate the risk of hip instability.

Preoperative Planning

- A detailed history and physical examination are essential. In particular, assessing the patient's baseline function, cognition, ambulatory status, living environment, medical comorbidities, anticoagulation, and additional injuries are paramount to planning.
- Preoperative planning should include assessment and optimization by the medical team, pain management, and establishing the level of care or documentation of an advanced directive.

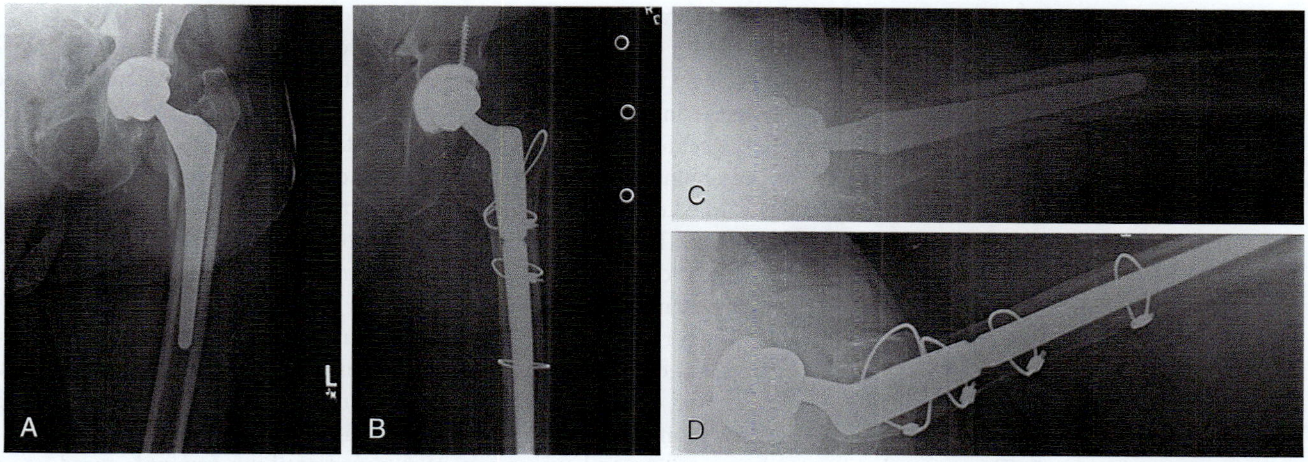

Figure 12.2 I Radiographs of a failed cementless total hip replacement in a 77-year-old man (A, C) due to early periprosthetic femur fracture and 5-year radiographs post treatment of the periprosthetic fracture using a modular taper fluted stem (B, D).

- Radiographs should be studied to determine the fracture morphology, femoral and acetabular bone quality, and presence of preexisting arthritis. Occasionally, notable external rotation of the limb may preclude accurate assessment of the fracture (femoral neck versus basicervical). Repeat radiographs with gentle traction and internal rotation of the leg may facilitate a more accurate diagnosis and consequent planning.
- Templating for femoral and acetabular component sizes and position is encouraged. Oftentimes, it is easier to template using the contralateral hip, which is typically well positioned on the radiograph and more accurately portrays the patient's anatomy.

Bone, Implant, and Soft Tissue Techniques

- Position and drape the patient according to the surgeon's preference and approach. If performing a hemiarthroplasty, extra care is needed to avoid damaging the labrum during exposure.
- Removal of the femoral head
  - Following deep exposure, the femoral neck fracture should be readily visible by rotating the limb to expose the fracture. The head may be removed by tapping a corkscrew extractor into the center of the neck and then screwing it into the head fragment. Use the contralateral thumb to stabilize the head while inserting the corkscrew.
  - If exposure to the fracture is limited, use the oscillating saw to cut the neck at the desired level and remove the interposed bone. This will facilitate exposure of the head fragment.
  - With the corkscrew securely seated, lever the head out of the acetabulum. Occasionally, the ligamentum teres will need to be cut using curved Mayo scissors.
- Acetabular preparation (for total hip replacement)
  - Standard exposure and acetabular preparation according to the surgeon's preference using a cementless hemispherical component with supplemental screw fixation. Note that the nonarthritic acetabular bone usually is very soft and great care must be taken to avoid reaming the socket excessively deep.
- Femoral preparation
  - Prepare the proximal femur according to the desired and templated stem. Remember the bone often is weak and at risk for fracture.
  - Perform a trial reduction to ensure hip stability, limb length restoration, and impingement-free range of motion. Note the approximate depth of the stem and desired anteversion, which will need to be replicated during stem insertion. While trialing, be careful to avoid forceful motions which could lead to greater trochanteric fracture.
- Cementing technique
  - Advise the anesthesia team that cementation will be performed shortly to ensure that the anesthetist is present and that the patient is well hydrated and oxygenated.
  - Insert an appropriately sized cement plug approximately 1 to 2 cm below the stem's tip (use the broach or stem as a reference).

    - Prepare the canal using pulse lavage.
    - A small catheter may be placed into the femoral canal followed by packing with epinephrine-soaked Ray-Tec sponges. Leave a trailing end of each sponge outside the femur to ensure each one is removed later. Dry sponges can then replace the wet sponges, and suction may be applied to the catheter immediately before cementation to dry the bone interface.
    - Place a sponge into the acetabulum to collect any cement extruded during stem insertion.
    - Vacuum-mixed cement is injected into the canal from distal to proximal once the cement has reached a doughy consistency. The authors routinely add 1 g of antibiotics (typically vancomycin or a powdered aminoglycoside) into a single batch of cement. This is an off-label medication use. Two batches of cement are needed for most femora.
    - Cement pressurization using a rubber adapter may be performed cautiously. Patients who are at high risk of cardiorespiratory complications probably are best treated without pressurization.
    - The stem is then slowly inserted to the desired position. A thumb may be placed over the calcar to increase cement pressurization during stem insertion (if desired).
    - The stem is held securely in position and excess cement removed until the cement is cured.
    - Ensure that there are no cement pieces in the acetabulum before hip reduction.
- Closure
    - Make every attempt to close and repair the capsule, which is often torn at the time of injury.

Postoperative Care

- Weight bearing as tolerated and early mobilization with physical therapy.
- Hip precautions depending on approach and surgeon preference.
- Initiate workup and treatment for osteoporosis.

Chapter 13
Failed Previous Hip Fracture

DANIEL J. BERRY

Key Concepts

- The main reasons to consider hip arthroplasty after failed treatment of a hip fracture are fracture nonunion or failure of internal fixation, osteonecrosis of the femoral head, or progression of hip joint arthritis. The first 2 typically occur early after the fracture; the latter often occurs late.
- Patients with failed hip fractures typically are very disabled, and effective operative means of salvaging the problem are essential.
- Failed hip fractures can be divided intellectually into 4 main groups: (1) failed femoral neck (FN) fractures in younger patients, (2) failed FN fractures in older patients, (3) failed intertrochanteric (IT) fractures in younger patients, and (4) failed IT fractures in older patients.
- Failed FN in younger patients often may be salvaged with head sparing procedures, most commonly valgus producing IT osteotomy that puts the fracture in compression and allows healing. Good results can be obtained, even if moderate-sized areas of femoral head osteonecrosis are present.
- Failed FN fractures in older patients and those with notably compromised bone are usually best treated with conversion to hip arthroplasty.
- Failed IT fractures in younger patients typically are treated with repeat open reduction and internal fixation using rigid fixation, autologous bone grafting as needed, and deformity correction.
- Failed IT fractures in older patients most commonly are treated with conversion to hip arthroplasty, although in some patients with good remaining bone and a good remaining hip joint another attempt at internal fixation may be indicated. Stronger indications for conversion to hip arthroplasty are poor bone quality, loss of bone in key areas needed for stability and fixation, damage to the acetabulum by screw cut out or arthritis, advanced hip arthritis or femoral head osteonecrosis. Advantages of arthroplasty are fracture healing is not required because the fracture is excised and rapid mobilization is possible (which is important to many elderly patients who have already been immobilized owing to the failed fracture for a period of time).
- Most patients having hip arthroplasty for failed hip fracture have had previous internal fixation. Before conversion to hip arthroplasty, infection should be excluded. History of wound healing problems, drainage, or systemic symptoms should raise concern as should physical findings of erythema or wound drainage. Most patients should be screened with erythrocyte sedimentation rate and C-reactive protein. If findings are concerning, advanced imaging and/or hip aspiration may be considered.
- Patients having conversion arthroplasty after fracture often have weak bone (typically this is why the fracture occurred in the first place, and disuse osteopenia as the fracture fails exacerbates this problem). This places patients at risk for intraoperative and postoperative fracture (of the acetabulum and femur) and also at risk for implant loosening (of the acetabular and femoral components). Cemented implants can reduce the risk of fracture and early loosening, particularly for the femur.
- Conversion to hemiarthroplasty or total hip arthroplasty (THA) both are options. Hemiarthroplasty is a high stability bearing and is a smaller operation than THA; however, pain relief is less reliable. Hemiarthroplasty may be considered for very infirm or minimally ambulatory patients. For most other patients, THA, which is associated with more reliable pain relief, is preferred.

- Patients having conversion arthroplasty after fracture commonly are at high risk for hip instability owing to age, cognitive factors, neuromuscular or balance factors, or anatomic abnormalities such as compromise of the greater trochanter (GT) in patients with previous IT fractures. High stability bearings such as large-diameter femoral heads (36 mm or greater) or dual mobility implants may be considered.
- If hardware is in place, understand what hardware is present (including the manufacturer) and the specifics of how to remove the hardware. Make sure the instruments, which may be manufacturer specific, are available for hardware removal.

Sterile Instruments/Implants

- Routine hip arthroplasty instrumentation. If cementation is anticipated, have all the needed materials for cementation, including cement guns and cement restrictors.
- Hip arthroplasty implants for the planned procedure. If an uncemented cup is planned, have available cups that allow for cup fixation screw augmentation. For failed FN fractures have available cemented or uncemented femoral implants (depending on surgeon preference—see following text), typically of standard length. For failed IT fractures, extended neck implants, calcar replacing implants, or distally fixed implants that allow the surgeon to compensate for deficient proximal bone usually are needed. Have available implants that can bypass screw holes in the proximal femur.
- Instrumentation to remove the hardware that is in place. This often is manufacturer specific.
- Broken screw removal instruments, including trephines and reverse thread screw extractors.
- Cerclage cables and wires.
- High-speed burrs with various sized tips.
- Have intraoperative radiography or fluoroscopy available as needed.

Positioning

- Lateral decubitus or supine as per surgeon preference.
- Make sure to include access to most of the femur in the operative field, including any areas that need to be accessed for hardware removal.
- For cases that will be more difficult consider placement of a Foley catheter.

Surgical Approaches

- For most failed FN fractures conversion to arthroplasty can be done via posterior, anterolateral/direct lateral, or direct anterior approach based on the surgeon's preference. However, cementation of the femoral component is preferred for many of these patients with very poor bone (owing to risk of femoral loosening and postoperative fracture with uncemented implants) and cementation is more difficult to do well through the direct anterior approach.
- For failed IT fractures, the operative approach often is dictated by the anatomy of the GT. If the GT is malunited in a position that impedes access to the femoral canal, or nonunited (Figure 13.2A), a trochanteric slide (see Chapter 4) or extended greater trochanteric osteotomy may be indicated. If this is not the case, a routine posterior or anterolateral/direct lateral approach may be used.
- The operative approach should provide for access to the hardware that will require removal.
- Usually some or all of the scar from previous internal fixation may be used, but this is dependent on the previous scar position and the planned new operative approach. Try to avoid parallel scars very close to one another to avoid devascularization of a skin bridge.

Preoperative Planning

- Discuss medical issues (often present in these cases) with internal medicine and anesthesia teams.
- Failed FN fracture: template for acetabular and femoral components, including implant size and position. If the leg is shortened template to restore leg length: plan how any existing hardware will be removed.
- Failed IT fracture: template for acetabular and femoral components, including implant size and position. If the leg is shortened, template to restore leg length: typically there is more calcar bone loss than is obvious, and implants that make up for bone in this area often are needed. Consider stem length: in most older patients plan to bypass holes or defects left in the proximal femur by a distance equal to about 2 femoral canal diameters. Plan how any existing hardware will be removed.

Bone/Implant/Soft Tissue Techniques

Failed Femoral Neck Fracture

- Perform the desired operative approach to the hip.
- Dislocate the hip once before attempting to remove the hardware. The initial hip dislocation maneuver usually places the highest torsional loads on the femur, so performing this maneuver with the hardware in place reduces risk of an intraoperative spiral femur fracture.
- Even when dislocating the hip with the hardware in place, be cautious during the dislocation and make sure sufficient soft tissue releases have been performed to avoid high torsional loads on the femur.
- Relocate the hip and remove existing internal fixation hardware using manufacturer-specific instrumentation as needed.
- Prepare the acetabulum (unless a hemiarthroplasty is being performed—see "Key Concepts"): remember the acetabular bone will be soft and often is very weak. These patients usually have osteopenia as the reason for their fracture and additionally usually do not have the harder subchondral bone typical of osteoarthritis. It is easy to ream too deeply and too medially. Just ream until the cartilage of the acetabulum has been removed, and try to preserve the subchondral bone; often it is the best bone. Ream to allow a moderate, not excessive, press fit of the component when an uncemented implant is planned. Too much press fit risks fracture; too little risks fixation problems.
- Prepare the femur: if screws have been present in the lateral femur, remember these create stress risers that place the GT at risk for fracture.
- Perform trial reductions and make sure leg length and hip stability have been optimized.
- Implant the acetabular component. For surgeons who are experts at cemented acetabular fixation, this is a reasonable indication for that type of implant. Most North American surgeons have less experience with cemented implants and prefer uncemented implants. Uncemented implants also usually provide more high stability options, which are helpful in many of these patients (Figure 13.1). When placing uncemented cups, a moderate press fit, usually about 1 mm, is best in these patients. When impacting the shell be careful to avoid very high forces that can lead to fracture of the weak bone. Augmenting cup fixation with screws is wise in most of these patients who have poor-quality bone.

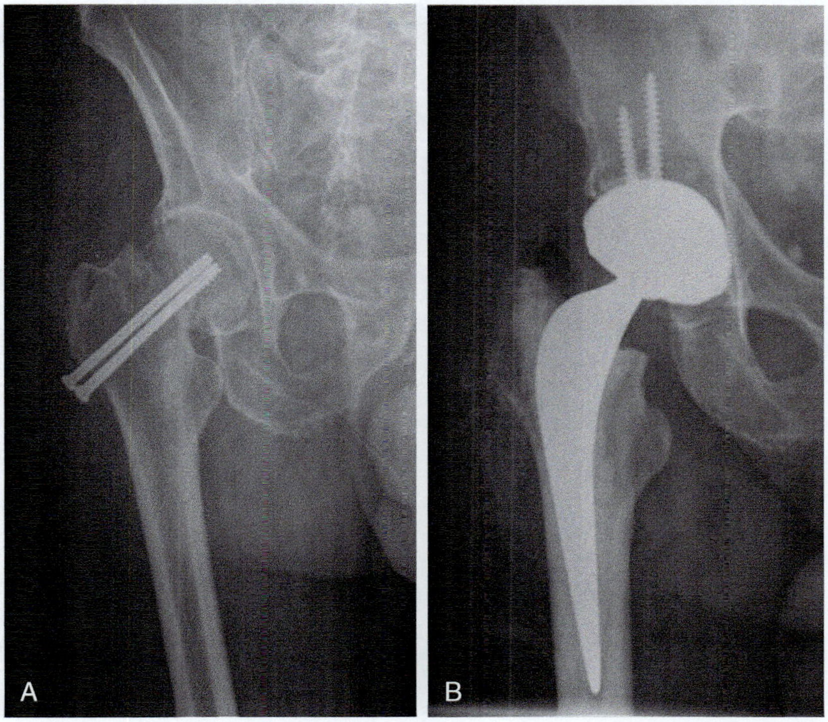

Figure 13.1 | A, Radiograph of nonunited femoral neck fracture. B, Postoperative radiograph after reconstruction with hybrid THA and high stability dual mobility acetabulum.

- Implant the femoral component. For older patients a cemented implant is preferred owing to lower risk of reoperation for loosening or postoperative femur fracture (see Figure 13.1). If cement is used, avoid extrusion through lateral holes in the femur, blocking the holes with finger pressure. Alert the anesthesia team before cementation so they can make sure the patient is well oxygenated and volume replete.
- Perform trial reductions and choose an optimal bearing. Remember, these patients are at risk for hip instability and a high stability bearing such as a large femoral head diameter or dual mobility bearing may be advantageous (see Figure 13.1).
- Use autogenous bone graft from the patient's femoral head to graft remaining screw holes in the femur.
- Perform careful capsular and muscle repair, depending on the operative approach.
- Close the wound in layers.

Failed Intertrochanteric Fracture

- Perform the desired operative approach to the hip. If the GT is nonunited or malunited in a varus position impeding access to the femoral canal, consider a GT slide (Figure 4.2) or extended GT osteotomy (Chapter 23) (see Figure 13.2).
- Dislocate the hip once before attempting to remove the hardware. The initial hip dislocation maneuver usually places the highest torsional loads on the femur, so performing this with the hardware in place reduces risk of an intraoperative spiral femur fracture.
- Even when dislocating the hip with the hardware in place, be cautious during the dislocation and make sure sufficient soft tissue releases have been performed to avoid high torsional loads on the femur.
- Relocate the hip and remove existing internal fixation hardware using manufacturer-specific instrumentation as needed.
- Removing existing internal fixation devices may be more difficult than expected. When removing intramedullary devices, finding the proximal aspect of the rod beneath the abductors may be challenging. Intraoperative fluoroscopy can be used. Avoid badly damaging the abductors searching for the proximal aspect of intramedullary rods. Broken screws in the diaphysis are common and may not be visible on the radiograph (Figure 13.3). Use dedicated broken screw removal instruments,

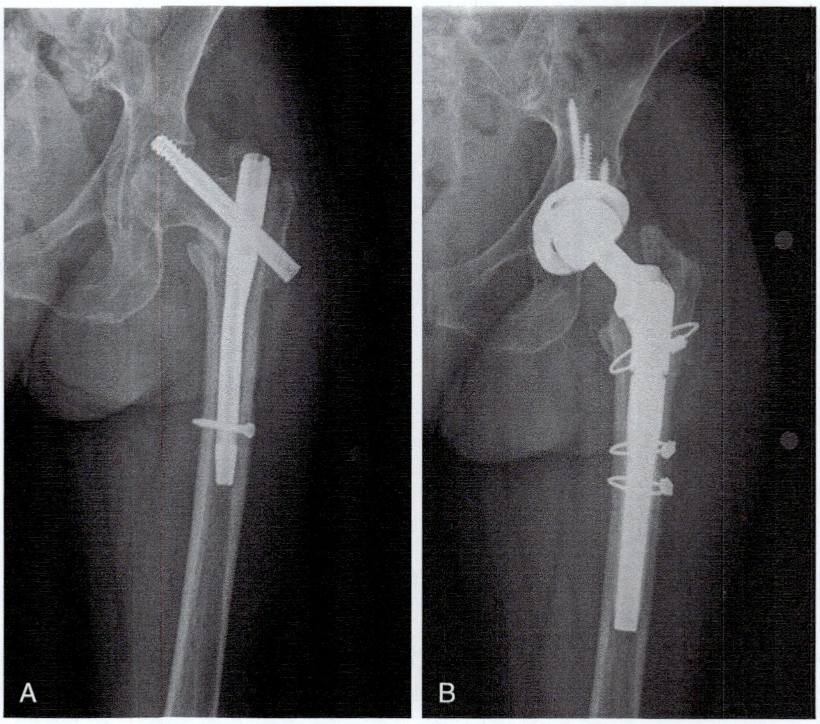

Figure 13.2 | A, Radiograph of patient with intertrochanteric hip fracture nonunion and greater trochanter overhanging the canal. B, Postoperative radiograph after reconstruction using extended greater trochanteric osteotomy approach.

including small trephines and reverse thread screw removal instruments. Fluoroscopy also can be used to find broken screws. Some broken screws that are not accessible, but that will preclude hardware removal or femoral component placement, may be pushed out the medial side of the femur or pushed down the femoral canal (Figure 13.4).

Prepare the acetabulum (unless a hemiarthroplasty is being performed—see "Key Concepts"): remember the acetabular bone will be soft and often is very weak. These patients usually have osteopenia as the reason for their fracture and additionally usually do not have the harder subchondral bone typical of osteoarthritis. It is easy to ream too deeply and too medially. Just ream until the cartilage of the acetabulum has been removed, and try to preserve the subchondral bone; often it is the best bone. Ream to allow a moderate, not excessive, press fit of the component when an uncemented implant is planned. Too much press fit risks fracture; too little risks fixation problems.

- Implant the acetabular component. For surgeons who are expert at cemented acetabular fixation, this is a reasonable indication for that type of implant. Most North American surgeons have less experience with cemented implants and prefer uncemented implants. Uncemented implants also usually provide more high stability options, which are helpful in many of these patients. When placing uncemented cups, a moderate press,fit, usually about 1 mm, is best in these patients. When impacting the shell be careful to avoid very high forces that can lead to fracture of the weak bone (Figure 13.5). Augmenting cup fixation with screws is wise in most of these patients who have poor-quality bone (Figure 13.6).
- Prepare the femur for the planned implant. Use an implant that will make up for bone loss that often extends to or below the lesser trochanter—such implants are needed to restore leg length and optimize hip stability. Use an implant that will bypass screw holes or other defects in the proximal femur, usually by 2 femoral canal diameters. Cemented and uncemented femoral components may be used. Cemented implants have the advantage of immediate secure fixation and often are preferred in older patients with poorer bone (Figure 13.7). In physiologically younger patients with a longer life expectancy uncemented implants may be preferred (see Figure 13.2). When the previous hardware was an intramedullary device, the cancellous bone may be damaged and this may be a relative indication for use of an uncemented implant. When using uncemented implants, diaphyseal fixation

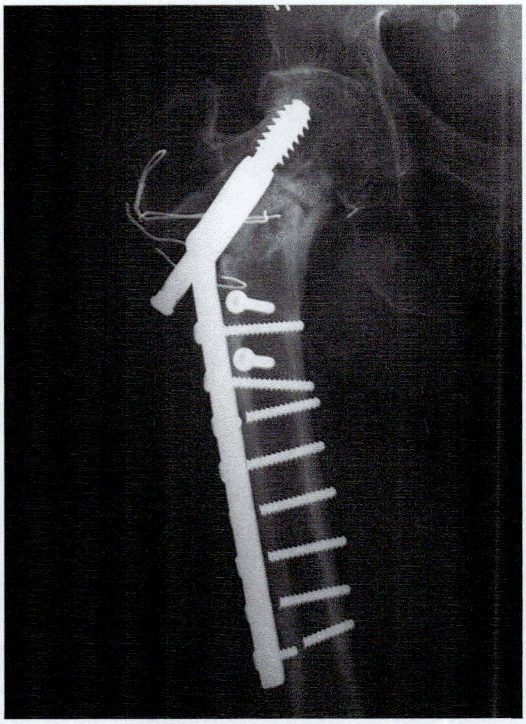

Figure 13.3 | Radiograph showing broken screws, which are common in failed hip fracture.

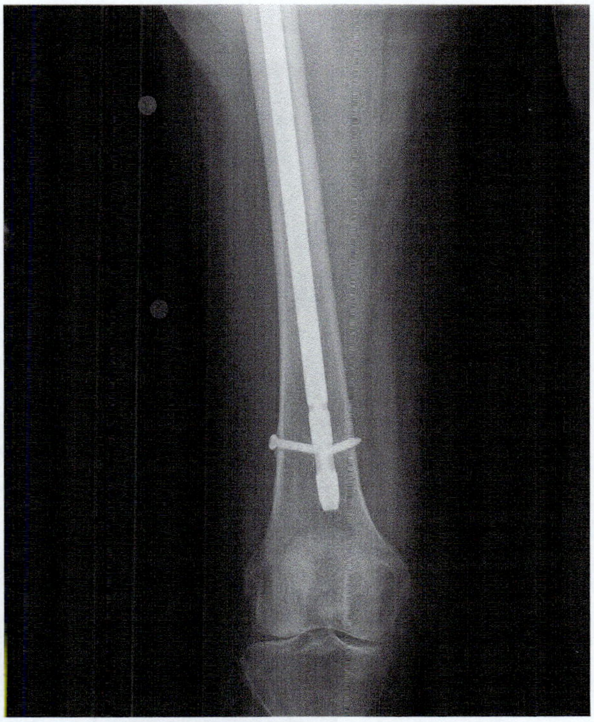

Figure 13.4 | Radiograph of broken interlocking screw in patient with arthritis after intertrochanteric hip fracture. The broken medial portion of the screw was pushed through the rod percutaneously with a Steinmann pin to allow rod extraction.

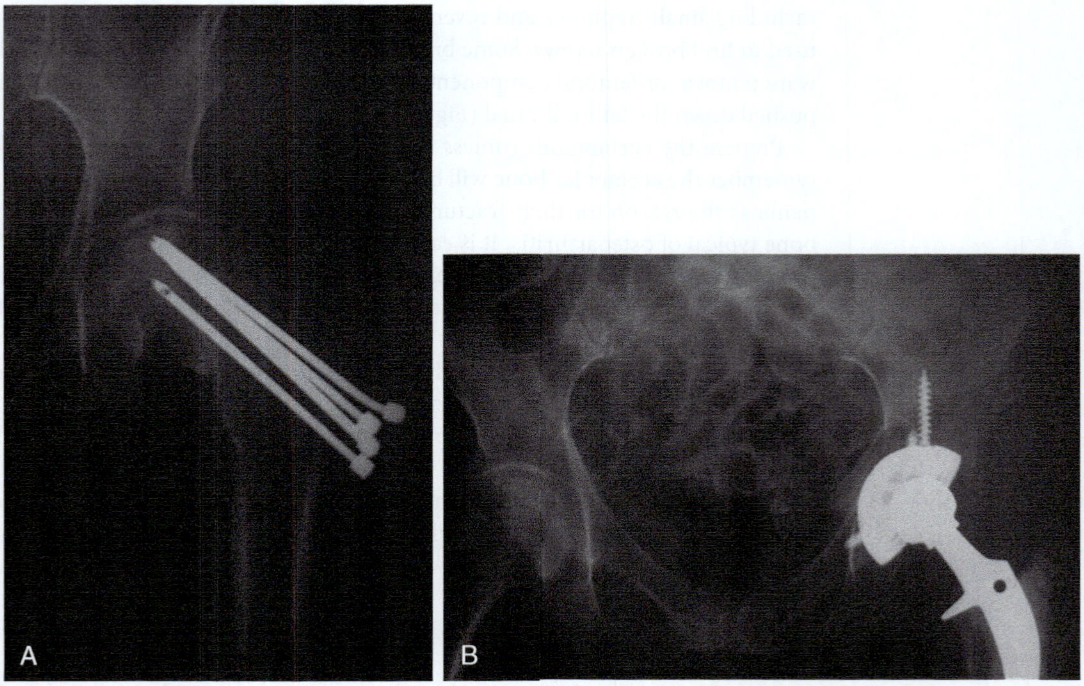

Figure 13.5 | A, Radiograph of patient with nonunited femoral neck fracture. B, Postoperative radiograph demonstrating fracture of the medial wall that occurred with cup insertions. The cup was fixed with screws and was stable.

is preferred in many cases in which the proximal metaphyseal bone is compromised (Figure 13.2). When the metaphyseal bone is good, implants that allow for bone preparation with reamers rather than with broaching provide advantages because the bone often is sclerotic and difficult to prepare with broaches (that can lead to fracture) (Figure 13.8).

- Have high-speed burrs available to aid in femoral bone preparation. The bone in the IT area around the fracture often is sclerotic and difficult to prepare.

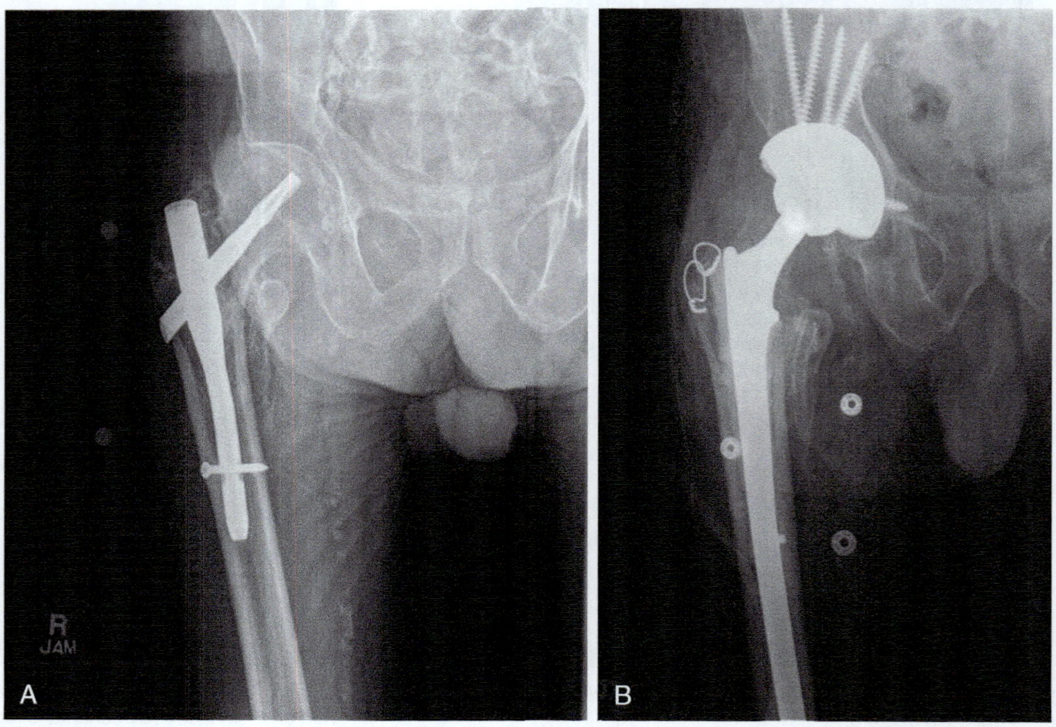

Figure 13.6 | A, Radiograph of patient with nonunited IT fracture. Intraoperatively the acetabulum bone quality was very poor. B, Postoperative radiograph demonstrating highly porous cup fixed with multiple screws.

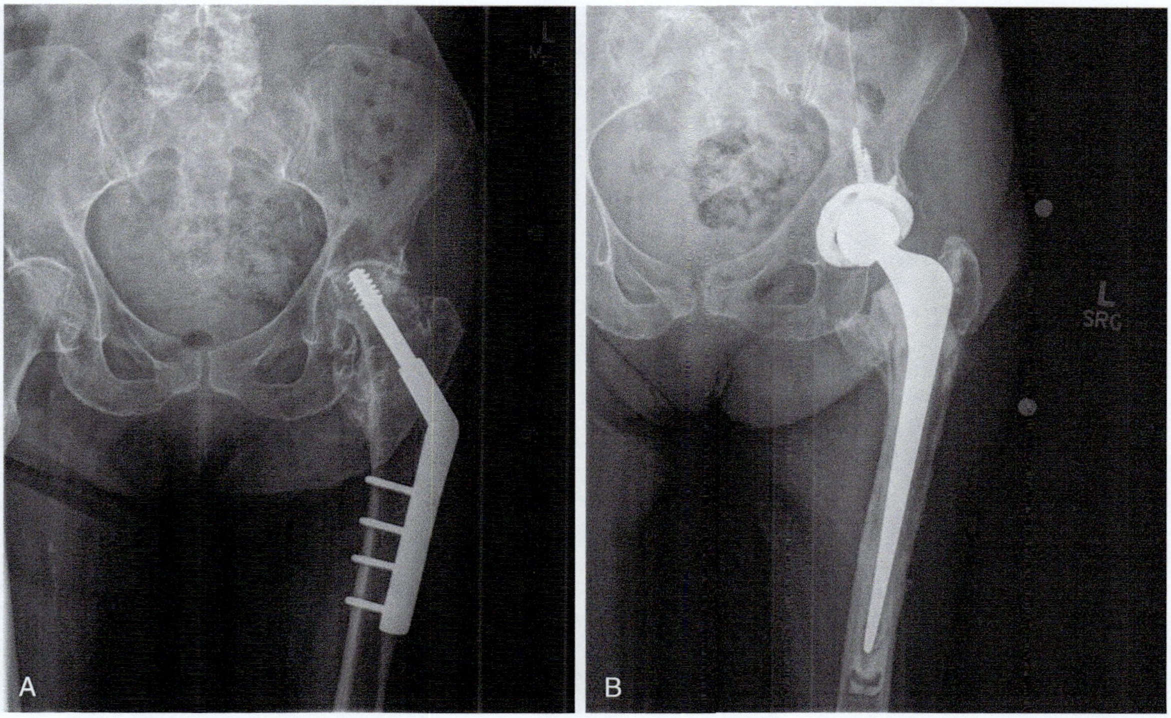

Figure 13.7 | A, Radiograph of failed intertrochanteric hip fracture in elderly patient. B, Radiograph after reconstruction with cemented stem.

- If the femoral anatomy is deformed, intraoperative fluoroscopy may be used during femoral preparation to avoid femoral bone damage or perforation. An intraoperative radiograph with trial implants in place can help optimize implant sizing and orientation.
- When uncemented diaphyseal fixation stems will be used, consider prophylactic cerclage wire/s or cable/s around the femur in areas of weakness where previous screws have been removed (Figure 13.9). This tactic can reduce the risk of intraoperative femur fracture.

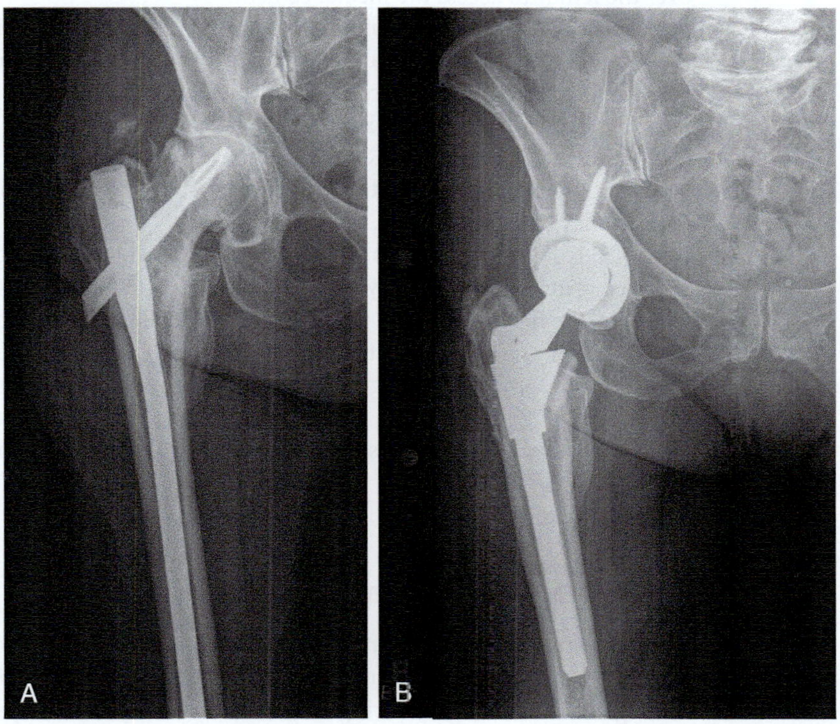

Figure 13.8 | A, Radiograph of a patient with osteoarthritis of hip, status post open reduction and internal fixation IT hip fracture with an intramedullary nail. B, Radiograph after THA using uncemented THA with ream-only femoral preparation.

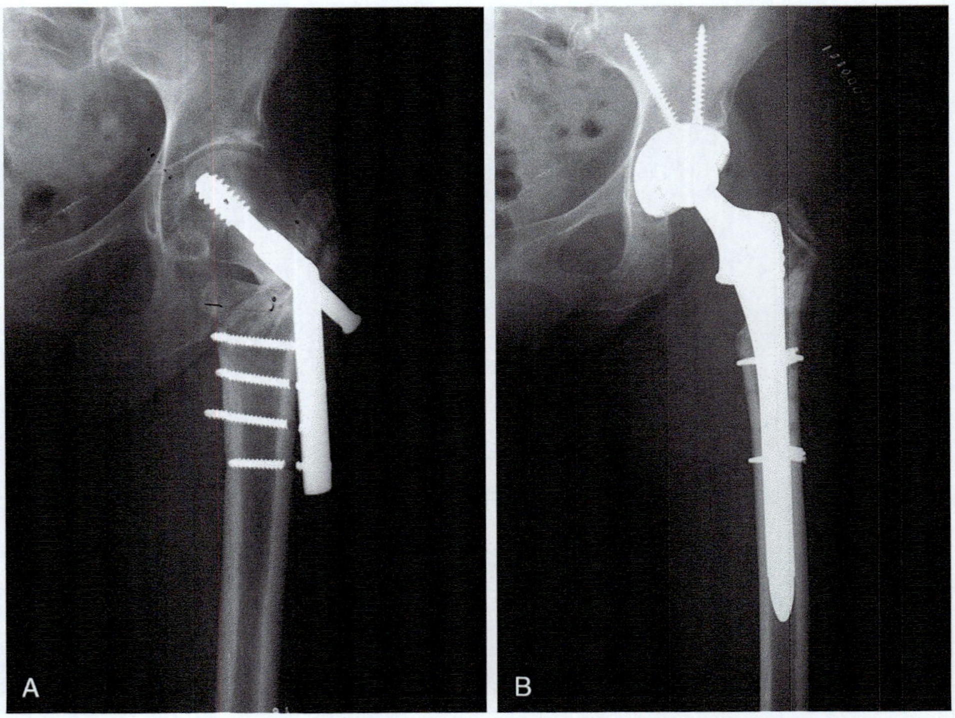

Figure 13.9 | A, Radiograph of nonunited intertrochanteric hip fracture. B, Postoperative radiograph after reconstruction with uncemented extensively coated stem. Prophylactic cables were placed around the diaphysis to avoid intraoperative fracture.

- When a cemented stem is used, occlude lateral empty screw holes with fingers to avoid cement extrusion. An alternative is to place temporary unicortical screws in the lateral screw holes. Be aware cement can also extrude medially through screw holes. Often soft tissues prevent this, but it is wise to take an intraoperative radiograph before wound closure to make sure cement has not extruded medially; if it has, manual removal is possible by lifting the vastus lateralis and dissecting anteriorly over the femur to access the medial cement.
- Perform trial reductions and make sure leg length and hip stability have been optimized. Be aware that deformity of the proximal bone can lead to extraarticular impingement by the GT against the pelvis in hip flexion/internal rotation. If this occurs, some of the anterior GT, deep to the abductor muscle attachments, may be excised.
- Choose the optimal bearing. Remember, these patients are at risk for hip instability, especially if the GT is not united, and a high stability bearing such as a large femoral head diameter or dual mobility bearing may be advantageous.
- If the GT is not united, assess whether there is a viable bed of bone for reattachment and consider whether reattachment is likely to lead to union. If there is a reasonable chance of union, function will likely be better and pain may be less. Rigid GT fixation with wires, claw, and cable or other devices may be considered. If there is little chance of bony union, fixation with sutures to try to gain fibrous union, without risking metal debris that is likely to form if rigid internal fixation fails, may be preferable.
- Close the capsule and/or muscles around the hip joint meticulously to optimize hip stability and function.
- Close the wound in layers.

Postoperative Care

- Weight bearing as tolerated typically is allowed for hybrid and cemented hip arthroplasty constructs. Weight bearing after uncemented constructs may be individualized based on bone quality. If GT healing is needed, weight bearing may be restricted to touch or partial weight bearing for 8 weeks.
- Particularly if GT healing is needed, a hip guide brace with a flexion stop (usually at 45-60°) and a hip abduction of 15° may be considered.

Chapter 14
Previous Acetabular Fracture

DAVID G. LEWALLEN

Key Concepts

- Posttraumatic degenerative changes of the hip are common after acetabular fracture.
- Fracture sequelae can include residual deformity due to malreduction and/or malunion.
- Nonunion or resorption of original fracture fragments can result in major segmental or cavitary defects.
- Retained hardware from prior fracture fixation can impinge on the joint or the acetabular preparation and may require removal in part (preferred) or less often in total.
- Partial hardware removal can be facilitated by metal cutting tools.
- Extensive hardware removal can place soft tissue and neurovascular structures at risk and is usually only indicated in the case of deep infection when a 2-stage reconstruction is planned.
- Heterotopic bone formation can be a challenge at the time of arthroplasty and can complicate postoperative course.
- Obtaining durable long-term fixation can be challenging, and consequently extra socket fixation often is needed.

Sterile Instruments and Implants

- Standard hip arthroplasty instruments and retractors.
- Extra-large or deep retractors for obese patients.
- Proper screw drivers for retained hardware removal or "universal" screw driver sets with multiple heads can be very helpful.
- Carbide cutting tools or high-speed burrs for sectioning metal screws or plates.
- Sterile ultrasound gel to trap metal debris when burring.
- Multihole highly porous acetabular components are preferred to allow 3 to 6 screws for secure cup fixation and encourage reliable bone ingrowth.
- Large-diameter heads (36 mm or greater) to reduce dislocation risk.
- Optional sciatic nerve monitoring if there is prior sciatic nerve dysfunction or complete removal of posterior column plate or posteriorly located heterotopic bone is required.
- A second surgical assistant many times is helpful.

Surgical Approaches

- The posterolateral approach is commonly used, especially if a prior Kocher-type posterior incision was used for internal fixation of the acetabular fracture originally and especially when complete removal of posterior column hardware is required.
- The direct lateral (and less often the direct anterior) approach can also be used, and both are preferred by some surgeons for some or even most cases. Partial hardware removal may be employed to manage any encroaching screws or hardware, generally using intra-acetabular access to those portions of the hardware encroaching on the joint or encountered during acetabular preparation.

- Rarely trochanteric osteotomy or supplemental ilioinguinal approaches may be required when truly extensile exposure is needed for removal of large masses of heterotopic bone or for complete removal of extensive hardware present on the inner table or going well up onto the iliac wing posteriorly.
- Complete hardware removal is not routine and is generally reserved for cases with associated deep infection.

Preoperative Planning

- Careful preoperative planning is important to anticipate special hardware removal needs as discussed earlier or to anticipate deformity or bone deficiency that might compromise implant fixation leading to cup loosening or cup malposition and associated hip instability.
- An anteroposterior (AP) radiograph of the pelvis and AP and cross-table lateral radiographs of the affected hip are required views (Figure 14.1A-C).
- Obturator and iliac oblique x-rays (Judet views) can also be very helpful in assessing bone defects and hardware location in some cases.
- Selective use of axial imaging with computed tomography or magnetic resonance imaging can provide additional help in visualizing the 3-dimensional relationships around the acetabulum of bone defects and hardware, or heterotopic bone location (Figure 14.2).
- It is important to rule out deep infection in all cases treated with prior surgery and especially those with retained hardware in place.
- Laboratory assessment and aspiration for culture may be reassuring when negative but can fail to reveal a low-grade infection present in the hip.
- Rarely technetium bone scanning and companion indium-labeled white blood cell scans are obtained when clinical suspicions of deep infection are still present after the standard infection workup is negative.

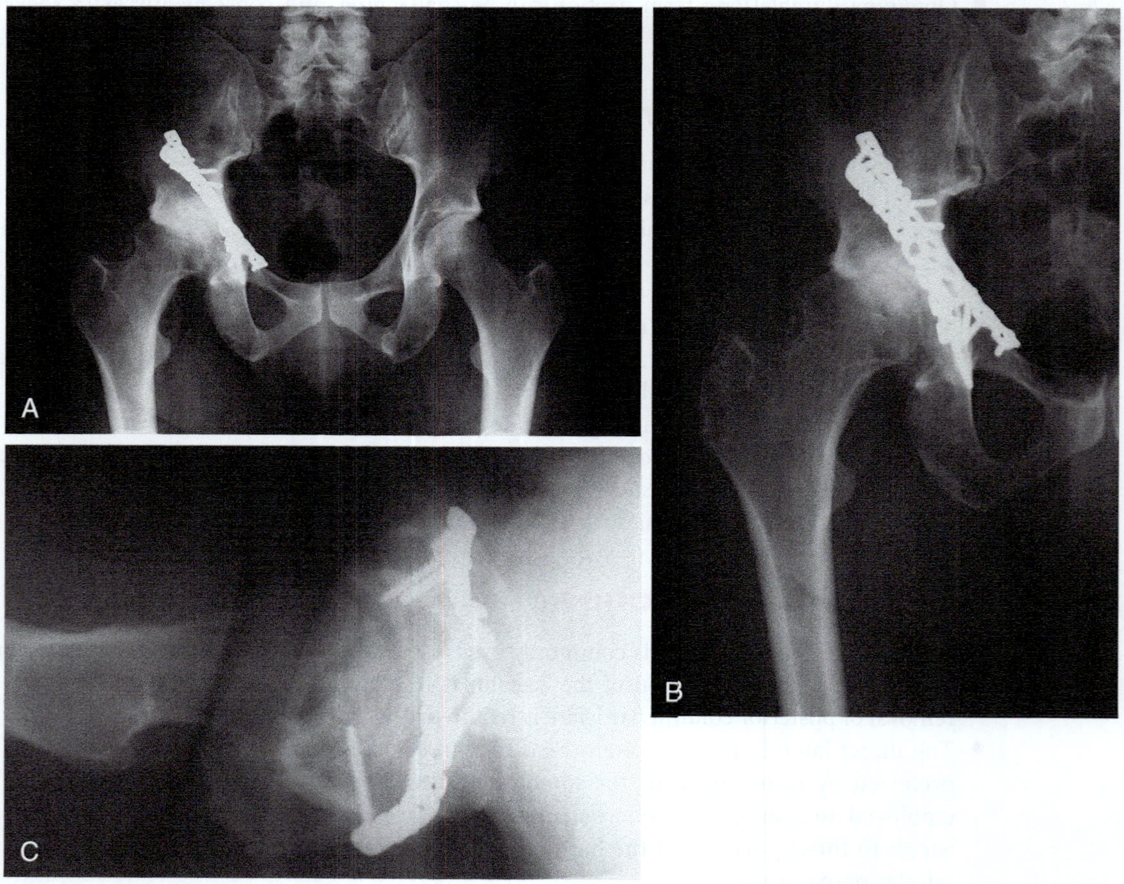

Figure 14.1 | Radiographic views of the hip following prior fracture should include an AP view of the pelvis (A), an AP view of the involved hip (B), and a cross-table lateral of the hip, which is properly exposed so as to show the posterior column in relief (C)

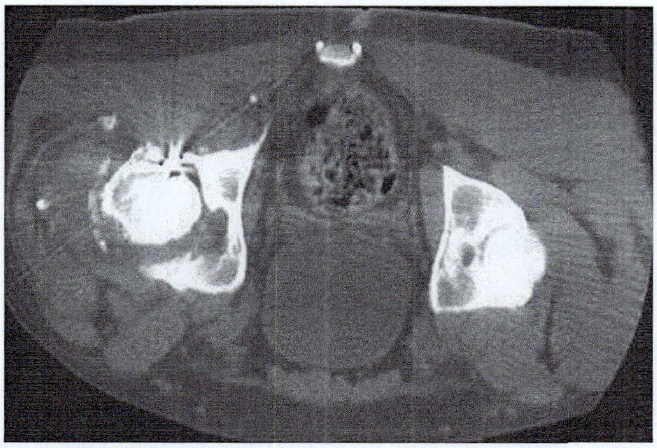

Figure 14.2 | One selected cut from a computed tomography scan of a hip with prior internal fixation for acetabular fracture showing intra-articular encroachment by screws.

- When infection is established before arthroplasty, usually a 2-stage approach is taken with removal of all hardware, complete debridement and resection of any dead bone (i.e., avascular Necrosis of the head) followed by placement of a temporary antibiotic-impregnated articulating hip spacer.
- Following appropriate intravenous (IV) antibiotic therapy specific to the infecting organism, the second stage of the procedure is done 8 to 12 weeks later to remove the articulating spacer, repeat the debridement, and place permanent implants.

Bone, Implant, and Soft Tissue Techniques

- Regardless of the surgical exposure chosen, plan on a longer than usual incision and exposure challenges more akin to revision hip surgery.
- Variable but sometimes excessive blood loss can occur with difficulty in gaining adequate exposure owing to scarring or heterotopic bone.
- Use of a cell saver to scavenge lost blood and avoid the need for homologous transfusion is worthy of consideration in more complex cases.
- Sciatic nerve palsy may already be present (partial or complete) due to the original fracture or prior surgery and is a higher risk following total hip arthroplasty after prior acetabular fracture.
- Formal sciatic nerve exploration (with or without nerve monitoring) may be required to allow safe exposure, necessary hardware removal, or extensive posterior heterotopic ossification excision.
- If difficulty in dislocation of the head is encountered because of excessive scarring or intrapelvic migration of the head into the deformed acetabular cavity, an in situ osteotomy of the femoral neck and separate removal of the head with a cork-screw extractor can be a safe alternative that reduces the risk of femoral or acetabular rim fracture.
- Retract the femur following osteotomy of the neck and expose the entire bony rim of the acetabulum to avoid reaming errors.
- Three or more intraoperative tissue cultures should be sent in all cases.
- After removal of scar and fibrous tissue from the acetabular cavity assess the pattern and extent of bone loss and burr away any encroaching hardware within the joint (Figure 14.3).
- Persistent fracture nonunion may be present involving the acetabular rim, a wall, or column or may cause residual pelvic discontinuity. Such nonunions may require bone grafting (cancellous or structural, typically using the patient's own femoral head), supplemental internal fixation of the bone (such as column plate), and/or added fixation of the cup (such a cup-cage construct).
- Progressively larger reamers are used carefully and slowly to enlarge the acetabular cavity and achieve as close as possible to a hemispherical bleeding bone surface for contact and support of an acetabular component.
- Take care to ream at the orifice of the original acetabulum with the goal of cup placement as close to an anatomic position as possible. This is especially important in cases of residual acetabular protrusion deformity due to the fracture.
- Altered cup placement of around 1 cm proximal or medial can be accepted and compensated for on the femoral side or with lateralized polyethylene cup inserts.

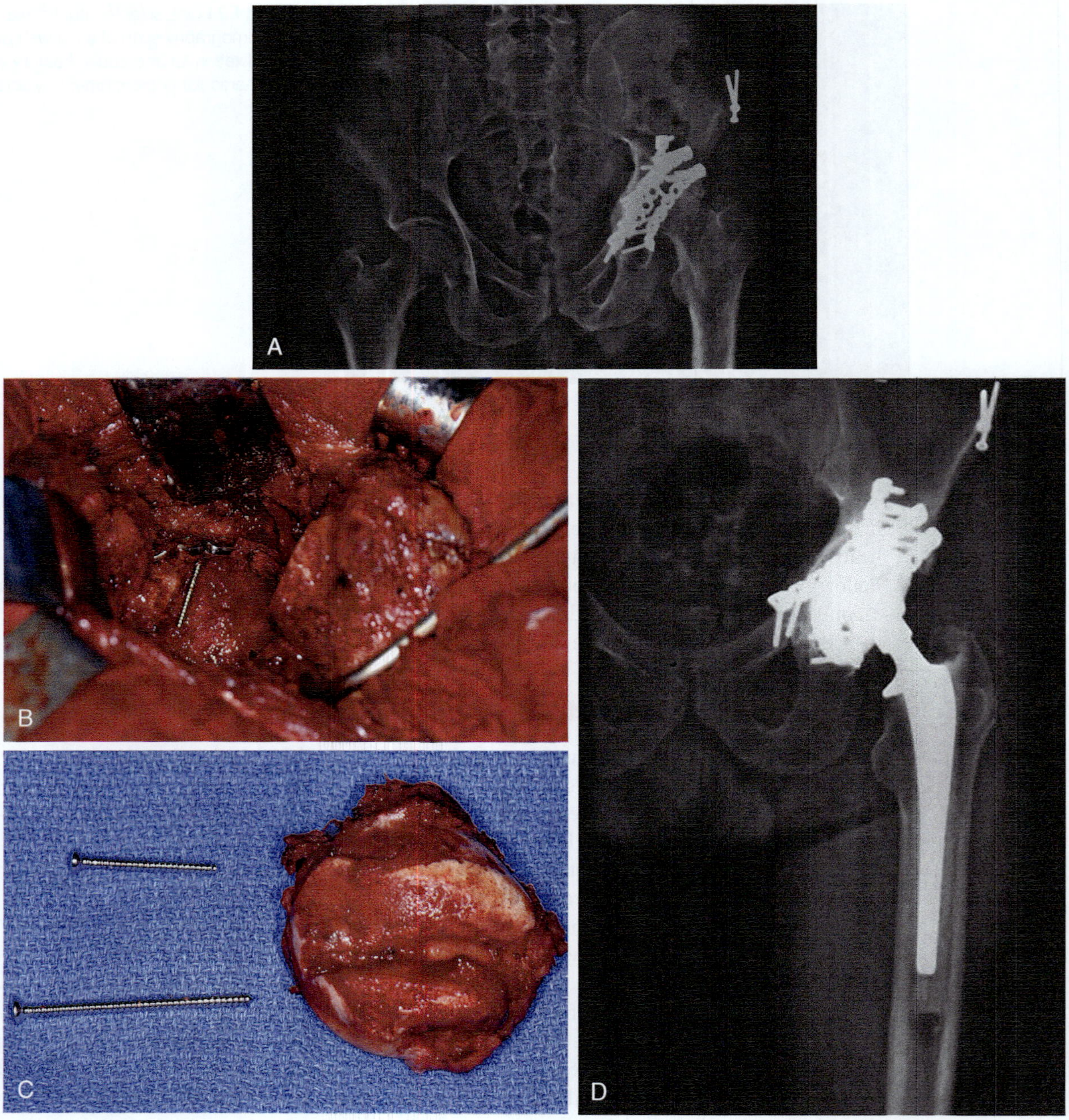

Figure 14.3 | Radiographic view of posttraumatic arthritis due to prior acetabular fracture (A) and intraoperative appearance at the time of surgery showing intra-articular hardware (B). Partial removal of the hardware using a burr along with the damaged femoral head (C) allows total hip arthroplasty to be performed without the need to remove all of the hardware about the hip (D).

- Larger deviations in cup placement from the anatomic hip center should be avoided by the use of acetabular augments or bone graft to reconstruct critical bone defects or, when this is not possible, by using special techniques or implants to compensate on the femoral side for the altered cup position.
- Excessive translation of the cup proximal or medial from the anatomic position can adversely affect hip stability, hip function, and implant survivorship.
- Establish stable cup support with as much host bone contact as possible.
- Use multiple screws to fix an uncemented porous metal cup in place as securely as possible. When bone quality is poor or there is notable bone loss, use a highly porous metal cup if possible.
- Depending on bone defects and host bone quality, typically 3 to 6 screws are used in as close to a 180° spread as possible to ensure a secure and motionless cup bone interface to facilitate bone ingrowth.
- Use an array of screws across the dome, and into the posterior column, ending at the posterior inferior rim of the cup (Figure 14.4A).

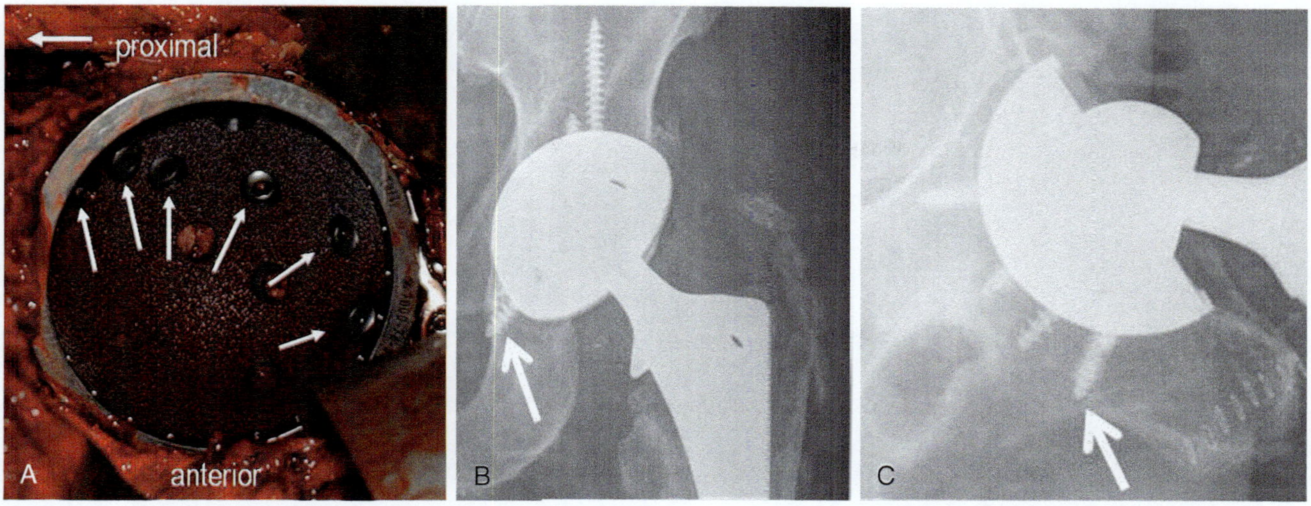

Figure 14.4 | Optimal acetabular component fixation is provided by an array of screws across the dome and down to the base of the ischium (A), with the most inferior screw shown on AP radiograph (B) and on a cross-table lateral view (C) extending out the quadrilateral surface or ilioischial line as viewed on the AP view. This provides critical zone 3 fixation and helps resist cup migration when bone support and bone quality is compromised.

- The most inferior screws extend into the base of the ischium and into the quadrilateral surface, which is visible as the ilioischial line on the AP x-ray of the hip (Figure 14.4B and C).
- When major bone defects, residual nonunion, or discontinuity precludes stable support for a hemispherical cup alone, use of large structural grafts, acetabular augments, or cup-cage constructs may be needed (see chapters on these specific techniques for reference).
- Large-diameter femoral heads (36 mm or greater) or dual mobility articulations can be used to reduce the risk of hip instability especially when there has been damage to the surrounding soft tissues or muscle innervation from the original injury or fracture treatment.
- Femoral component choice and implantation can be routine unless extra length is needed to compensate for a high or displaced hip center on the acetabular side.

Postoperative Care

- Antibiotics are continued after surgery until intraoperative cultures are reported as negative. If more than 1 of the 3 or more cultures sent at the time of surgery come back positive for the same organism, then 6 weeks of IV therapy is usually recommended followed by prolonged oral antibiotic suppression.
- Patients are mobilized with either partial weight bearing or weight bearing as tolerated on crutches or walker depending on the severity of bone defects treated and the quality of implant fixation achieved.
- Prophylaxis against heterotopic bone is routinely used in those with prior HO formation or selectively in patients at risk: those requiring extensive exposure or having other comorbidities that might increase the risk of heterotopic bone formation.
- Standard prophylaxis against heterotopic bone can be used with either a single dose of low-dose radiation with shielding of the ingrowth portions of the hip implants or with 2 to 3 weeks of oral indomethacin (or an alternative nonsteroidal anti-inflammatory drug).

Chapter 15
Hip Dysplasia

ADAM HART
DANIEL J. BERRY

Key Concepts

- Hip dysplasia entails a spectrum of deformity, which must be evaluated preoperatively and addressed at the time of surgery.
  - The acetabulum is shallow, typically deficient anteriorly and superiorly, and may have additional bone loss or erosion from a subluxated femoral head.
  - The femur often, but not always, has excessive anteversion and may also have posterior overhang of the greater trochanter, coxa valga, and a narrow canal (especially in the medial-lateral plane).
- Goals of surgery include:
  - In most cases, restore the hip's true center of rotation thereby improving the abductor lever arm and locomotive kinematics and minimizing joint reactive forces.
  - Implant an acetabular component that is supported as well as possible by host bone and that gains good long-term fixation (typically with an uncemented implant).
  - Select an appropriate femoral implant that accommodates the patient's anatomy and provides sufficient hip stability.
  - Minimize complications, chiefly overlengthening and traction injury on the sciatic nerve, loosening of the acetabular or femoral components, and nonunion of an osteotomy.
- The Crowe classification system subdivides dysplastic hips by the level of hip subluxation (Figure 15.1) and provides a practical framework by which the surgeon can systematically assess, plan, and execute the reconstruction.
  - Crowe 1 (Figure 15.2A): An uncemented acetabular component in the true acetabular region with slight medialization and a cemented or uncemented stem based on patient age, bone quality, and bone geometry.
  - Crowe 2-3 (Figure 15.2B and C): An uncemented component at or near the true acetabular region, if necessary with autograft augmentation or high hip center or component medialization. A cemented or uncemented stem based on patient age and bone geometry.
  - Crowe 4 (Figure 15.2D): An extra-small uncemented acetabular component in the true acetabular region with an uncemented stem and usually shortening subtrochanteric osteotomy (refer to Chapter 16).

Sterile Instruments and Implants

- Perioperative: Consider having intraoperative electromyography (EMG) monitoring for the sciatic nerve (if potentially lengthening more than 3 cm or 10% the length of the femur), cell saver and tranexamic acid, Foley catheterization, general anesthesia without paralysis or spinal anesthesia, and intraoperative fluoroscopy or radiography as needed.
- Implants: Uncemented acetabular components with multiple screw holes and available in small diameters (in addition to small-diameter femoral heads). Femoral components that can best

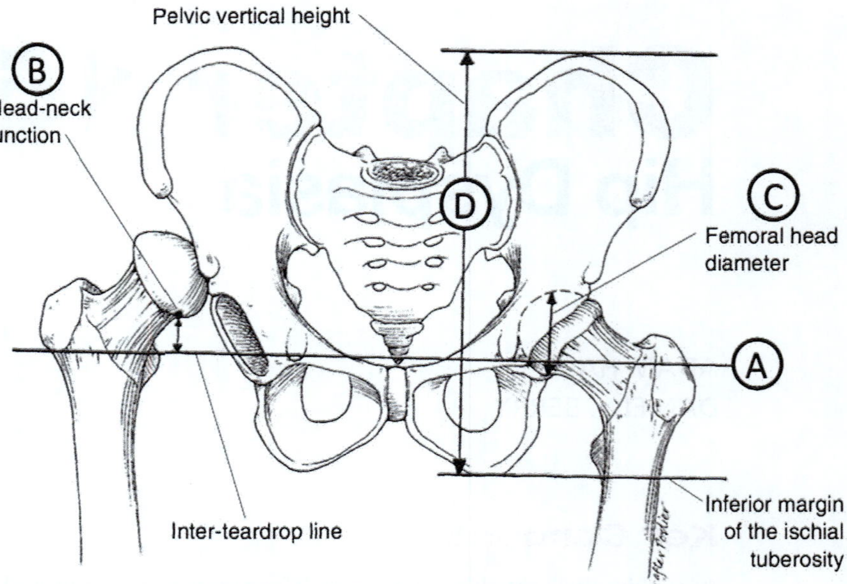

Figure 15.1 | Crowe classification: draw the inter-teardrop line (A), then take the ratio of (B/C) to determine percent dislocation: I for 0 to 50%, II for 50 to 75%, III for 75 to 100%, and IV for >100%. If the femoral heads are significantly deformed, one can use the pelvic height (D/5) to approximate (C). Used with permission of Mayo Foundation for Medical Education and Research. All rights reserved.

accommodate the patient's anatomy such as a monolithic conical or modular stem with a proximally coated triangle and distal fluted body versus a small cemented stem. Uncemented fixation is typically preferred in younger patients (Figure 15.3).
- Extras: High-speed burr with 6.5-mm round tip, 4.5-mm screws, and cables or cerclage wires.

Surgical Approaches

- Anterolateral or posterolateral based on surgeon preference.
- When femoral shortening is required, there are 2 options:
    - A transtrochanteric approach with sequential proximal femoral resection provides excellent exposure but has the disadvantage of advancing the trochanter onto a progressively narrow and tubular proximal femur. There is a high risk of trochanteric nonunion with this technique.
    - Combining an anterolateral or posterolateral approach with a subtrochanteric osteotomy (this is the authors' preferred technique and is discussed in detail in Chapter 16).

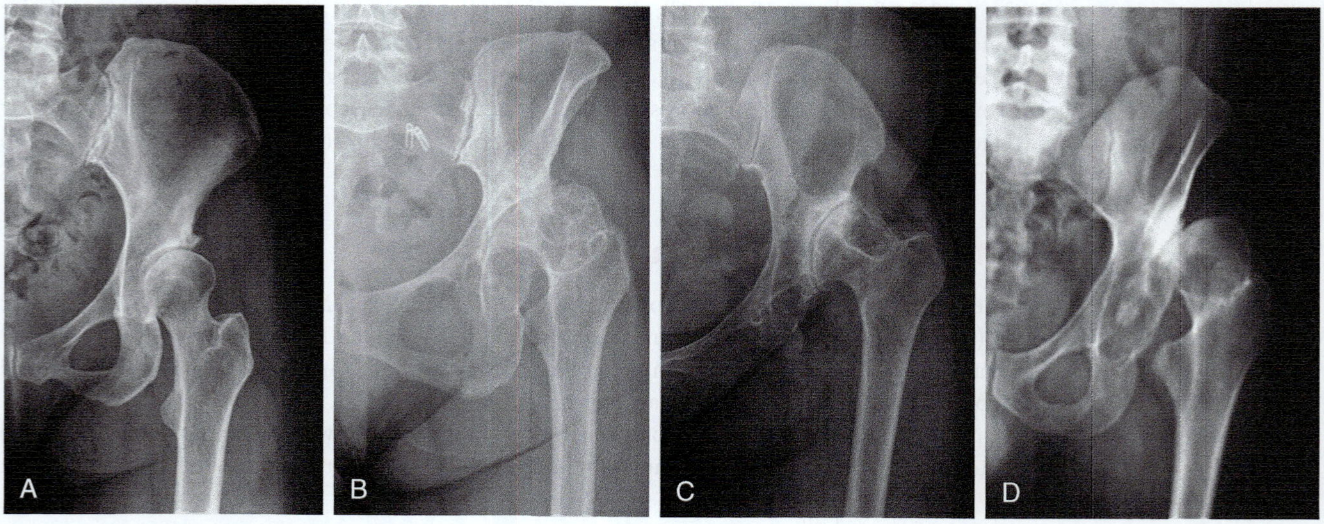

Figure 15.2 | Radiographic examples of dysplastic hips with Crowe 1 (A), 2 (B), 3 (C), and 4 (D) classification.

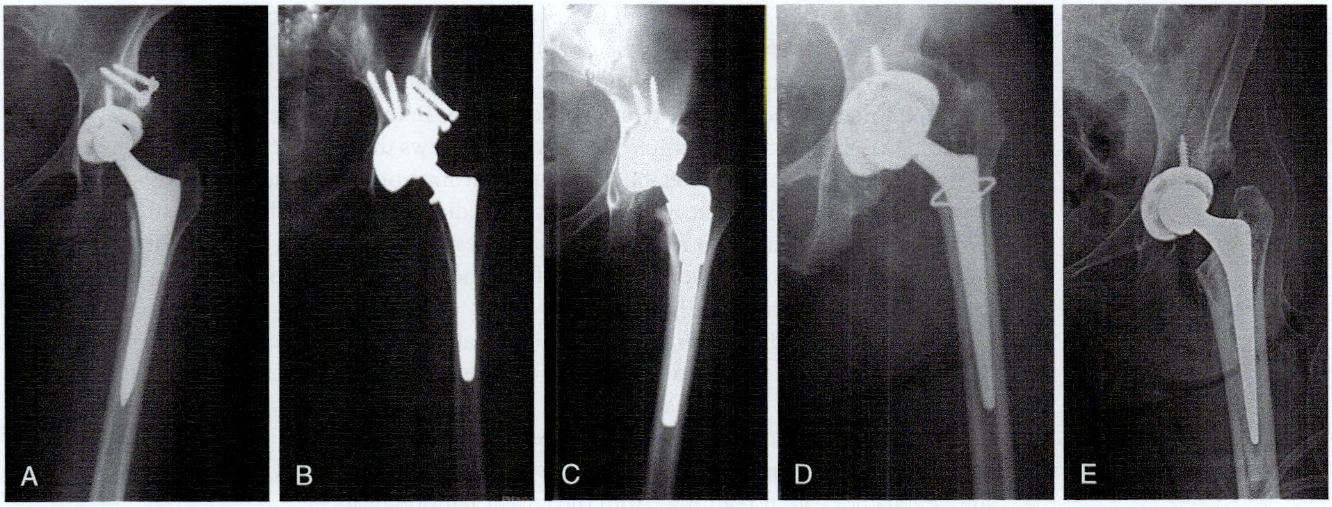

Figure 15.3 | Select the femoral component that best accommodates the patient's anatomy and bone quality. Options include proximally coated tapered (A), fully porous coated cylindrical (B), modular (C), fluted tapered (D), and cemented (E) stems.

Preoperative Planning

- Review the radiographs and template the implants to determine:
  - The amount of lengthening that would occur if the cup and stem are placed at the desired location (generally, a shortening osteotomy should be considered for anticipated lengthening greater than 3 cm).
  - Access bone defects superiorly and available bone medially to estimate the size of the acetabular component.
  - Ensure the availability of femoral components that are adequately suited for the patient's anatomy (canal diameter and proximal femoral morphology).
- Special considerations for patients with bilateral hip dysplasia:
  - Given that most patients will require a period of partial weight bearing after surgery, simultaneous bilateral hip replacements are not recommended.
  - If both sides are of similar severity, stage the procedures and start with the most symptomatic side. Any bone removed (e.g., the femoral head) from the first hip may be conserved (frozen) for the second hip.

Bone, Implant, and Soft Tissue Techniques

- Place the patient in the lateral decubitus position with solid pelvic supports (ideally radiolucent) and drape a wider-than-usual field to facilitate greater exposure demands.
- Perform the desired approach to the hip. Note that the femur may be located more proximally than usual under the fascia.
- Perform the femoral neck osteotomy, and preserve the femoral head for potential bone grafting.
- The acetabular reconstruction with an uncemented hemispherical component involves a series of steps and methods to negotiate between optimal cup placement at the true hip center, adequate fixation of the implant, and avoiding overlengthening the extremity.
  - The first and most important step is to gain adequate exposure of the acetabulum and to identify the true hip center. After exposing the anterior and posterior walls, the acetabular fovea and "teardrop" become essential internal landmarks to guide cup placement. In subluxated hips, the fovea will become more apparent after the initial reaming and should be identified using a curette between sequential reamings. Typically there is adipose tissue in the fovea.
  - Crowe 1: In these hips with mild subluxation, there is usually sufficient host bone stock to accommodate the acetabular component. Tips to optimize fixation of the cup are to (1) intentionally medialize the cup slightly to gain more rim support superiorly and circumferentially, (2) avoid overreaming the anterior column (as this is typically deficient), (3) take an intraoperative radiograph to assess the position of the acetabular trial, and (4) in most cases fix the cup with multiple screws for additional stability.

- Crowe 2-3: Subluxation of the femoral head without complete dislocation usually results in lateral acetabular bone deficiency because of (1) the underlying developmental deficiency and (2) subsequent erosion by the femoral head. These acetabuli are therefore the most challenging to reconstruct. Uncemented cups are typically used, and as in the case of revision surgery with compromised bone, fixation with multiple supplemental screws through the cup is routine.
  - In most cases, satisfactory acetabular component fixation can be achieved with slight component medialization, to but not through the medial wall. The medial wall can be identified during reaming because the medial bone becomes more cortical in nature. If there is uncertainty as to the thickness of remaining medial bone, a 2-mm drill hole can be made and bone thickness judged with a depth gauge.
  - Mild elevation (less than a centimeter) of the acetabular center of rotation also may be needed in some hips to gain adequate component coverage. The component is adequately covered if it is inherently stable in the reamed socket and does not seem at risk for lateral "spin out." A modest amount of lateral uncoverage of the cup is well tolerated in most cases, particularly if good supplemental cup fixation with screws is obtained. Small lateral defects may be filled with autogenous bone graft reamings from the cup or femoral head.
  - If adequate component coverage cannot be obtained with the combination of mild medialization and superiorization of the hip center, one of the below techniques may be considered.
  - Acetabuloplasty: intentional overreaming slightly to (but usually not through) the medial wall to medialize the socket providing increased lateral coverage of the acetabular component (Figure 15.4).

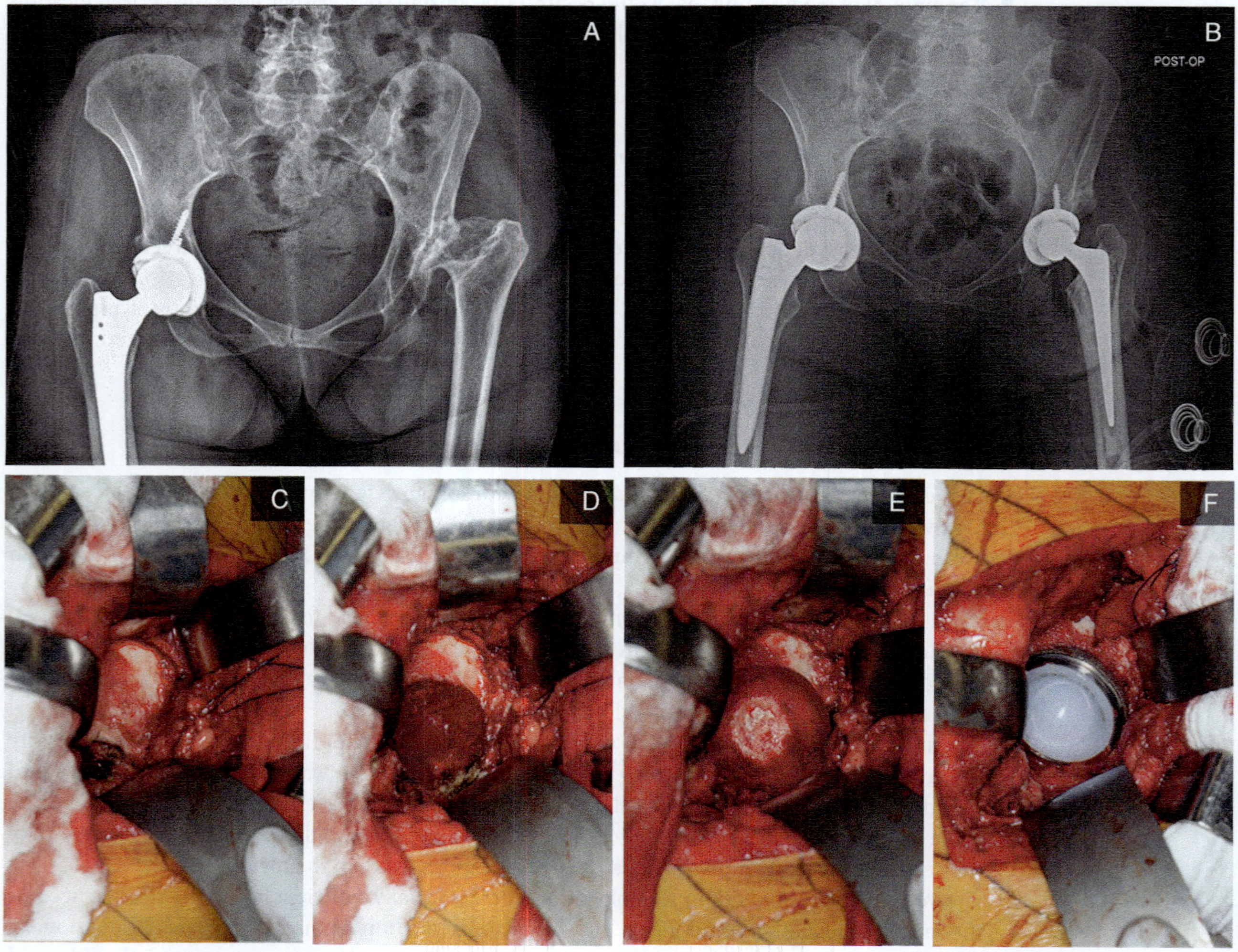

Figure 15.4 | A, Radiograph of patient with left hip dysplasia. B, Postoperative radiograph after total hip arthroplasty. The cup was medialized to the medial wall to provide sufficient cup support and lateral cup coverage. C, Intraoperative picture of dysplastic acetabulum before reaming. D, Intraoperative picture during reaming. Note the center of hip rotation is chosen to optimize cup coverage after reaming. E, Intraoperative picture showing reaming to but not through the medial wall at completion of reaming. F, Intraoperative picture after cup placement. Note the cup is well covered laterally.

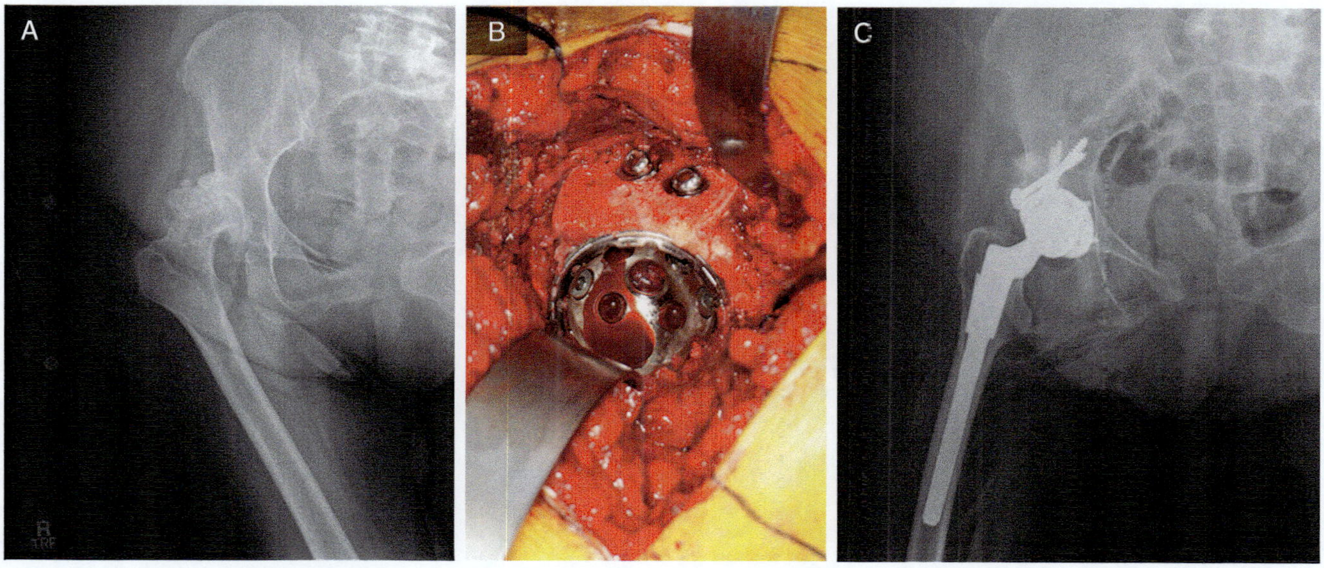

Figure 15.5 | Preoperative radiograph of a Crowe 2 hip with significant erosion of the superolateral acetabulum (A), intraoperative photograph of a superolateral autograft using the resected autogenous femoral head (B), and postoperative radiograph demonstrating restoration of the hip's true center of rotation, and well supported acetabular component with the bulk autograft and modular stem (C).

- Superolateral bulk autogenous femoral head graft: acetabular augmentation by structural grafting may be used when the cup has insufficient superolateral support (Figure 15.5). In addition to supplemental cup fixation in the short term, the graft restores bone stock in the long term. After reaming of the acetabulum, the bone is decorticated in the deficient area to a bleeding bed. A step cut is made in the neck of the resected femoral head and shaped to provide an intimate fit with the superolateral acetabulum in the area of bone deficiency (Figure 15.6A). The graft is held in place with smooth K wires or Steinman pins while it is being fixed with screws (Figure 15.6B). The graft is fixed onto the acetabular rim with 2 to 3 partially threaded 4.0- or 6.5-mm (depending on graft size) cancellous screws with washers (Figure 15.6C). Make sure to place the screws sufficiently proximally so they will not interfere with the final reaming process. A burr is then used to fashion the approximate contour of the acetabulum followed by reapplication of the final reamer and placement of the definitive component (Figure 15.6D). Figure 15.7 demonstrates the steps of the procedure.
- High hip center: Placing the acetabular component superior to its true anatomic location improves coverage with native bone superiorly and may also shorten the extremity (therefore potentially obviating the need for a shortening osteotomy). Unfortunately, this technique

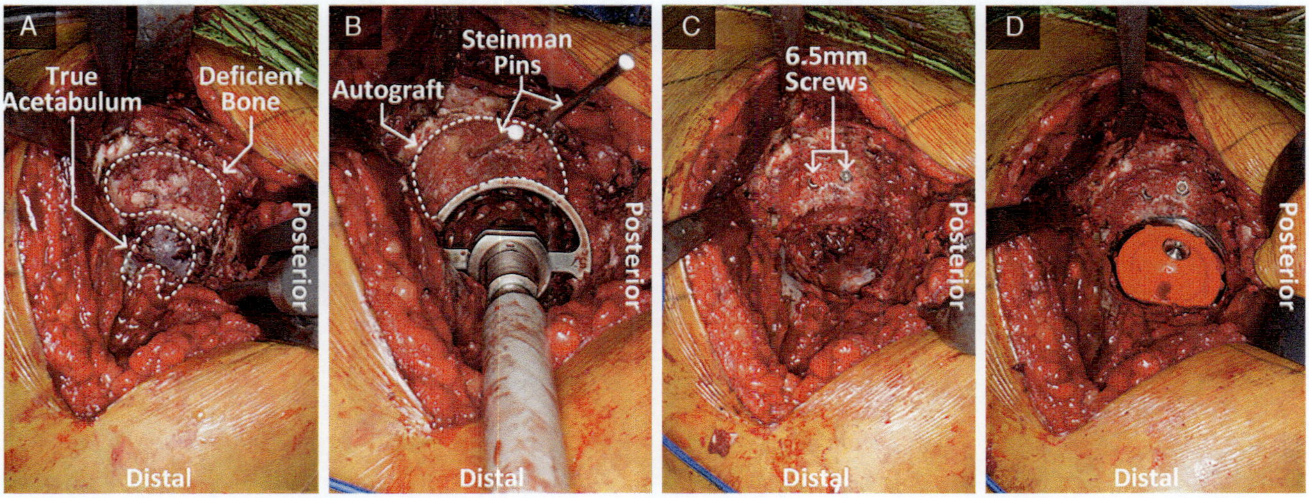

Figure 15.6 | Intraoperative photographs demonstrating exposure of the true acetabulum and deficient superolateral rim (A), placement of the femoral head autograft secured with two Steinman pins (B), replacement of the pins with 6.5-mm partially threaded cancellous screws (C), and final cup placement (D).

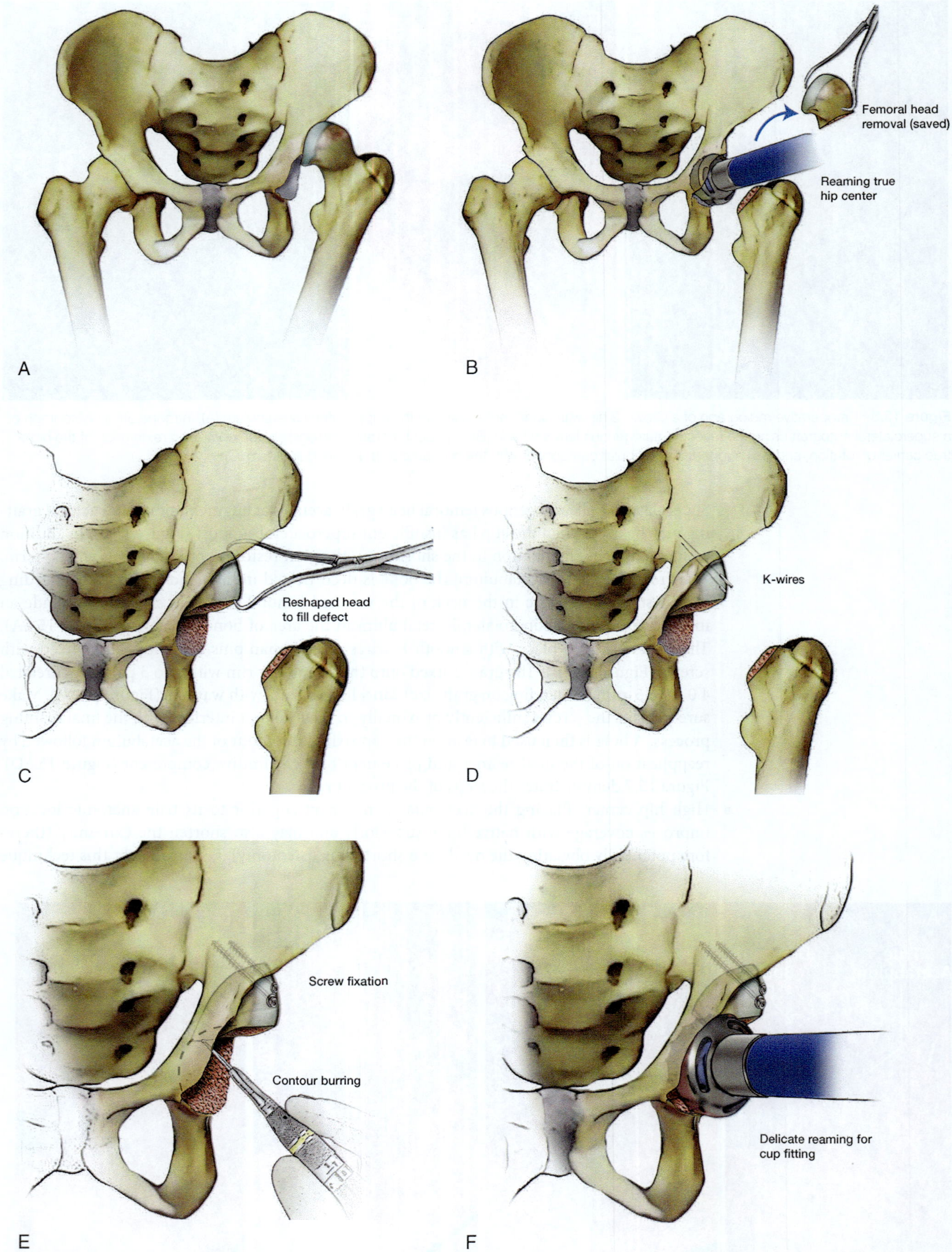

Figure 15.7 | Technique of autogenous femoral head bone grafting of the acetabulum in dysplastic hip. A, Depiction of Crowe 3 hip. B, Acetabular preparation at desired hip center of rotation. C, The autogenous femoral head is contoured to fit into the lateral acetabular bone defect. D, The femoral head is provisionally fixed with smooth pins. E, The graft is definitively fixed with 2 screws with washers. Partially threaded cancellous screws are preferred. The fixed graft is contoured with a burr. F, The fixed graft is reamed again gently with the last several reamers until the graft contour matches the previously reamed cup contour.

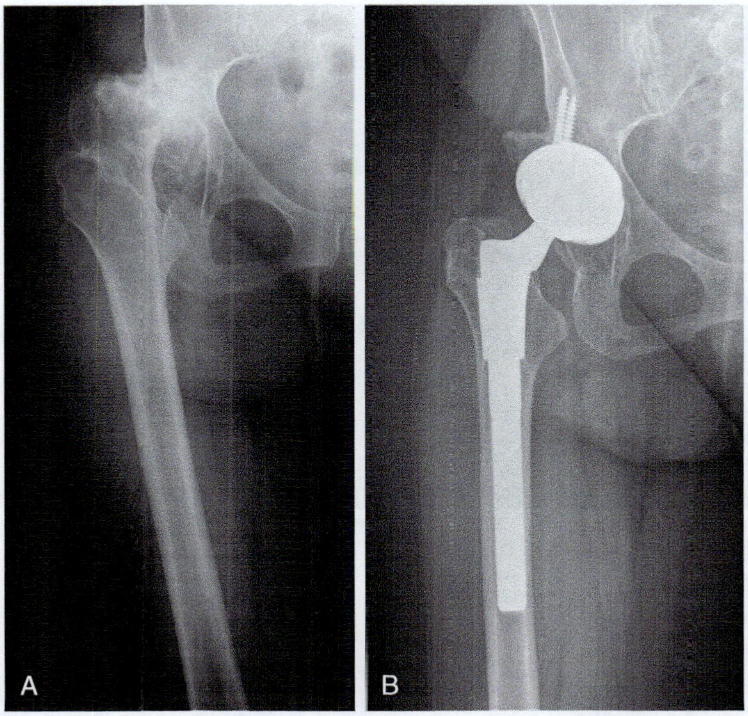

Figure 15.8 | A, Radiograph of a patient with Crowe 3 level hip dysplasia. B, Radiograph after placement of uncemented cup at moderately elevated hip center.

compromises hip biomechanics and may result in impingement with the ischial tuberosity or anterior inferior iliac spine promoting hip instability. The authors therefore recommend limited and judicious use of this technique (Figures 15.8A,B and 15.9A-D).

- Crowe 4: In most cases of high dislocation, the acetabulum can be reconstructed with an extra-small acetabular component at the anatomic hip center without bone grafting (discussed in detail in Chapter 16).

- With the acetabulum prepared, the patient's new hip center is established, which will guide the subsequent femoral reconstruction. The following tips are recommended during femoral preparation:
  - The surgeon should remain cognizant of tension placed on the sciatic nerve, which is commensurate to the amount of lengthening performed. As permitted, the knee should be kept bent and the hip semi-extended. The nerve often can be palpated under the gluteal sling and intraoperative EMG may warn of undue traction.
  - Although a subtrochanteric shortening osteotomy (as described in Chapter 16) is sometimes unavoidable to prevent overlengthening and associated sciatic nerve injury, the added time and complexity as well as the potential for fracture and nonunion pose additional risks with an osteotomy. In some cases, "cheating" the femoral component distally by using a small-diameter stem and a low neck cut may provide sufficient shortening to obviate an osteotomy.
  - Femoral component choice in dysplastic patients is important because the femoral anatomy typically deviates from the norm. Many (but not all) dysplastic patients have extra femoral anteversion. They may also have other abnormalities of metaphyseal anatomy, mismatch in size between the metaphysis and diaphysis, and very small bone and/or small diaphyses. Because most patients are young, when possible, uncemented fixation is preferred by most North American surgeons.
  - Two types of uncemented implants are especially helpful to accommodate the anatomic challenges: modular stems with a modular proximal triangle to fit the metaphysis and fluted cylindrical diaphyseal section that fits the metaphysis and diaphysis independently (see Chapter 9) (Figure 15.10) and short fluted tapered monoblock conical stems (see Chapter 10). The modular stem allows the fit of the porous triangular sleeve in the metaphysis to be established and the stem to be placed in optimal anteversion independent of the sleeve position, which allows management of most anteversion abnormalities and many metaphyseal deformities. Short conical stems

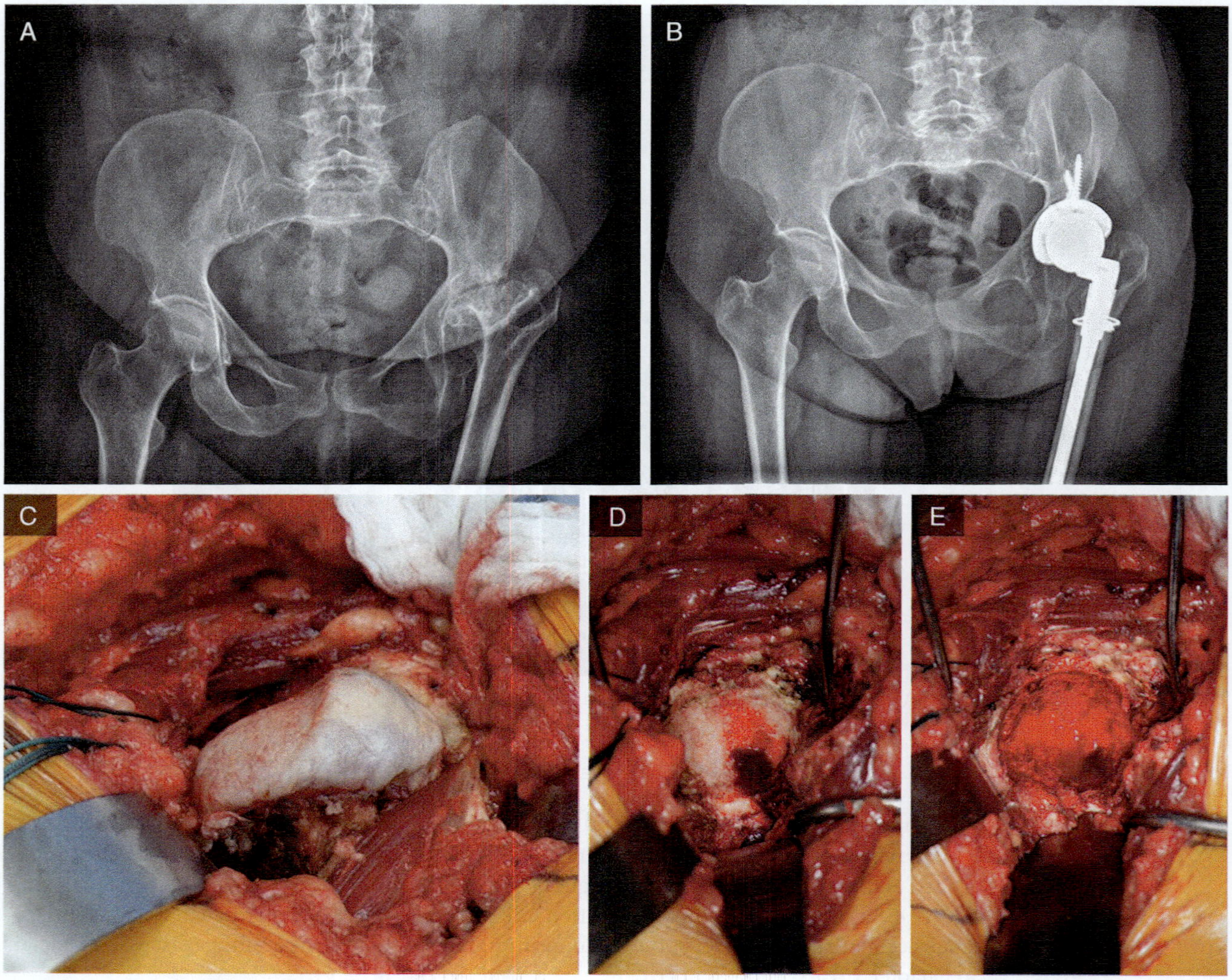

Figure 15.9 | Preoperative (A) and postoperative (B) radiographs of a Crowe 3 hip with significant erosion of the superolateral acetabulum, intraoperative photographs of the dislocated deformed femoral head (C), exposure of the acetabulum (D), and preparation for the acetabular component with a high hip center (E).

allow fixation in the diaphysis and placement of the stem in optimal anteversion independent of host metaphyseal shape and anteversion. Such stems are particularly valuable when metaphyseal deformity is severe (Figure 15.11).

- Using the stem of choice (see techniques in Chapters 9 and 10), prepare the proximal femur. With trials in place, obtain a radiograph and assess the limb lengths, test for impingement, and ensure sufficient stability. Generally, the leg should be lengthened the minimum amount required to reestablish reasonable function and hip stability.

- Before final implant placement, carefully assess hip stability. Be conscious that extra-articular impingement due to abnormal pelvic and femoral anatomy is possible and should be mitigated if possible. Also be conscious that with smaller-diameter cups, smaller-diameter femoral heads may have been used, and hip instability is a greater risk.
- Perform standard wound closure in layers, place a drain (optional), and position the knee in flexion (with a pillow) to help alleviate tension on the sciatic nerve (can be left in place for 1-2 days).

Postoperative Care

- Depending on the bone quality, amount of host bone support for components, and need for bone grafting, we typically restrict patients to toe-touch or partial weight bearing for 8 weeks.
- Standard hip dislocation precautions (per approach and surgeon's preference).

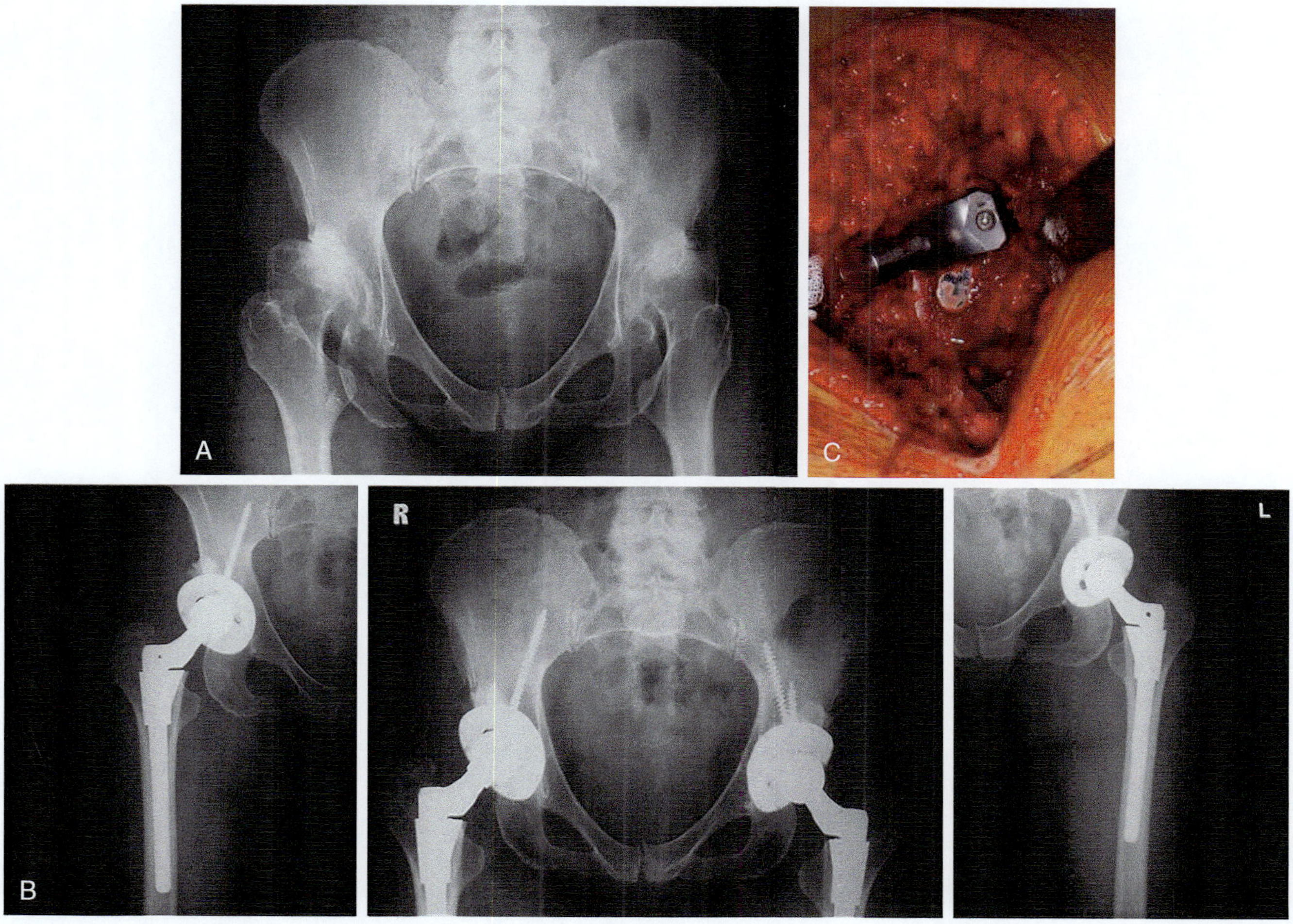

Figure 15.10 | A, Radiograph of patient with hip dysplasia. B, Postoperative radiograph after treatment with modular stems that allows correction of anteversion and management of metaphyseal diaphyseal mismatch. C, Intraoperative photo of a patient with approximately 80° of femoral anteversion. The modular implant sleeve is placed to fit the metaphysis, and the stem is placed in approximately 15° of anteversion.

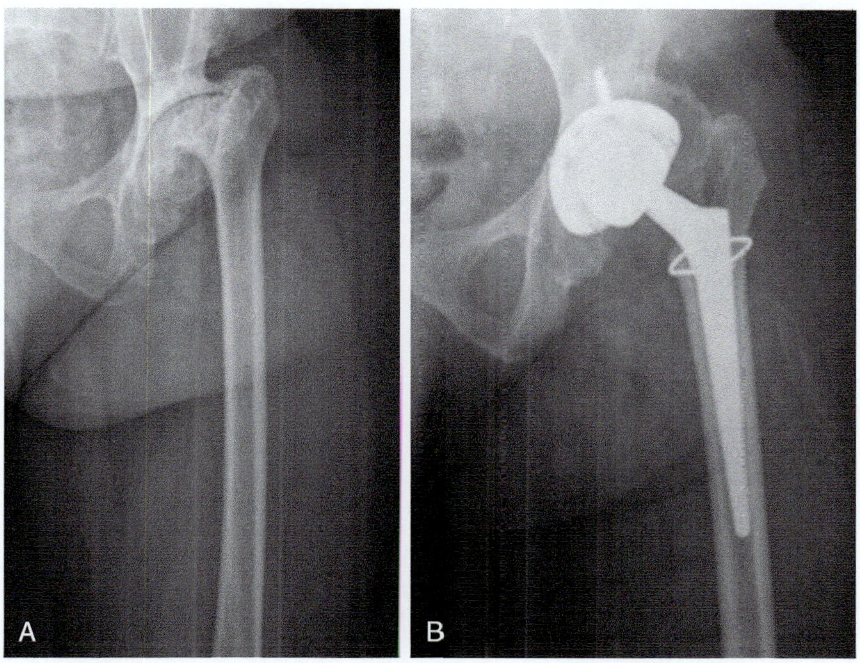

Figure 15.11 | A, Radiograph of a patient with hip dysplasia. B, Postoperative radiograph after treatment with uncemented fluted tapered cone-shaped stem that allows correction of anteversion and fixation in the diaphysis.

Chapter 16
High Hip Dysplasia

DANIEL J. BERRY

Key Concepts

- In high hip dislocation the femoral head is in a false acetabulum superior to the true acetabulum (Figure 16.1A).
- The goal is to place the acetabular component in the true acetabulum; this is where the best acetabular bone is, and it optimizes hip biomechanics. The true acetabulum is small, so small components are needed, including small-diameter femoral head sizes.
- Once the acetabular component is placed in the true acetabulum, reduction of the hip is difficult, and the sciatic nerve is at risk for stretch injury, unless further measures are taken.
- The most common modern method of achieving safe reduction is shortening subtrochanteric osteotomy (Figure 16.1B and C). Other methods including (1) greater trochanteric osteotomy along with proximal femoral shortening and (2) prolonged skeletal traction without shortening have been described but have drawbacks and are less commonly used today.
- Different subtrochanteric osteotomy configurations have been described, but a transverse osteotomy is the simplest, allows both shortening and rotational correction, and can be fixed rigidly by the implant if implants that provide rotational fixation of the proximal and distal fragments of bone are chosen (Figure 16.2).
- The femoral bone typically has a small diameter; therefore, small-diameter implants need to be available (see Figure 16.1).
- Most patients are young, so uncemented implants are preferred, particularly because they work well in conjunction with subtrochanteric osteotomy.

Sterile Instruments and Implants

- Routine hip retractors
- Narrow (1-cm) ribbon retractors
- Large pointed bone reduction forceps
- Serrated bone reduction forceps
- Large and small oscillating saws
- Power burr
- Cerclage cables
- Uncemented acetabular component components (with instrumentation): include very-small-diameter cups down to 40 mm or below.
- Uncemented femoral components (and instrumentation) that have a proximal triangle for fixation of the proximal fragment and also have flutes, sharp corners, or extensive porous coating to provide firm rotational control of the distal fragment.

Positioning

- Lateral decubitus position.
- Drape to allow access to proximal pelvis and entire femur.
- If desired affix sciatic nerve monitoring equipment to limb before draping.

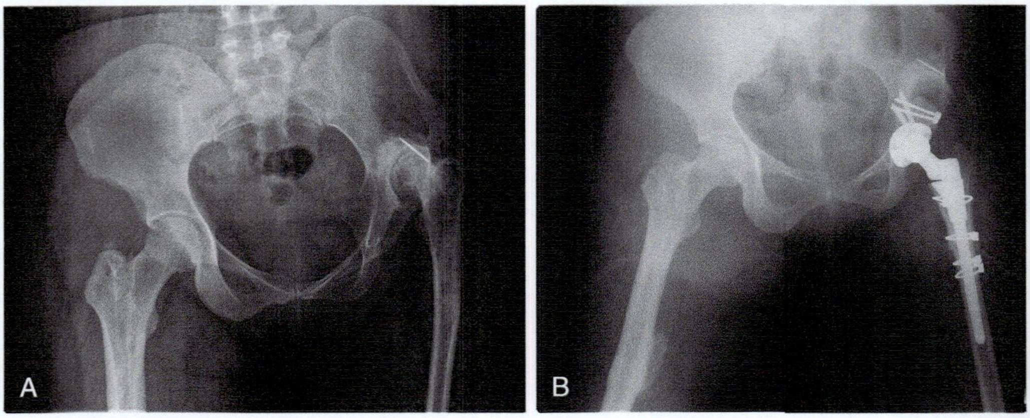
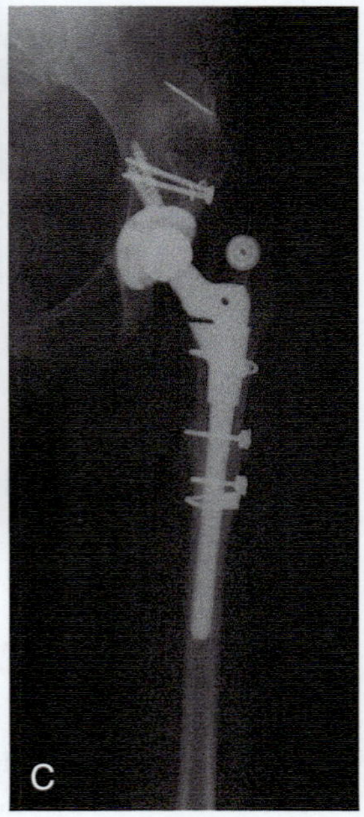

Figure 16.1 I A, Radiograph of patient with high hip dislocation. Note the characteristic findings of high hip center in false acetabulum, small but preserved true acetabulum, and small femoral bone diameter. B, Postoperative radiograph after total hip arthroplasty with concomitant shortening subtrochanteric femoral osteotomy. C, Five years postoperatively after osteotomy healing.

Surgical Approaches

- Posterior approach to the hip is preferred (the abductor attachments and vascular supply to the proximal femoral fragment is left undisturbed). Anterolateral approaches also are acceptable.
- Femur at level of the osteotomy will be exposed by elevating a small section of vastus lateralis from femur.

Preoperative Planning

- Know patient's preoperative leg length discrepancy.
- Template cup size and position.
- Template femoral component size.

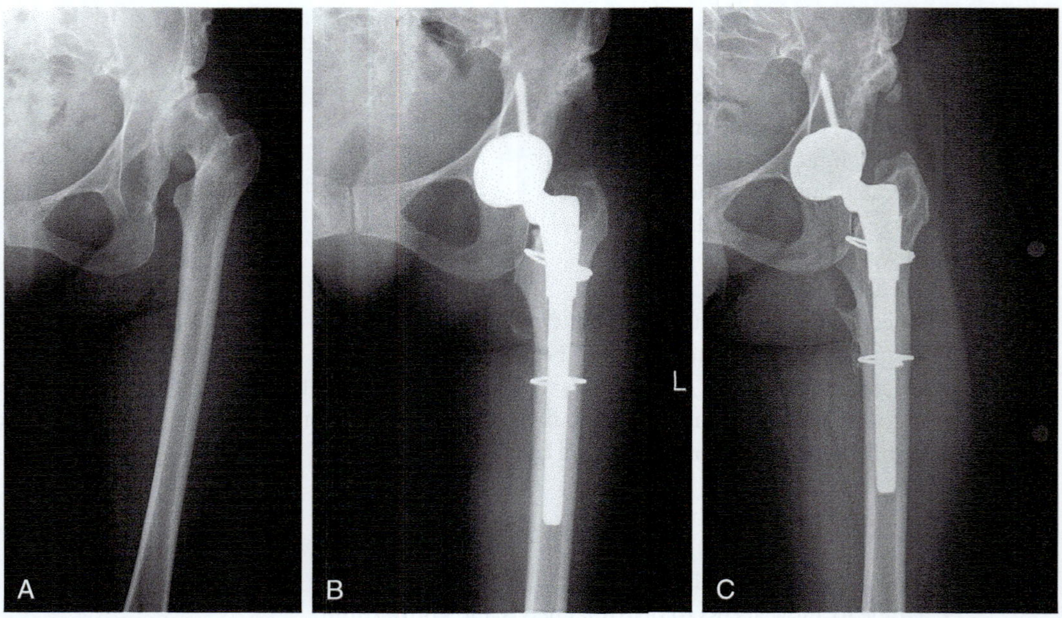

Figure 16.2 I A, Radiograph of patient with high hip dislocation. B, Radiograph immediately after total hip arthroplasty with shortening subtrochanteric osteotomy. C, Radiograph after osteotomy healing.

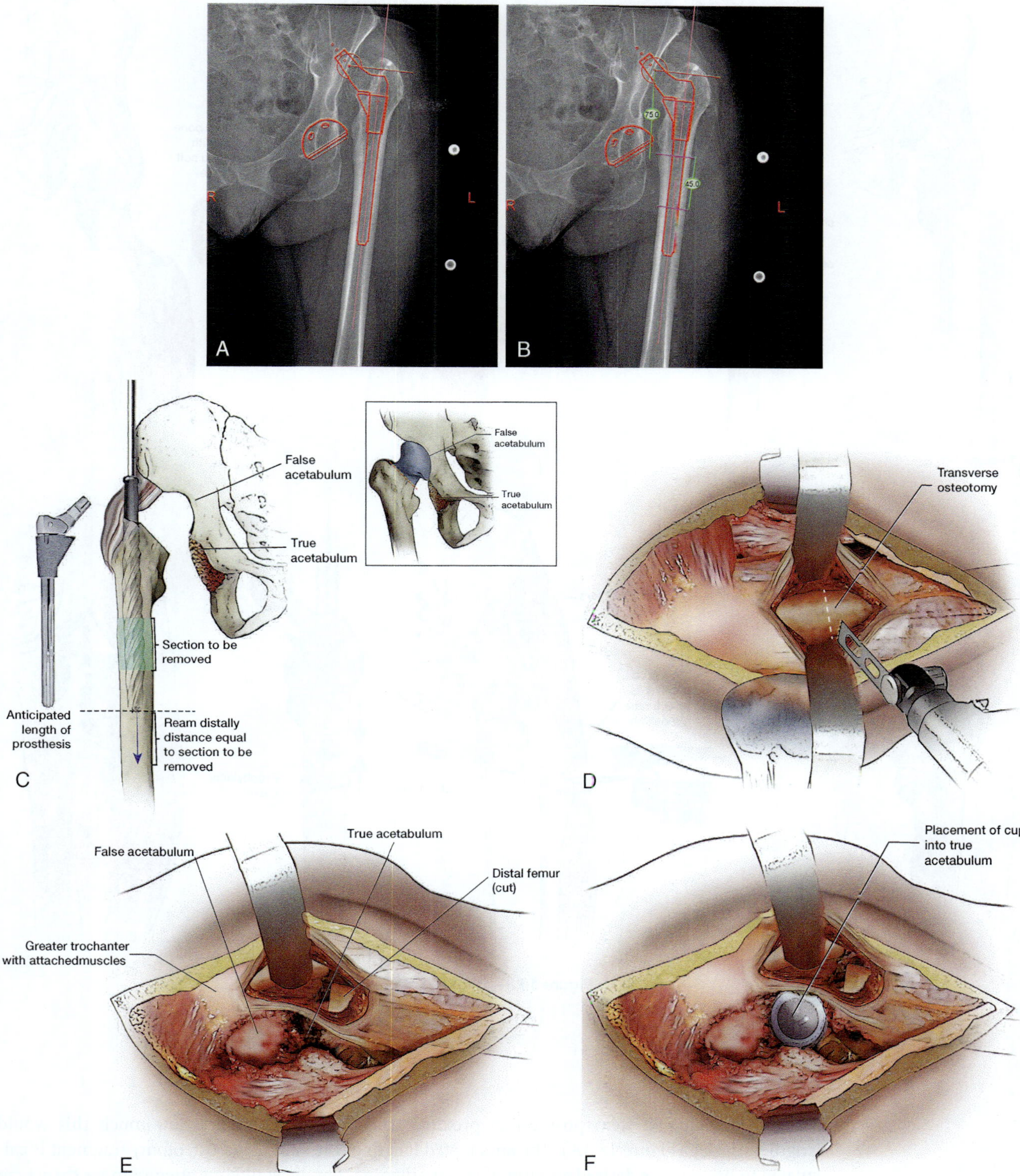

Figure 16.3 | A, Templating showing the amount of leg lengthening that would occur without femoral shortening. The templating allows calculation of the desired amount of shortening and also of the location of the osteotomy (below the flare of the proximal prosthesis but allowing for sufficient distal fixation). B, Templating allows calculation of the desired level of the proximal osteotomy. It should be below the proximal flare of the prosthesis, but allow for sufficient distal fixation of the osteotomy by the implant. C, After exposure of the hip and false acetabulum, and femoral neck osteotomy, ream and proximally prepare the proximal femur. D, Perform the transverse osteotomy at the preplanned level. E, Translate the femur anteriorly to expose the true acetabulum. F, Insert the cup into the true acetabulum. G, Perform trial reduction with the trial only in the proximal fragment. H, Traction on the limb provides estimate of the amount of subtrochanteric shortening required and should be correlated with the preoperative plan. I, The distal osteotomy is performed. J, The subtracted osteotomy fragment is kept vascular and split longitudinally with a saw. K, Trial reduction of hip and osteotomy. L, The osteotomy is trimmed as needed to perfect bone apposition. M, Placement of the real implants. N, Use of vascular strut to provide extra fixation and healing potential.

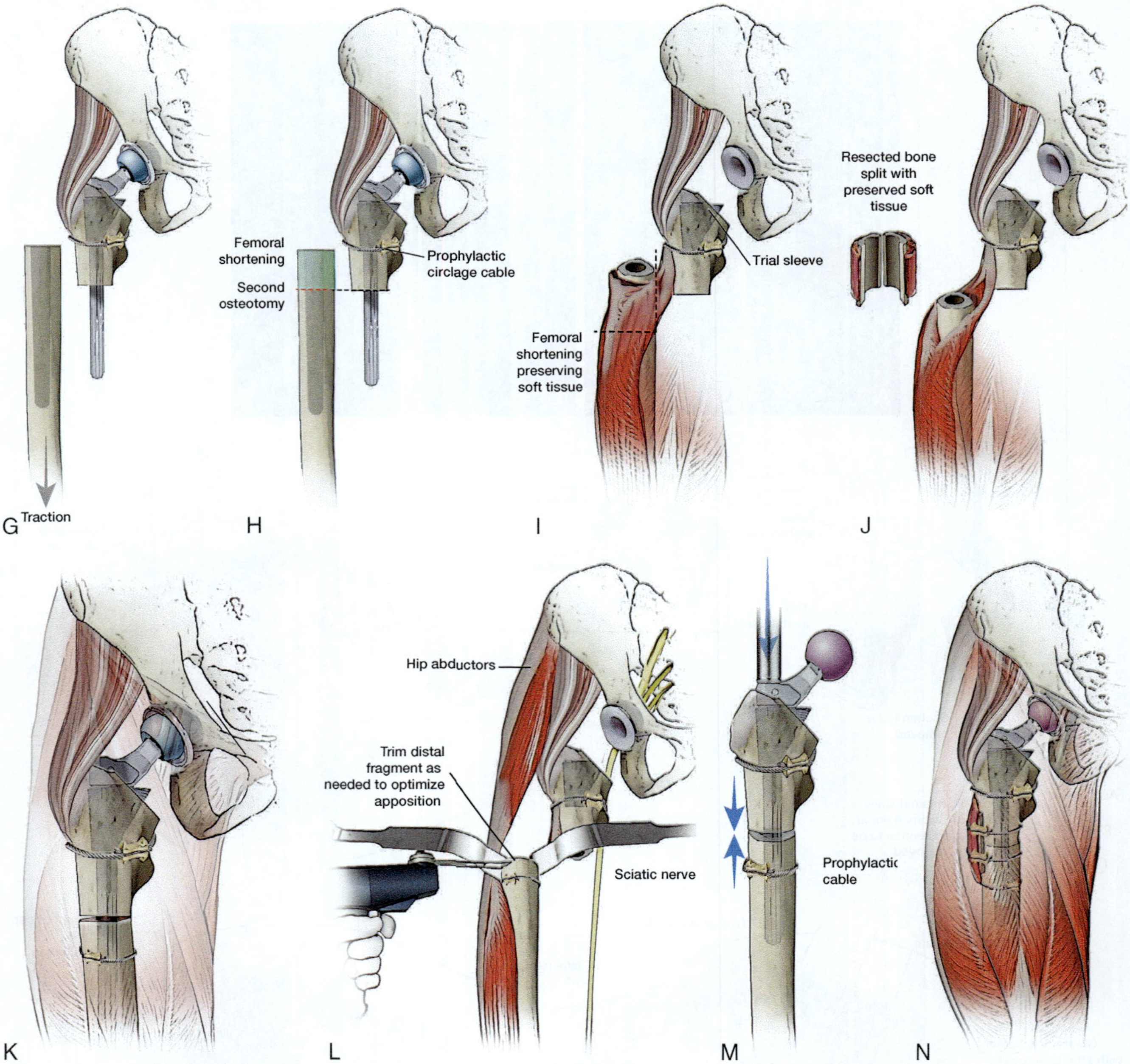

Figure 16.3—Cont'd

- Template anticipated stem position in proximal fragment and measure how much this would lengthen the leg (Figure 16.3A). The anticipated length of the subtracted osteotomy fragment is calculated to provide the desired amount of leg lengthening. Rarely would one attempt more than 4 cm of lengthening. The typical length of the subtraction osteotomy (the amount of femoral shortening) usually is about 4 cm.
- Measure the distance from the tip of the trochanter to planned osteotomy level. The osteotomy should be below the level of the triangular flare of the proximal implant, yet proximal enough to allow good fixation of the distal fragment by the implant (Figure 16.3B).

Bone/Implant/Soft Tissue Techniques

- Perform the desired approach to the hip joint (the author prefers a posterior approach in these cases).
- Perform the femoral neck osteotomy.

- Perform preliminary reaming of the femur with implant-specific instrumentation (Figure 16.3C). If there is notable proximal femoral deformity, for example, from a previous osteotomy, then this step cannot be performed until after the subtrochanteric osteotomy. However, when possible, it is easier to perform initial femoral preparation, particularly of the proximal bone, before the osteotomy. Often it is best to wait on final reaming of the distal bone until after the osteotomy because more precise sizing to fit the femoral canal can be chosen under direct vision.
- Place a prophylactic cerclage cable around the proximal femur just above the lesser trochanter. This helps prevent a longitudinal fracture of the proximal fragment, which is difficult to fix.
- Measure the distance from the greater trochanter tip to planned proximal osteotomy level.
- Expose femur at the level of planned proximal osteotomy by splitting the posterior aspect of vastus lateralis. Avoid devascularizing the bone with excessive muscle stripping.
- Mark starting rotation of the limb with 2 longitudinal parallel cautery marks that will cross the osteotomy. One mark may not guarantee rotational alignment.
- Place ribbon retractors around the femur at the planned osteotomy level.
- Perform a transverse osteotomy with a small oscillating saw taking care not to burn the bone (irrigate during osteotomy) (Figure 16.3D).
- The proximal fragment may now be translated anteriorly to expose the true host acetabulum (Figure 16.3E). To translate the fragment anteriorly, some soft tissue, including the gluteus maximus tendon, typically needs to be released from the posterior aspect of the proximal fragment. The true acetabulum will look small and often has bone partially overgrowing the socket. Follow the internal dimensions of the hip capsule, which is often like a tunnel, down from the pseudoacetabulum to the real acetabulum (Figure 16.4). Finding the inferior aspect of the fovea also helps with orientation. If you are not certain about the anatomy, obtain an intraoperative radiograph to confirm before initiating reaming.
- Prepare the acetabulum for an uncemented hemispherical component. The dimensions will be very small, and sometimes opening the socket with a power burr is helpful. Ream to the floor of the fovea or slightly deeper if needed. Avoid reaming through the medial wall. Thickness of the remaining medial wall can be checked if needed with a small-diameter drill and depth gauge. Typically, the best bone is in the posterior column and biasing reaming into the posterior column can provide improved cup coverage and also protect the anterior wall. The bone quality often is poor, and reaming the bone in "reverse" for the last few reamers can compact the bone and increase density while still creating the proper dimensions.
- Trial and insert the final cup (Figure 16.3F). Fix cup with screws in most cases. Small cups have few screw hole options, so orient screw holes optimally before insertion. Place trial acetabular liner.

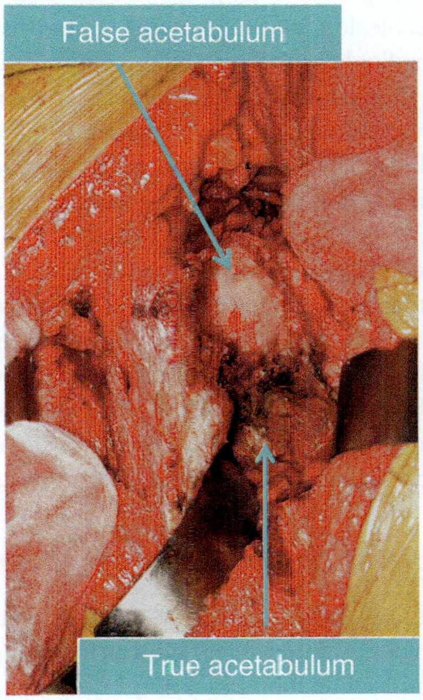

Figure 16.4 | Intraoperative picture showing false acetabulum and false acetabulum in patient with high hip dislocation.

- Next, place a trial stem into only the proximal fragment of femoral bone and attempt reduction of the hip (Figure 16.3G). If this is not possible, then shorten the neck cut and reprepare the proximal fragment as necessary. Usually the abductors will be somewhat tight. Often reduction is aided by removing scar or tight capsule from beneath the abductors. If necessary, the psoas tendon can be released from its insertion at the lesser trochanter.
- Once the proximal fragment is reduced put traction on the limb and determine the amount of overlap between distal and proximal fragments (Figure 16.3H). This provides a general estimate of how much distal bone will need to be resected to allow hip reduction once the osteotomy is closed. Avoid initial overresection.
- Based on the estimate described earlier and on preoperative planning, determine the level of the inferior transverse femoral osteotomy and expose lateral femur at that level. Carry the 2 parallel longitudinal marks to just below the level of the planned osteotomy; this helps estimate any rotational corrections or changes.
- Perform the distal transverse osteotomy with a small oscillating saw being careful to avoid burning the bone (Figure 16.3I).
- Split the subtraction osteotomy longitudinally in the mid-coronal plane creating an anterior and posterior fragment with muscle and vascular supply intact (Figure 16.3J). These fragments can later be used as vascularized cortical strut grafts to add extra rotational stability and biologic healing potential to the osteotomy site.
- Under direct vision complete preparation of the distal fragment. A tight fit of the implant in the distal fragment is necessary to provide excellent rotational stability of the transverse osteotomy, which is needed for healing.
- Place the trial implant through the proximal and distal fragments of the femur and reduce the osteotomy (Figure 16.3K). Rotational control of the proximal fragment at this stage can be challenging but is important. Pointed or serrated bone reduction clamps are useful for this purpose. If desired, rotation of the proximal fragment can be changed from the previous rotation to correct anteversion of the proximal fragment and to minimize posterior impingement of the greater trochanter against the pelvis.
- Determine if the hip can be reduced, and test hip stability. If the hip cannot be reduced, shorten the distal fragment sequentially as needed with "salami" slices. Make sure the sciatic nerve is not excessively taut by palpation and/or by nerve monitoring; if it is too taut, further shorten the distal fragment as noted earlier.
- Once length and rotation are optimized, carefully evaluate the osteotomy site and trim as needed to optimize bone apposition—excellent bone apposition is needed for prompt osteotomy healing (Figure 16.3L).
- Place a prophylactic cable around the distal femoral fragment just below the osteotomy. Without such a cable, longitudinal fractures of the distal fragment are common.
- Place the final desired acetabular component liner.
- Impact the real uncemented femoral component into place (Figure 16.3M). As this is being done, hold the proximal and distal fragments in the chosen and ideal rotational alignment. Axial pressure on the knee often is needed to prevent distraction at the osteotomy site.
- Perform a trial reduction, and ensure hip stability is good. Place the real femoral head and reduce the hip.
- If desired, fix one or both of the subtraction osteotomy fragments around the transverse osteotomy as vascularized strut grafts using cables or cerclage wires (Figure 16.3N). Pack the area around the osteotomy with host cancellous bone from the acetabular reamings or host femoral head.
- Close the capsule of the hip joint. Often it is redundant and some needs to be excised.
- Close the vastus lateralis and then close the wound in layers.
- Send the patient to the recovery room with a pillow to flex the knee and relax the sciatic nerve. The pillow can be kept in place for a day or two after the operation if desired.

Postoperative Management

- Patients are typically made toe-touch weight bearing for 8 weeks, then partial weight bearing for 4 more weeks or until radiographic osteotomy healing is visible.
- A hip guide abduction brace may be used for 8 weeks after surgery to protect the hip if desired.

Chapter 17
Acetabular Protrusio

MATTHEW P. ABDEL

Key Concepts

- Acetabular protrusio is an intrapelvic displacement of *both* the acetabular fossa and femoral head so that the femoral head projects medial to the ilioischial line (i.e., Kohler line) (Figure 17.1A-C).
- In contrast, in coxa profunda, only the acetabular fossa is medial to the ilioischial line (and often considered a "deep acetabular socket").
- The etiology of acetabular protrusio can be primary (e.g., osteoarthritis in middle-aged women) or secondary in nature (e.g., Paget disease, psoriatic arthritis, rheumatoid arthritis, osteogenesis imperfecta, trauma, ankylosing spondylitis).
- Good exposure is key to completing an optimal total hip arthroplasty (THA) in such patients, with many THAs requiring an in situ femoral neck cut for safe exposure.
- The patient's femoral head should be kept and used for autogenous acetabular bone graft.
- The patient's acetabulum should be sequentially reamed at the introitus, gradually increasing the reamer diameter until there is a rim fit with punctate bleeding bone.
- The urge to medialize the acetabular reamer, as during routine primary THAs, should be strongly resisted.
- Cancellous autogenous bone graft obtained from the patient's femoral head should then be reverse reamed in the acetabulum to fill the defect between the medial wall and trial acetabular component at the introitus of the acetabular fossa.
- One may freshen the unreamed surfaces of the sclerotic medial wall with a small reamer or a burr or use a 3.5-mm drill to create punctate bleeding. Avoid weakening the already thin medial wall.
- Intraoperative imaging is helpful with a trial acetabular component in place to determine restoration of the hip center of rotation, as well as acetabular component inclination and version.

Sterile Instruments and Implants

Instruments

- Routine hip retractors
- Single-sided reciprocating saw for an in situ femoral neck cut
- Cork screw for femoral head removal
- Small-diameter acetabular reamers to ream the autogenous femoral head and acetabular fossa
- Intraoperative imaging capability
- 3.5-mm drill bit or power burr to freshen floor of acetabulum before grafting

Implants

- Autogenous femoral head
- Allograft bone chips (rare)
- Metal acetabular augments (rare)
- Appropriately sized acetabular components with supplemental screws
- Appropriate femoral components, polyethylene inserts, and femoral heads at the surgeon's discretion

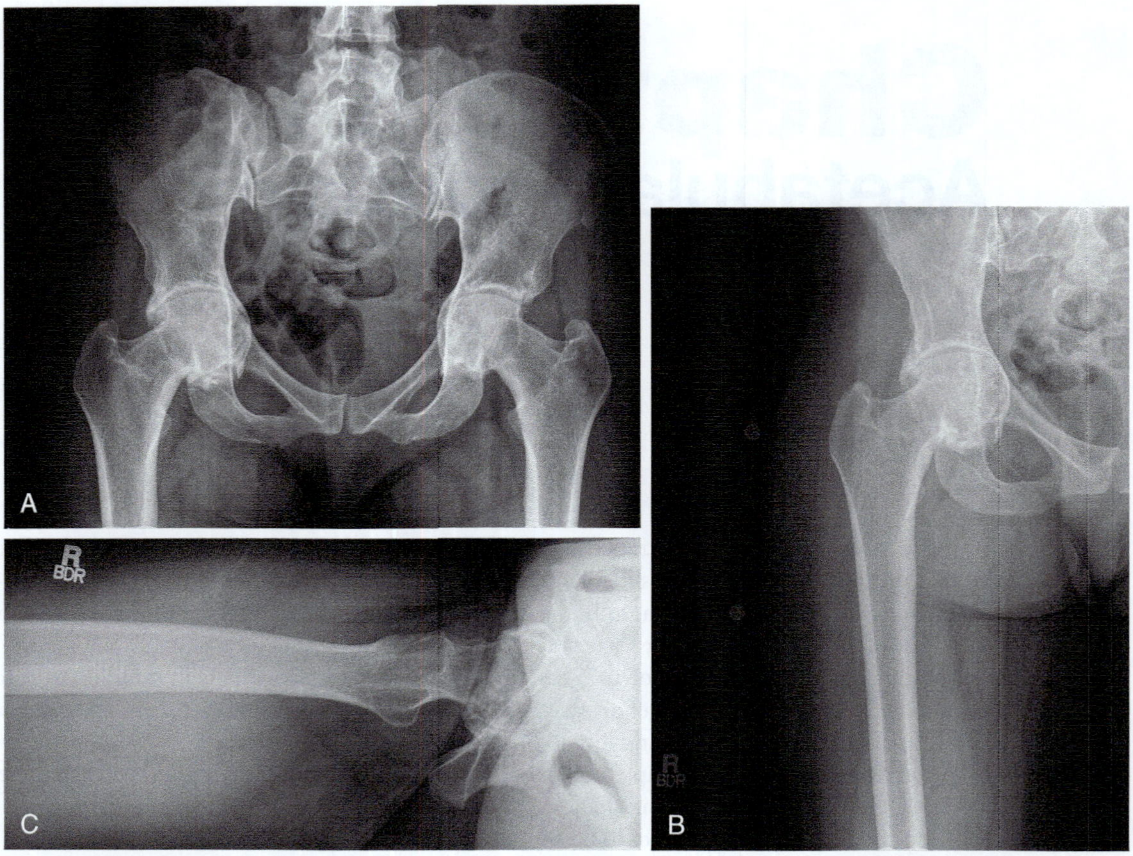

Figure 17.1 | Anteroposterior pelvis (A), anteroposterior hip (B), and cross-table lateral (C) radiographs demonstrating primary acetabular protrusio bilaterally in a 51-year-old woman as noted by intrapelvic displacement of *both* the acetabular fossa and femoral head, with the femoral head clearly medial to the ilioischial line (i.e., Kohler line).

Positioning

- Lateral decubitus position or supine at the surgeon's discretion

Surgical Approaches

- The author prefers a posterior approach, as it allows for an in situ femoral neck cut, as well as excellent acetabular exposure.
- Other operative approaches also are acceptable.

Preoperative Planning

- Utilize an anteroposterior radiograph of the hip with magnification correction to determine the appropriate hip center of rotation based on where the ilioischial line should be if acetabular protrusio were not present. Also determine the estimated acetabular component diameter (Figure 17.2). In protrusio cases the cup diameter is often a few millimeters larger than in routine primary cases in the same size patient, because this allows a "rim" fit of the cup, which avoids medial cup placement or subsequent medial migration.
- Evaluate the cross-table lateral radiograph for safe placement of acetabular screws (Figure 17.1C).

Bone/Implant/Soft Tissue Techniques

- Perform an approach to the hip based on surgeon's preference; the author prefers a posterior approach.
- An in situ femoral neck osteotomy frequently is needed because hip dislocation often cannot be achieved without the risk of acetabular rim or femoral fracture. The osteotomy may be completed with single-sided reciprocating saw at the subcapital level.

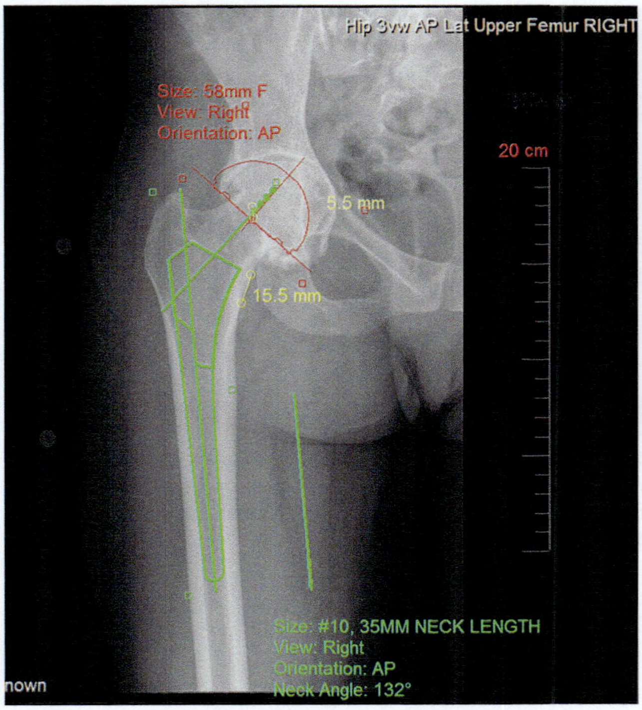

Figure 17.2 | This preoperative template with accurate magnification markers is utilized to place the acetabular component at the appropriate hip center of rotation based on where the ilioischial line should be if acetabular protrusio were not present.

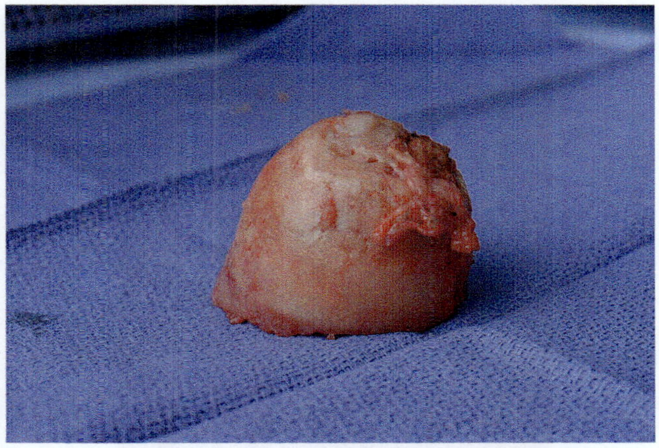

Figure 17.3 | Regardless of the bone quality, the patient's femoral head should be retained after the femoral neck osteotomy for autogenous bone grafting, which is often required in the acetabular fossa.

- The femoral shaft can then be retracted anteriorly, and the femoral head can be removed from the acetabular fossa with a corkscrew device or by quartering the femoral head with a small saw if it is incarcerated.
- The patient's femoral head should then be kept (Figure 17.3) and reamed from the subcapital region (Figure 17.4A) to the subchondral bone (Figure 17.4B) to provide autogenous bone graft.
- Occasionally, additional allograft bone chips and/or acetabular augments (Figure 17.5) are needed as a medial footing. Also, the femoral head may be used as a bulk structural graft in rare instances.
- If the femoral neck cut is long after the in situ subcapital femoral neck cut, an additional "napkin ring" of bone can be removed from the femoral neck to create the appropriate neck length as determined based by preoperative templating (Figure 17.3). This will assist with acetabular exposure.
- Starting with an intermediate diameter reamer, the patient's acetabulum should be sequentially reamed at the introitus, gradually increasing the reamer diameter by 2-mm increments until there is a rim fit with punctate bleeding bone. The key is to create a chamfered ring of bone at the introitus

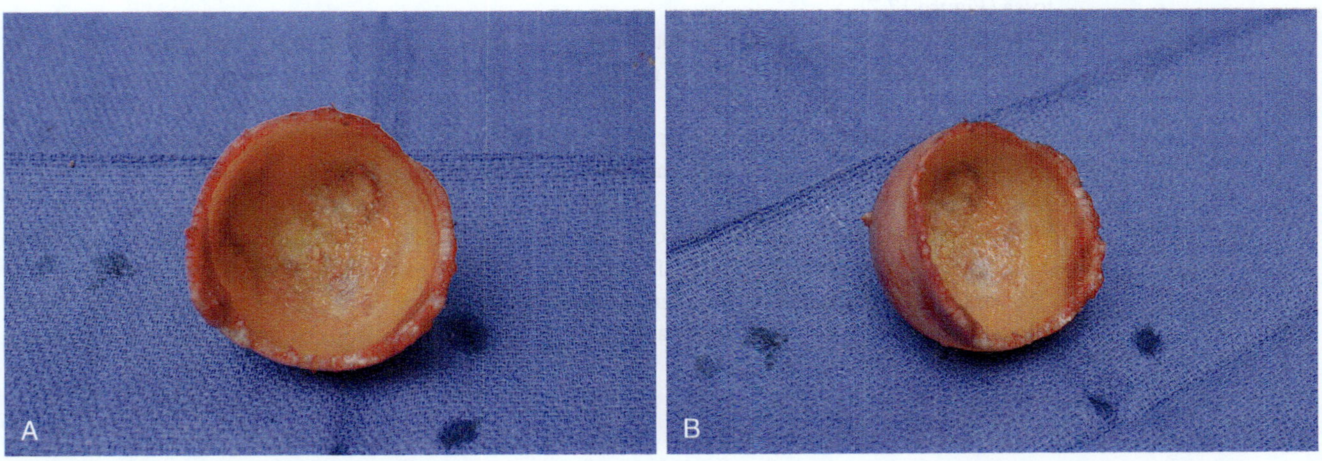

Figure 17.4 | The femoral head should be reamed from the subcapital region (A) to the subchondral bone (B) starting with a small-diameter reamer to create cancellous autogenous bone graft.

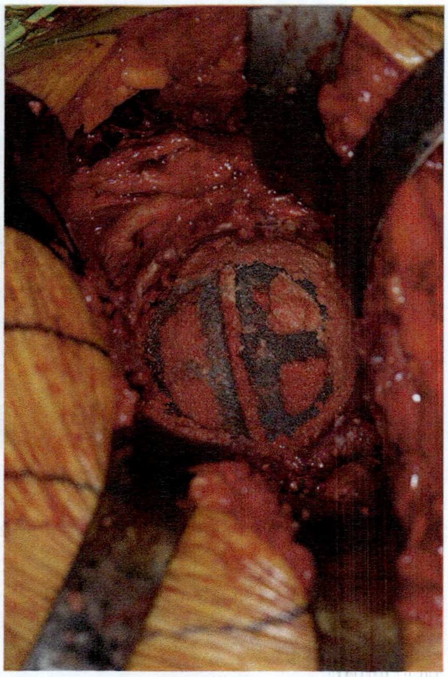

Figure 17.5 | An intraoperative picture of a 75-year-old man with acetabular protrusio and complete avascular necrosis of the femoral head. As such, allograft bone chips as well as 2 acetabular augments as medial footings were required for restoration of the anatomic hip center of rotation.

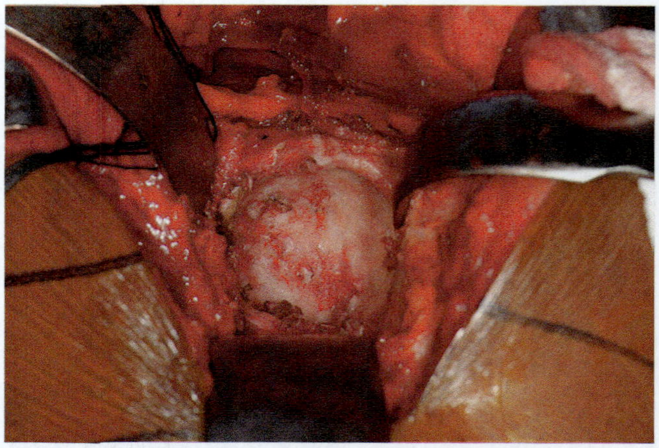

Figure 17.6 | The surgeon must strongly resist the urge to ream medially (even though the bone is very sclerotic there) as during routine primary THAs because the native acetabular fossa is medial to the ilioischial line.

of the acetabulum that will provide "rim" support of the cup. Reaming too deeply will create a tunnel that will lead to an overly medially placed cup.

- The surgeon must strongly resist the urge to ream medially (even though the bone is very sclerotic there) as during routine primary THAs because the native acetabular fossa is medial to the ilioischial line (Figure 17.6) and is not an appropriate anatomic landmark for acetabular reaming or acetabular component placement.
- Stop reaming when there is a good supportive rim of reamed bone of sufficient strength and surface area to support and provide fixation for an uncemented cup.
- Use a burr or small reamer to freshen the bone surface of the sclerotic medial wall. One may also use a 3.5-mm drill bit to create punctuate bleeding surfaces of the medial wall. Avoid weakening the already thin medial wall.
- The autogenous bone graft should then be packed into the cup and reverse reamed to densely fill the defect between the medial wall and a trial acetabular component at the introitus of the acetabular fossa (Figure 17.7).
- Intraoperative imaging should be considered with a trial acetabular component in place to determine restoration of the hip center of rotation, as well as acetabular component inclination and version (Figure 17.8).
- The real acetabular component is then placed with a secure rim fit at the introitus of the acetabular fossa. Supplemental screws are then placed through the acetabular component into host bone (Figure 17.9A and B).
- Femoral preparation and femoral component choice usually are routine and based on surgeon preference. In some extreme protrusio cases the femoral neck will have remodeled and be narrow from anterior to posterior. This pattern of remodeling may favor use of certain uncemented femoral component designs with narrow anterior to posterior dimensions or use of a cemented femoral component.

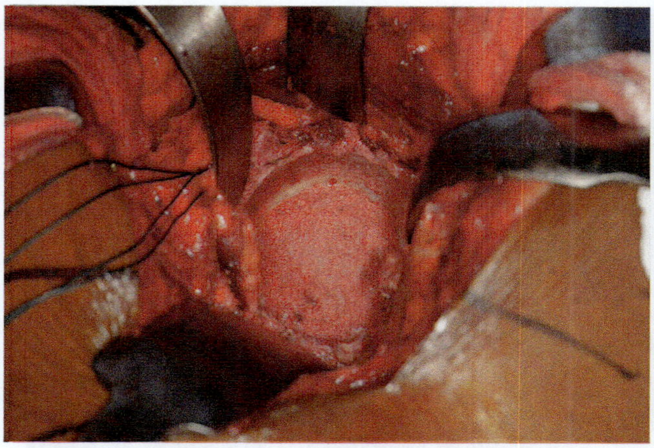

Figure 17.7 | Autogenous bone is packed medially by reverse reaming to a depth that allows placement of the acetabular component at the introitus via a rim-fit technique. The bone graft should not be placed at the rim where the acetabular component will garner a rim fit.

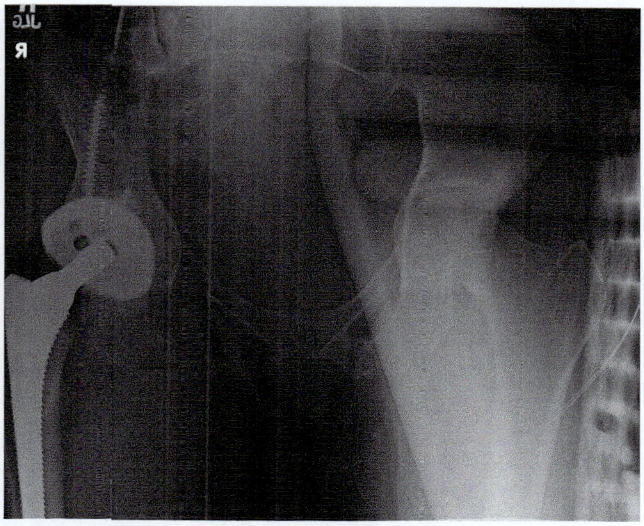

Figure 17.8 | A single intraoperative image can be very helpful to determine if the acetabular component is placed at the appropriate depth to restore hip center of rotation.

Postoperative Care

- Most patients are made weight bearing as tolerated if secure acetabular fixation is achieved with a solid rim fit and adjuvant screw fixation. If the bone is very deficient, weight bearing may be limited to toe touch or partial for 6 to 8 weeks postoperatively.
- This allows for loading of the bone graft and consolidation over the next several months and years (Figure 17.10A-C).

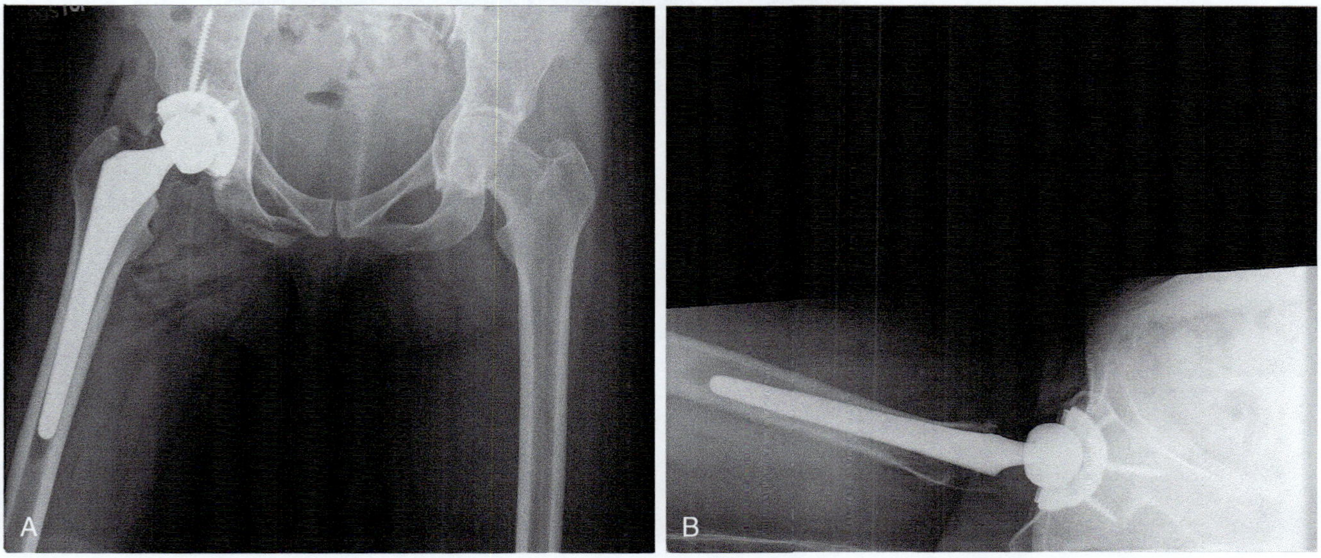

Figure 17.9 | Postoperative anteroposterior pelvis (A) and cross-table (B) radiographs of the 51-year-old woman in Figure 17.1 status post an uncemented total hip arthroplasty with a 58-mm acetabular component, autogenous bone grafting, 3 supplemental screws, and a proximally porous coated femoral component.

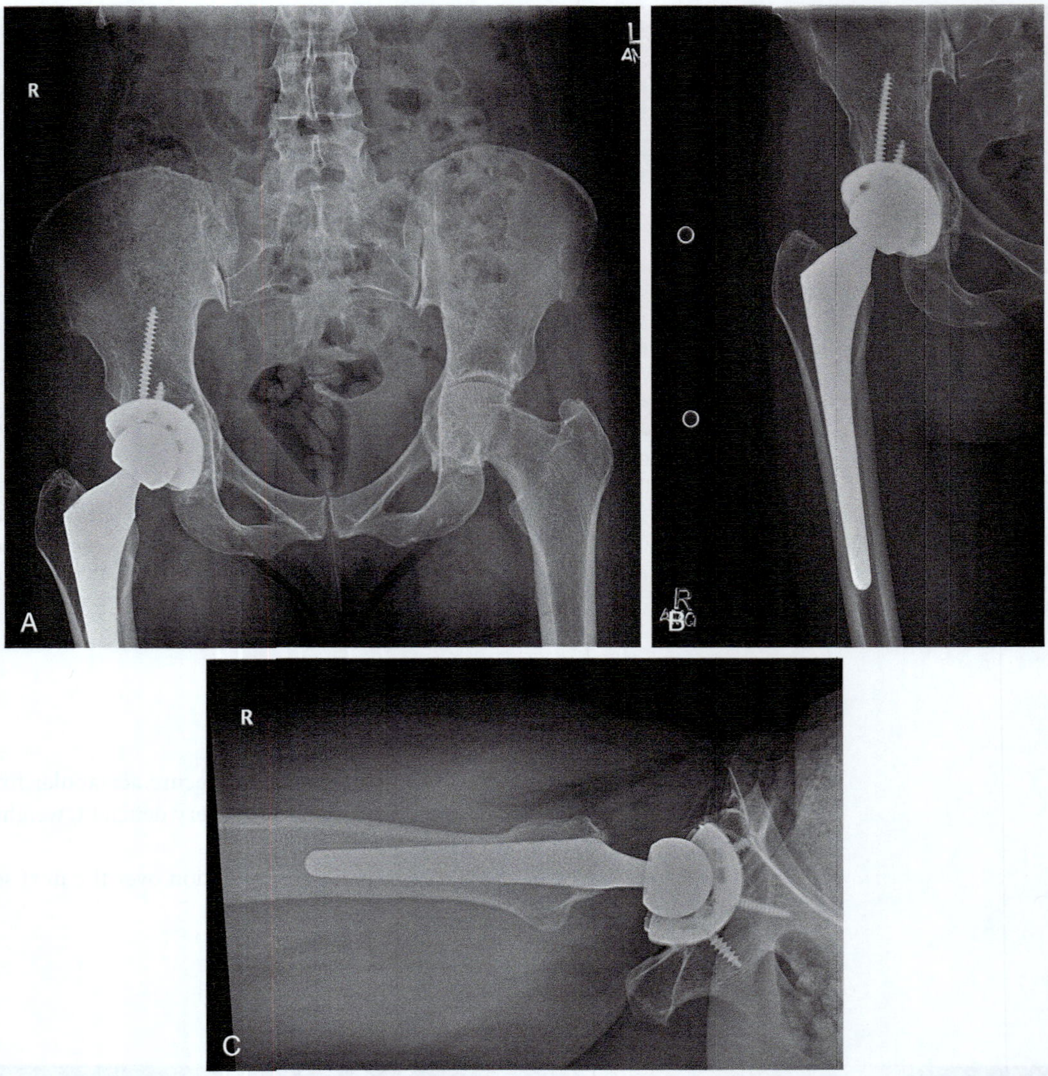

Figure 17.10 | With adequate acetabular fixation, autogenous bone grafting, and physiologic loading, the bone graft will incorporate as noted in the above-mentioned patient on these anteroposterior pelvis (A), anteroposterior hip (B), and cross-table lateral (C) radiographs at 2 years.

Chapter 18
Proximal Femoral Deformity

DANIEL J. BERRY

Key Concepts

- The most common reasons for total hip arthroplasty (THA) in the presence of proximal femoral deformity include posttraumatic conditions, previous proximal femoral osteotomy, developmental abnormalities, and metabolic abnormalities.
- Proximal femoral deformities make THA more difficult because of the challenges in fitting a femoral component into the femoral canal, challenges in accessing the femoral canal, and challenges in creating optimal hip biomechanics to provide good function and hip stability.
- Key goals of THA in the presence of deformity are (1) to avoid allowing the deformity to create circumstances that lead to poor hip biomechanics or (2) avoid problems with femoral component short- or long-term fixation.
- Deformities may be categorized in different ways: according to the etiology, the anatomy of the deformity, or the location of the deformity.
- For technical purposes the most valuable methods of categorization involve identifying the site of the deformity and the anatomy of the deformity. A practical method of doing this is to consider 3 main sites (levels) of deformity (Figure 18.1): proximal femoral deformity, subtrochanteric deformity (Figure 18.2), and more distal deformities (Figure 18.3). Each presents different challenges and can be treated differently.
- Most proximal deformities can be managed with implants that allow satisfactory implant position and fixation despite the deformity or by using implants that allow the deformity to be excised.
- Most more distal deformities, that is, those that occur below the stem tip level, can be ignored.
- Subtrochanteric deformities are the most difficult to manage. Strategies for management, including use of special implants and corrective femoral osteotomies, are discussed in this chapter.
- This chapter will not concentrate on 2 types of deformity that are covered in more detail elsewhere in this text: deformity mainly involving the greater trochanter (see Chapter 5) and rotational (anteversion) deformities of the femur (see Chapter 15).
- Deformities mainly involving the greater trochanter typically are most problematic when the greater trochanter is positioned to impede access to the femoral canal. Such deformities when mild may be managed with femoral implants that can be inserted by more medial access to the canal, or for more severe deformities, with trochanteric osteotomy (conventional or slide) or extended greater trochanteric osteotomy (Figure 18.4) (both discussed in Chapter 23).
- Rotational abnormalities of the proximal femur are most common in hip dysplasia, and management is discussed in detail in Chapter 15. Most can be managed with cemented components or uncemented components that provide for femoral component anteversion adjustment independent of the rotational relationship between the femoral metaphysis and diaphysis (such as modular stems or conical tapered fluted stems). Rarely derotational osteotomy is needed (discussed in this chapter).
- Preoperative planning in proximal femoral deformity cases is essential to choose the best techniques to manage the specific deformity.

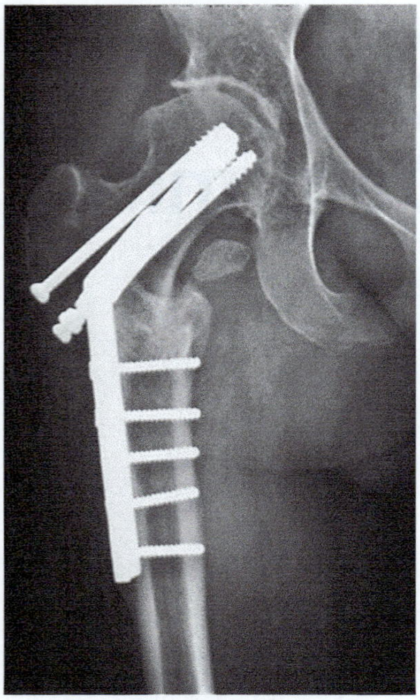

Figure 18.1 | Proximal level proximal femoral bone deformity.

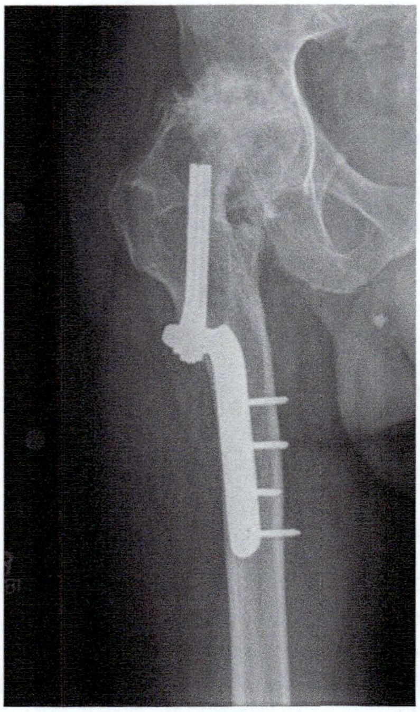

Figure 18.2 | Subtrochanteric level proximal femoral deformity.

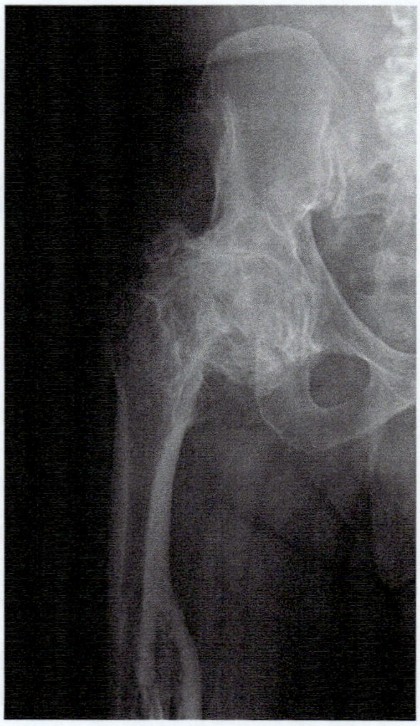

Figure 18.3 | More distal level proximal femoral deformity.

Sterile Instruments/Implants

- Routine hip instrumentation for the planned prosthesis (based on careful preoperative planning).
- If diaphyseal femoral osteotomy is planned:
  - Small oscillating saw
  - Narrow ribbon retractors
  - Pointed and serrated jaw bone clamps

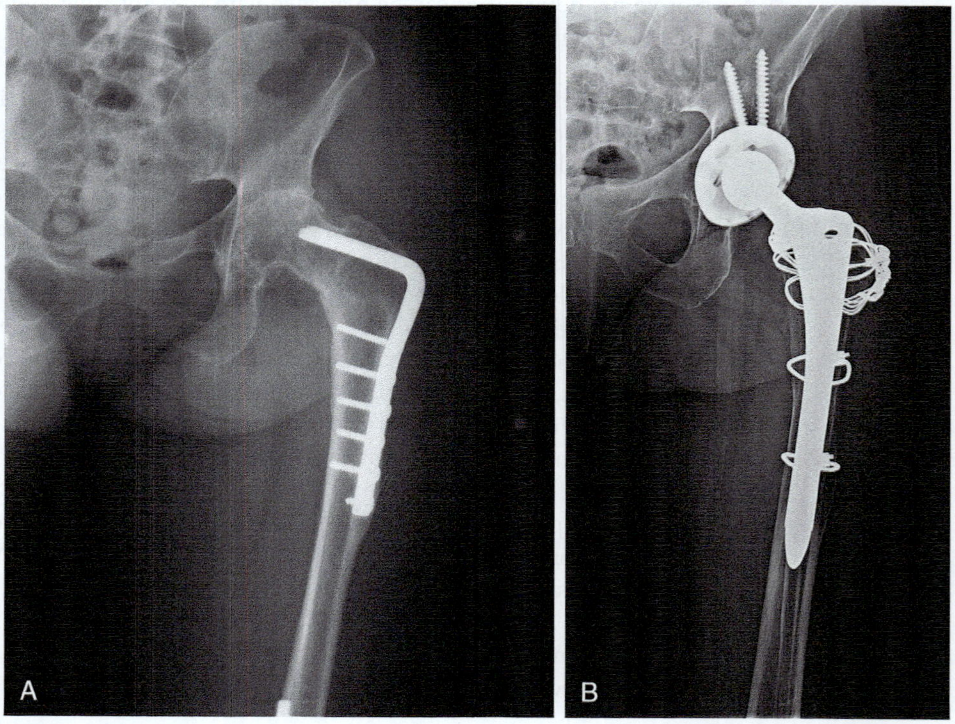

Figure 18.4 | A, Radiograph of patient with proximal femoral deformity and greater trochanter overhanging the femoral canal. B, Postoperative radiograph after exposure using greater trochanteric osteotomy.

- Cerclage wires or cables
- Intraoperative radiography and/or fluoroscopy
- Choose a femoral implant system that provides fixation in the proximal and distal fragments of the femur. This is essential to the success of the procedure. Typically, the component should be one that provides good rotational control of the proximal fragment with a triangle or sleeve that fits in the metaphysis and good rotational control of the distal fragment with flutes, very sharp corners, or extensive porous coating. Implants that have a round proximal geometry typically will not provide good rotational control of the proximal fragment. The implant chosen must be long enough to gain good fixation in the distal fragment below the planned osteotomy level.

Positioning

- Lateral decubitus or supine depending on surgeon preference and planned operative approach.
- Drape the hip to provide wide access to most of the femur to the knee.
- For complex cases, insert a Foley catheter and consider having a red blood cell salvage system (cell saver) available.

Surgical Approaches

- Posterior, anterolateral, and direct lateral approaches are versatile for these cases. Some simpler cases may be manageable with a direct anterior approach but not if femoral osteotomy is planned or may be needed.

Preoperative Planning

- Careful and thorough preoperative planning is essential to successful management of these problems.
- Understand the level and anatomy of the deformity. Typically, anteroposterior and lateral radiographs are sufficient, but occasionally computed tomography scan with 3-dimensional reconstruction is helpful to understand the deformity better (Figure 18.5). In most cases, having full length radiographs of the femur is helpful.
- Template the femur with various appropriate implants to determine whether conventional implants can be used to fit the deformity or whether special implants are needed. Determine implant design, size, and length. Cemented implants may provide more flexibility in sizing and bone preparation (Figure 18.6). Certain uncemented femoral implants, such as modular implants and fluted tapered cone-shaped implants allow the surgeon to adapt the implant to a wide range of metaphyseal anatomies.

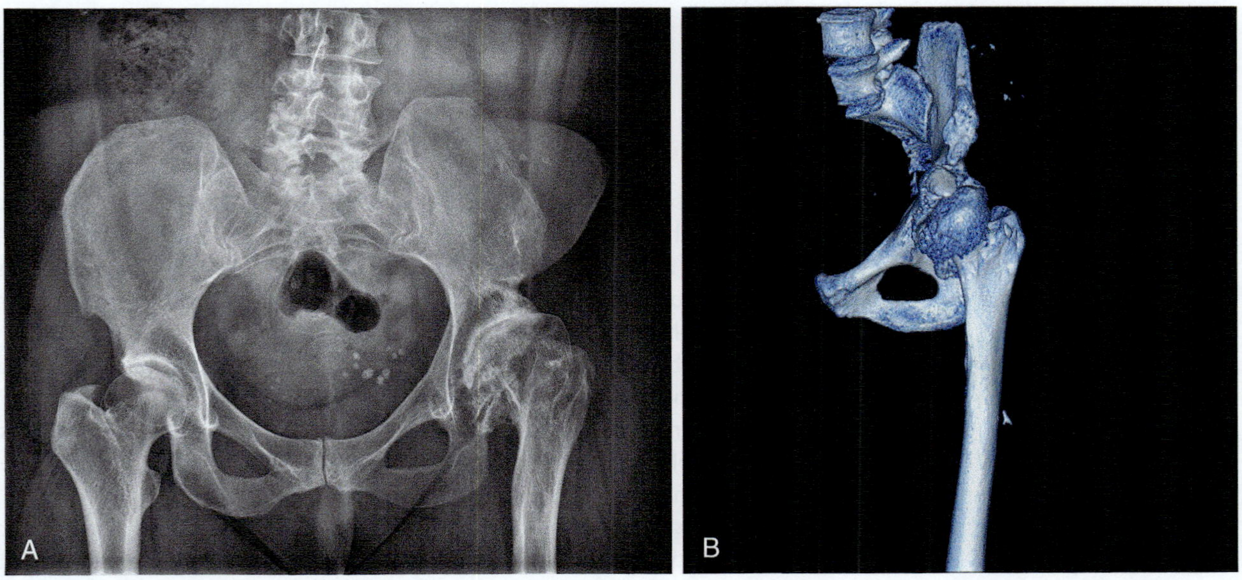

Figure 18.5 | A, Radiograph of patient with proximal femoral deformity. B, Three-dimensional reconstruction of proximal femur to define the 3-dimensional anatomy of the deformity.

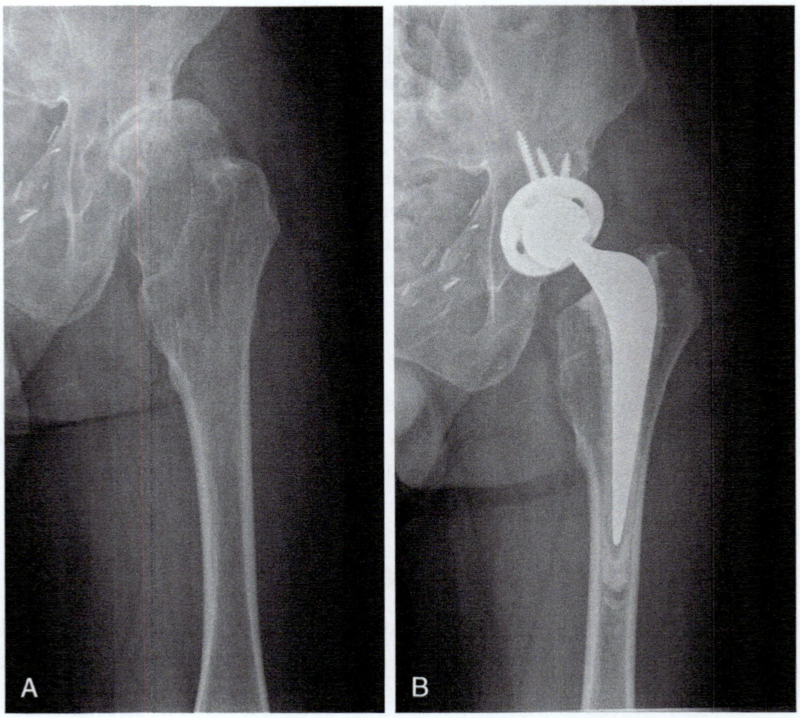

Figure 18.6 | A, Radiograph of patient with proximal femoral deformity from familial exostoses. B, Postoperative reconstruction with cemented stem, which accommodated the deformity.

- If the deformity is in the subtrochanteric area, determine whether a corrective osteotomy is likely to be needed. If so, draw out the anticipated correction to determine the precise level of the osteotomy and to determine the shape of closing wedges likely to be needed. Choose and template for a femoral implant system that will provide good rotational and angular control of both the proximal and distal fragments of the femur after the osteotomy. In the great majority of cases uncemented femoral components are preferred because cement tends to extrude through the osteotomy site. To reiterate the aforementioned comments: the component should be one that provides good rotational control of the proximal fragment with a triangle or sleeve that fits in the metaphysis and good rotational control of the distal fragment with flutes, very sharp corners, or extensive porous coating. Implants that have a round proximal geometry typically will not provide good rotational control of the proximal fragment. The implant chosen must be long enough to gain good fixation in the distal fragment below the planned osteotomy level.

Bone, Implant, and Soft Tissue Techniques

Proximal Level Deformities

- Perform the preferred operative approach based on the considerations discussed earlier.
- Osteotomize the femoral neck at the level chosen by templating and prepare the acetabulum.
- Prepare the femur for the chosen implant. During this process make sure the implant will fit satisfactorily without causing fracture or perforation during canal preparation and component implantation. Use intraoperative radiographs or fluoroscopy to asses during preparation as needed.
- A prophylactic cerclage wire or cable may be placed around the proximal femur during bone preparation if the shape of the femur places it at risk for fracture.
- As noted earlier, cemented implants may provide more flexibility in sizing and bone preparation. Certain uncemented femoral implants, such as modular implants and fluted tapered cone-shaped implants allow the surgeon to manage a wide range of metaphyseal anatomies.
- Place trial implants and test hip stability and biomechanics. Test for extra-articular impingement related to the bone deformity. If present, remove impingement sources by excising bone or create more space between the femur and pelvis with implants that provide more length or femoral offset.
- Implant the definitive components.

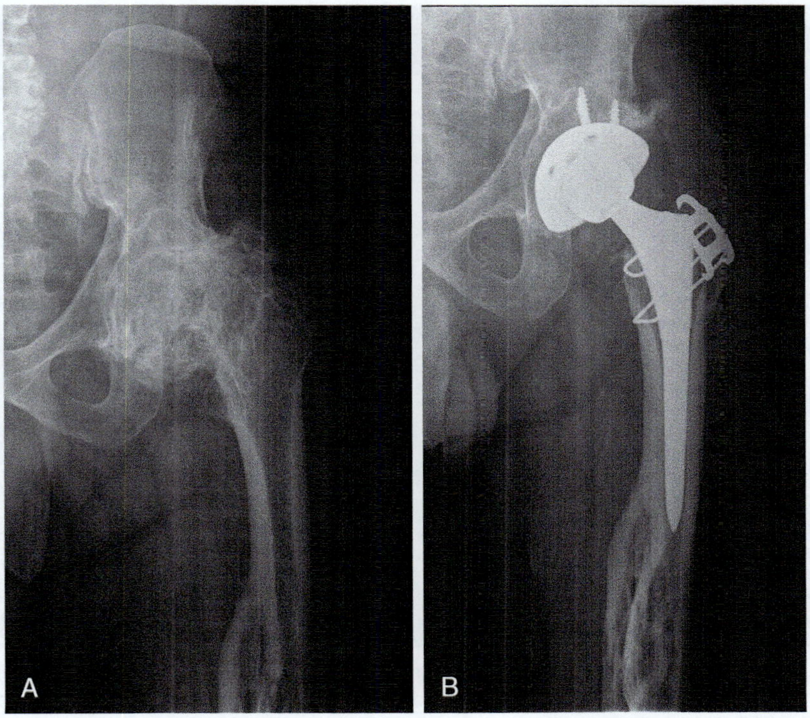

Figure 18.7 | A, Radiograph of patient with proximal femoral deformity distal to the anticipated level of conventional femoral implant stem tip (based on templating). B, Postoperative radiograph after reconstruction with standard length femoral stem.

Distal Level Deformities

- Preoperative planning should identify the level of the deformity. Most distal deformities can be ignored so long as preoperative planning allows choice of an implant that will terminate proximal to the deformity and so long as that implant will gain adequate fixation (Figure 18.7).

Subtrochanteric Level Deformities

- Use preoperative planning to determine whether the deformity will be managed with a special implant or with a corrective osteotomy (Figure 18.8A).
- In some cases an implant that terminates above the deformity may be considered, thereby obviating the need for an osteotomy. Such implants include "stubby" short uncemented metaphyseal fixation implants and hip resurfacing implants (Figure 18.8B).
- If a short implant is chosen, make sure during canal preparation that it will fit adequately proximal to the deformity. Use intraoperative fluoroscopy or radiographs as needed.

If a Corrective Osteotomy Will be Utilized (Figure 18.9)

- Expose the hip through a posterior or anterolateral/direct lateral approach, perform a femoral neck osteotomy of the desired configuration at the desired level, and expose and prepare the acetabulum. Save acetabular reamings and the femoral head to provide autogenous bone graft for the femoral osteotomy.
- Measure the distance from the tip of the greater trochanter to the level of the planned osteotomy based on preoperative templating. The level of the planned osteotomy typically will be at the apex of the deformity.
- Expose a short section (less than 5 cm) of the femur at the level of the planned osteotomy by splitting the vastus lateralis (Figure 18.10A).
- Remeasure the distance from the tip of trochanter to the planned osteotomy, and mark this point on the femur with electrocautery. If desired, confirm that the level of the osteotomy is at the apex of the deformity with fluoroscopy.

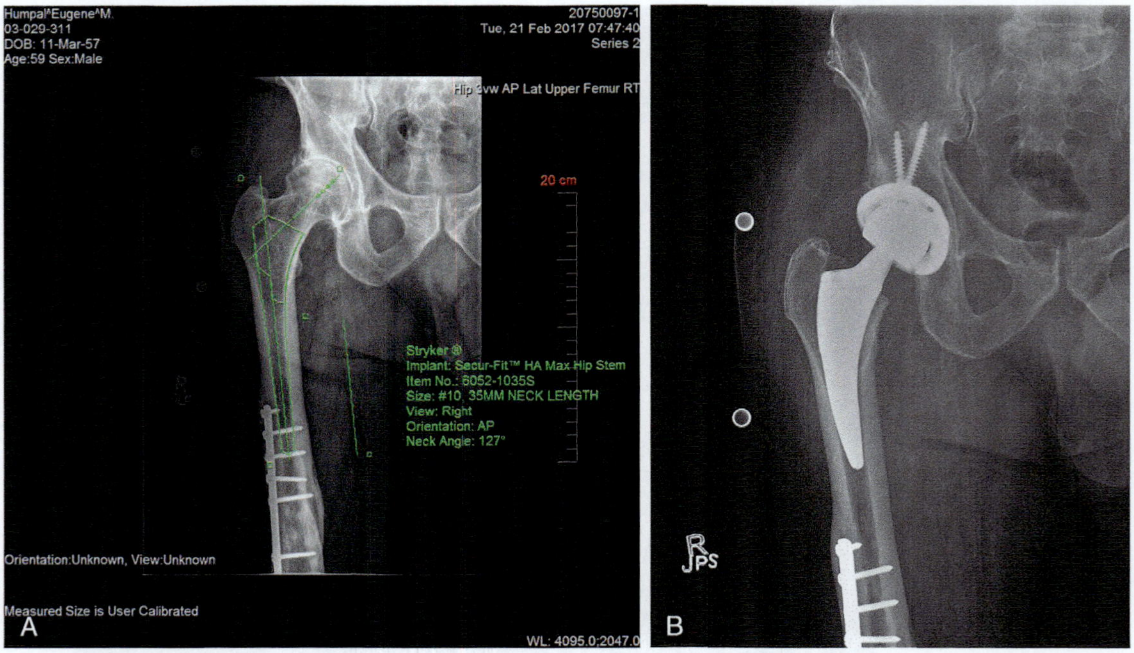

Figure 18.8 | A, Preoperative templating demonstrating femoral deformity and retained buried hardware is not amenable to standard length femoral component. B, Postoperative radiograph after reconstruction with short "stubby" femoral component, which avoided conflict with the deformity and internal fixation devices.

- Expose a narrow band of the femur circumferentially with a periosteal elevator and place narrow (1-cm) ribbon retractors anteriorly and posteriorly around the femur.
- Using a small oscillating saw, and irrigating frequently to avoid burning the bone, make a transverse osteotomy of the femur perpendicular to the axis of the femur proximal to the deformity (Figure 18.10B).
- Roughly line up the distal fragment of the femur parallel to the proximal fragment of the femur, and remove a wedge of bone from the distal fragment that will provide the desired correction.

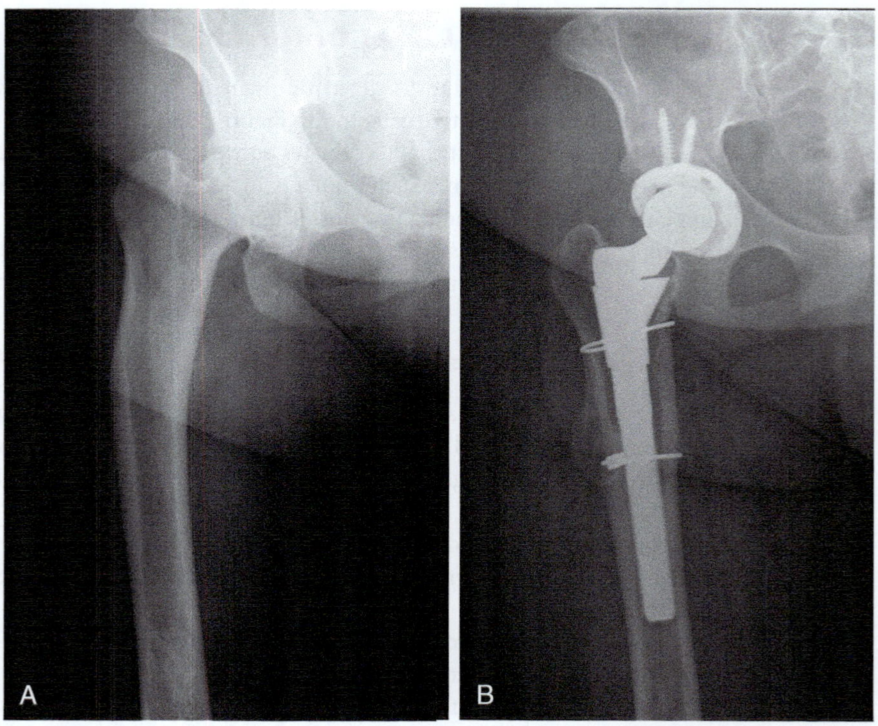

Figure 18.9 | A, Preoperative radiograph of patient with subtrochanteric level femoral deformity. B, Postoperative radiograph after THA with corrective subtrochanteric osteotomy. The osteotomy has healed.

Typically, the subtracted bone will be wedge shaped tapering to a minimal resection on its thin side and the osteotomy will be roughly parallel to the axis of the distal fragment of the femur (Figure 18.10C). As a double check, the osteotomy should match the dimensions and angle predicted from the preoperative plan.

- Prepare the proximal fragment with the instrumentation for the planned femoral component. To do this effectively, pointed bone holding clamps or serrated jaw bone holding clamps typically are needed to hold the proximal fragment rotation in appropriate alignment for bone preparation. Make sure preparation of the proximal fragment is done so that (1) the anteversion of the stem in the proximal fragment will be correct relative to the greater trochanter and (2) sizing is such that the implant will gain good fixation in the proximal fragment. A prophylactic cerclage wire or cable may be placed around the proximal fragment to prevent longitudinal fracture when the implant is placed (avoiding such fractures is important because they are difficult to manage if they occur).
- Prepare the distal fragment with the instrumentation for the planned component. Under direct vision, ensure that the sizing and fit in the femoral canal with final reamers appear appropriate. Gaining good rotational control of both the proximal and distal fragments with the implant is imperative for success of the procedure. Place a prophylactic cerclage wire or cable around the most proximal aspect of the distal fragment to prevent fracture during trial or final component implantation.

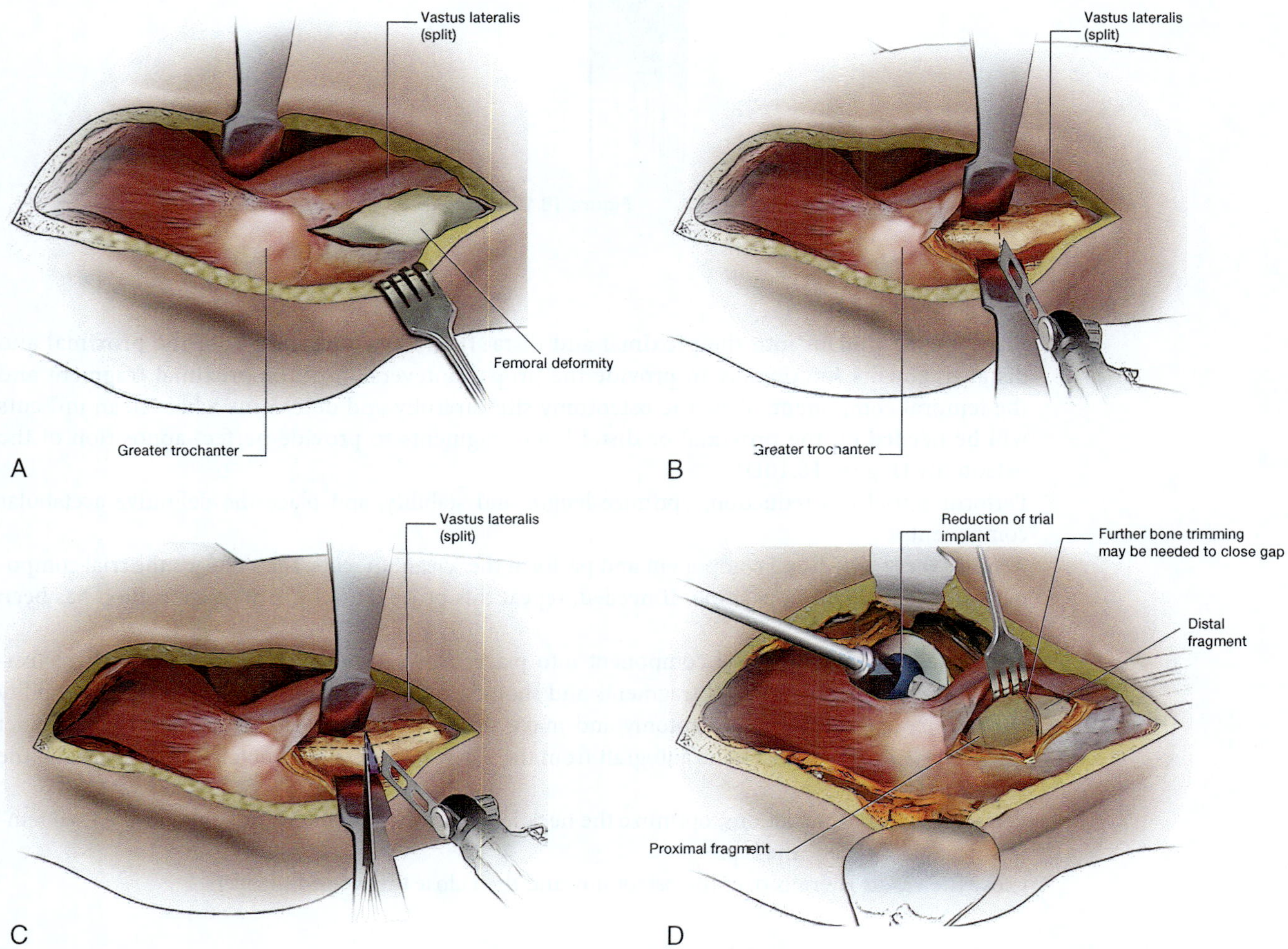

Figure 18.10 | A, The lateral femur is exposed at the apex of the deformity by splitting the vastus lateralis. B, The first osteotomy is made perpendicular to the proximal femur superior to the deformity. C, The second osteotomy is made perpendicular to the distal femur inferior to the first osteotomy. Unless shortening is desired, the osteotomy should be shaped like a wedge. D, With trial implants in place assess osteotomy apposition and calculate the "clean up" cuts required to get perfect bone apposition. E, The final components are implanted. The osteotomy should be well opposed and very stable angularly and rotationally. Autologous bone graft is packed around the osteotomy.

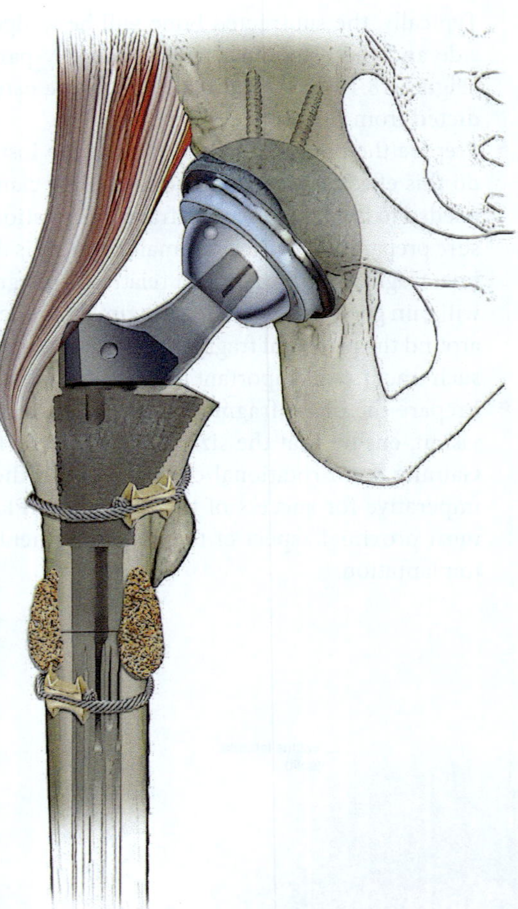

Figure 18.10—Cont'd

- Place a trial implant into the proximal and distal fragments and align both the proximal and distal fragments rotationally to provide the proper anteversion of the proximal fragment and the femoral component. View the osteotomy site carefully and determine what "clean up" cuts will be needed on the proximal or distal bone fragments to provide perfect apposition of the osteotomy (Figure 18.10D).
- Perform a trial hip reduction, optimize length and stability, and place the definitive acetabular component.
- Remove the trial femoral component and perform the "clean up" cuts, then replace the trial component and check bone apposition. If needed, repeat this process until the bone apposition has been optimized.
- Impact the definitive femoral component into place. This component should gain excellent fixation in the proximal and distal fragments and should provide rigid angular and rotational stability of the osteotomy. View the osteotomy and make sure it is well opposed with good bone contact (Figure 18.10E). Pack host bone autograft from the femoral head or acetabular reamings around the osteotomy.
- Perform final trial reductions, optimize the neck length of the modular head, implant the final femoral head, and reduce the hip.
- Close the vastus lateralis over the osteotomy and then close the wound in layers.

Postoperative Management

- Weight bearing typically is restricted to toe touch until radiographic osteotomy healing is identified; typically this takes about 8 weeks. Thereafter progressive weight bearing is allowed.

Chapter 19
Previous Hip Fusion

JOSHUA S. BINGHAM
DANIEL J. BERRY

Key Concepts

- Conversion of a hip fusion to a total hip arthroplasty (THA) is a technically demanding procedure with variable outcomes and should not be undertaken without careful consideration by both the surgeon and the patient.
- The most common indications for conversion of an arthrodesed hip include malposition, pseudarthrosis, ipsilateral knee pain, and disabling low back pain.
- Patients may also seek conversion related to the disability associated with an immobile hip or before undergoing an ipsilateral knee replacement.
- Important technical considerations include adequate exposure, removal of hardware if present, careful identification of bony landmarks to ensure proper implant orientation, and maintenance or restoration of hip biomechanics.
- Surgical exposure is often dependent on the fused hip position, boney anatomy, and presence and location of hardware but commonly requires a more extensile approach.
- Acetabular bone quality may be poor, and when uncemented cups are used, supplemental screw fixation is commonly needed.
- Hip fusion takedowns can provide significant improvement in pain and function for patients with good survivorship at 10 years but generally do not achieve the same reliable outcomes as primary THA (Table 19.1).
- The best outcomes are seen in patients whose abductors have not been violated during the hip fusion and in patients with a spontaneous arthrodesis.
- Patients with poor abductor function after surgery may become cane dependent for life.

Sterile Instruments and Implants

Instruments

- Routine hip retractors
- Metal cutting burr
- Sagittal saw
- Hardware removal instruments
- Broken screw removal set
- Intraoperative fluoroscopy

Implants

- In addition to an uncemented acetabular component, in cases with distorted anatomy or significant bony defects, autogenous bone graft from the arthrodesis site, supplemental screw fixation, and metal augments may be required.
- On the femoral side uncemented femoral components most commonly are used. Proximal fixation may be used if the metaphyseal bone is of good quality and there is no significant proximal femoral deformity requiring correction. Distal fixation is preferred if the proximal metaphyseal bone is distorted or significantly compromised by a deformity or prior hardware.

Table 19.1 | Ten-year Survivorship After Hip Fusion Conversion to Total Hip Arthroplasty

Author (y)	No. of Hips	Age at Conversion (Range) (y)	Follow-up Years (Range)	Surgical Approach	Spontaneous Versus Surgical Fusion	Ten-year Survivorship (%)
Kilgus et al. (1990)	41	53 (24-75)	7 (2-16.5)	Transtrochanteric	Higher failure rate in the surgical fusion patients	96
Joshi et al. (2002)	208	51 (20-80)	9.2 (2-26)	Transtrochanteric	Spontaneous fusion had better functional results	96.1
Richard et al. (2011)	26	49 (25-74)	9 (2-21)	Transtrochanteric or direct lateral	Not reported	74.2
Fernandez-Fairen et al. (2011)	48	50 (31-68)	17 (10-29)	Anterolateral (21); transtrochanteric (15); posterolateral (12)	18 spontaneous; 30 surgical	93

- Large-diameter femoral heads (36 mm or larger) in combination with ultrahigh-molecular-weight polyethylene liners are the preferred bearing surface. Dual mobility constructs may also be considered, particularly when there are abductor deficiencies or severe spine degeneration and deformity.

Positioning

- If a posterior, anterolateral, or transtrochanteric approach is planned, the patient is placed in a lateral decubitus position, which allows for a more extensile exposure if needed.
- A supine approach may be used if a direct anterior approach is preferred or required to remove anteriorly placed or intrapelvic hardware.
- Draping should allow for adequate access to the proximal pelvis and entire femur.

Surgical Approaches

- The skin incision may be influenced by previous incisions and location of hardware that may need to be removed.
- Commonly an extensile posterior or anterolateral approach is used in conjunction with an in situ neck cut.
- A transtrochanteric approach may be required if an in situ neck cut is not possible or to reduce additional trauma to the abductors (Figure 19.1A-D).
- Any hardware present over the trochanter and proximal femur is removed after the surgical approach, if possible.
- In rare cases with significant proximal femoral deformity requiring correction, an extended trochanteric osteotomy can be performed to correct the deformity, improve exposure, and aid in hardware removal.
- Soft tissues around the arthrodesis and proximal femur should be adequately cleared to identify the femoral neck and other bony landmarks.

Preoperative Planning

- Routine preoperative radiographs (anteroposterior [AP] pelvis, AP hip, and cross-table lateral) are usually sufficient.
- If there is distorted anatomy or unusual hardware placement, a preoperative computed tomography scan can be helpful to better define the anatomy, localize hardware, and identify anatomic landmarks.
- Abductor function can be evaluated preoperatively by asking the patient to try to abduct the hip and determining by palpation whether the abductor muscles contract. Further evaluation with electromyography or magnetic resonance imaging may be performed but is not routinely required.

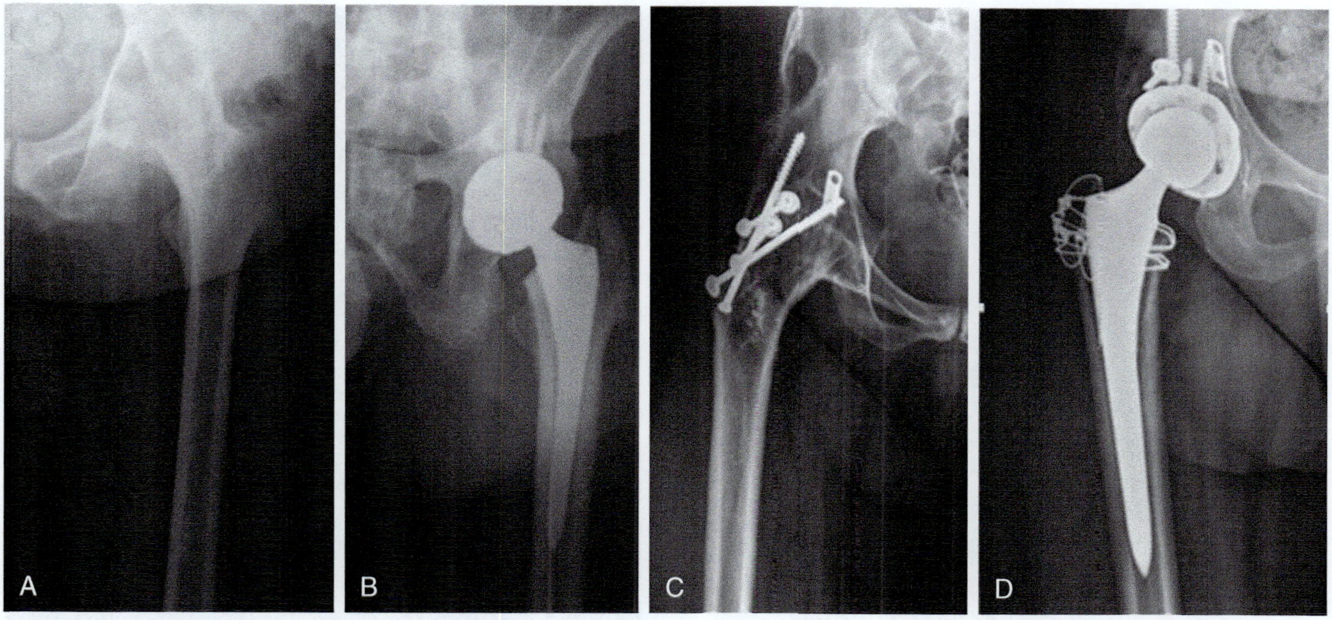

Figure 19.1 | A, Preoperative radiograph of a spontaneously ankylosed hip where an in situ neck cut is appropriate. B, Postoperative radiograph after an in situ neck cut. C, Preoperative radiograph of a surgical arthrodesis where a transtrochanteric approach is required. D, Postoperative radiograph after a transtrochanteric approach.

- The surgeon should be familiar with the technique that was used for the arthrodesis, as this may influence the exposure and the need for bone removal, particularly with an extra-articular arthrodesis.

Bone, Implant, and Soft Tissue Techniques

- After the desired surgical approach has been performed based on preoperative planning, the femoral neck osteotomy can be performed either in situ or through a transtrochanteric approach.
- Identification of bony landmarks (greater and lesser trochanter) and intraoperative fluoroscopy are useful to help determine the correct level and angle of the femoral neck cut (Figure 19.2).
- Be careful to avoid angulation of the saw that leads the osteotomy into the pelvis bone.
- A slightly lower neck cut can provide additional exposure for acetabular preparation if needed.
- Further release of soft tissue around the femur will improve exposure.

Acetabular Preparation

- Bony preparation begins on the acetabular side. The anatomy often is difficult to interpret, and finding key landmarks, including the ischium and the lateral ileum, before reaming is valuable.
- An intraoperative radiograph or fluoroscopy can help identify the ischium, ilium, teardrop, and fovea in preparation for acetabular reaming.
- Often some extra bone from the old femoral head and neck will be needed to be removed as the reaming is initiated. This may be done with burr.
- Retractors placed anteriorly over the anterior wall and posteriorly in the ischium are helpful in maintaining orientation and exposure. Once exposure and orientation have been achieved, the acetabulum is carefully deepened and widened with reamers using the fovea as a guide (if it is present) and a radiograph or fluoroscopy for confirmation (Figure 19.3).
- Often, in cases of spontaneous fusion, as the acetabulum is deepened, soft tissues can be visualized (transverse acetabular ligament and remnants of the ligamentum teres) in the floor of the acetabulum. Be careful to avoid overly medial or lateral acetabular component placement.
- Careful attention to the thickness of the anterior and posterior walls is necessary during preparation of the socket.
- Once the acetabulum is prepared, a trial acetabular component can be used to check stability and position (Figure 19.4).
- Acetabular cup fixation should be treated like a revision THA with an uncemented cup, and supplemental screw fixation usually is advisable (Figure 19.5).

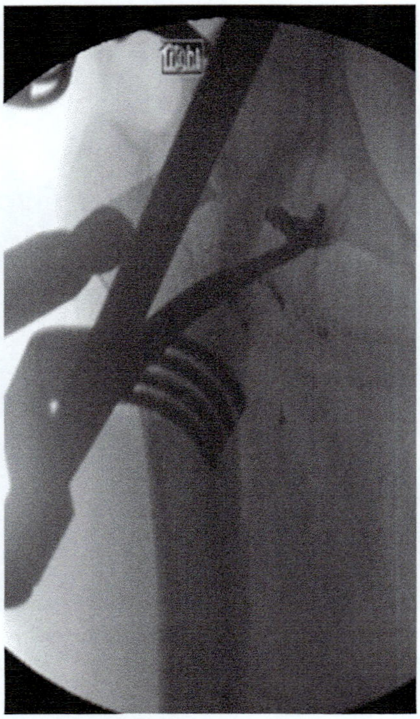

Figure 19.2 | Intraoperative fluoroscopy used to confirm the correct level and angle of the in situ femoral neck cut.

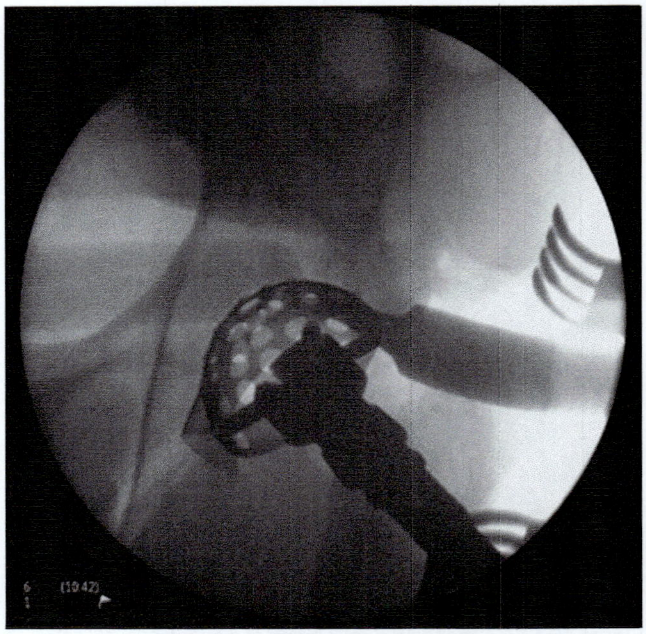

Figure 19.3 | Intraoperative fluoroscopy to confirm the appropriate acetabular cup position during reaming.

Femoral Preparation

- Release of capsular tissue around the proximal femur can facilitate femoral exposure if needed.
- Femoral prosthetic selection depends on several factors including the patient's bone quality, the presence of cortical defects, stress risers related to hardware removal, and any proximal femoral deformity requiring correction.

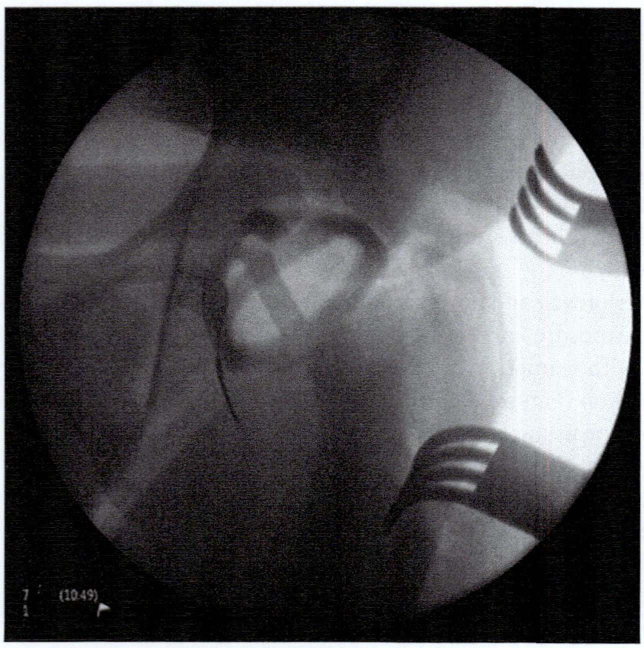

Figure 19.4 | Intraoperative fluoroscopy with an acetabular trial in place.

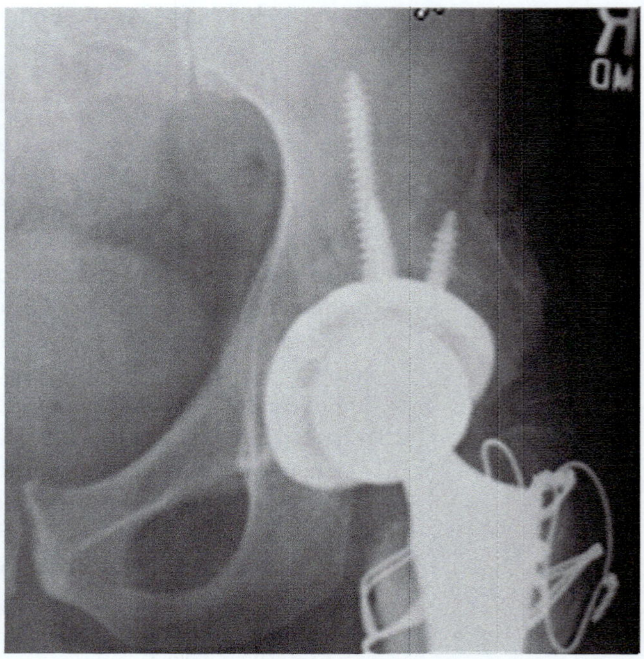

Figure 19.5 | Postoperative radiograph of an acetabular component after takedown of a surgical arthrodesis with a well-fixed, well-oriented cup against the tear drop.

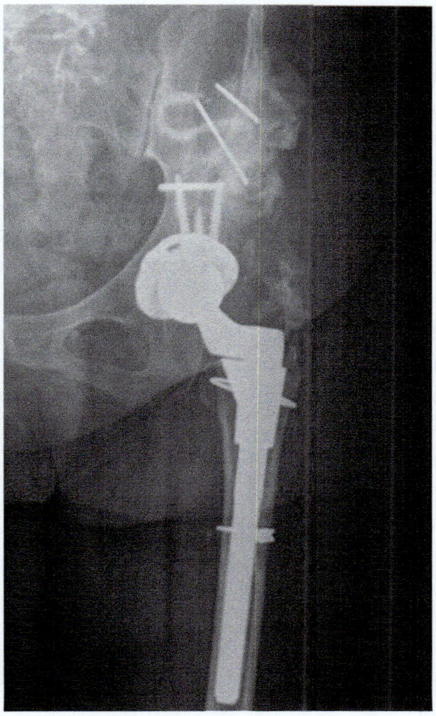

Figure 19.6 | Postoperative radiograph of a surgical arthrodesis takedown with a modular femoral stem.

- Proximal fixation may be used if the proximal metaphyseal bone is of good quality; however, distal fixation should be used if the proximal metaphyseal bone is distorted or an extended trochanteric osteotomy is required for exposure or correction of a deformity (Figure 19.6).
- If hardware was removed resulting in multiple stress risers, a longer stem to bypass the defects should be considered to avoid risk of postoperative fracture.
- A large-diameter femoral head and liner (36 mm or larger) is preferred, especially if the abductors are deficient. If the patient is at high risk for postoperative instability, a dual mobility articulation should also be considered.

Trialing

- Before final component implantation, a trial reduction is performed to determine the appropriate neck length for soft tissue tension and leg lengths.
- Palpation of the sciatic nerve should be performed to ensure that it is mobile with the hip slightly flexed and the knee extended. If excess tension on the nerve is noted, the neck length or the femoral component position may need to be adjusted.
- The risk of stretching the sciatic nerve and associated palsy is dependent on both the age of the patient and the amount of shortening at the time of arthrodesis. Excessive lengthening (>4 cm) at the time of THA should be avoided.
- Before closure, the hip should be placed through a range of motion to assess stability and inspect for any bone or soft tissue impingement. Be particularly aware that extra bone around the acetabulum from the fusion can cause extra-articular impingement, which can lead to hip instability. Any impinging or potentially impinging structures should be removed. Increased motion over time may result in impingement, which can lead to both pain and instability.
- Hip abduction should also be evaluated, and if limited, an adductor tenotomy can be performed.

Wound Closure

If a trochanteric osteotomy was performed, the greater trochanter is fixed with wires or cables.

If the trochanter is absent, the abductors or lateral scar tissue may be sutured to the proximal femur and closed to the posterior soft tissue sleeve. Alternatively, the tensor fascia lata may be tenodesed to the trochanter or the proximal femur to improve abductor function.

If the patient's extremity was significantly lengthened, a pillow should be placed to flex the knee and take tension off the sciatic nerve for the first several days postoperatively.

Postoperative Care

- Weight bearing after conversion depends on the presence of an osteotomy, the type of implants used, implant fixation, and the surgeon's preferences regarding weight bearing after THA.
- If a trochanteric osteotomy was performed, touch weight bearing should be maintained for 6 to 8 weeks after surgery. Once the trochanteric osteotomy is well healed, active abduction exercises should be started.
- Patients with severely deficient or absent abductors are at an increased risk of dislocation. These patients may be braced with a hip abduction orthosis, restricting flexion and adduction for 6 to 12 weeks.
- Prophylaxis against heterotopic ossification is not necessarily required. However, if the arthrodesis occurred spontaneously, or if the patient has other risk factors for the development of heterotopic bone, prophylaxis with anti-inflammatory medications and/or radiation therapy is indicated.

Chapter 20
Total Hip Arthroplasty for Oncologic Conditions

STEPHEN M. PETIS
MATTHEW P. ABDEL

Key Concepts

- The majority of pelvic girdle and femoral bone tumors are bony metastases. Primary bone tumors may occur in the pelvic girdle in up to 15% of cases.
- Bone tumors can create large segmental bone deficits, which makes stable implant fixation to host, nonpathologic bone challenging.
- Preoperatively, patients should be medically optimized to address anemia and other anomalies such as hypercalcemia. Cases should be staged locally and systemically and evaluated and treated in corroboration with a multidisciplinary oncology team.
- Radiographs and cross-sectional imaging should be carefully assessed to map out planned resections and predict residual bone defects that require reconstructions.
- Oftentimes, bone loss is much greater than anticipated, and pathologic pelvic discontinuities frequently are present.
- These cases necessitate a wide armamentarium of implants to manage bone defects—cemented and cementless implants, allograft-prosthetic composites, tantalum acetabular components and augments, supplemental cages, megaprostheses, and structural allografts.
- Surgical approach and exposure are dictated by the location of the tumor. An approach should be selected that allows complete resection of the tumor if primary in nature or adequate visualization of bone defects for stable reconstruction if metastatic.
- There will be 2 main focuses of this chapter:
  1. Acetabular reconstructions for periacetabular lesions, with emphasis on 2 groups:
     a. Primary periacetabular lesions: Wide excision *and* acetabular reconstruction are needed
     b. Metastatic periacetabular lesions: Only acetabular reconstruction is needed
  2. Femoral reconstructions for femoral lesions, with emphasis on 2 groups:
     a. Primary femoral lesions: Wide excision *and* femoral reconstruction are needed
     b. Metastatic femoral lesions: Only femoral reconstruction is needed

  For primary periacetabular lesions, there are 4 types of resections and reconstructions:
- Type I: Resection at sciatic notch (Figure 20.1)
- Type II: Supra-acetabular resection (Figure 20.2)
- Type III: Posterior column preserved (Figure 20.3)
- Type IV: Anterior column preserved (Figure 20.4)

Sterile Instruments and Implants

Instruments

- Routine hip retractors
- Saws (reciprocating and oscillating) for bone resection
- Wide range of sizes of acetabular reamers to accommodate various bone defect sizes and morphologies

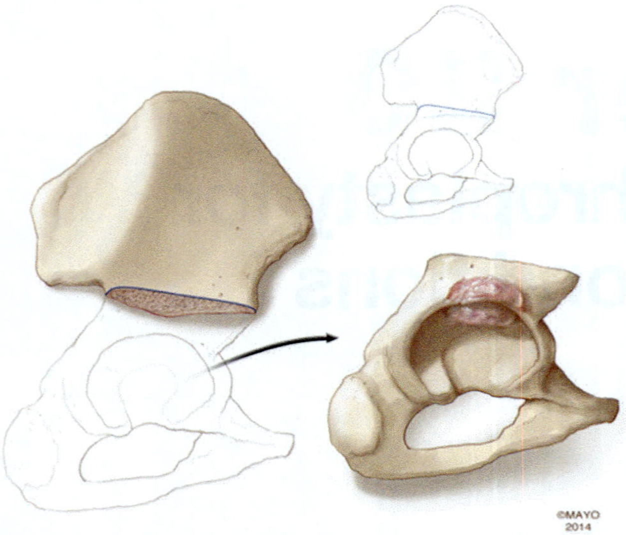

Figure 20.1 | Illustration depicting a Mayo type I resection at the level of the sciatic notch, mandating the most difficult acetabular reconstruction on the ilium. (Used with permission of Mayo Foundation for Medical Education and Research. All rights reserved.)

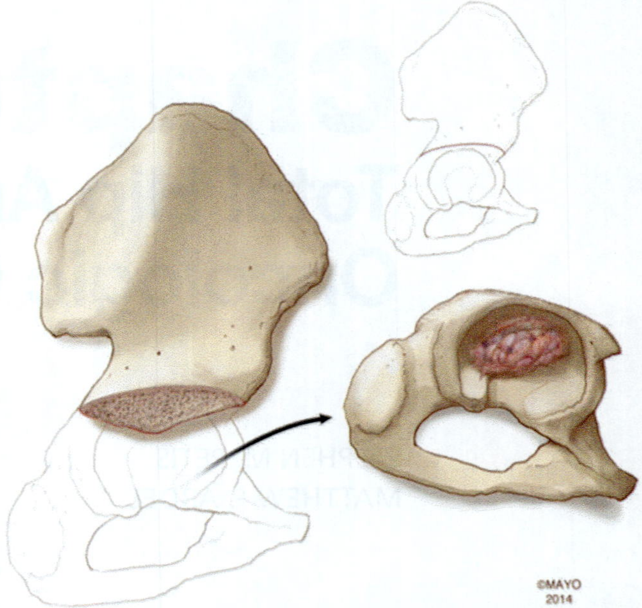

Figure 20.2 | Illustration depicting a Mayo type II supra-acetabular resection mandating a large acetabular reconstruction on the ilium. (Used with permission of Mayo Foundation for Medical Education and Research. All rights reserved.)

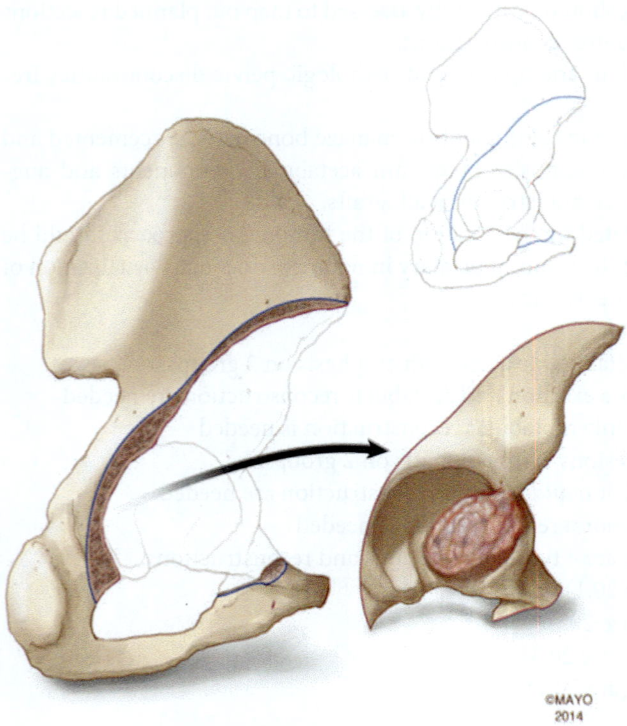

Figure 20.3 | Illustration depicting a Mayo type III resection where the posterior column is preserved and utilized for the acetabular reconstruction. (Used with permission of Mayo Foundation for Medical Education and Research. All rights reserved.)

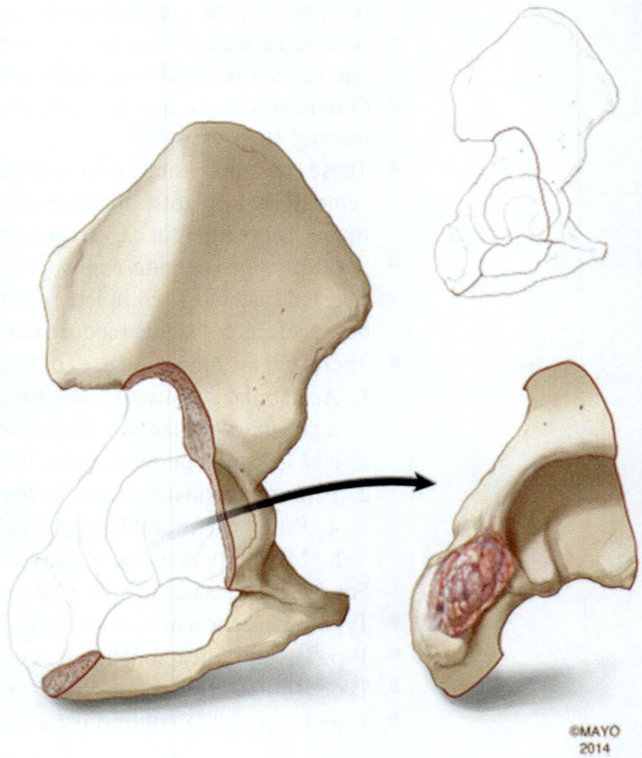

Figure 20.4 | Illustration depicting a Mayo type IV resection where the anterior column is preserved and utilized for the acetabular reconstruction. (Used with permission of Mayo Foundation for Medical Education and Research. All rights reserved.)

- Metal-cutting burr
- 6.5-mm burr
- Flexible reamers to bypass complex defects during femoral preparation
- Intraoperative imaging
- 3.5-mm drill bit

Acetabular Implants

- Allograft bone
- Highly porous metal acetabular component
- Highly porous metal augments
- Supplemental acetabular cages for cup-cage constructs
- Cementless or cemented femoral components
- Megaprostheses
- Occasionally, a custom acetabular component will be required (see Section II-D, Chapter 6).

Femoral Implants

- Cemented stems of various lengths are needed depending on the location of the metastatic disease.
- Modular, fluted tapered stems of various lengths and diameters can be utilized for primary lesions requiring proximal resection.
- Megaprostheses with either cemented or uncemented distal fixation can be considered for primary lesions requiring proximal resection.

Positioning

- Lateral decubitus position

Surgical Approaches

- A posterolateral or anterolateral approach may be appropriate for most periacetabular lesions requiring acetabular reconstruction, as well as most femoral reconstructions.
- More complex surgical approaches, such as an extended iliofemoral approach, may be required for more extensive bone resections and acetabular reconstructions.

Preoperative Planning

- The anteroposterior (AP) pelvis, AP hip, and lateral hip radiographs are used for preoperative templating (Figure 20.5A-C). This includes identifying the location of tumor, planning for management of bony deficiencies, and anticipating implant choice and sizes of implants.
- Judet views can supplement standard radiographs to determine the bone stock available for acetabular fixation, as well as the presence of pelvic discontinuity (Figure 20.5D and E).
- Cross-sectional imaging, including computed tomography, magnetic resonance imaging, and positron emission tomography (PET) scans (Figure 20.5F and G), can be helpful in planning resection and/or acetabular reconstruction.

Bone/Implant/Soft Tissue Techniques

- Surgical approach is dictated by the location of the tumor, planned resection, as well as the surgeon's preference. The approach should allow adequate visualization of the acetabulum and femur for reconstruction, while permitting access to bone tumors for resection if necessary.
- The hip is dislocated and a femoral neck osteotomy is made based on preoperative templating.
- The acetabulum is exposed. Adequate exposure is critical to assess bone deficiency caused by pathological bone loss or bone loss due to tumor resection.
- At this point, the reconstructive surgeon should identify remaining bone, as well as the quality of that bone.

Cup-Cage Construct

- Standard acetabular reaming of host bone is performed in an effort to obtain capture of the socket within remaining intact portions of the acetabulum.
- Oftentimes, supplemental acetabular augments will be needed superiorly and/or medially (Figure 20.6A-C) to make up for large acetabular defects.
- These are secured to host bone with supplemental screws if placed superiorly. If metal augments are placed medially, the acetabular component is placed against the augments and unitized to them with bone cement.

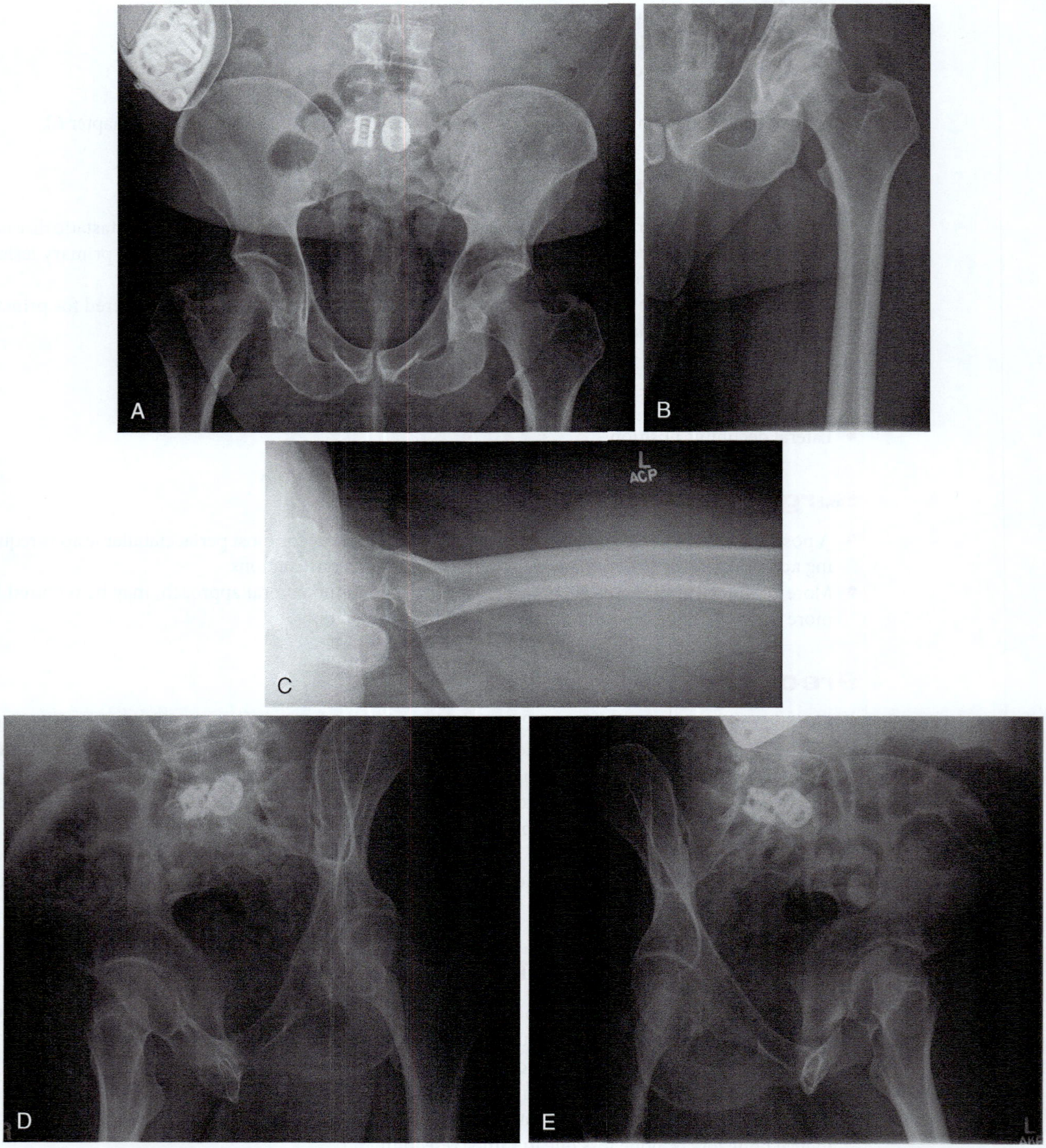

Figure 20.5 | AP pelvis (A), AP hip (B), and cross-table (C) lateral radiographs of a 44-year-old man with a large left periacetabular lesion secondary to metastatic adenoid cystic carcinoma. Judet radiographs, including an obturator oblique (D) and iliac oblique (E), were suspicious for a pelvic discontinuity. The large periacetabular lesion was confirmed on PET scans (F and G).

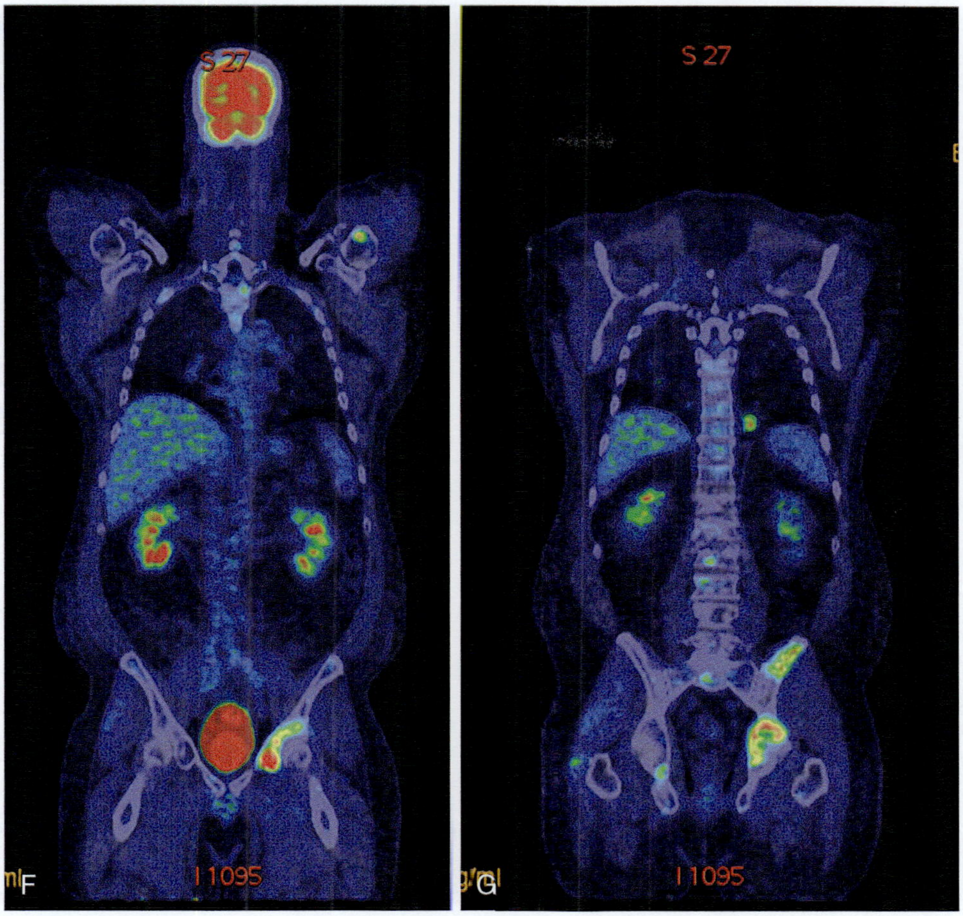

Figure 20.5—Cont'd

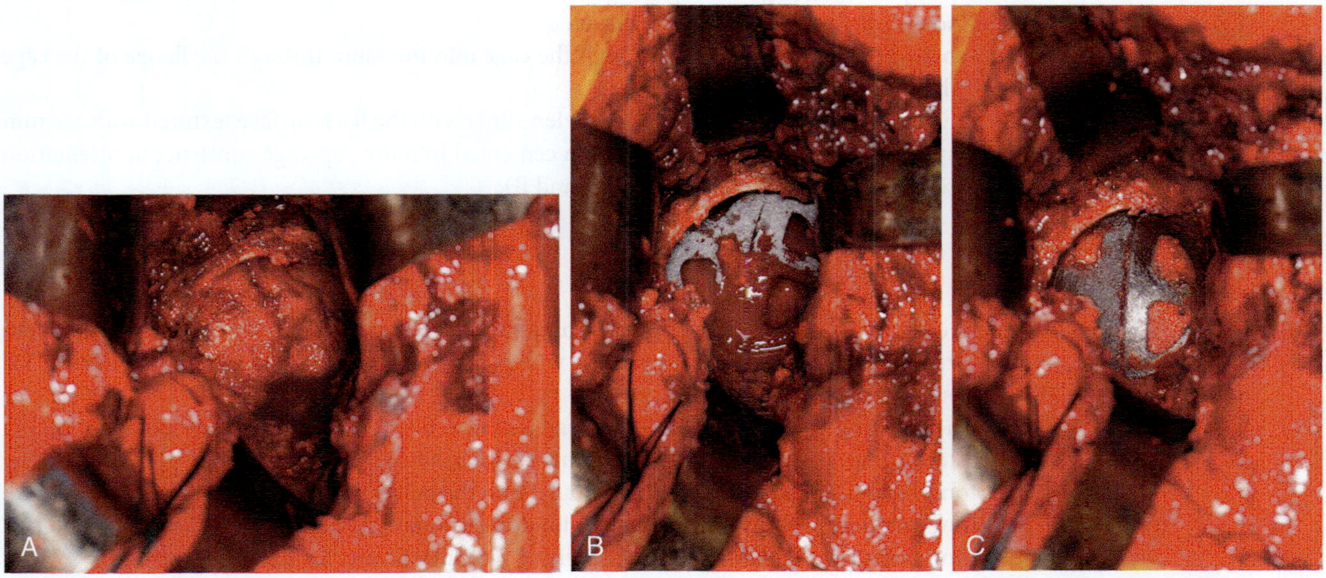

Figure 20.6 | Intraoperative images of the patient from Figure 20.5 with a pathologic pelvic discontinuity (A) treated with 2 medial augments (B) and allogenic bone graft (C) before implantation of an acetabular component.

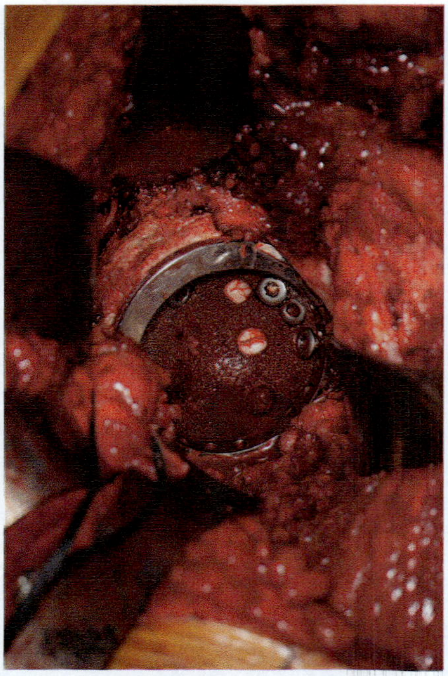

Figure 20.7 I Intraoperative image of the patient from Figure 20.5 after placement of a highly porous acetabular component with supplemental screw fixation.

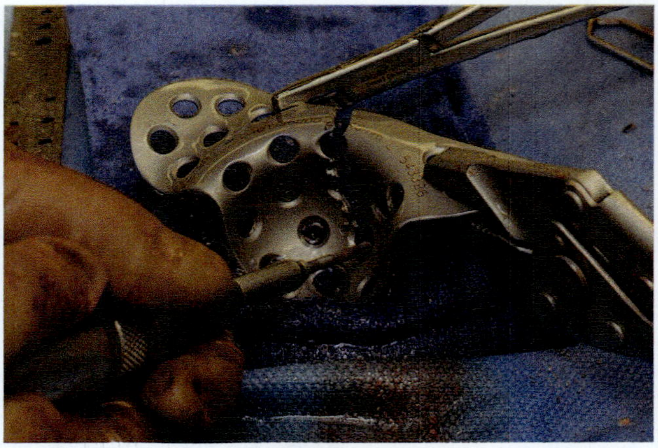

Figure 20.8 I Intraoperative image of the patient from Figure 20.5 showing a supplemental cage having the inferior flange removed.

- After the acetabular component is placed, supplemental cup fixation screws are placed superiorly and inferiorly (Figure 20.7).
- Thereafter, a supplemental cage (usually "half-cage" with the ischial flange removed; Figure 20.8) is placed over the acetabular component. The ischial flange can be removed with a metal cutting burr. This is utilized if there is not excellent primary capture of the acetabular component that provides rigid stability, if there is >40% bone loss due to the periacetabular lesion (regardless of primary implant stability), and/or if there is notably compromised acetabular bone quality due to the periacetabular lesion and/or adjuvant treatment such as pelvic radiation.
- Before cage placement, one screw may be removed from the acetabular component. Subsequently a screw may be placed through the cage, and the acetabular component, and into host bone (following the same screw track) to unitize the construct.
- About 3 to 4 screws are then placed through the cage into the ilium through the flange of the cage above the hemispherical cup.
- An all-polyethylene cup or a modular polyethylene liner with the back surface textured with a 4-mm burr in a spiderweb pattern for cement is then cemented into the cup-cage construct in orientation to optimize hip stability (Figure 20.9, 20.10A and B).

Custom Components

- Although custom constructs are not the senior author's preferred construct because bone loss and quality varies at the time of surgery in patients with periacetabular lesions, there is a growing role for custom constructs (Figure 20.11).
- After the acetabulum is reamed, prominent bone is removed with a 6.5-mm burr to allow optimal fit of the custom component using a sterile 3-dimensional model as a guide.
- The custom acetabular component is then rotated into the pelvis underneath the abductors.
- The custom component is fixed to the ilium with dome compression screws and then to the inferior ischium and pubis (if present), and then remaining proximal screws are placed in the ilium.
- Initially, cancellous screws are utilized to compress the implant to the bone.
- Thereafter, locking screws are placed in the remaining holes.
- Usually, 9 to 13 screws are utilized (Figure 20.12A-D).

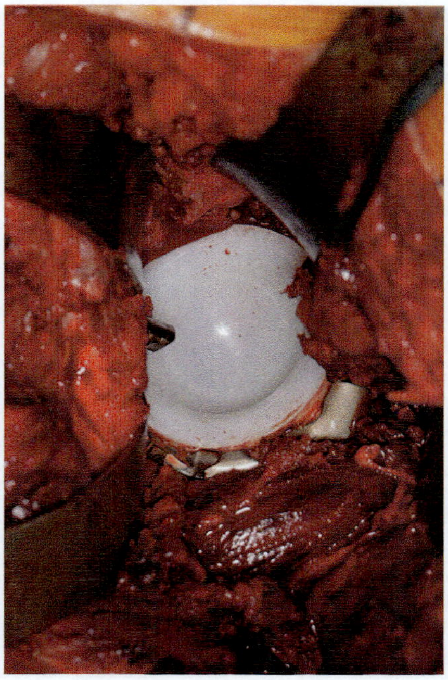

Figure 20.9 I Intraoperative image of the patient from Figure 20.5 after a polyethylene liner is cemented into place.

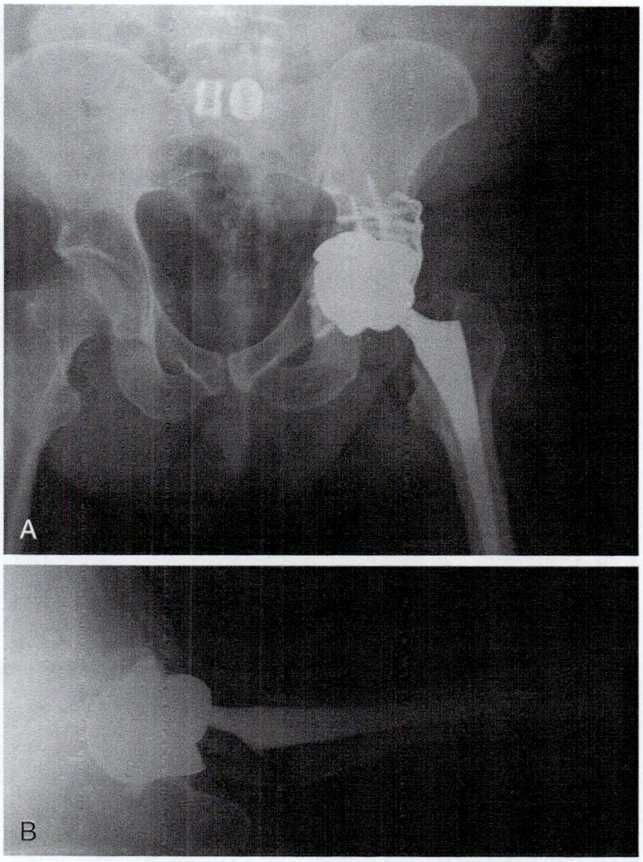

Figure 20.10 I Postoperative AP (A) and lateral (B) radiographs of the patient from Figure 20.5.

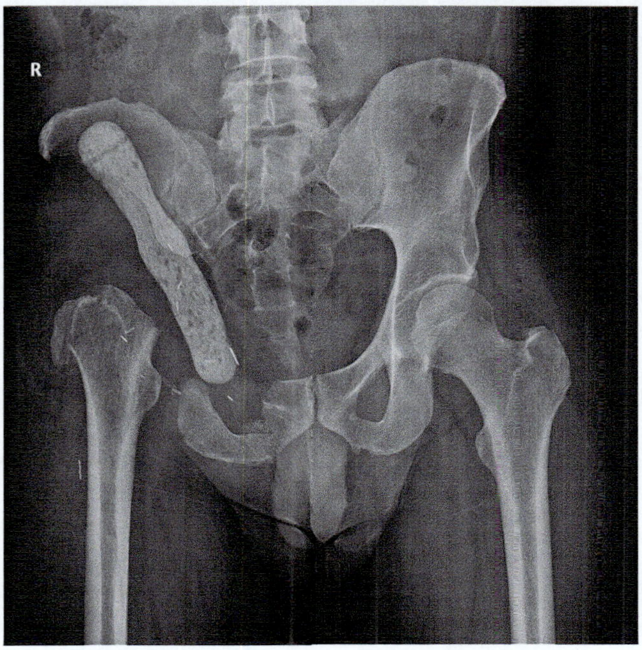

Figure 20.11 I AP radiograph of a 43-year-old man after a large internal hemipelvectomy for chondrosarcoma that was not amenable to a cup-cage construct. As such, a cement spacer was fashioned and a custom acetabular component was fabricated and subsequently implanted 4 months later.

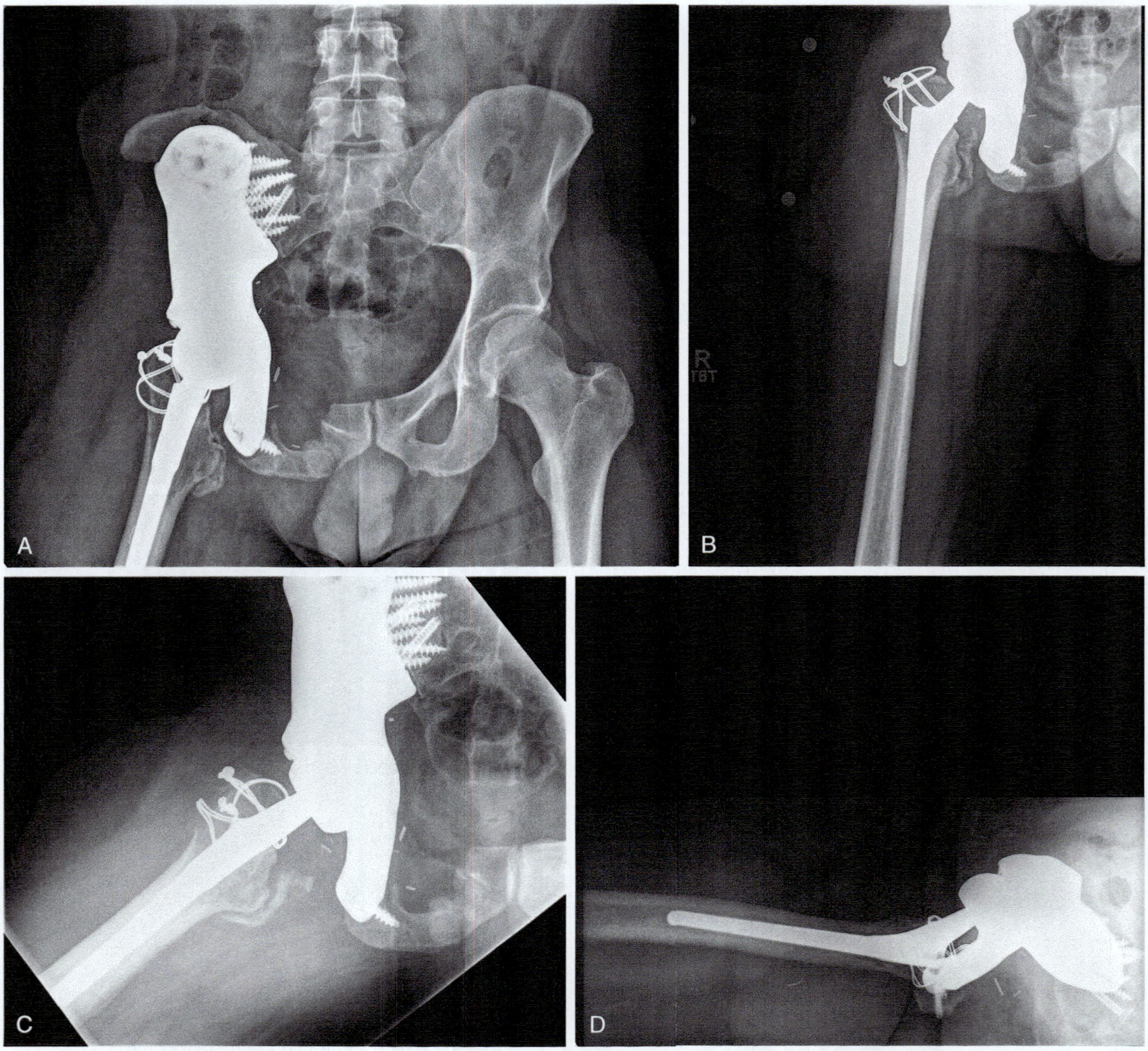

Figure 20.12 | Postoperative AP pelvis (A), AP hip (B), oblique (C), and lateral (D) radiographs of the patient from Figure 20.11 after implantation of the custom acetabular component.

Femoral Reconstruction for Metastatic Lesions

- In most cases that involve metastatic disease of the femur, a cemented stem is the best option to mitigate the risk of intraoperative periprosthetic femur fracture while also allowing immediate full weight bearing without concern for subsidence or failure of biologic fixation (Figure 20.13).
- For metastatic lesions that are proximal, a standard-length cemented stem can be utilized with a cement plug, but without pressurization of the canal.
- Typically the metastatic lesion is not removed.
- For metastatic lesions that are distal or encompass the entire femur, a long and curved cemented stem can be utilized. However, the patient must be well hydrated by the anesthesia team, on 100%

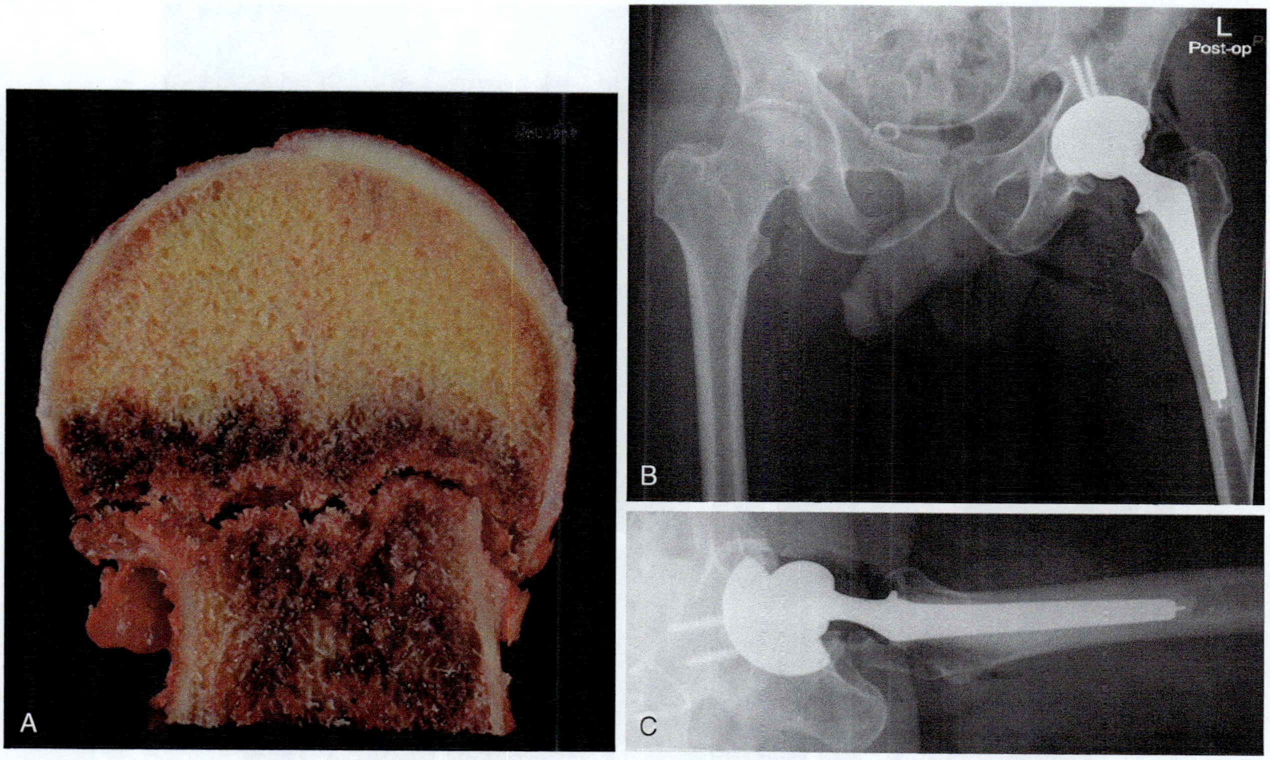

Figure 20.13 | A 61-year-old man with metastatic disease and a left pathologic femoral neck fracture (A) treated with a hybrid total hip arthroplasty (B and C).

FiO_2, and the distal femur should be vented with a 3.5-mm drill hole to reduce the risk of fat embolism syndrome in this situation.

- Moreover, the cement should be placed in the canal very wet and via a cement gun with a long cement nozzle. If the femoral canal diameter is small, a small-diameter nozzle (such as a cement nozzle for cementing humeral prostheses) may be used.
- The canal should not be pressurized.
- Occasionally, when the femoral canal has been violated of cancellous bone, modular, fluted tapered stems may be utilized for the femoral reconstruction (Figures 20.14 and 20.15).

Femoral Reconstruction for Primary Lesions

- After an adequate oncologic resection for primary lesions in the proximal femur, femoral reconstruction is reliant on distal fixation.
- For Dorr A and B bone, a modular, fluted tapered stem or uncemented proximal femoral replacement may be utilized.
- For Dorr C bone, a cemented proximal femoral replacement may be utilized, although frequently a modular, fluted tapered stem can be utilized for these canals as well.
- Regardless of stem choice, an attempt should be made to fix the remaining greater trochanter to the lateral aspect of the prosthesis with the use of wires or heavy nonabsorbable sutures.
- If the trochanter is compromised, high-stability bearings, such as a dual-mobility construct can be utilized.

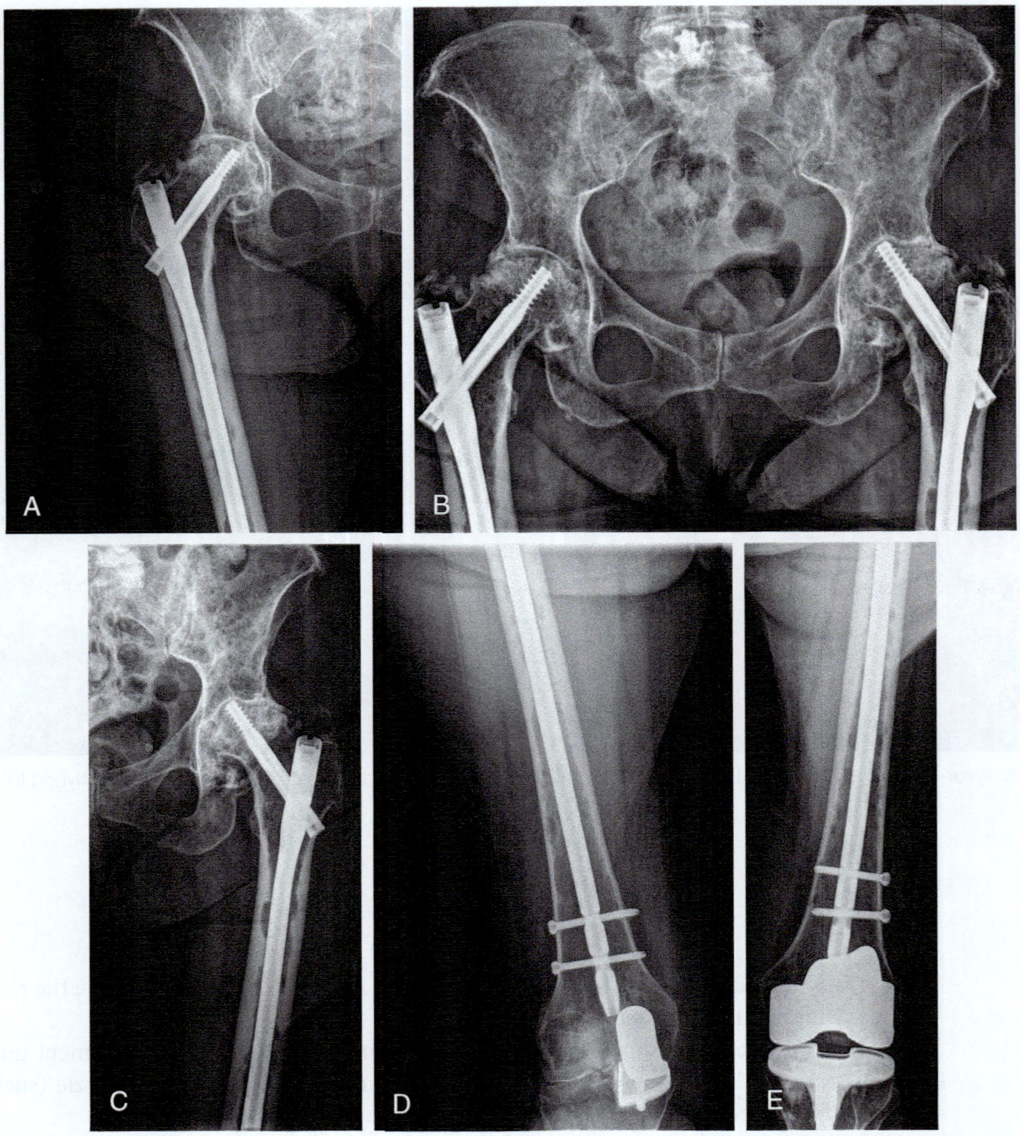

Figure 20.14 I Preoperative imaging (A-E) of a 73-year-old woman with advanced multiple myeloma treated with bilateral prophylactic cephalomedullary nails who now presents with end-stage arthritis of both hips.

Postoperative Care

- Based on the bony resection and fixation of the acetabular component, some patients will be weight bearing as tolerated. However, most patients are toe-touch weight bearing for 8 to 12 weeks postoperatively.
- Given the high risk of dislocation with such acetabular reconstructions, most patients are placed in an abduction brace for 6 weeks postoperatively.

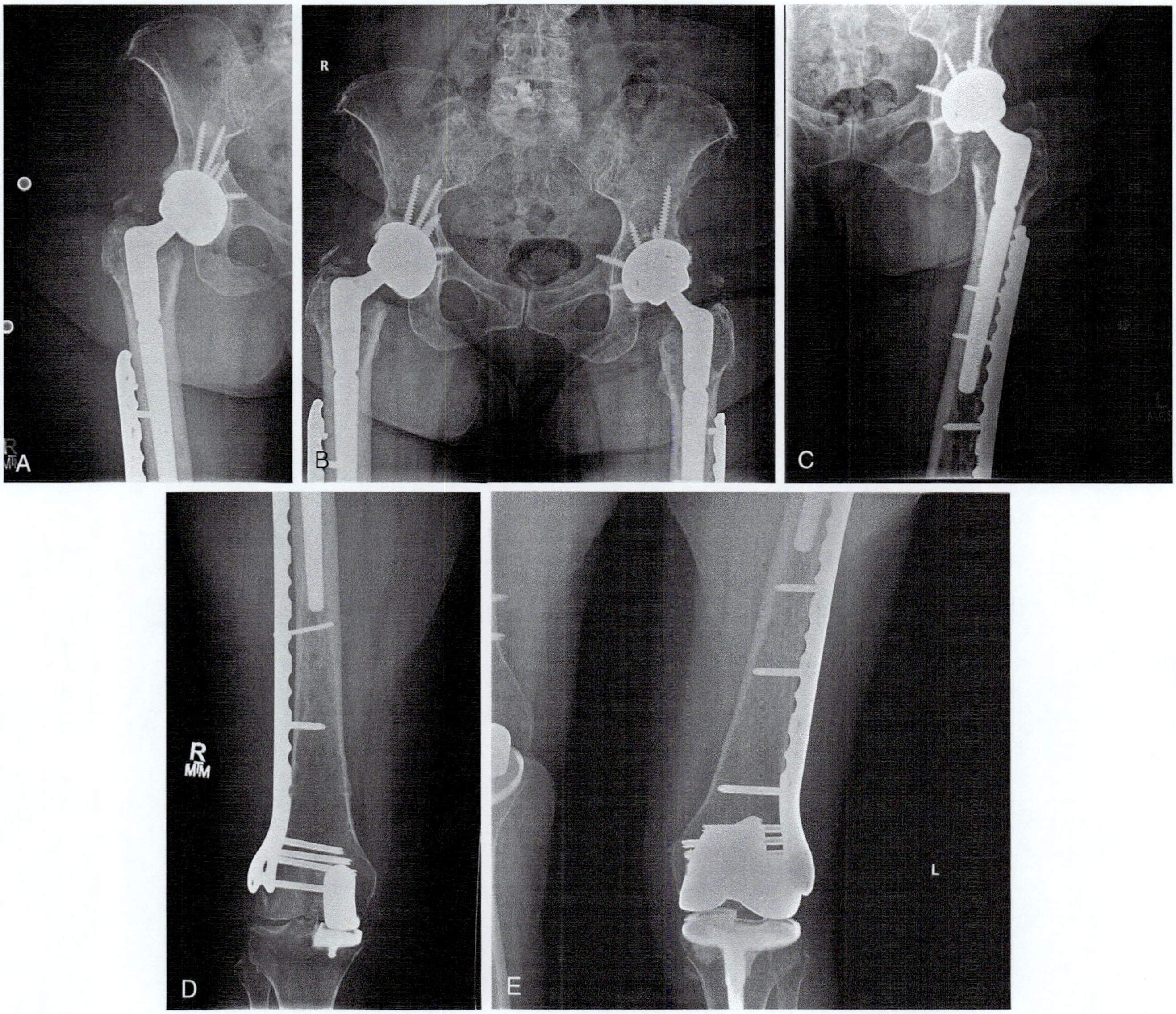

Figure 20.15 | The above patient was treated with staged bilateral conversion to total hip arthroplasties with modular fluted tapered stems and prophylactic plating of both femora (A-E).

Suggested Reading

1. Brown TS, Salib CG, Rose PS, Sim FH, Lewallen DG, Abdel MP. Reconstruction of the hip after resection of periacetabular oncological lesions: a systematic review. *Bone Joint Lett J*. 2018;100-B(1 Supple A):22-30.
2. Abdel MP, von Roth P, Perry KI, Rose PS, Lewallen DG, Sim FH. Early results of acetabular reconstruction after wide periacetabular oncologic resection. *J Bone Joint Surg Am*. 2017;99(3):e9.
3. Sculco PK, Ledford CK, Hanssen AD, Abdel MP, Lewallen DG. The evolution of the cup-cage technique for major acetabular defects: full and half cup-cage reconstruction. *J Bone Joint Surg Am*. 2017;99(13):1104-1110.
4. Viste A, Perry KI, Taunton MJ, Hanssen AD, Abdel MP. Proximal femoral replacement in contemporary revision total hip arthroplasty for severe femoral bone loss: a review of outcomes. *Bone Joint Lett J*. 2017;99-B(3):325-329.

Part II
Revision Total Hip Arthroplasty

Chapter 21
Preoperative Evaluation, Planning, and Templating for Revision Total Hip Arthroplasty

STEPHEN M. PETIS
DANIEL J. BERRY

Preoperative Evaluation

- Create a differential diagnosis for possible etiologies that explain the cause of total hip arthroplasty (THA) failure, and use patient history, physical examination, and investigations to determine the most likely diagnosis.
- Anticipate challenges related to exposure, implant removal, bone reconstruction, and hip instability.
- The goal is to treat the cause of failure, while minimizing further complications. A successful revision THA will have well-fixed implants in good position, bone deficiencies have been addressed, and a hip can move through a functional range of motion without subluxating or dislocating, while avoiding complications of the revision operation.
- Use templating to determine which implants provide the best reconstruction options and also to determine anticipated implant sizes. Use templating to predict intraoperative challenges and solutions to problems such as bone deficiencies and bone deformities.

History

- Understand the indication for the initial surgery (i.e., primary osteoarthritis, posttraumatic arthritis), as this may help predict reasons for failure.
  - Was there a period of time when the hip was functioning well and pain-free? If not, rule out periprosthetic joint infection as a cause for ongoing pain.
  - Elicit any history of hip instability and any previous treatment attempts (i.e., closed or open reductions).
  - The location of the patient's pain may help delineate which implant has failed—groin and buttock pain most commonly is associated with a failed acetabular component or synovitis, whereas thigh pain most commonly is associated with a failed femoral component.
- Obtain and review previous operative reports.
- Obtain "stickers" to confirm brand and size of implants in place.

Physical Examination

- Inspect the patient's gait—look for signs of antalgia or a Trendelenburg or Duchenne gait suggestive of abductor insufficiency. Evaluate abductor strength to help detect insufficiencies.

- Inspect old surgical incisions: are there any signs of infection? If there are multiple incisions, choose the one that will allow treatment of as many problems as possible and provide the most intraoperative flexibility.
- Evaluate and document hip range of motion.
- A painful resisted straight leg raise often is associated with hip pathology.
- Evaluate and document neurovascular status, particularly the sciatic nerve.
- Rule out any preexisting lumbar spondylosis or radiculopathy, as well as pelvic or intra-abdominal pathology that may cause referred pain to the hip.

Radiographs

- Obtain anteroposterior pelvis views and anteroposterior with shoot-through lateral views of the involved hip. Make sure radiographs are of sufficient scope to show the entire hip prosthesis and any bone likely to be instrumented during the revision surgery.
- Judet views are useful in assessing acetabular bone loss and to assess for pelvic discontinuity (Figure 21.1).
- A computed tomography scan with metal suppression can be a helpful adjunct to assessing bone deficiencies.
- Magnetic resonance imaging with metal suppression is useful to evaluate adverse local soft tissue reactions related to wear of metal-metal bearings on taper corrosion.
- Full-length femur views should be obtained when long revision stems will be used to ensure there is no aberrant distal femur morphology or other implants distally in the femur.

Tests

- A baseline complete blood count, erythrocyte sedimentation rate, and C-reactive protein can help rule out infection.
- Arthrocentesis of the hip joint should be performed to rule out infection before further reconstruction if serologic tests are abnormal or if other factors (such as radiographic findings or unexplained

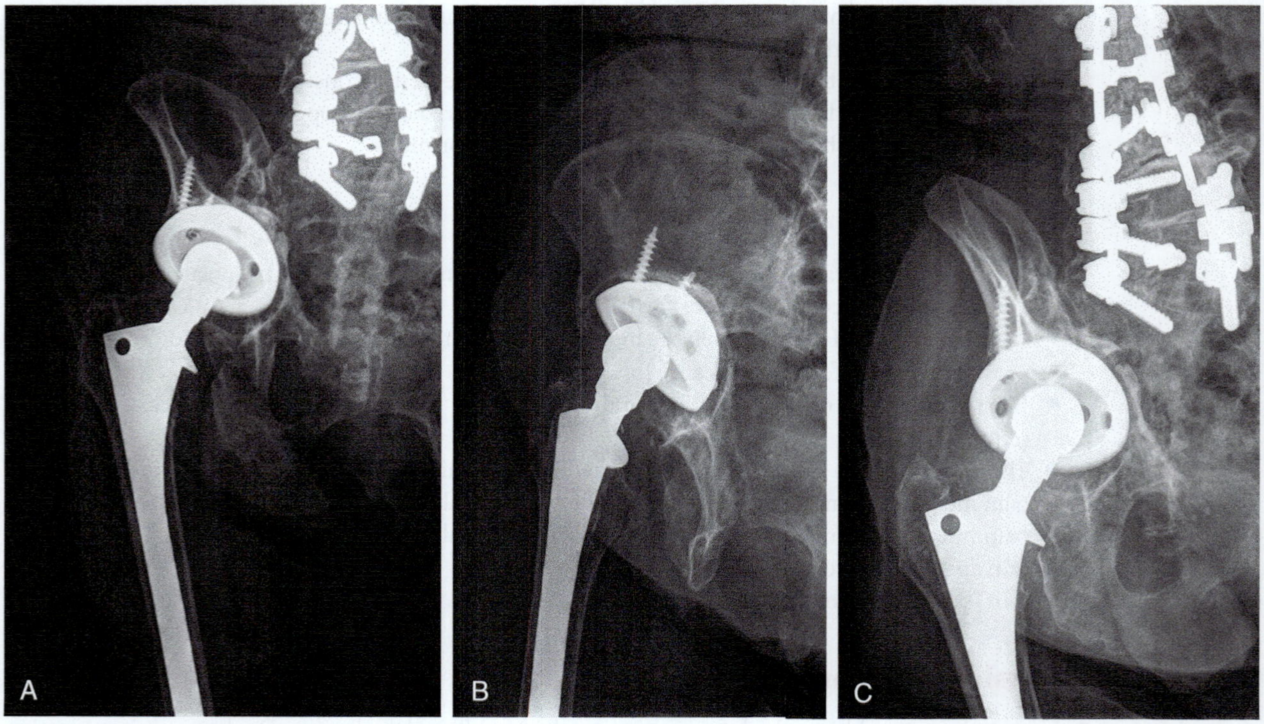

Figure 21.1 | A, Radiograph of patient with loose cup and Paprosky 3b acetabular bone loss. The anteroposterior films are not diagnostic of pelvic discontinuity, but a medial wall fracture is seen. B, C. Judet oblique films of the pelvis demonstrate fractures of both the anterior and posterior columns, indicative of pelvic discontinuity.

early failure) are present. The fluid should be sent for culture, cell count, and differential. If adverse local soft tissue reaction to metal is suspected, a manual cell count and differential should be performed because automated cell counts are unreliable in these circumstances.

- Nucleated cell count >3000; polymorphonuclear neutrophil (PMN) >80% → suggestive of chronic periprosthetic joint infection (PJI).
- Nucleated cell count <10,000; PMN >90% → suggestive of acute PJI.
- Synovial fluid alpha defensin may provide further information about infection in equivocal circumstances.

Preoperative Planning

- It is imperative to anticipate unforeseen complications at the time of surgery. Ensure that implants are available that can address varying levels of complexity (i.e., hip constraint, length of femoral stems, head and liner options, cup fixation, metal augments).
- Operative approach: the workhorse approaches for revision THA are either the posterolateral or anterolateral approach.
- Implant removal: ensure extraction devices are available, and be prepared to utilize extensile exposures.
  - Femur: high-speed burr, Moreland osteotomes, ultrasonic instruments to remove cemented implants, metal cutting burr to section stems, trephines to remove distally well-fixed uncemented stems.
  - Cup: Acetabular size-specific self-centering, curved osteotome system, screws to disengage polyethylene inserts.

Bone Reconstruction

- Femur—reconstruction depends on the quality of the proximal metadiaphyseal bone, the femoral isthmus, and defects left over from implant removal.
  - Typically a diaphyseal-engaging stem is preferred, with proximal modularity to address limb length and femoral offset.
  - Presently, many surgeons favor modular fluted-tapered stems.
  - Other options include conical stems, cement-in-cement technique when the cement mantle remains well fixed, proximal femoral replacement, and allograft prosthetic composites.
- Acetabulum—requires careful preoperative and intraoperative assessment of remaining bone.
  - Key is to optimize host bone contact to avoid creating further bony defects and to optimize the center of hip rotation.
  - Generous supplemental screw fixation is recommended in the revision setting.
  - Constructs include multihole shells, highly porous multihole shells, cup-cage constructs, custom triflange constructs, and allograft reconstruction.

Hip Stability

- Anticipate when there is likely a need for an increased level of constraint.
- Minimize damage to the abductor muscles during exposure.
- Be critical of implant position (femoral and acetabular version and cup abduction angle).
- Ensure there is no intra-articular or extra-articular impingement (femoral neck, malunited bone, heterotopic bone).
- Modularity: head length options, femoral and liner offset options, lipped/face-changing liners, dual-mobility implants, constrained liners.

Closure

- Osteotomies should be anatomically reapproximated to optimize healing, hip biomechanics, and implant fixation.
- Posterior approach: joint capsule should be reapproximated to bone to mitigate postoperative instability.
- Lateral approach: sturdy anatomic repair of the abductors is critical to optimize hip function and reduce the risk of postoperative instability.

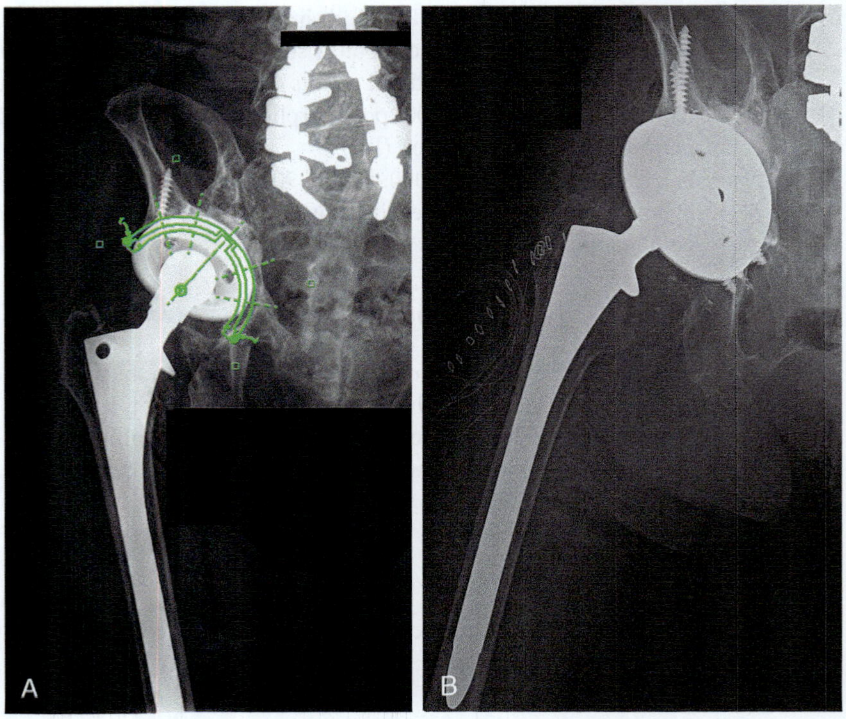

Figure 21.2 | A, Templating of the acetabular component of the same patient as in Figure 21.1 for a large hemispherical cup. B, Postoperative radiograph of the same patient demonstrating reconstruction similar to that planned on the radiograph. Because a pelvic discontinuity was present and a distraction technique was utilized, the cup diameter was slightly larger than that templated.

Templating

- Acetabulum—anticipate zones of bone loss after templating a shell that will optimize host bone contact.
  - Determine whether a hemispheric shell will be sufficient to gain implant fixation. If so, template shell size to provide good support on host bone and to optimize hip center of rotation (Figure 21.2).
  - If major bone deficiencies are present, anticipate the need for metal augments, bone grafting, or alterative reconstruction methods (Figure 21.3).
  - Use the templating methods described in Chapter 1 to optimize leg length, femoral offset, and hip biomechanics.
- Femur—anticipate length and implant diameter, attempting to engage quality host bone with cementless fixation (Figure 21.4).
  - Choose implant length based on need to bypass bone defects and based on need to engage sufficient bone for implant fixation.
  - Choose implant diameter based on fixation needs in the diaphysis to obtain an intimate fit if a diaphyseal fixation stem is being used.
  - Be mindful of offset options needed to restore hip stability.

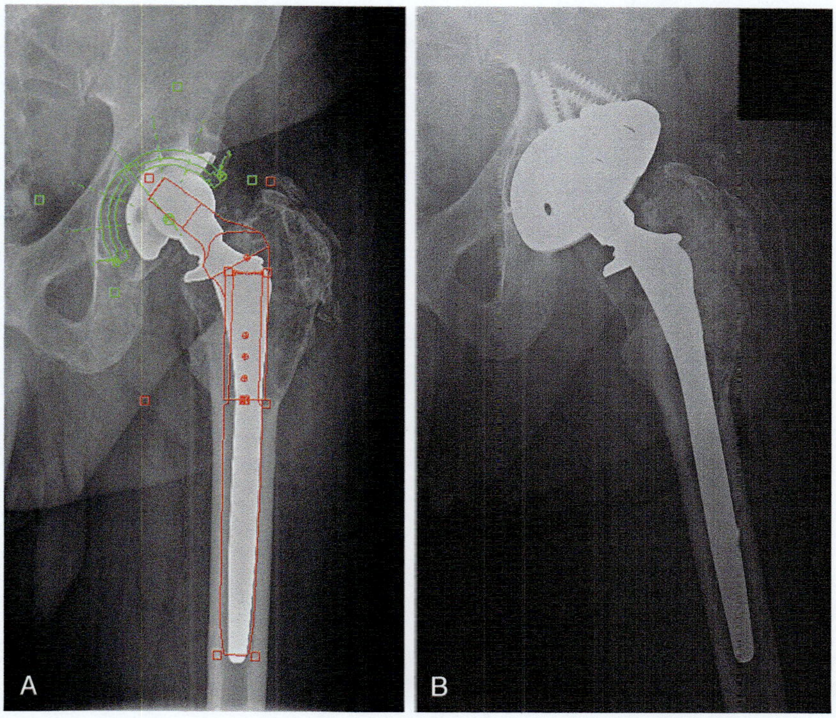

Figure 21.3 | A, Radiograph of patient with acetabular component loosening and severe osteclysis. Templating with a hemispherical cup demonstrates residual superolateral bone loss not filled by the cup. A superolateral metal augment was planned. The femur was templated for reconstruction only if required. B, Radiographs of the same patient after acetabular revision with hemispherical cup and superolateral metal augments. The femoral component was retained.

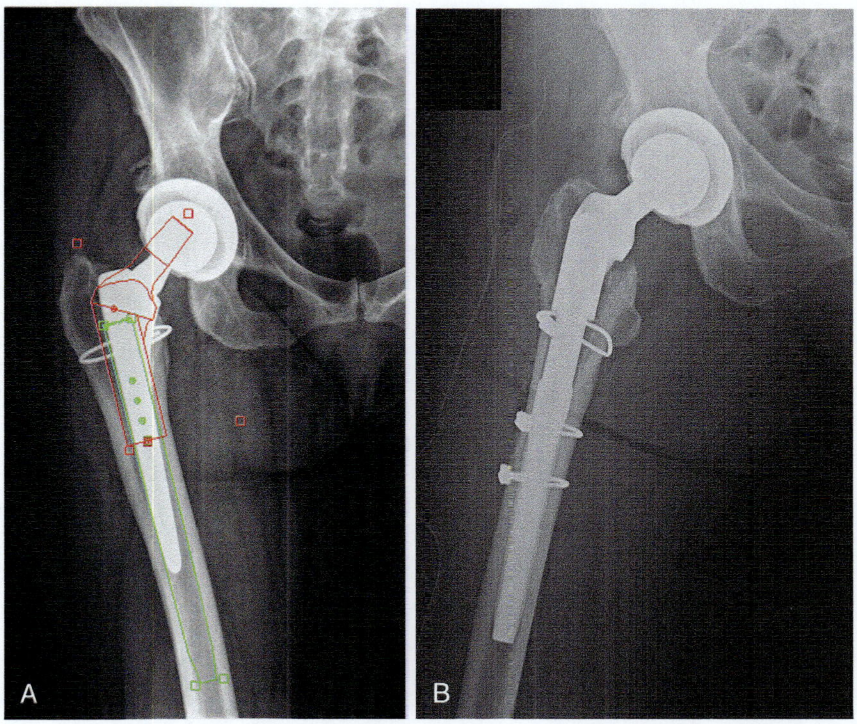

Figure 21.4 | A, Radiograph of patient with failed THA due to adverse local tissue reaction to metal corrosion of dual modular neck implant. The stem is well fixed, and an extended greater trochanteric osteotomy was planned. Templating shows planned stem length diameter and offset. Note the predicted conflict between the proximal modular stem body and proximal bone. This helped predict the need for a shorter proximal body. B, Postoperative radiograph after reconstruction with fluted tapered modular uncemented stem through an extended greater trochanteric osteotomy as planned from the preoperative templating.

Chapter 22
Choosing the Exposure

ASHTON H. GOLDMAN
MICHAEL J. TAUNTON

Key Concepts

- Choice of operative exposure in revision total hip arthroplasty (THA) has a strong influence on how well and how efficiently the rest of the procedure can be performed.
- Surgeon experience and preference plays an important role in operative approach choice.
- However, specific revision scenarios are better suited to one exposure than another.
- Each exposure has specific advantages and disadvantages in terms of how extensile the exposure is and also the risks and potential complications associated with that exposure.
- Some exposures allow conversion to a more extensile approach more easily than others.

Sterile Instruments and Implants

Instruments

- Routine hip retractors
  - Specialized hip retractors for direct anterior approach (DAA).
- A full set of revision THA instruments, including:
  - Cup explant system
  - Femoral component explant system instruments and tools
  - High-speed burrs (short and long pencil-tip burrs, 6.5-mm round burr)
  - Osteotomes (straight, curved, flexible)
  - Cement removal instruments if cement is present
  - Ultrasonic cement removal device if available and if cement is present in femur
  - Curettes
  - Cobb elevators
  - Drill, drill bits, threaded drill guides, depth gauge
- In the event of a trochanteric osteotomy:
  - Cabling device/wire passers (also for prophylactic use during femoral component revision)
  - Oscillating saw

Implants

- Highly porous revision acetabular components
- Various acetabular liner options: standard, dual mobility, constrained
- Acetabular screws
- Porous metal augments
- Acetabular cages
- Revision femoral components (with trial stems)
- Femoral heads (with trial heads)
- Cerclage cables and wires
- Allograft bone chips

Positioning

- Lateral decubitus with hip positioners or supine based on approach.
- The operative limb should be draped out and sterilely prepared from the iliac crest to the distal thigh.

Surgical Approach

- The authors typically prefer a posterolateral approach, although an anterolateral, a direct anterior, or a transtrochanteric approach may be used. This discussion on approach will be the focus of this chapter.
- A trochanteric osteotomy can facilitate femoral component removal and/or relieve tension when exposure of the ilium could risk traction injury to the superior gluteal nerve.

Preoperative Planning

Record Review

- Obtaining the outside operative report and implant stickers is essential.

Laboratory Workup

- Assess for infection preoperatively with inflammatory markers and fluoroscopically guided hip aspiration as indicated.

Imaging

- Preoperative imaging is imperative and includes the following:
  - Anteroposterior (AP) pelvic radiograph
  - AP hip radiograph
  - Cross-table lateral hip radiograph
- Additional views in cases of extreme bone loss or fracture may include the following:
  - Judet radiographs (obturator and iliac oblique views)
  - Thin-slice computed tomography (CT) scan with 3-dimensional reconstruction
- The above-mentioned imaging should be used to determine:
  - The extent and location of acetabular bone loss, including the presence of a pelvic discontinuity (separation of the ilium from the ischiopubic segment).
  - The extent and location of femoral bone loss and to determine if there is enough diaphysis to obtain a stable fixation of a revision femoral stem.

Indications

- Revision THA is appropriate in situations of symptomatic THA in which the surgeon has identified one of known THA failure modes as a reason for the failure and has a concrete plan to solve that problem.

Exposure Options: Approaches

Direct Anterior Approach

Advantages

- Some recent studies have demonstrated improved early perioperative functional recovery in the primary setting.
- The supine position allows for improved use of intraoperative fluoroscopy and assessment of leg lengths postoperatively.
- The posterior capsule and external rotators are left intact leading to improved posterior stability.
- The abductors are not cut leading to reduced chance of permanent muscle deficiency or denervation.

Disadvantages

- In revision surgery, the need for extensile exposure usually outweighs the advantages of a tissue sparing approach.
  - There are methods to make the DAA more extensile, and it may be suitable in certain revision situations.
- The neurovascular bundle to the vastus lateralis is at risk when making femoral osteotomies.
- Risk of denervation or neuropraxia of the lateral femoral cutaneous nerve and the femoral neurovascular bundle from overretraction anteriorly.

Suitable Situations

- Head and liner exchange may be performed through the DAA because a limited revision through this approach may decrease the risk of instability.
- Revision of a loose femoral stem to a diaphyseal engaging stem is possible through this approach by surgeons very experienced with the approach, but there are some caveats:
  - If the tensor fascia lata muscle is left attached to the iliac rim, exposure to the femoral canal with a straight reamer is very difficult and sometimes impossible.
  - The anterior 1 cm of the tensor fascia lata origin may be taken down off the iliac rim to allow for access to the longitudinal axis of the femoral diaphysis.
  - Others have proposed an iliac rim osteotomy.
- Removal of a well-fixed femoral stem through an osteotomy.
  - The neurovascular bundle to the vastus lateralis, which runs just distal to the lesser trochanter, must be managed while performing osteotomies.
  - The author would typically extend the approach superficially and split the fascia distally. The vastus lateralis is lifted off of the femur from the linea aspera. A Bennet retractor is placed to retract the vastus lateralis.
  - The distal aspect of the anterior limb of an extended trochanteric osteotomy is made with an oscillating saw. Then attention is turned superior to the vastus lateralis and the anterior limb is created proximally.
  - The osteotomies are connected with a narrow osteotome using care not to disrupt the neurovascular supply to the vastus lateralis. This "episiotomy" can be widened with a wide osteotome without creating a formal extended trochanteric osteotomy (ETO) (Figure 22.1).
  - Combined with a pencil tip burr and flexible osteotomes, even some well-fixed stems may be removed through this technique.
  - However, if the stem still cannot be removed, the distal limb may be made and the wide osteotomes may be used to crack the posterior cortex to complete the ETO.
  - The external rotators should be left attached to the medial limb, and the osteotomized fragment can be translated anterior-medially for access to the femur.
- Acetabular revision
  - If the tensor fascia lata muscle is released 1 to 2 cm off of the anterior iliac rim and the rectus femoris is taken off the anterior inferior iliac spine, there is considerably increased exposure to the acetabulum (Figure 22.2).
  - Exposure to the posterior column is limited.
  - Surgeons should be very familiar with revisions through traditional approaches and familiar with performing complex primaries and simpler revisions through DAA before attempting complex acetabular revisions through the DAA.

Anterolateral Approach

Advantages

- The anterolateral, Harding, Watson-Jones, or other variations of a laterally based abductor splitting approach have been employed.
- The anterolateral approach (ALA) has a demonstrated long history of a very low hip instability rate.
- The ALA has versatility, from small to very extensile exposure.
- The posterior capsule and external rotators are left intact leading to low risk of posterior hip instability.

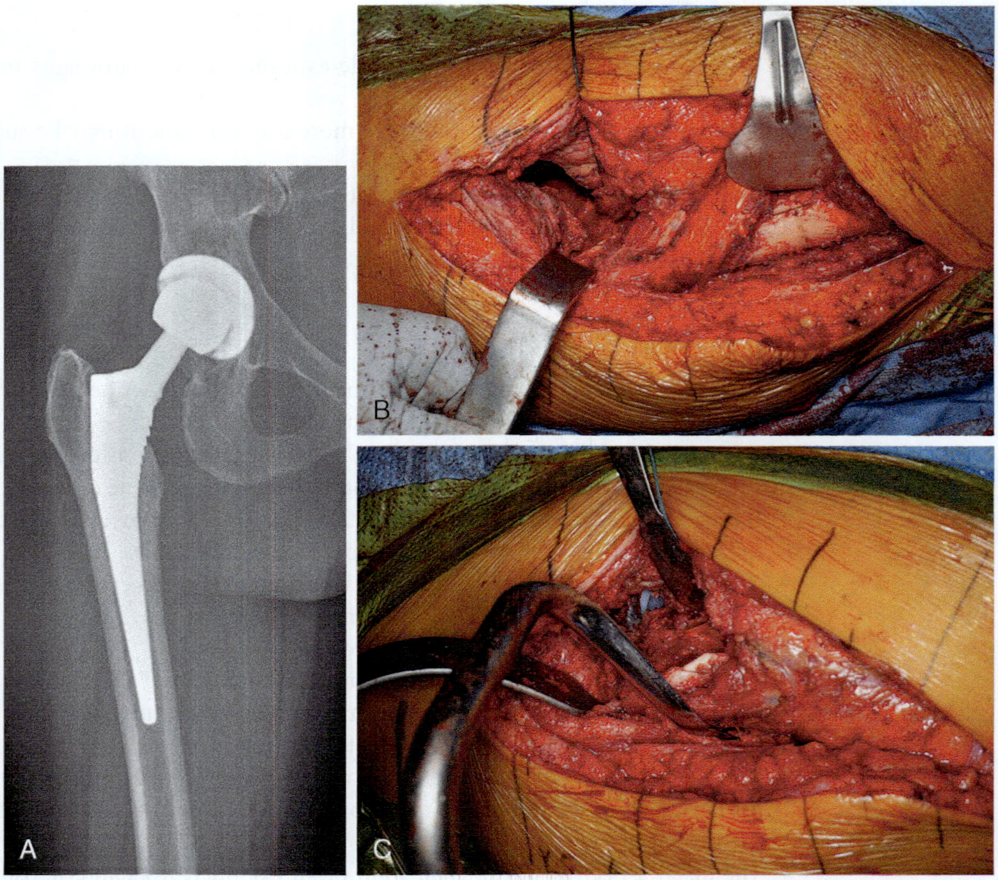

Figure 22.1 | A, AP femur radiograph demonstrating septic loosening of an uncemented hydroxyapatite-coated stem. A clinical photograph (B) demonstrates that an extensile direct anterior approach has been carried out distally. The vastus lateralis has been translated medially, while preserving its neurovascular bundle. An anterior osteotomy has been made distal and proximal and completed underneath the vastus to aid in removal of the stem. Once the stem is removed, the osteotomy can be reapproximated with a cable and the femur elevated for preparation for a diaphyseal engaging stem. A specialized table with a bed attachment hook is seen aiding in the elevation of the femur (C).

Disadvantages

- The abductors are cut leading to an increased chance of permanent muscle deficiency or denervation.
- Risk of injury to the superior gluteal neurovascular bundle when extending the abductor split proximally.
  - Typically, if the abductors are split more than 2 cm above the acetabular rim, or 5 cm or more above the tip of the greater trochanter, the surgeon should watch out for the bundle.

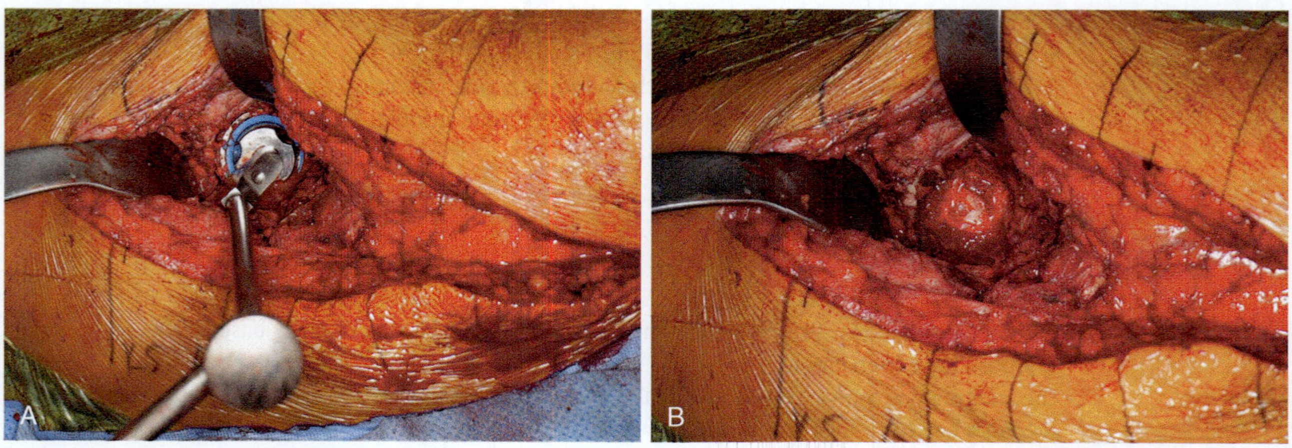

Figure 22.2 | A, Clinical photograph of the direct anterior approach with exposure of the acetabulum. The posterior retractor is directed toward the sciatic notch, and the anterior retractor is on the anterior wall below the psoas tendon to protect the femoral neurovascular bundle. The component was removed with minimal bone loss (B).

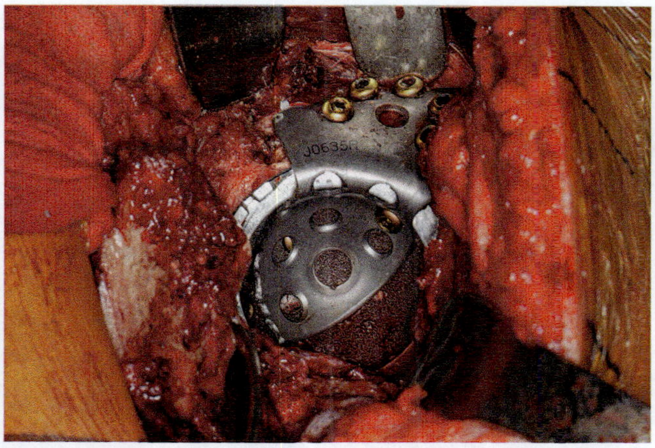

Figure 22.3 I Clinical photographs of the extensile exposure that is obtained through the anterolateral approach. Here a trabecular metal cup has been placed, with a cage that has been overlaid and fixed to the ilium superiorly.

- Risk for denervation or neuropraxia of the femoral neurovascular bundle from over-retraction anteriorly.
- Although some surgeons are able to ably manage issues with the posterior column through the ALA, most find it more difficult to directly manage posterior column fractures and defects through the ALA and would prefer the posterolateral approach (PLA) in this setting.

Suitable Situations

- Many surgeons who use the ALA as their primary approach of choice would scarcely use another approach for revision unless for certain situations.
- A complete view of the rim may be obtained without osteotomy, and there is a favorable angle achieved for screw placement in the anterior and posterior columns (Figure 22.3).
  - As mentioned previously, care must be taken to avoid injury to the superior gluteal neurovascular bundle if the exposure is extended proximally on the ilium.
- One particular situation in which we typically utilize an ALA is if we are performing a head and liner exchange or other revision where we are planning on retaining an underanteverted acetabular component where we are concerned that a PLA would lead to instability and force an acetabular component revision.
  - An overly anteverted acetabular component that is planned to be retained may be an example of a contraindication for ALA.
- Femoral revision may be carried out through the ALA favorably as well.
  - Access to the femur allows for a reasonable starting position for femoral diaphyseal preparation especially with larger amounts of anterior femoral bow.
  - An anterior-based extended greater trochanteric osteotomy (Wagner style osteotomy) goes through a similar muscular interval as the ALA but keeps muscle attached to bone.
  - However, if an osteotomy is needed after an ALA is completed, that anterior osteotomized fragment is stripped of muscle attachment.

Posterolateral Approach

Advantages

- The PLA is the workhorse revision approach the author prefers.
- It allows extensile exposure on the femoral and acetabular sides.
- PLA allows easy conversion to a femoral osteotomy on the femoral side if needed
- The abductors are not cut leading to reduced chance of permanent muscle deficiency or denervation.

Disadvantages

- The PLA has the highest risk for postoperative hip instability.
- Risk for denervation or neuropraxia of the sciatic nerve through retraction or direct injury posteriorly.

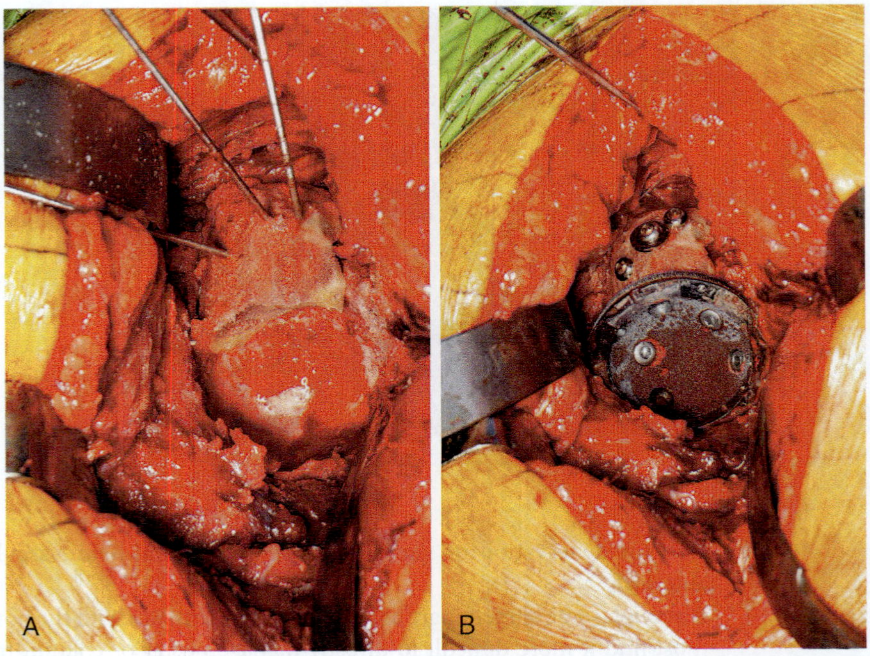

Figure 22.4 | A, Clinical photograph of the extensile exposure that is obtained through the posterolateral approach. A deficient posterior column and wall is encountered necessitating a structural femoral head allograft provisionally fixed with Steinman pins. B, A trabecular metal cup was placed with multiple screws, and the pins were exchanged for partially threaded cancellous screws.

Suitable Situations

- Many surgeons who use the PLA as their primary approach of choice would scarcely use another approach for revision expect in certain situations in which osteotomy is needed.
- The posterior column, wall, and ischium are best visualized through this approach.
- A complete view of the acetabular rim may be obtained without osteotomy, and there is a favorable angle achieved for screw placement in the anterior and posterior columns (Figure 22.4).
  - As mentioned previously, care must be taken to avoid injury to the sciatic nerve with retraction posteriorly.
- One particular situation in which we typically utilize a PLA is if we are performing a head and liner exchange or other revision where we are planning on retaining an overly anteverted acetabular component and we are concerned that an ALA would lead to instability and force an acetabular component revision.
  - An underanteverted acetabular component that is planned to be retained may be an example of a contraindication for PLA.
- Femoral revision may be carried out through the PLA favorably as well.
  - The position of the femur allows for a reasonable starting position for femoral diaphyseal preparation especially with varus femoral remodeling.
  - If a laterally based extended trochanteric osteotomy is needed to appropriately place the stem, the PLA is most conducive (Figure 22.5A-C).

Conventional Trochanteric Osteotomy

Advantages

- Allows the abductors and the greater trochanteric fragment to be reflected proximally to expose the joint and thereby protects the superior gluteal nerve.
- Can keep the posterior capsular tissues intact to the distal fragment.

Disadvantages

- Possibility of trochanteric nonunion and chronic abductor insufficiency and gait disturbance.
- Proximal migration of the trochanteric fragment is more likely than in a trochanteric slide.
- May be difficult to regain bony contact of osteotomy after femoral revision.

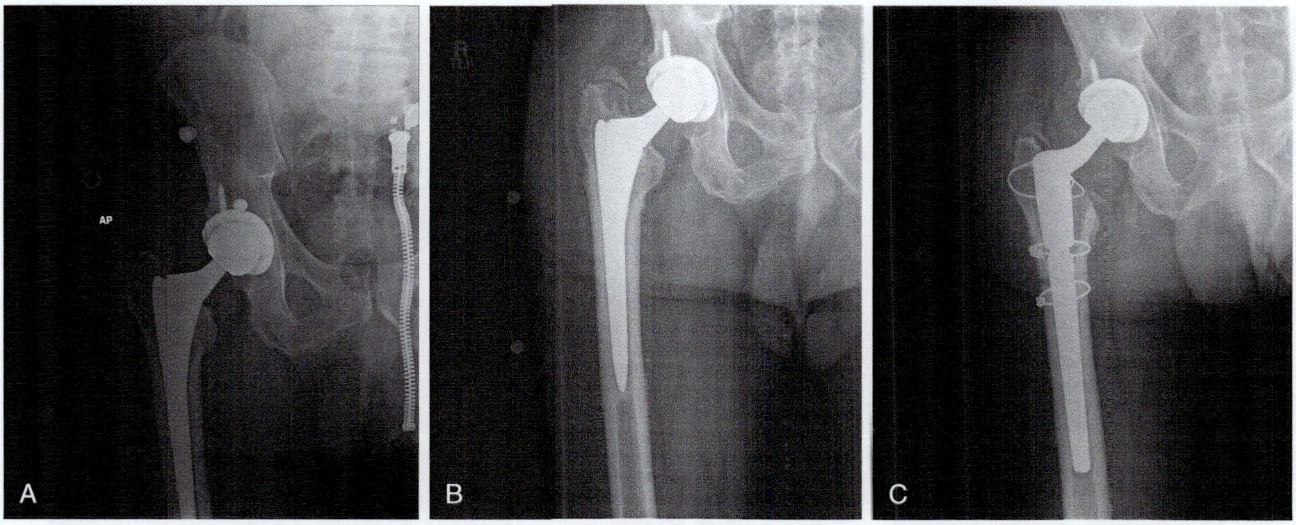

Figure 22.5 I Immediate postoperative AP femur radiograph of the right hip (A) demonstrating a dual tapered uncemented stem that is slightly undersized. At 1-year follow-up, an AP femur radiograph demonstrates the femoral component has aseptically loosened and subsided. The proximal femur has remodeled into a varus configuration, and the greater trochanter is overlying the femoral implant, preventing safe removal from the top. (B) A laterally based extended trochanteric osteotomy was performed to allow safe removal of the stem and placement of a new fluted tapered diaphyseal engaging stem as demonstrated in this postoperative AP femur radiograph. (C) Note the prophylactic cable placed distal to the osteotomy and the cable and wire utilized to fix the osteotomized fragment.

Suitable Situations

- Very useful in extremely stiff hips, as it allows immediate exposure to the entire joint from anterior to posterior.
  - Excellent for fusion take-downs or in situations of extreme heterotopic ossification.
  - Useful in some acetabular revisions when there is a need for a large exposure of the iliac face and there is risk to the superior gluteal neurovascular bundle that is not adequately managed with other techniques.

Trochanteric Slide Osteotomy

Advantages

- Allows for exposure of the joint while keeping the abductors, the greater trochanteric fragment, and the vastus lateralis in continuity.
- The approach leaves the posterior structures entirely intact.

Disadvantages

- There is a possibility of fragmentation or nonunion for the trochanteric fragment.
- Need for fixation of the trochanteric fragment to the proximal femur.
  - May be difficult to regain bone contact of the osteotomy after femoral revision.

Suitable Situations

- Useful in cases of extremely stiff hips, cases of heterotopic ossification.
- More useful in difficult primary situations.

Laterally Based Extended Trochanteric Osteotomy

Advantages

- A reliable and reproducible osteotomy providing extensile exposure to the femoral diaphysis.
- Best osteotomy for femurs with varus remodeling or excessive coronal bow (Figure 22.5).
- Low rate of nonunion.

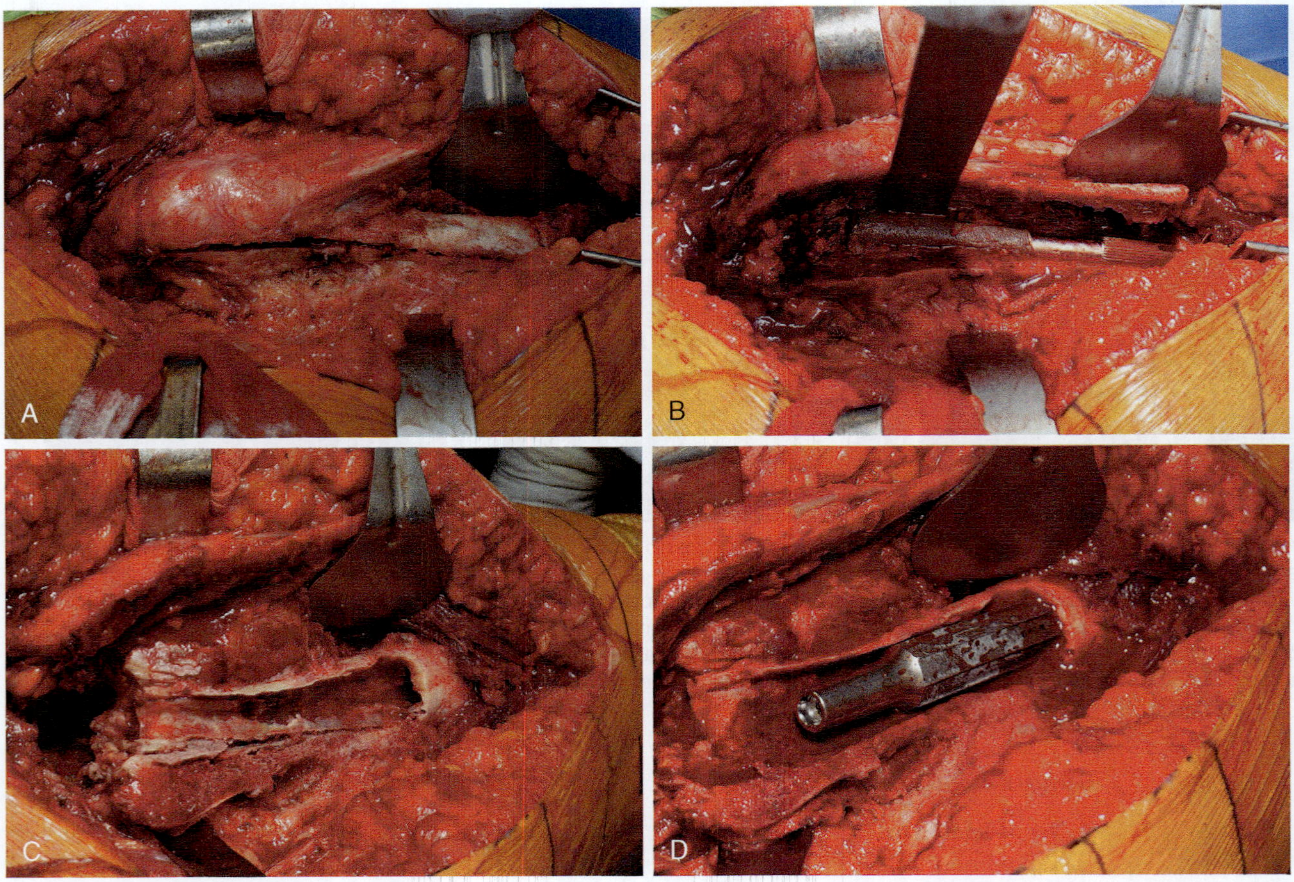

Figure 22.6 | A, Intraoperative photograph demonstrating a completed laterally based extended trochanteric osteotomy. B, Wide osteotomes are distributed along the osteotomy to perform osteoclasis on the anterior cortex and provide one large laterally based osteotomy fragment. C, The resultant osteotomy provides enhanced exposure to the acetabulum and excellent exposure to the femoral diaphysis for preparation and removal of debris. D, This intraoperative photograph demonstrates a diaphyseal engaging modular fluted tapered stem that has been placed properly with the assistance of the osteotomy. (Photos courtesy of Matthew P. Abdel, MD.)

- May be performed as part of the initial approach or after a PLA has been performed with no devascularization of bone fragment.
- Provides additional exposure to the acetabulum.

Disadvantages

- Potential for fracture of the osteotomy fragment.
  - If fracture occurs at the vastus ridge, there is a potential for trochanteric escape.
- Potential for nonunion.
- Need for reduced weight bearing while osteotomies heal.

Suitable Situations

- The laterally based ETO is particularly useful in cases of varus remodeling of the proximal femur (Figure 22.6).
  - The osteotomized fragment allows for a straight shot for placing the diaphyseal engaging stem in the mid-diaphysis.
  - The trochanter is reapproximated to the lateral aspect of the stem.
  - The proximal medial cortex may be approximated to the stem through osteoclasis.
- The laterally based ETO is the workhorse osteotomy for the removal of well-fixed uncemented and cemented stems.
  - Excellent visualization for removal of cement.
  - Complete cement removal needed in prosthetic joint infection.

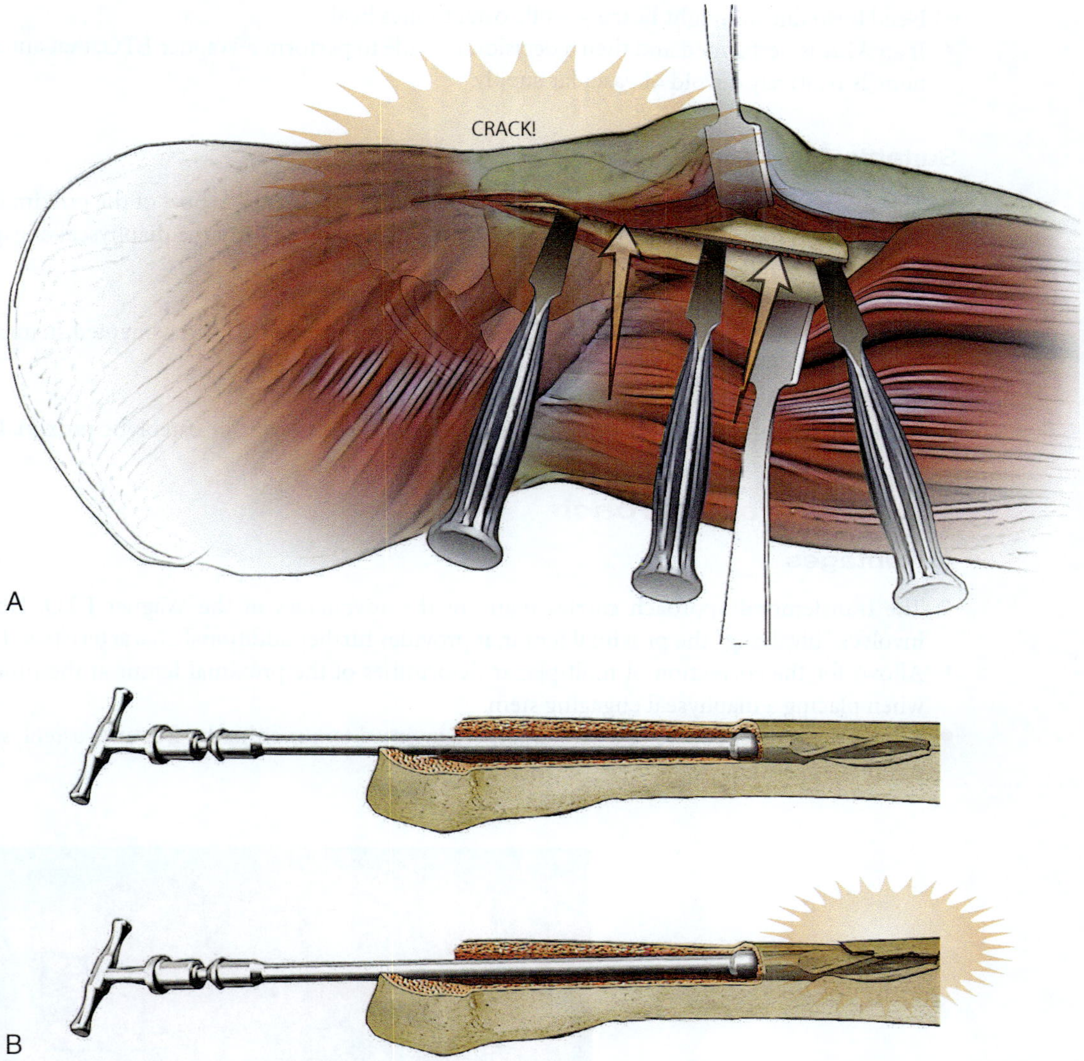

Figure 22.7 | A, Illustration demonstrating the Wagner osteotomy. The abductor mechanism is split from the mid-lateral aspect of the vastus lateralis to the middle of the abductors. The osteotomy is centered over the trochanter and is carried out from lateral to medial angling slightly anteriorly. A retractor is placed under the vastus lateralis anteriorly so that the distal osteotomy is made safely with the hip externally rotated. Osteotomes are then utilized to crack the medial cortex. B, The Wagner osteotomy is advantageous in patients with an increased sagittal bow. Surgeons must remember to raise their hand when reaming to avoid perforating the anterior cortex.

Wagner (Anterior-Based) Extended Trochanteric Osteotomy

Advantages

- A reliable and reproducible osteotomy providing extensile exposure to the femoral diaphysis.
- Best osteotomy for femurs with excessive sagittal femoral bow (Figure 22.7).
  - Direct access to the diaphysis with straight reamers.
- Low rate of nonunion.
- Provides additional exposure to the acetabulum.
  - Easy to retract the anterior femur out of the way.
- Posterior structures intact, leading to potential improvement in hip stability.
- In the case of a osteolytic femur, the Wagner ETO may be a "safer" osteotomy than the lateral ETO:
  - If the anterior piece of bone fractures, there is less downside.
  - If the lateral piece fractures in lateral ETO, more likely to lead to trochanteric escape.

Disadvantages

- Many of the same disadvantages of the ALA.
  - Need to split the abductors and the vastus lateralis. The osteotomy is basically a "bony ALA."
- Potential for fracture and/or nonunion of the osteotomized fragment.

- Need for reduced weight bearing while osteotomies heal.
- If an ALA is performed and then a decision is made to perform a Wagner ETO, that anterior piece of bone is relatively devoid of vascular supply.

Suitable Situations

- The Wagner ETO is particularly useful in cases of increased sagittal bow of the proximal femur.
  - The osteotomized fragment allows for a straight shot for placing the diaphyseal engaging stem in the mid-diaphysis.
  - Helps prevent anterior perforation of the femur.
- A workhorse osteotomy for the removal of well-fixed uncemented and cemented stems.
  - Excellent visualization for removal of cement.
  - Complete cement removal needed in prosthetic joint infection.
- Particularly useful for femoral revision in extremely osteoporotic or osteolytic proximal femora.

Transfemoral Approach

Advantages

- The transfemoral approach carries many of the advantages of the Wagner ETO. However, as it involves "bivalving" the proximal femur, it provides further additional characteristics (Figure 22.8).
- Allows for the correction of multiplanar deformities of the proximal femur at the time of revision when placing a diaphyseal engaging stem.
- Allows for wide exposure of a proximally fragmented femur either by fracture, osteolysis, infection, or other situations.

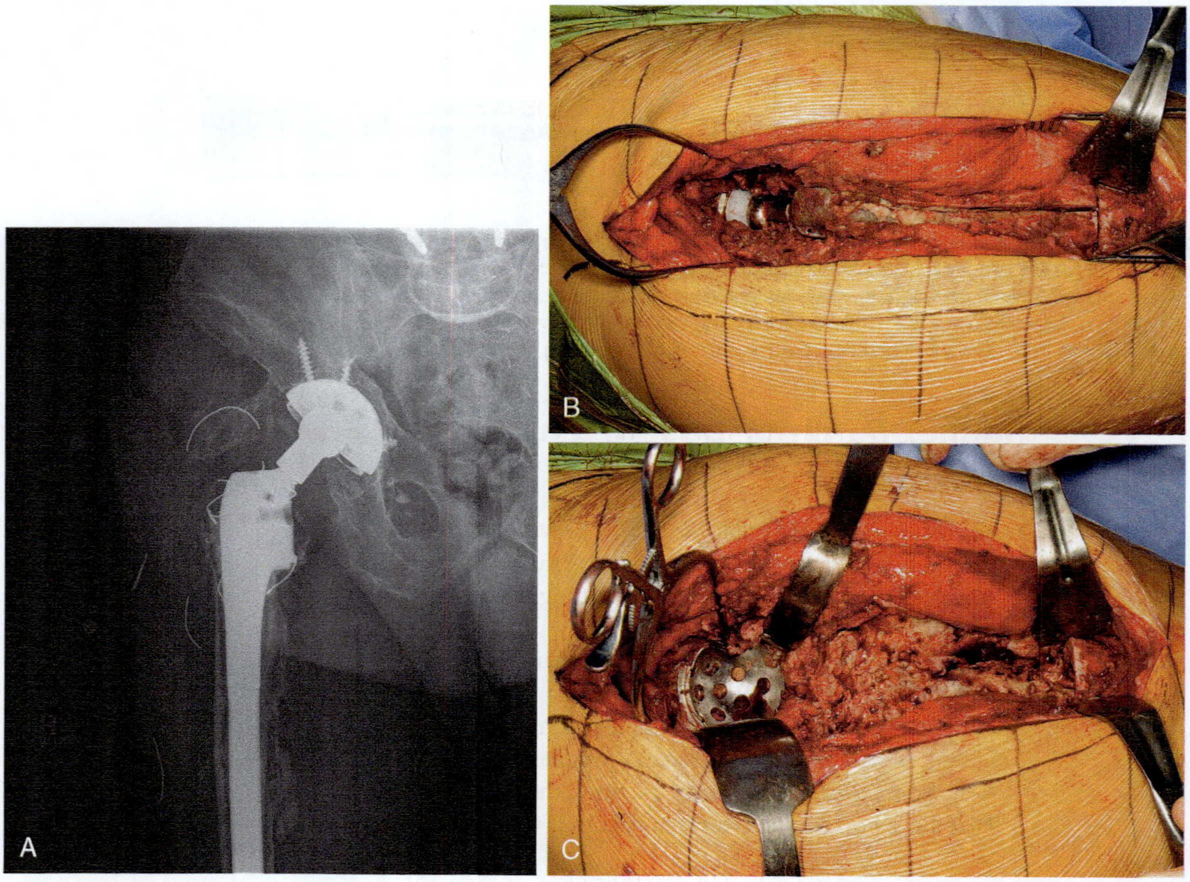

Figure 22.8 | A, AP radiograph of the proximal right femur demonstrates massive osteolysis involving the entire proximal femur. B, The greater trochanter has fractured. The only femoral implant fixation will be distal. An intraoperative photograph demonstrates the transfemoral approach to the femur. The abductors are split proximally, and the femur is split laterally to a point distally where good bone is encountered. A transverse osteotomy is made at that location. C, This provides a wide exposure of the acetabulum with maintenance of the posterior structures and continuity of the soft tissue sleeve despite the chronic greater trochanteric nonunion.

Disadvantages

- The proximal femur is completely detached from the distal femur, allowing for potential of some relative proximal fragment migration, although the tissues are typically kept as a continuous sleeve.
- Many of the same disadvantages of the ALA.
  - Need to split the abductors and the vastus lateralis.
- Potential for fracture and/or nonunion of the osteotomized fragment.
- Need for reduced weight bearing while osteotomies heal.
- If an ALA is performed and then a decision is made to perform a transfemoral osteotomy, that anterior piece of bone is relatively devoid of vascular supply.
- Situations in which a transfemoral osteotomy is needed are often situations of massive bone loss and/or soft tissue disruption. The surgeon should have concern for instability at the front of the decision-making process.

Suitable Situations

- Periprosthetic fractures of the proximal femurs with comminution. A transfemoral osteotomy and soft tissue split can be made through common planes in the fracture to provide excellent exposure for revision.
- Prior cemented THA with massive proximal femoral osteolysis indicating a proximal femoral replacement.
- Need for femoral revision with a biplanar proximal femoral deformity.
- Wide exposure in prosthetic joint infection.

Revision Scenarios

The prior operative report should be obtained before any hip revision. It is important to know the prior approach utilized as it may affect the choice of the revision approach or implant selection. Although it is important to have a plan for approach before the case, it is important to be flexible as the approach may need to change based on pathology encountered intraoperatively.

Insert Exchange for Wear/Instability

Favored Operative Approaches

- Insert exchanges typically involve little morbidity, but instability is a risk. Approaches that reduce the risk of instability for the individual patient are favored. Circumstances may be altered by the patient's prior operative approach, component positioning, spinal deformity, or other factors. However, an approach that can keep as many stabilizing structures intact as possible while safely performing the liner exchange is favored. The author prefers the direct anterior approach for most liner exchanges for favorable recovery and reduced risk for instability.
- The femoral head diameter should be maximized, and a face-changing liner may be utilized to improve stability. If stability is not achieved with liner exchange, revision of the acetabular component may be considered for improved position or to facilitate dual mobility bearing placement.

Contraindicated Approaches

- It would typically be unadvisable to do a limited liner exchange through a posterior approach with an underanteverted acetabular component or an anterolateral approach with an overanteverted acetabular component. Osteotomies typically are not required for limited exchanges.

Straight Forward Acetabular Component Revision

Favored/Acceptable Approaches

- The decision about which approach to use to perform a straight forward acetabular revision will be based primarily on the operative surgeon's preference.

- However, factors that impact that decision involve:
  - The prior operative hip approach
  - The status of the abductors
  - Position of the acetabular component being revised
  - Position of the femoral component
  - Whether the femur will or will not be revised
- If the patient had a prior anterolateral approach, and on examination the patient has abductor weakness, there are likely deficient abductors.
  - The surgeon should plan an anterolateral approach for acetabular revision and perhaps attempt an abductor repair or augmentation.
- If the patient has had a prior posterior approach, and has a fairly overanteverted femoral stem, it would be best to go back through the posterior approach,independent of the operative surgeon's preference.
- For a simple acetabular revision for failure of ingrowth, the author would consider the direct anterior approach for revision.
  - However, if there is a high likelihood that the procedure will be a complex revision (osteoporosis, osteolysis, segmental bone loss, etc.), the preference is the posterior approach.

Contraindicated Approaches

- Any approach that limits the surgeon's ability to fully expose the entirety of the acetabulum to carry out a complete acetabular revision.
- The approach should be extensile enough so that the entire rim is visualized to ensure an excellent press fit.
- As earlier, if the femoral component should be inspected.
  - Retroverted femoral stem—consider no PLA
  - Overanteverted femoral stem—consider no ALA

Complex Acetabular Revision

Favored/Acceptable Approaches

- Any extensile approach is favored for a complex acetabular revision.
- Iliac exposure:
  - The ALA can provide excellent iliac exposure, but it is important to note that the superior gluteal neurovascular bundle is at risk.
- The PLA provides excellent exposure to the posterior column and ischium and exposure for posterior plating.
- Trochanteric and all ETOs generally relieve tension off of the abductors and mobilize the femur, providing the surgeon enhanced exposure, particularly in cases in which a cage or a custom triflange is required.

Contraindicated Approaches

- Any approach that is not able to be made extensile is not appropriate for complex acetabular revision. The surgeon has to be comfortable with making the specific approaches extensile as well.
- The trochanteric slide osteotomy is not a great option for complex acetabular reconstruction, as its extensile nature is limited, and if the fragment fractures, the fixation is significantly compromised.
- Most surgeons would be advised to avoid complex acetabular revision through a DAA.

Additional Comments

Femoral Revision: Loose Stem/Mild Bone Loss

Favored/Acceptable Approaches

- The author's favored approach for a loose stem with mild bone loss is the PLA if the patient has had a prior PLA.
- The ALA or DAA would also be acceptable.

- The surgeon should be familiar with the approach used as well as the revision system as it relates to the approach.
- When reaming the diaphysis through a PLA with the femur in the usual position in a lateral decubitus position, the surgeon should drop his or her hand, to avoid damaging or perforating the anterior cortex.
- When reaming through an ALA, the surgeon should raise his or her hand to avoid the anterior cortex.

Contraindicated Approaches

- Unless there is a massive amount of cement to be removed or a femoral deformity, there should be no need for an osteotomy in these situations.

Femoral Revision: Well-Fixed Cemented Stem

Favored/Acceptable Approaches

- The author's favored approach for a well-fixed cemented stem with good bone stock is a laterally based ETO at the time of approach.
  - This allows the posterior structures to remain attached to the medial fragment of the femur, enhancing stability.
  - Osteotomy is continued at least 13 to 14 cm.
  - This aids in removing cement efficiently.
  - Further femoral preparation typically is easy through the osteotomy.

Contraindicated Approaches

- The DAA is not well suited for removal of cement.
  - It can be done, but it is much harder than a standard laterally based ETO and offers no benefit.
- A conventional trochanteric osteotomy or trochanteric slide osteotomy is contraindicated as another ETO will likely be needed to aid in cement and/or stem removal.

Femoral Revision: Well-Fixed Uncemented Stem

Favored/Acceptable Approaches

- The favored approach to revise a well-fixed stem is the PLA if the patient has had a prior PLA.
- The ALA or DAA would also be acceptable.
- The type of stem widely changes the approach.
  - Removal of a blade-type stem often does not require an osteotomy.
  - The author may use a DAA in this circumstance. Dual-tapered ream and broach stems and fully porous coated cylindrical stems are examples of stems that typically are most safely removed with an ETO.
- Usually the stem can be "worked" from above with a pencil-tipped burr, thin flexible osteotomes, specialized femoral removal osteotomes, and femoral explant tools.
- If those methods are not successful, the posterior limb (if through PLA) or anterior limb (if through DAA) of the laterally based ETO can be made with a microsagittal saw. The osteotomy is opened with a wide osteotome.
  - The implant often can then be removed with a femoral disimpactor without the need of a formal ETO.
- If that is not successful, the full osteotomy may be completed.
- If the author is planning to remove a well-fixed femoral stem and is planning on the ALA, he prefers to go straight to a Wagner osteotomy to avoid devascularizing the anterior fragment.

Contraindicated Approaches

- The direct anterior approach is best limited to removing loose stems, short stems, or blade-style stems. If there is a need to remove a long stem, or a stem that is known to be difficult to be removed, another approach is much more versatile in this situation.
- The conventional and trochanteric slide osteotomies provide no additional benefit over the extended osteotomies or approaches in the majority of situations.

Femoral Revision: With Femoral Bone Deformity

Favored/Acceptable Approaches

- In this situation, the transfemoral osteotomy is favored. This osteotomy allows for immediate correction of multiplanar deformities.
- The laterally based ETO is the favorite for correcting limited varus remodeling of the proximal femur.
- The anterior-based Wagner ETO is the favorite for accommodating limited sagittal bowing of the femur especially when utilizing diaphyseal engaging stems.

Contraindicated Approaches

- In the author's limited experience, the DAA is contraindicated in cases of femoral deformity.
- Any approach that does not accommodate for the deformity in the correct plane is contraindicated.
- The common mistake is the failure to template and thus failure to recognize that the greater trochanter is sitting over the top of the femoral canal in the case of a varus remodeling of the proximal femur. This would be an indication to consider using a laterally based osteotomy.

Bone, Implant, and Soft Tissue Techniques

- After implantation of the femoral and acetabular components a trial reduction is performed.
- An intraoperative AP pelvic radiograph is obtained to verify acceptable implants positioning and acetabular screw lengths and positions.
- Hip stability and leg lengths are assessed.
- The modular insert is placed.
- In patients with poor abductor function (denervation, detachment, or an absent greater trochanter), a constrained or dual mobility liner may be used. In other cases, large femoral head diameters are utilized.
- If a trochanteric osteotomy was done, the fragment is reduced and fixed with cables below the level of the lesser trochanter, and if needed, Luque wires above the level of the lesser trochanter.
- Wound closure in layers is performed after thorough wound irrigation. Closure of any remaining capsular structures is attempted. Muscle is reapproximated if elevated from bone. A deep subfascial drain often is placed to avoid postoperative hematoma. Use of vacuum-assisted wound closure may be considered in patients at increased risk of wound complications.

Postoperative Care

- Patients generally are made toe-touch weight bearing for 6 to 8 weeks postoperatively and particularly if an osteotomy has been performed, a complex acetabular revision has been performed, or if bony or soft tissue fixation was tenuous. Weight bearing can be progressively advanced over the next 1 to 2 months based on clinical examination and serial radiographs demonstrating the absence of component migration. In patients with pelvic discontinuity, weight-bearing restrictions may be extended until the surgeon appreciates reconstitution of the posterior column.
- A hip abduction brace can be used at the surgeon's discretion for patients believed to be at high risk for dislocation or for protection of a healing trochanteric osteotomy. This is not routinely used in our practice.

Suggested Reading

1. Berry DJ. Anterior extended greater trochanteric osteotomy. *Semin Arthro.* 2004;15:126-129.
2. Paprosky WG, Perona PG, Lawrence JM. Acetabular defect classification and surgical reconstruction in revision arthroplasty: a 6-year follow-up evaluation. *J Arthroplasty.* 1994;9:33-44.
3. Miner TM, Momberger NG, Chong D, Paprosky WL. The extended trochanteric osteotomy in revision hip arthroplasty. *J Arthroplasty.* 2001;16(8 suppl 1):188-194.

Chapter 23
Extended Greater Trochanteric Osteotomies

ALAN K. SUTAK
DANIEL J. BERRY

Key Concepts

- Extended greater trochanteric osteotomies provide wide access to the femoral canal and hip joint. The most common indications are in revision total hip arthroplasty (THA) procedures with well-fixed or broken femoral implants that require removal, extensive bone cement that requires removal, or bone deformity limiting safe longitudinal access to the femoral canal (Figure 23.1A-F).
- Most commonly extended greater trochanteric osteotomies are used to facilitate removal of well-fixed cemented or uncemented femoral components. Additional indications include access to the femoral canal when the greater trochanter overhangs the implant or circumstances in which an osteotomy is needed to correct proximal femoral deformity.
- There are two main categories of extended trochanteric osteotomies (ETOs): those that elevate the lateral one-third of the circumference of the femur and those that elevate the anterior one-third of the circumference of the femur (Figures 23.2 and 23.3).
- For all types of ETO, to maximize healing potential, preserve the blood supply of the ETO fragment by retaining muscle (abductor and vastus lateralis) attachments to most of the fragment.
- Preoperative templating is critical. Plan the length of osteotomy and account for any proximal femoral deformity. Make sure the osteotomy is long enough to gain enough exposure to remove implant or cement mantle and yet leave sufficient diaphysis to allow for solid fixation of a the planned revision femoral component.
- If the patient has a notable anterior bow of the femur or if you are planning insertion of a very long straight stem, consider an anterior osteotomy as this will allow straight access to the femoral canal and minimize risk of distal anterior perforation

Sterile Instruments and Implants

- Thin oscillating saw
- Broad osteotomes and narrow osteotomes
- Power burr with fine side cutting tip
- Cerclage cables and wires
- Bennett retractors

Surgical Approaches

The type of surgical approach is dictated by the type of ETO.

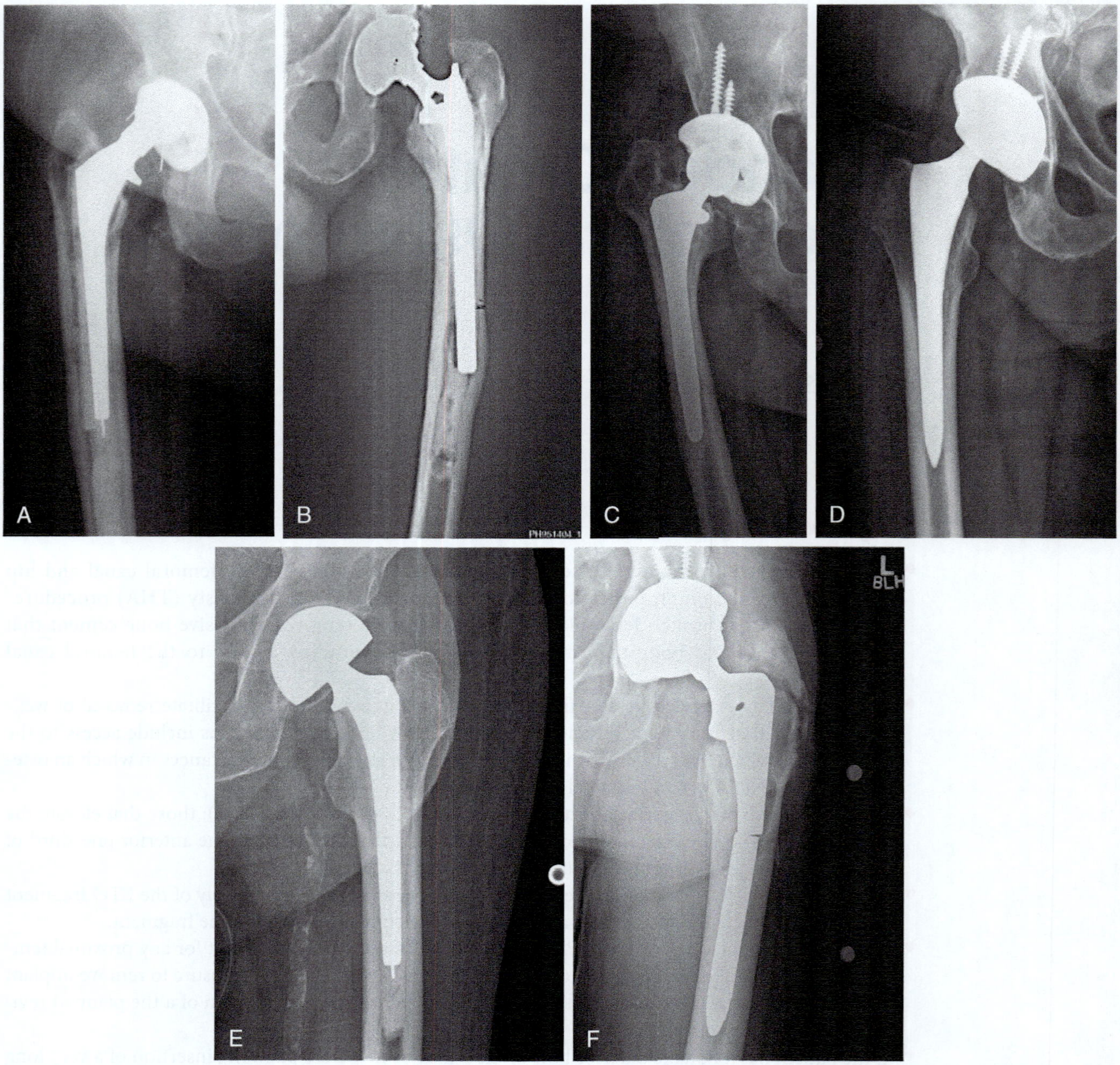

Figure 23.1 | Indications for extended trochanteric osteotomy (ETO). Distal cement mantle (A). Proximal femoral deformity (B). Stem subsidence with overhanging greater trochanter (C). Well-fixed uncemented stem requiring removal (D). Well-fixed cemented stem requiring removal (E). Broken femoral stem (F).

Preoperative Planning

- Template choice of stem, typically a long uncemented stem, either fluted tapered or fully porous coated.
- Plan the length of the osteotomy and measure the distance from the tip of greater trochanter (usually 12-18 cm) for intraoperative reference. Make sure the osteotomy is long enough to allow safe removal of the stem or cement mantle but also leaves enough diaphyseal bone to allow for solid implant fixation. If an extensively porous-coated cylindrical stem is being removed, it is important to extend the planned osteotomy to a point where the stem is cylindrical to allow for trephines to pass over the stem for easier removal.

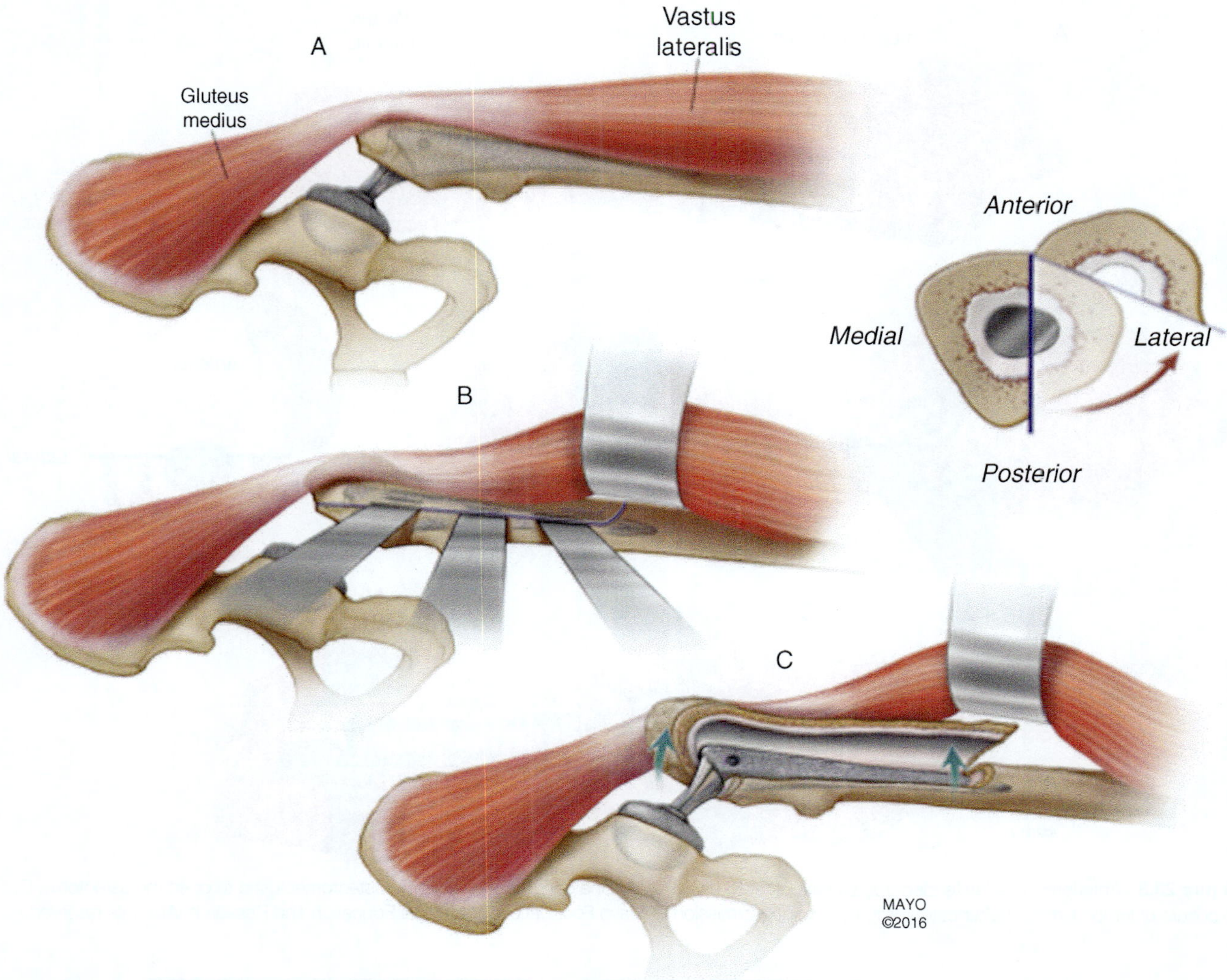

Figure 23.2 | Laterally based extended trochanteric osteotomy (ETO). A, Femur with well-fixed stem requiring removal. B, Osteotomes used to open the osteotomy. C, Exposure of the femoral implant after osteotomy. (Used with permission of Mayo Foundation for Medical Education and Research. All rights reserved.)

Bone, Implant, and Soft Tissue Techniques

Lateral Extended Trochanteric Osteotomy

- Position patient in a lateral decubitus position and perform posterior approach to the hip up to but not including opening the pseudocapsule.
- If the proximal canal is not filled by the implant, the posterior hip capsule can be kept intact (thereby optimizing hip stability) and the hip dislocated anteriorly. To use this technique there must be sufficient space between the implant and lateral femur (Figure 23.4A and B) to perform the proximal anterior longitudinal limb of the osteotomy by sliding a saw from posterior to anterior. If there is not sufficient lateral bone to allow this technique (Figure 23.5A and B), complete a formal posterior approach to the hip and dislocate the hip posteriorly.
- Identify the vastus lateralis and divide the posterior portion of the vastus lateralis longitudinally just anterior to the linea aspera. There will often be deep perforating vessels coming through the septum posteriorly. These vessels should be ligated or cauterized to minimize excessive bleeding. Use a ruler to mark the level of the transverse limb of the osteotomy by measuring the distance from the tip of the greater trochanter. The length of the osteotomy is usually at least 12 cm and rarely more than 16 cm. At this level, elevate a small amount of vastus lateralis (about 2-3 cm wide) from the lateral

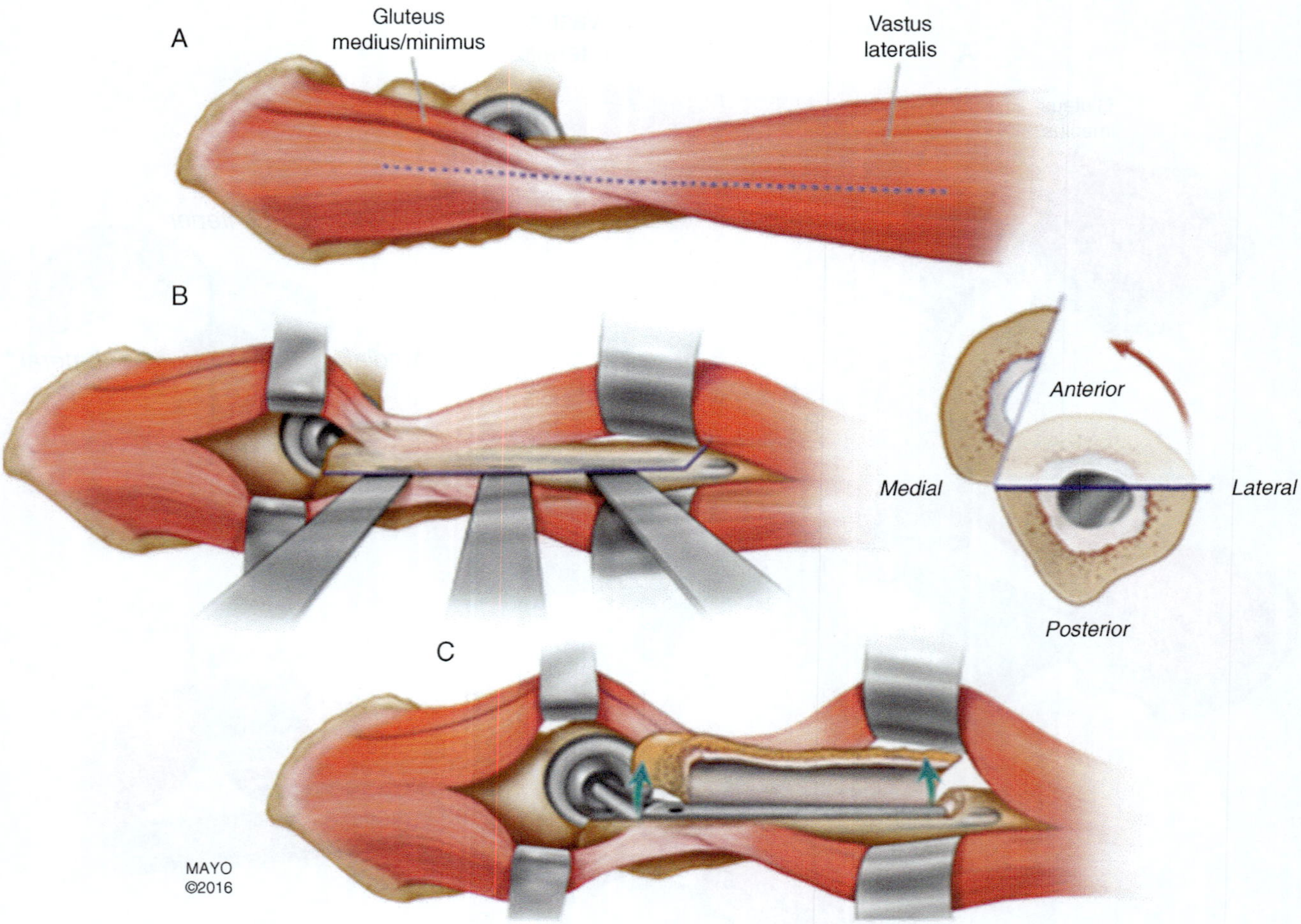

Figure 23.3 | Anteriorly based extended trochanteric osteotomy (ETO). A, Line of muscle splitting. B, Osteotomes used to open the osteotomy. C, Exposure of femoral implant after osteotomy. (Used with permission of Mayo Foundation for Medical Education and Research. All rights reserved.)

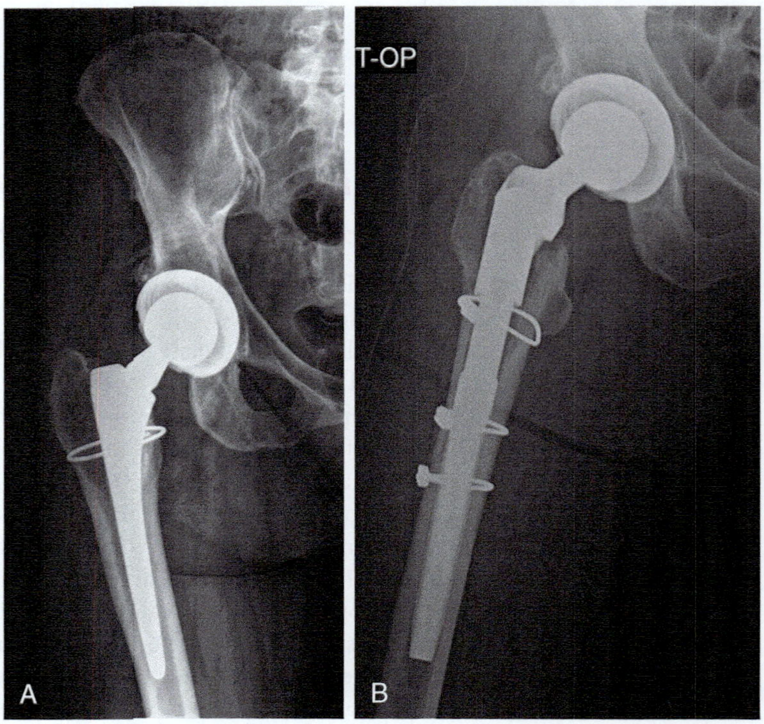

Figure 23.4 | A, Preoperative radiograph of patient with well-fixed dual modular neck femoral stem requiring removal. There is sufficient thickness of lateral bone to allow the proximal anterior longitudinal osteotomy to be made with a saw from posterior to anterior without first dislocating the hip. B, Postoperative radiographs after revision with laterally based extended trochanteric osteotomy (ETO).

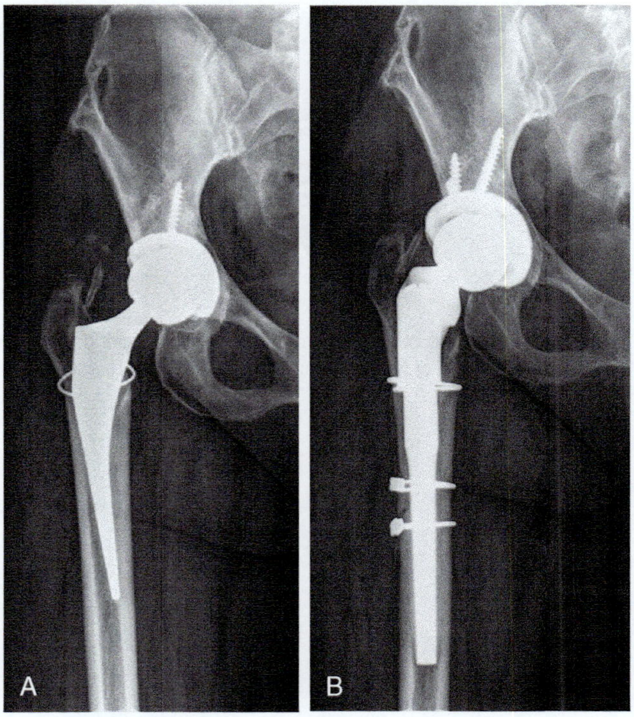

Figure 23.5 | A, Preoperative radiograph of patient with well-fixed, infected total hip arthroplasty (THA) requiring removal as part one of a two-stage procedure. The bone laterally is too thin to allow the anterior longitudinal limb of the osteotomy to be made from posterior to anterior, so the hip must be first dislocated and the anterior longitudinal limb of the osteotomy is then made separately under direct vision with the hip in a dislocated position. B, Postoperative radiographs after the second stage of the operation (reimplantation).

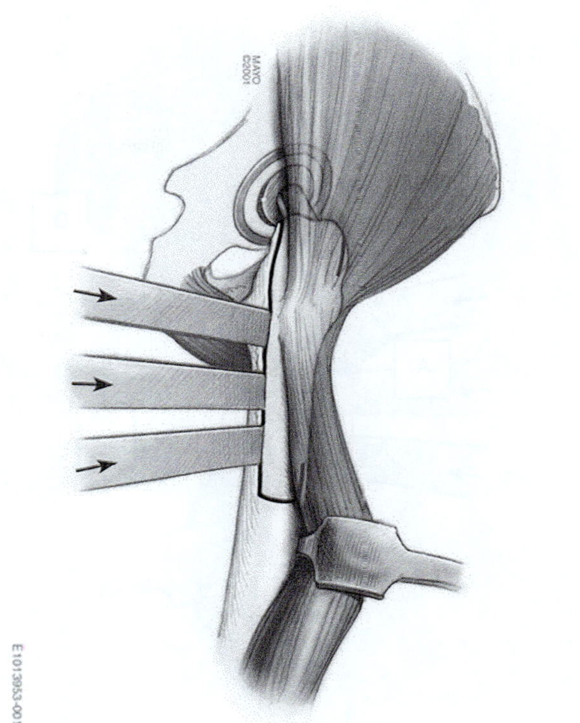

Figure 23.6 | A Bennett retractor is placed to expose the site of the distal transverse osteotomy and the anterior distal longitudinal osteotomy. (Used with permission of Mayo Foundation for Medical Education and Research. All rights reserved.)

femur working posterior to anterior. This will be the level of the distal and transverse aspect of the osteotomy. Once the vastus lateralis is elevated in this small section, a blunt retractor (such as a Bennett retractor) can be placed to retract the vastus lateralis anteriorly (Figure 23.6).

- Use a cautery or marking pen to mark the lines for the osteotomy. There are four aspects of the osteotomy: the posterior longitudinal limb, the proximal anterior longitudinal limb, distal anterior longitudinal limb, and the distal transverse limb (Figure 23.7A-D).
- Posterior limb (Figure 23.7A):
  - Use an oscillating saw along the planned osteotomy going from posterior to anterior. If stem is present, ensure saw goes through posterior cortex and stops against the stem. Continue the osteotomy along the posterior femur according to the length determined by the preoperative plan. Stop this osteotomy slightly short of the planned transverse osteotomy.
- Transverse limb (Figure 23.7B):
  - Using a small oscillating saw or high-speed burr, make a transverse osteotomy about one-third the circumference of the femur. Making this osteotomy beveled from distal to proximal provides more surface area for contact and prevents the osteotomy fragment from falling into the open femur if a resection arthroplasty is being performed. External rotation of the femur can help facilitate exposure for this part of the osteotomy. Be careful not to extend this transverse osteotomy beyond the boundaries of the longitudinal posterior or the planned anterior osteotomy, which can make a stress riser and risk an unplanned fracture.
- Anterior limb (Figure 23.7C and D):
  - The proximal anterior osteotomy (Figure 23.7D) can be made with a burr, small saw, or osteotome for a short distance which will allow for a controlled fracture between the distal end of the anterior longitudinal limb and the proximal aspect of the anterior distal limb, beneath the muscle. If the canal is empty (stem has been removed) or if the stem is not canal filling in this zone, the proximal anterior limb can be made with the saw going from posterior to anterior, perforating both cortices. If stem is present and the anterior bone cannot be cut by passing a saw from posterior to anterior just

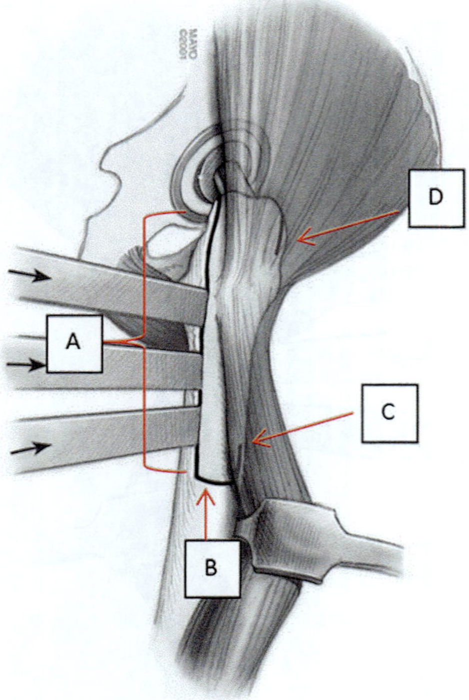

Figure 23.7 | Posterior longitudinal limb of osteotomy (A). Distal transverse osteotomy (B). Short distal longitudinal anterior osteotomy (C). Proximal anterior longitudinal osteotomy (D). (Used with permission of Mayo Foundation for Medical Education and Research. All rights reserved.)

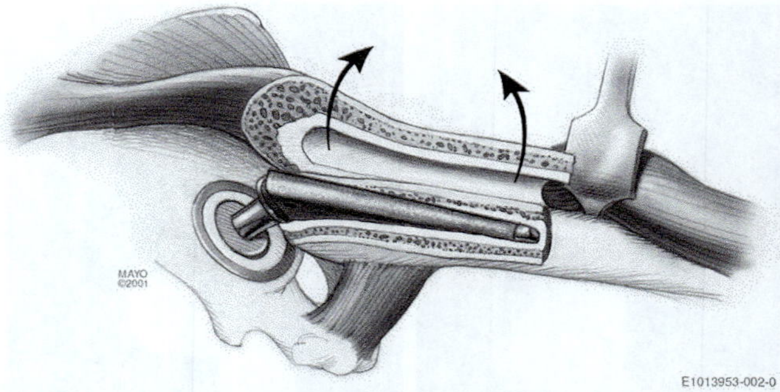

Figure 23.8 | Elevation of the osteotomized fragment anteriorly. (Used with permission of Mayo Foundation for Medical Education and Research. All rights reserved.)

lateral to the shoulder of the implant, make the proximal anterior osteotomy limb from inside out with a high speed thin side-cutting burr with the hip in a posteriorly dislocated position.

- Make a distal longitudinal anterior osteotomy (Figure 23.7C), to create an osteotomy fragment that encompasses about one-third the circumference of the femur. Make this osteotomy about 2 to 4 cm in length using a small oscillating saw. Be careful to keep vastus lateralis attached to femur.
- Connect the distal posterior and distal anterior longitudinal osteotomies to the transverse distal osteotomy using a thin side cutting high-speed burr. Round the corners of the osteotomy to reduce the stress riser effect.

- Once the osteotomy limbs are complete, insert several broad osteotomes along the posterior osteotomy and gently lever the osteotomy open until a controlled fracture occurs between the proximal anterior limb of the osteotomy and the distal anterior limb of the osteotomy, in the area covered by the intact vastus lateralis. Once the fragment is elevated, there may be some anterior hip capsule proximally tethering the fragment which can be released to allow for full retraction. Place one or two blunt Bennett retractors to retract the osteotomized fragment anteriorly.

Removal of Stem

- After the osteotomy is elevated and retracted anteriorly, access is gained to implants in the femoral canal (Figure 23.8). A pencil-tipped burr, small flexible osteotomes, or a Gigli saw can be used to separate the bone-implant or bone-cement interface of well-fixed implants. The stem will then be free and can be removed.
- If a distal cement mantle remains, an ultrasonic device or manual cement osteotomes can be used to clear out the remaining cement.
- Once the canal is clear and before reaming the canal for reimplantation, it is important to place a cerclage wire or cable about 1 cm distal to the osteotomy. This will help minimize fracture risk during reaming and stem insertion.
- The acetabulum can be accessed by retracting the proximal femur posteriorly or distally.

- While preparing the femur and acetabulum save any autogenous bone reamings to graft the osteotomy site at closure.
- Do not remove cement or membrane from the inner surface of the osteotomized fragment until just before closing the osteotomy. This reduces bleeding and reduces risk of fracture of the osteotomy fragment during acetabular and femoral preparation.

Closure of an Extended Trochanteric Osteotomy

- Once the canal has been prepared and the stem implanted, the osteotomized fragment can be reduced and prepared for fixation.
- Often, some bone from the inner aspect of the osteotomized fragment may need to be removed to facilitate closure around the new stem. This can be done using a 6.5-mm high-speed burr.
- If the bulk of the stem precludes the osteotomy from perfect anterior and posterior contact with the femur, despite internal contouring of the osteotomy fragment with a burr, the osteotomy fragment may be reduced along the posterior longitudinal limb and a small gap accepted along the anterior limb. Autogenous particulate bone graft from acetabular or femoral reamings may be used to fill this defect.
- Sharp rakes are helpful instruments to reduce the fragment.
- Once adequate reduction is obtained, cables or wires may be passed circumferentially around the proximal fragment and tightened. Cables provide stronger fixation than wires and have higher friction against the fragment, thereby resisting proximal migration of the fragment. Usually two cables are sufficient; the proximal cable is placed just distal to the lesser trochanter and distal cable about 1 to 2 cm proximal to the distal aspect of the osteotomy (Figure 23.4B). The distal cable is on cortical bone and can be tightened very vigorously; caution should be exercised not to over tighten the proximal cable because there is a risk of the cable cutting through the lateral femur just below the vastus ridge and fracturing the osteotomy fragment. If the osteotomy fragment seems prone to proximal migration a double Luque wire cerclage wire may be passed through a hole drilled in the lesser trochanter and over the superolateral greater trochanter (Figure 23.9).
- Use autogenous particulate bone graft from reamings from the femur or acetabulum, if available, to graft along the osteotomy site.

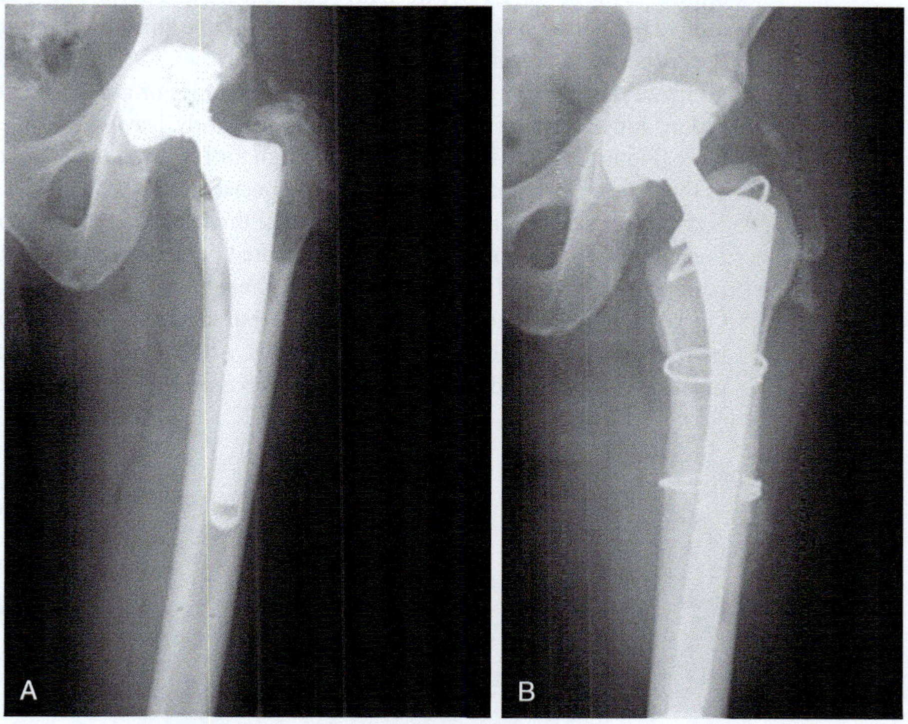

Figure 23.9 I A, Preoperative radiograph of patient with well-fixed uncemented patch porous-coated stem with osteolysis requiring revision. B, Postoperative radiograph showing a double Luque wire passed over the superior greater trochanter to provide extra resistance to proximal migration of the osteotomy fragment.

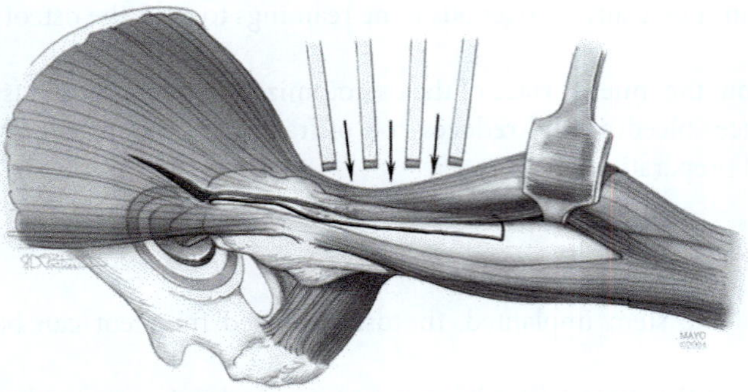

Figure 23.10 I The proximal longitudinal anterior limb of an anteriorly based extended trochanteric osteotomy (ETO) can be made with multiple narrow osteotome cuts. The osteotomes are carefully passed through the intact muscle. (Used with permission of Mayo Foundation for Medical Education and Research. All rights reserved.)

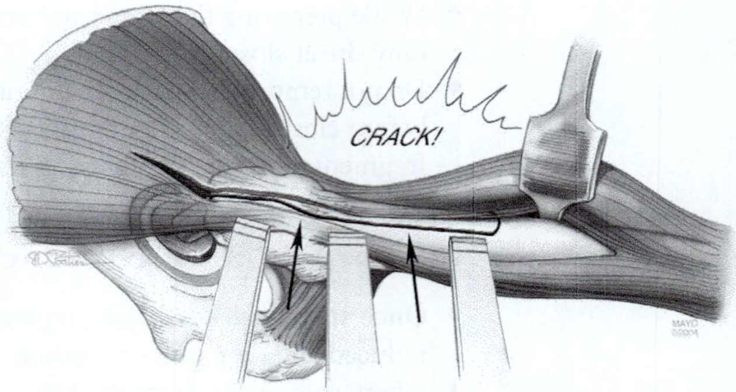

Figure 23.11 I Completing the anteriorly based osteotomy by elevating the fragment with several broad osteotomes. A controlled fracture, of the anterior cortex, beneath the intact muscle, occurs through the previously made distal longitudinal saw cut and the osteotome cuts. (Used with permission of Mayo Foundation for Medical Education and Research. All rights reserved.)

Anterior Extended Osteotomy

See comments in the above description, many of which are also relevant to an anterior extended osteotomy (Figure 23.2).

- Identify the gluteus medius muscle and the vastus lateralis.
- Make a longitudinal split in the middle of the abductor mass beginning proximally and following the line of the muscle fibers (extending no more than 4-5 cm proximal to the tip of the greater trochanter), through gluteus medius, minimus, and capsule. Extend this split down the vastus lateralis on the lateral aspect of the femur to the level of the planned osteotomy. Be careful to maintain continuity of the abductor and vastus lateralis sleeve on either side of the split. Do not elevate any muscle away from the femur.
- Next, use an oscillating saw to make the longitudinal osteotomy along the length of the lateral femur to a distance identified on your preoperative plan. Proximally, the osteotomy should exit the femur in the mid coronal plane at the tip of the greater trochanter.
- Similar to the lateral ETO, externally rotate the leg and perform the distal transverse osteotomy using a small oscillating saw or high-speed burr about one-third the circumference of the femur. Rounding the corners will prevent a stress riser.
- To make the anterior osteotomy, narrow osteotomes or a drill can be used to make multiple perforations longitudinally through the muscle anteriorly, leaving the anterior vastus lateralis attached to bone (Figure 23.10). Getting anterior enough for the osteotomy to encompass the requisite one-third of the femoral circumference can require special effort.
- Next, insert several broad osteotomes along the lateral osteotomy to create a controlled fracture of the anterior femur along the previously created perforation line (Figure 23.11). The osteotomy fragment can be retracted anteriorly to expose the femoral canal (Figure 23.12).
- Once the stem has been removed, canal prepared, and the new stem implanted, the osteotomy can be reduced and closed using cables or wires. At the greater trochanter, the anterior and posterior portions can be closed with wires or sutures passed through the bone of the greater trochanter.

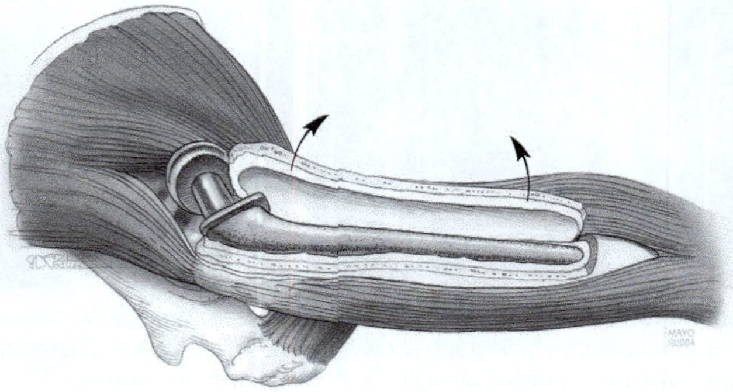

Figure 23.12 I The anteriorly based osteotomy is opened anteriorly providing access to the joint and the intramedullary canal. (Used with permission of Mayo Foundation for Medical Education and Research. All rights reserved.)

Postoperative Care

- Toe touch weight bearing on operative extremity for 6 to 8 weeks to allow for bone healing.
- Teach total hip precautions to minimize risk of dislocation, including limiting adduction and internal rotation of the hip.
- Healing of the longitudinal limbs of the osteotomy typically occurs well before radiographic healing of the transverse limb of the osteotomy. If the osteotomy fragment has not moved in the first 8 weeks after the operation, the longitudinal limbs typically will be healing well.

Chapter 24
Implant Removal

TIMOTHY S. BROWN
DAVID G. LEWALLEN

Key Concepts

- The importance of efficient and bone-sparing implant removal cannot be overemphasized. Care and efficiency with this part of the procedure sets the reconstructive portion of the procedure up for success. Likewise, problems that develop in this portion of the procedure will echo throughout the procedure, often causing further problems.
- Successful removal of implants in total hip arthroplasty (THA) requires careful preoperative planning.
- In all cases, every attempt should be made to obtain the outside hospital records. This is useful for sizing, for determining the need for standard equipment (for example, hexagonal head versus cruciate head screwdrivers), for identifying the need for specialized extraction tools, and for predicting otherwise unsuspected intraoperative difficulties.
- Preoperative radiographs should be carefully evaluated and can often help predict areas at risk for bone damage or bone loss on both the pelvic and the femoral side of the hip.

Sterile Instruments and Implants

- Implant-specific removal tools (when the design of existing implant is known)
- Large bone tamp
- Drill bit and 50-mm 6.5-mm cancellous bone screw and companion drill bit
- Curved osteotomes designed for cup extraction
- Special curved blade cup removal tool (for example, Explant system, Zimmer Biomet, Warsaw, Indiana)
- Small sagittal saw
- Gigli saw and handles
- High-speed burr with standard and pencil tips, metal-cutting burr
- Universal stem extractor
- Long-handled hip osteotomes (i.e., Moreland osteotomes, Depuy Synthes, Warsaw, Indiana)
- Ultrasonic cement removal system (i.e., Oscar, Orthofix Inc., Lewisville, Texas)
- Trephines
- Large drill bit from femoral nail set
- Broken hardware removal set (if broken screws are present)
- Universal hardware removal set (if implant/screws are of unknown design)

Preoperative Planning

- A key to successful removal of implants in THA is understanding the specific features of the implants that are coming out (Figure 24.1).
  - Obtain implant records from prior operations if at all possible.
  - Specific implant extraction tools are available for most designs, particularly for femoral components (Figure 24.2).
  - Certain constructs require special planning:
    - Well-fixed cemented femoral components
    - Well-fixed extensively porous coated femoral components

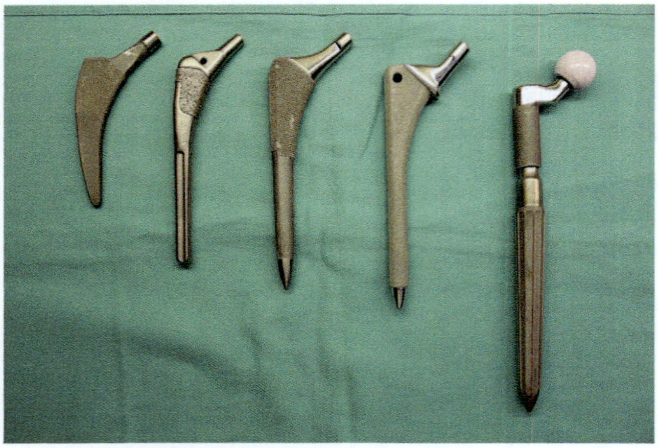

Figure 24.1 | Variety of femoral implants.

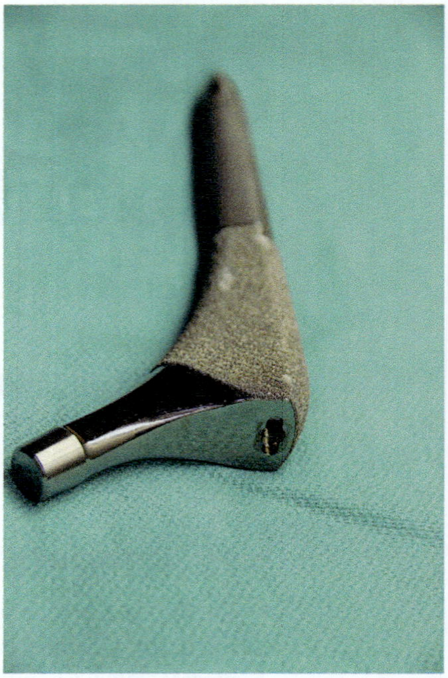

Figure 24.2 | Threaded area of proximal implant for extraction/insertion.

        - All polyethylene components
        - Monoblock acetabular components
        - Modular dual-mobility cups with metal liners
        - Stems with dual-modular femoral necks (Figure 24.3)
- By examining the radiographs try to identify areas of bone loss and predict areas where the bone will be weak and at risk for fracture.
    - Pelvis
        - Anteroposterior (AP) pelvis, Judet oblique view, cross-table lateral radiographs. Perform careful evaluation of each zone of the acetabulum for osteolytic lesions (Figure 24.4).

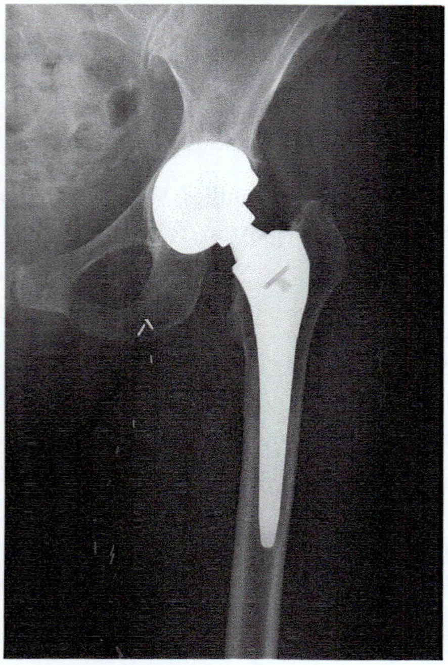

Figure 24.3 | Dual-modular femoral neck implant that requires specialized extraction tool.

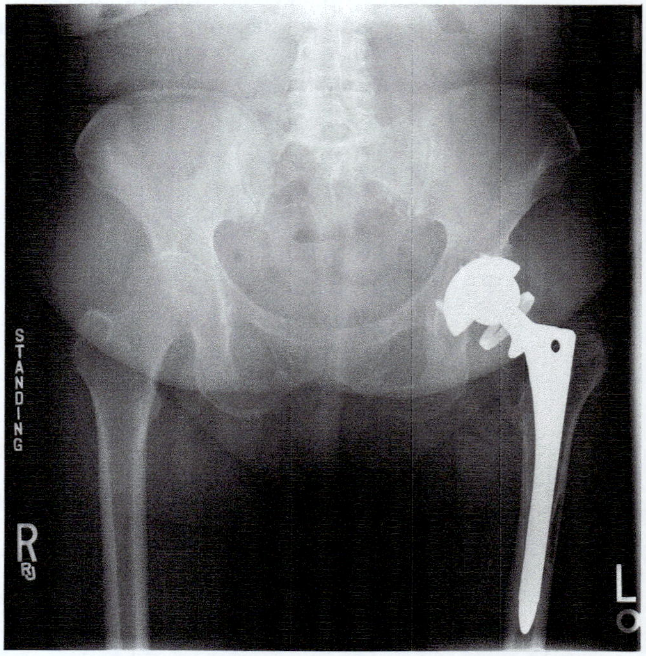

Figure 24.4 | Total hip arthroplasty with failure due to osteolysis and instability. Osteolysis medially was predicted from the radiograph and bone grafted at the time of revision THA.

  - Femur
    - AP hip, frog leg, or cross-table lateral radiographs of the femur. Careful evaluation of the proximal bone stock, femoral deformity, and stem alignment in both the coronal and sagittal planes are all important.
- Know the previous operations
  - Get operative reports
    - Surgical approach?
    - Any complications?

Bone, Implant, and Soft Tissue Techniques

- Any extensile approach to the hip joint can be used: anterolateral, posterolateral, or transtrochanteric, but understand how to perform each extensile approach when needed, including extended trochanteric osteotomy (ETO) (laterally based posterior to anterior, laterally based anterior to posterior, or anteriorly based [Wagner style] lateral to medial).
- The hip is dislocated, the femoral head disimpacted with a bone tamp and mallet, and the femur retracted to expose the acetabulum if only the acetabulum will be revised.

Acetabulum

- Circumferential exposure of the acetabulum is critical for safe and efficient implant removal.
- Use straight or curved pointed retractors (i.e., Hohmann) placed into the bone of the ilium superiorly and the base of the ischium inferiorly, along with a curved blunt retractor over the anterior wall just above the iliopsoas tendon. Alternative or additional retractors can be placed along the outer table of the posterior column just above or just below the posterior inferior iliac spine to expose the posterior wall and posterior column. Additional retractors are placed as needed to improve the exposure, and a hook around the neck of the femur can help pull it out of the field especially for isolated acetabular revision procedures. Generally at least 3 retractors are needed.

Cemented Polyethylene Cup

- If the cup is grossly loose, it may be removed with a rongeur (Figure 24.5).
- If the construct cannot be removed, then a small acetabular reamer is used to slowly remove the polyethylene from the cement mantle. All polyethylene reamings are carefully debrided and irrigated from the joint.
- Alternatively, the cup can be debonded from the underlying cement with osteotomes and removed.
- Once the cement is exposed, cement osteotomes are used to carefully break up the cement. The cement fragments are all removed, and the joint is irrigated to prevent subsequent third body wear problems. Well-fixed cement can be removed with a burr. In most cases, cement that has penetrated the medial wall of the pelvis is left in situ (unless infection is present).

Monoblock Cementless Cup

- Often a special curved blade cup removal system (Figure 24.6) may be used inside a well-fixed monoblock cup with intact polyethylene to circumferentially separate the cup from the host bone. Begin by gaining full circumferential exposure of the cup. Use a pencil tip burr to create a small trough circumferentially around the cup staying very close to the cup. This will help the curved blades (used next) to follow the correct track. Start with the smallest curved osteotome that will fit the external diameter of the existing acetabular component and introduce it carefully at the junction between the implant and the bone. Use the self-centering feature of the system by choosing a ball size that fits the internal diameter of the cup. Start with the shorter blades and graduate to the longer blades. Be careful when introducing the blades not to allow them to wander or to cause a fracture. Bone of the superior lateral wall, near the sciatic notch is at unique risk. After sequentially impacting the blade into the cup-bone interface all around the circumference of the cup, it is possible to rotate the handle and to complete the separation around the periphery of the entire cup. The longer blade osteotome is then used in the same fashion to divide any deeper more polar areas of bone attachment.

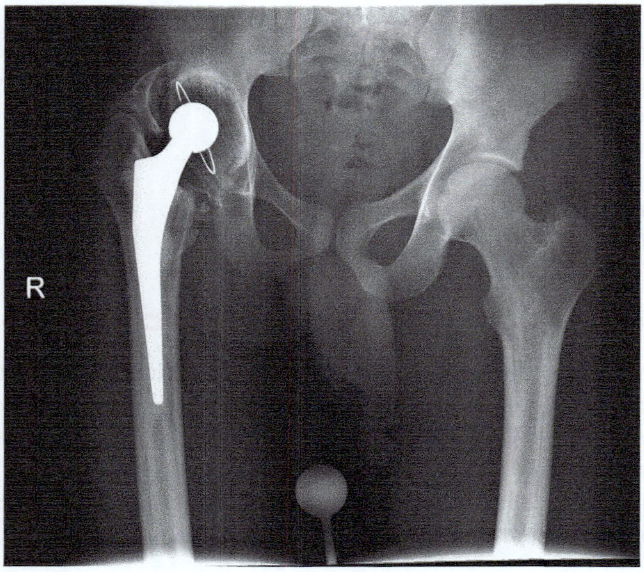

Figure 24.5 | Loose all polyethylene cemented acetabular component.

Modular Cementless Cup, Polyethylene Liner

- Use of the manufacturer's liner removal tool (when available and cup design is known) can be helpful. However, even when available, many of the various removal tools are bulky, difficult to position properly as a result, and can be ineffective and ultimately time consuming.
- Frequently liner removal can be quickly accomplished using a curved narrow osteotome and mallet. The osteotome is placed at the junction between the liner and the cup and impacted until just inside the locking mechanism. The osteotome is then levered medially to disengage the polyethylene liner. Some liners have locking retention rings or wires that can make liner removal difficult. Cutting the rim of the liner away from the shell with an osteotome can provide direct access to the locking wire, which can then be removed to facilitate liner removal.
- If attempted removal with the osteotome is unsuccessful, then a drill bit and matching 50-mm cancellous screw can be used either centrally in thicker polyethylene liners or at the periphery of the polyethylene especially with thinner liners to disengage the polyethylene from the locking mechanism.
- For monoblock designs in which polyethylene exchange is desired or for modular liners that do not come out easily with the above-mentioned maneuvers, a quick and effective alternative is to simply ream out the polyethylene with progressively larger acetabular reamers.

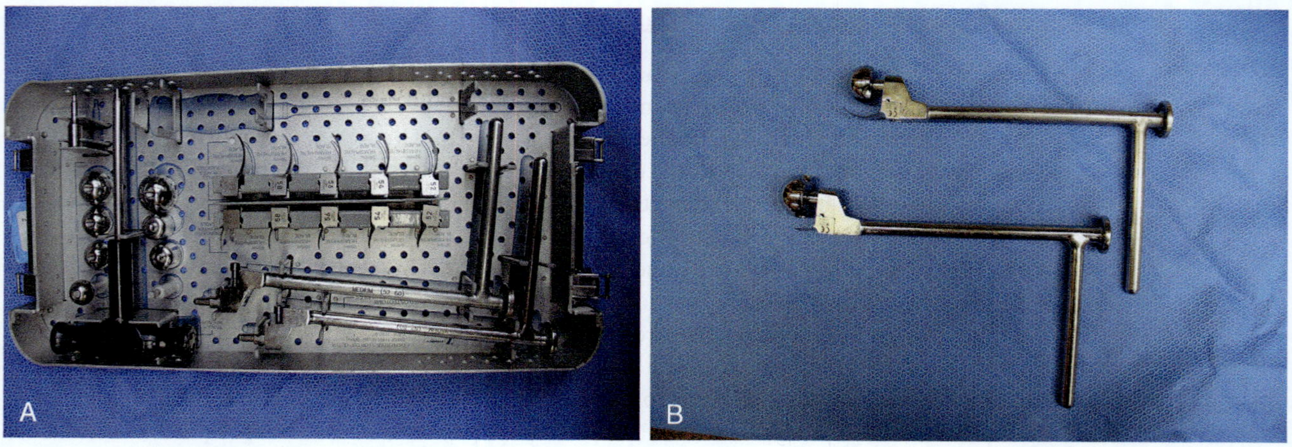

Figure 24.6 | A special curved blade cup removal system.

- Once the liner is removed, the cup is carefully cleaned and all screw heads are exposed. The appropriate screwdriver is then used to remove all screws. In the event of a stripped screw, or if no driver can be found, then the screw head can be destroyed with a metal cutting burr from within the cup (with screw removal after cup extraction).
- A trial liner can then be placed into the cup, and the Explant tool can be used as described earlier to separate the cup from the host bone.

Modular Cementless Cup, Metal Liner (Dual Mobility or Metal-on-Metal Articulation)

- Removal of the metal liner is often possible with impaction on the rim of the cup near the junction with the metal liner using specialized tools that vary by implant company. This may require many impactions and patience. Removal of the liner once it is loose may require grabbing it with a Kocher clamp or levering it out of the cup with a periosteal elevator.
- Similarly, a reciprocating saw loaded with no blade can be used to vibrate the edge of the cup and separate the metal liner from the cup.
- For monoblock metal-on-metal designs or those in which the liner will not come out, a trial bipolar head sized to the inner diameter of the acetabular component can be used with the Explant system as a self-centering device.

Femur

- Adequate exposure of the proximal femur is critical for safe implant removal.
- We use a wide Hohmann retractor placed above the lesser trochanter on the medial femoral neck and a Mueller retractor either anteriorly or posteriorly depending on surgical approach.
- A forceps and electrocautery are used to identify clearly the intersection of host bone with the femoral implant. Once the interval is clearly defined, implant removal can begin.
- When removing any stem, a helpful trick can be to create a divot in the stem's body with a metal-cutting burr. This can create an excellent spot for the bone tamp to facilitate retrograde disimpaction in stems of any design, especially for those implants without a fitting for a special removal tool or collar for direct impaction.

Cemented Femoral Stem

- The cement around the proximal aspect of the femoral stem and shoulder is removed with cement osteotomes and mallet. Clearing the superior-lateral shoulder of the stem of cement or bone that will be in the trajectory of the stem during extraction is essential to prevent fracture of the greater trochanter. If the stem has a threaded extraction device, the lateral aspect of the proximal femur is cleared for this device and it is threaded in place. Otherwise, a universal stem extractor is then placed around the femoral neck and the stem disimpacted from the cement mantle. If the stem is not easily removed from the cement mantle or if an extensive cement mantle is present, strongly consider an ETO.
- The cement mantle is then removed from host bone with a combination of osteotomes specially designed for cement removal (such as Moreland osteotomes), threaded cement removal devices, and/or ultrasonic devices. A helpful strategy is to create longitudinal cuts in the cement with an ultrasonic osteotome and then remove segments of the cement with curved cement-removal osteotomes. This strategy avoids hoop stresses caused by space-occupying osteotomes that can lead to femur fracture.
- Cement plug removal is best accomplished with the plug puller ultrasonic tip. Insert the plug puller under power, rotate it 90° under power, allow the cement to polymerize, and then disimpact the cement from the canal. If the cement is well fixed, only try to remove about a centimeter at a time. If the cement plug cannot be removed with an ultrasonic plug puller, create a hole in the cement with an ultrasonic instrument or drill and then remove the cement with back biting instruments or treaded taps.
- In many cases of well-fixed cemented stems or stems with a well-fixed, extensive cement mantle, an extended osteotomy is used to open the femur and remove the implant and cement under direct visualization.

Proximal Porous Coated Cementless Stem

- The specific shape and track record of each stem of this design should be understood before removal. For some designs it is possible to remove the stem from the top without an extended femoral osteotomy.
- In spite of a limited proximal porous coating, some stems will have distal ongrowth to areas of grit blasting or roughening that makes stem removal from above much more challenging; in these cases an ETO is preferred.
- A high-speed pencil-tipped burr is used to start the interval between the implant and bone and is worked distally as far as possible.
- Flexible osteotomes are then used to carefully continue this interval distally. Anteriorly and posteriorly osteotomes can be more easily and safely introduced. Depending on stem shape and size within the canal passage laterally and especially medially can be difficult and can risk femoral perforation or fracture. If in doubt an ETO reduces the risk of bone loss or uncontrolled fracture.
- The lateral shoulder is cleared and an extraction device (specific or universal) can be attached to the stem, and extraction attempted. The stem is pulled into varus as it is disimpacted to protect the greater trochanter from damage or fracture.

Extensively Porous Coated Stem

- Removal of a well-fixed, extensively porous coated stem can be challenging (Figure 24.7).
- Unless the stem is loose, these implants usually require an ETO for safe removal, with extension of the ETO down to the diaphyseal region, past the triangular portion and well into the cylindrical portion of the implant.
- After ETO the underlying stem is divided transversely with a metal cutting burr at the level at which it becomes uniformly cylindrical. Capture metal debris by carefully packing sponges to protect the surrounding soft tissues. Be careful not to past point with the metal cutting burr, which will damage the medial cortical bone.
- After the stem is cut, the upper portion is separated from the proximal bone with the use of pencil-tipped burr anteriorly and posteriorly. A Gigli saw is used for medial separation. Expect getting the Gigli saw started may be difficult and expect the Gigli saw will bind frequently and break. Have many Gigli saws available.
- The proximal stem is removed.
- The distal aspect of the stem is then removed with the appropriately sized trephines. Multiple trephines slightly larger than the stem diameter need to be available, as several are usually needed, and

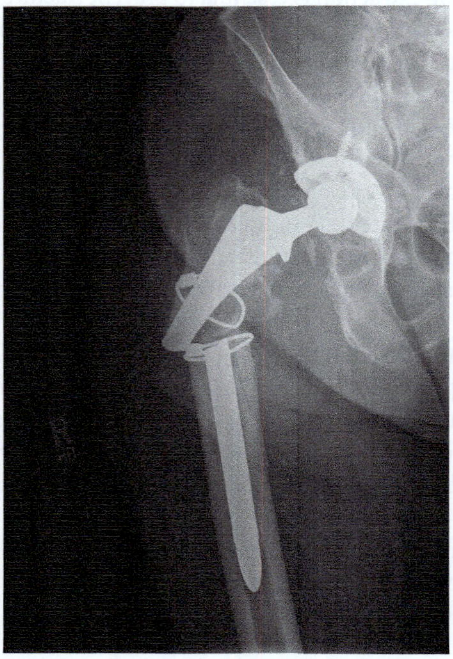

Figure 24.7 I Broken, well-fixed extensively porous coated stem.

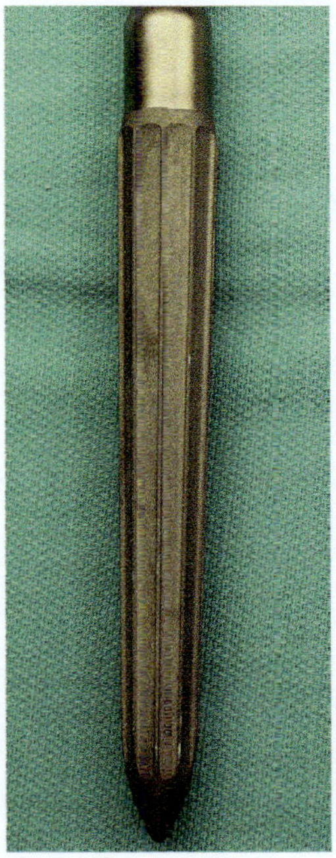

Figure 24.8 I Close up view of the flutes on a modular fluted tapered stem.

it is common for them to break or become dull during use. Remove the trephine frequently during reaming to prevent it from becoming hot and burning the bone. Each time the trephine is removed clean it carefully: adherent bone creates friction, which tends to bind the trephine. When the trephine reaches the end of the implant it will usually spin freely and the implant is removed with the trephine.

Monoblock Fluted Stem

- It is often helpful to have a long 3.5- to 4.0-mm drill bit for these stems, as the drill can be passed between each of the flutes to help separate the implant from the host bone.

Modular, Fluted, Tapered Stem

- Knowing the implant design helps as the modular components can be separated with the use of appropriate tools.
- The bolt connecting the proximal body to the stem is removed first, and the proximal body is removed after separating it from the host bone with flexible osteotomes and pencil-tipped burr.
- Drill bits are used to break up the bone between the flutes on the distal stem (Figure 24.8).
- Trephines or curved osteotomes can then be used distally around the stem. If the stem is "kinked" in shape it will need to be divided below the kink with a metal cutting burr before trephines are used.
- If trephines are used to remove a fluted tapered stem, they should be directly visualized while in use with a lateral view fluoroscopic image. This is critical to avoid the otherwise inevitable anterior cortex perforation related to the anterior bow of the femur and typical stem position just under that anterior cortex on the lateral projection.
- A specialized extractor or universal vice-grip extractor can then be used to remove the stem, or a notch can cut with a metal cutting tool on the side of the stem proximally to allow direct disimpaction.

Conclusion

- Knowing the size, make, and model of the implants that you are planning to remove can make the operation quicker and more effective.
- Preoperative planning for the operation follows the clinical work and prepares the surgeon for challenges faced in the operating room and allows special instruments, equipment, or revision components to be brought in beforehand. Barriers to exposure, possible bone loss, and implant removal needs can often be predicted before surgery.
- Safely and efficiently removing implants from the acetabulum and femur with minimal bone loss is the first key step to performing successful revision THA.

Section C
Revision THA Implants

Chapter 25
Uncemented Hemispherical Cups

JOSHUA S. BINGHAM
ROBERT T. TROUSDALE

Key Concepts

- Several options are available for acetabular reconstruction in the revision setting, including cementless hemispherical components, impaction grafting, reconstruction cages or rings, hemispherical cups with augments, cemented all-polyethylene components, and custom implants.
- Although multiple options are available, the great majority of acetabular reconstructions can be successfully performed using an uncemented hemispherical component with screw supplemental augmentation.
- This surgical technique is straightforward and should be familiar to most arthroplasty surgeons. The mid- and long-term results have been good.
- Excellent long-term results have been reported with uncemented hemispherical cups in the revision setting (Table 25.1).
- Highly porous metal implants with enhanced frictional coefficient against bone and high bone-ingrowth potential have expanded the indications for this form of reconstruction.
- Alternative forms of acetabular reconstruction should be considered in cases with severe segmental bone loss, in cases with a pelvic discontinuity, and in situations in which obtaining bone ingrowth is challenging.

Sterile Instruments and Implants

- Routine hip retractors.
- Hand-guided curved acetabular osteotomes for implant removal if required.
- A curved osteotome explant system for implant removal if needed.
- Broken screw removal set if screws are present in previous reconstruction.
- Power burr with pencil tip and carbide attachments.
- Sequential hemispherical reamers.
- Cancellous particulate allograft.

Implants

- Either a fully porous coated hemispherical multihole revision acetabular component (with instrumentation) or a highly porous titanium or tantalum cup. For complex revisions consider using a tantalum cup that allows the surgeon to bore supplement screw holes.
- Appropriately sized acetabular screws with a tap and instrumentation.
- Full array of bearing options including highly cross-linked polyethylene inserts of different inside diameters with different lateralized or elevated rim options. When instability is a concern, modular dual-mobility implants may be considered.

Table 25.1 | Results of Cementless Acetabular Reconstruction in Revision Total Hip Arthroplasty

Author (y)	No. of Hips	Follow-up in Years (Range)	Results
Della Valle et al. (2005)	138	17 (15-19)	2.2% of aseptic loosening, 96% survivorship at 15 y
Templeton et al. (2001)	61	12.9 (11.5-14.3)	3.5% were radiographically loose at last follow-up
Paprosky et al. (1994)	147	5.7 (3-9)	4.1% rate of failure, all failures in 3B acetabulums
Jamali et al. (2004)	63	11 (5-17)	5% rate of aseptic loosening
Hallstrom et al. (2004)	188	12 (10-17)	11% aseptic loosening, 96% survivorship at 12 y
Leopold et al. (1999)	138	10.5 (7-14)	1.8% radiographically loose at last follow-up
Silverton et al. (1996)	138	8.3 (7-11)	0.7% failure rate at last follow-up

Positioning

- The patient is placed in a lateral decubitus position, which allows for a more extensile exposure if needed.
- Draping should allow for adequate access to the proximal pelvis and entire femur.

Surgical Approaches

- The preferred approach of the authors in the majority of revision total hip arthroplasties (THAs) is a posterior approach. The posterior approach allows access to the posterior column and the ability to perform an extended femoral osteotomy if needed. However, anterolateral approaches also are compatible with this technique (as are direct anterior approaches for surgeons expert at the approach in very selected cases).
- The skin incision is partly dictated by the previous incisions, but ideally, a lateral incision is used, centered over the posterior trochanter and curving posteriorly proximally.
- A continuous soft tissue sleeve from the posterior border of the gluteus medius proximally to the gluteus maximus insertion distally is maintained. This continuous sleeve of tissue allows for an optimal soft tissue closure at the end of the procedure (Figure 25.1).

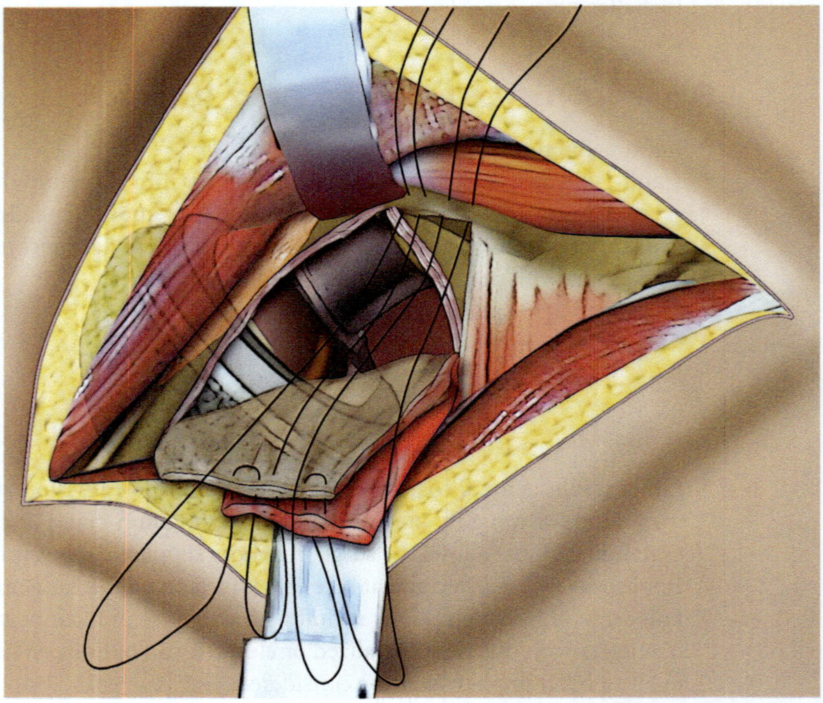

Figure 25.1 | A continuous soft tissue sleeve from the posterior border of the gluteus medius proximally to the gluteus maximus insertion distally for soft tissue closure at the end of the procedure.

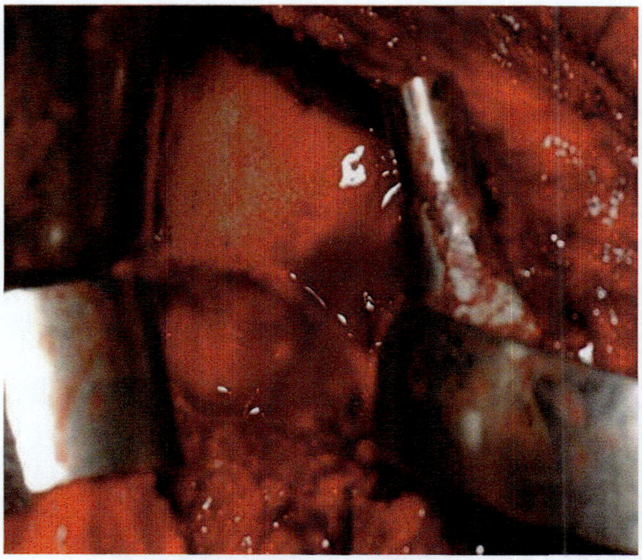

Figure 25.2 | An anterior soft tissue pocket allowing the trunnion to be translated anteriorly for complete exposure of the acetabulum.

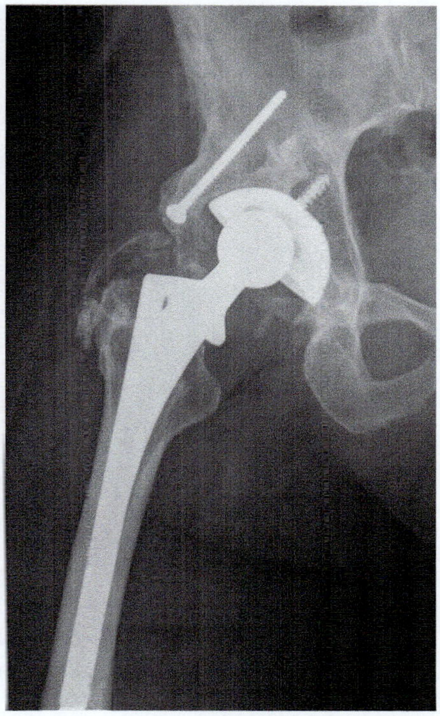

Figure 25.3 | Preoperative AP radiographs of an acetabular component with progressive osteolysis secondary to polyethylene wear.

- Once the prosthesis has been exposed, the hip is dislocated posteriorly and next the femoral component is extracted. If the femoral component is to be retained, a soft tissue pocket can be developed over the anterior superior acetabulum in which to place the trunnion (Figure 25.2).
- The entire rim of the acetabulum should be exposed to identify the interface between the host bone and existing acetabular component in preparation for component removal.
- A high-speed pencil-tipped burr can help define the interface between the implant and bone in preparation for use of osteotomes to cut the existing cup (if uncemented and well fixed) free of bone.
- Before using osteotomes, all the screws must be removed. If the screw head is stripped, a high-speed carbide burr can be used to remove the screw head to allow the curved osteotomes access to the bone-implant interface.

Preoperative Planning

- Routine preoperative radiographs (anteroposterior [AP] pelvis, AP hip, and cross-table lateral) are critical for appropriate surgical planning (Figure 25.3).
- A cross-table lateral, iliac oblique, or false profile view can be particularly helpful in evaluating the integrity of the posterior column and ischium.
- In cases with severe bone loss, oblique radiographs of the pelvis (Judet views) can help determine the amount of bone loss, including the anterior and posterior column, and the presence of a pelvic discontinuity. If a pelvic discontinuity is identified, alternative reconstruction options should be considered (cup-cage construct, distraction technique, or custom implant).
- Radiographic features of a pelvic discontinuity include transverse fracture lines on the AP or oblique pelvis radiographs, medial translation of the inferior hemi-pelvis with disruption of the ilioischial line, and asymmetry of the obturator ring compared with the contralateral side.
- A computed tomography scan can be helpful in certain situations but is not routinely performed.

Bone, Implant, and Soft Tissue Techniques

- After the desired surgical approach has been performed and the prior implants have been removed, the acetabulum must be carefully examined, including the anterior column, posterior column, acetabular roof, and medial wall.
- Adequate bone support must be present for an uncemented acetabular cup. If a pelvic discontinuity is identified, alternative reconstruction methods may be required.

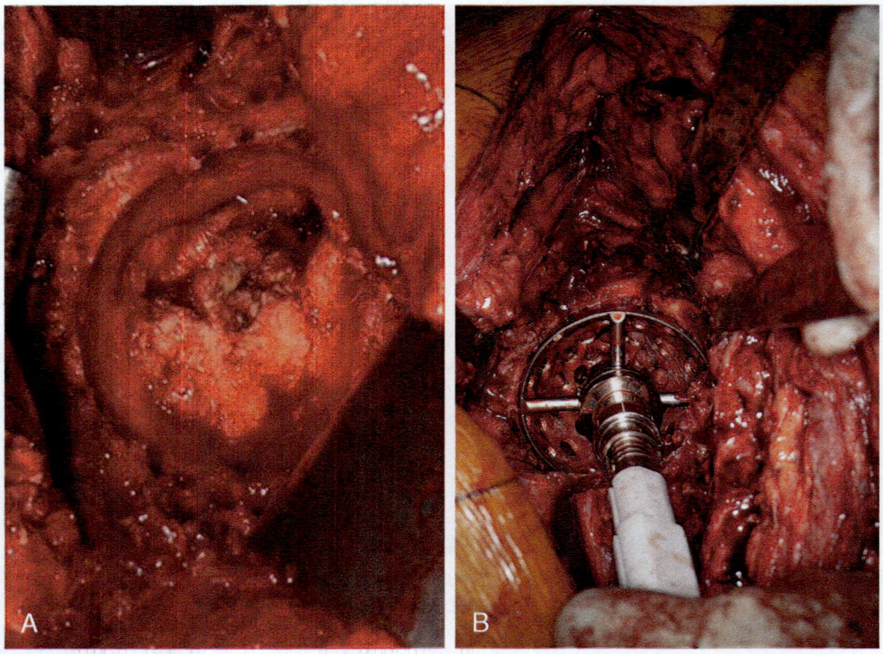

Figure 25.4 I A, Intraoperative photograph of a Paprosky IIC defect treated with an uncemented hemispherical cup. B, Sequential reamers being used in 45° of abduction and 20° of anteversion to recreate a hemisphere for a hemispherical uncemented acetabular component.

- Intraoperatively, a transverse fracture of the acetabulum with gross motion of the inferior aspect of the acetabulum is indicative of a pelvic discontinuity. Pushing on the ischium with an impactor to evaluate for motion is one way to assess for a pelvic discontinuity.
- Hemispherical reamers are used to sequentially ream the acetabulum until an adequate hemispherical bony bed is created for insertion of a revision acetabular component. Creating a supportive hemisphere of bone that provides optimal host bone contact with the implant and also restores the hip center of rotation is the goal. Overhanging areas of the rim of the acetabulum may be reamed away to provide a fully supportive hemisphere. The new cup is often 4 to 10 mm larger in diameter than the cup that is removed.
- Reaming should be performed in the same direction as the desired implant position (approximately 45° of abduction and 20° of anteversion) to create a hemisphere (Figure 25.4A and B).
- It is imperative to avoid damage to the posterior column (which is often the main supporting structure in the revision setting) with progressively larger reamers in an effort to create a hemisphere.
- Sacrificing a small portion of the anterior column to create a hemisphere may be necessary while preserving the posterior column (more common in smaller patients).
- Leaving the final reamer in place or placing a trial component can be helpful to determine the stability and amount of host bone contact that the revision hemispherical cup will obtain.
- Try to obtain a good “press-fit” of the cup with host bone because primary stability is required for bony ingrowth to occur. The trial must have stability when a posteriorly directed force is placed on it. If the construct is not inherently stable, alternative reconstruction techniques should be considered. Supplemental screws are used in almost all acetabular revisions; these screws can enhance primary cup stability in cases of deficient bone.
- In general, maximum host bone contact is desirable. No exact percentage of contact is required, and stability and bone-ingrowth potential depends on the location as well as surface area of bone contact.
- The acetabulum is usually reamed 1 to 2 mm smaller than the planned revision component.
- Any acetabular defects present should be packed with particulate cancellous allograft. The acetabulum should then be reverse reamed to fully impact the bone allograft into the defects. Care must be taken not to allow any interposition of allograft between the host bone and implant interface. A sponge can be used to clean off the host bone to ensure there is no interposition of allograft (Figure 25.5A-D).
- The hemispherical revision implant can now be impacted in the desired position (approximately 40°-45° of abduction and 20° of anteversion).

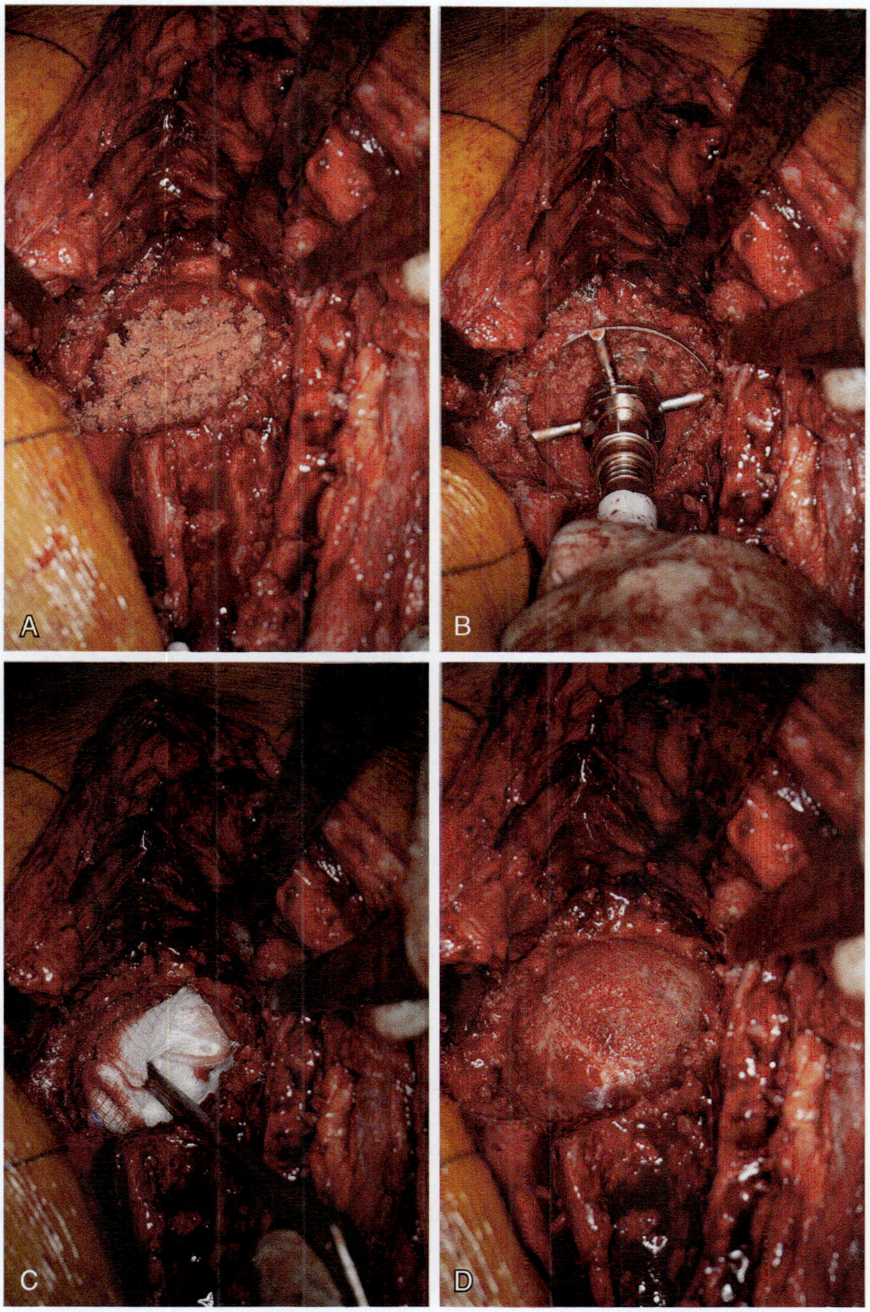

Figure 25.5 | A, Particulate cancellous allograft placed into the acetabular defects. B, Reverse reaming of the particulate cancellous allograft. C, A gauze sponge is used to ensure that there is no allograft interposed between the host bone and acetabular component. D, Compacted particulate cancellous allograft after reverse reaming.

- A revision cup with multiple holes should be utilized to allow for as many screws as reasonably possible to be inserted into the posterior-superior quadrant and ischium to augment the component stability (Figure 25.6).
- In cases with severe bone loss, additional screws augmentation outside the posterior-superior quadrant may be required. Care should be taken when placing these screws. Using an ischial screw can be helpful to prevent early cup failure by rotation to an abducted position.
- When using a porous tantalum acetabular component designed for polyethylene insert fixation with cement, a high-speed carbide burr can be used to bore through the porous tantalum material, allowing the surgeon to place a screw hole in any desired position. Additionally, with cementation of a polyethylene liner, the cement around the acetabular screws creates a fixed-angle locking screw.
- Screws should have adequate length to provide very secure purchase. Tapping can be performed before insertion, especially in sclerotic bone.

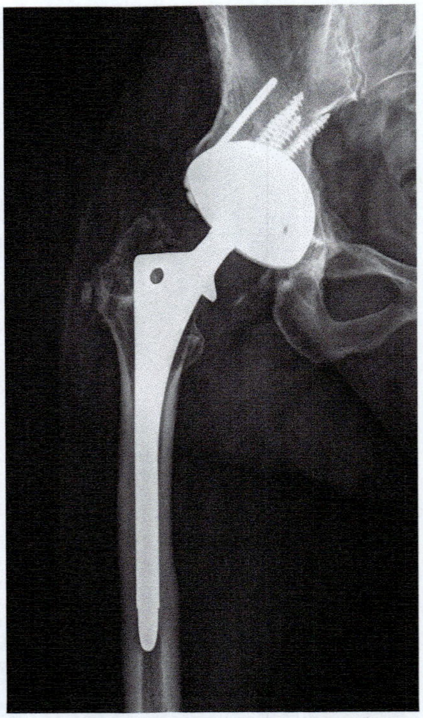

Figure 25.6 | Postoperative AP radiograph of a revision THA with an uncemented hemispherical cup and screw augmentation.

- The overall stability of the construct should be tested to ensure that sufficient stability has been achieved.
- A large-diameter (36 or 40 mm) femoral head or dual-mobility construct can be utilized in the revision setting for increased hip stability.

Postoperative Care

- Weight bearing after acetabular revision depends on the presence of a femoral osteotomy, the type of implants used, and the surgeon's preferences regarding weight bearing after THA. Most patients are treated with toe-touch weight bearing for about 8 weeks, and then weight bearing is gradually advanced.
- A hip abduction brace may be used in addition to hip precautions in patients at increased risk of dislocation based on the surgeon's discretion.

Chapter 26
Uncemented Cup With Metal Augments or Structural Graft

DAVID G. LEWALLEN

Key Concepts

- The goal of any uncemented acetabular revision procedure is to maximize stable implant contact against viable host bone to encourage bone ingrowth for long-term durability.
- When faced with irregularly shaped acetabular bone defects, simply reaming larger and larger to try to fill up the void can remove excessive amounts of remaining host bone and may destroy key rim or column support for the cup.
- Creation of an individualized irregularly shaped acetabular construct is possible by intraoperative assembly of a hemispherical acetabular component with one or more off-the-shelf highly porous acetabular augments.
- Acetabular augments can serve as a prosthetic structural bone graft alternative without the risk of late resorption.

Sterile Instruments and Implants

- Standard retractors and hip instruments.
- High-speed burr to contour bone to fit defects.
- Hemispherical acetabular component instruments and trials.
- Acetabular augment trials in a variety of sizes and thicknesses to aid in intraoperative assessment, sizing, and planning of final construct.
- Large plastic syringe to aid in placing cement precisely along the concave surfaces and edges of the augment where it contacts the revision cup.
- Cancellous bone graft to fill the fenestrations of the augment and any small remaining gaps or defects.

Surgical Approaches

- Any of the standard potentially extensile surgical approaches can be used per surgeon preference similar to any revision total hip arthroplasty (THA).
- Posterolateral and direct lateral approaches are the most commonly used at our institution either alone or in combination with an extended trochanteric osteotomy as needed to address the femoral side.

Preoperative Planning

- Careful assessment of the location and extent of acetabular bone defects is critical for the preoperative planning and preparation needed to ensure that the implants, instrumentation, and bone graft materials that might be needed are available for not only the planned procedure but also for potential alternative procedures or implant combinations, because intraoperative findings and events may require a change in plan.
- Radiographic assessment begins with the 3 standard views of the hip (anteroposterior [AP] pelvis, AP of the hip, cross-table lateral).

- In cases of major bone defects or suspected pelvic discontinuity, iliac and obturator oblique x-rays (Judet views) are extremely helpful and are recommended.
- Occasionally, if uncertainty about defect character, size, and location still exists after obtaining the above-mentioned 5 standard radiographs, a computed tomography (CT) scan with 3D reconstructions can assist in bone defect assessment.
- CT scans are used selectively as needed after careful study of the x-ray views because of the added cost and x-ray exposure to the patient.
- Although a general idea of whether and where an augment may be needed can be gained from preoperative review and planning, final implant sizing, orientation, and placement is based on intraoperative assessment of the deficient acetabulum and provisional use of cup and augment trials.

Bone, Implant, and Soft Tissue Techniques

- The initial goal of any acetabular reconstruction should be to achieve stable cup support on as large an area of host bone as possible.
- In more than 90% of cases, this can be achieved using a hemispherical cup and multiple screws and is the preferred reconstruction when possible.
- Maximal cup fixation is achieved with an array of screws across the dome of the acetabulum and down the posterior column into the base of the ischium (Figure 26.1).
- Major acetabular bone loss encountered at the time of revision surgery can threaten cup support and fixation, especially when uncontained or segmental bone loss has occurred as seen in Paprosky 3A ("up and out") or 3B ("up and in") bone defects.
- When bone defect location and size are severe enough, revision cup contact on host bone and the resulting fixation can be inadequate to provide mechanical cup stability under physiologic loads and to ensure a motionless interface for reliable bone ingrowth. These are the cases in which increased fixation for added mechanical support for the cup is required.
- Acetabular augments are one of the available options for improved mechanical support for the acetabular component in such instances and are particularly useful when segmental or very large cavitary defects are present.
- Designed as a prosthetic alternative to structural allograft, acetabular augments are made of highly porous metal but unlike structural bone graft are not at risk for resorption over time.
- Used as a prosthetic, structural bone graft substitute acetabular augments are employed in many of the same locations and configurations that structural bone grafts have been used historically.

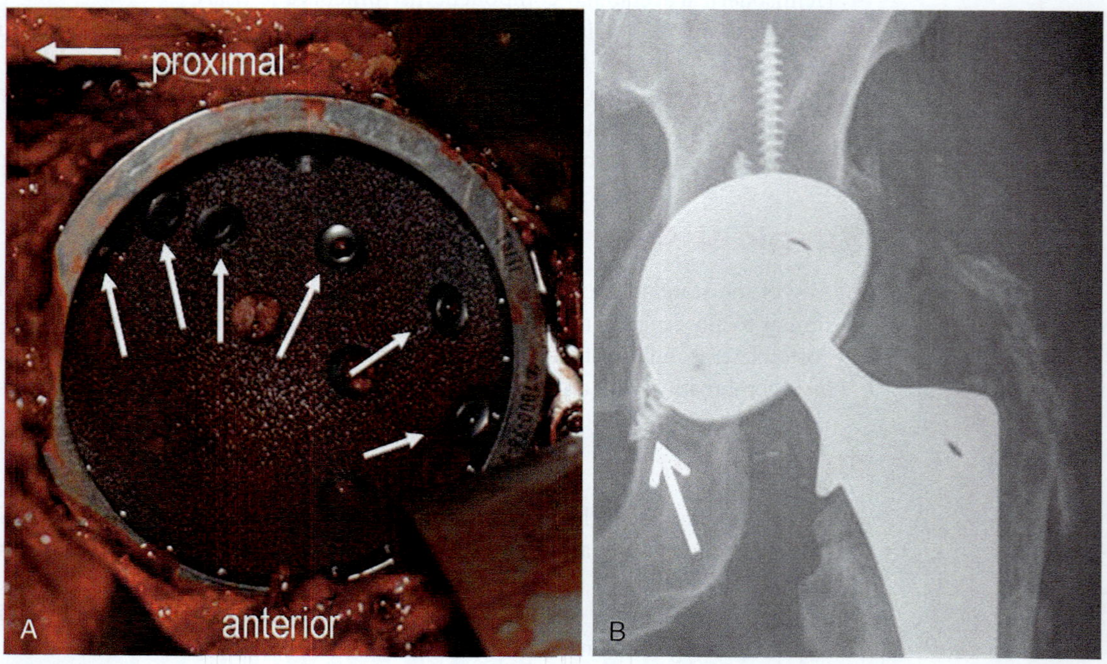

Figure 26.1 | A, Intraoperative view of acetabular component with 3 zone fixation using an array of screws across the dome (left hand arrow) and extending down the posterior column to the base of the ischium (right hand arrow) to maximize initial cup fixation and stability. B, AP x-ray of the same acetabular component with critical zone 3 screw (arrow) into the base of the ischium engaging the dense bone of the ilioischial line, which is the quadrilateral surface medial to the acetabulum.

- The location of bone defects and the quality of remaining host bone dictate when acetabular augments may prove helpful and in which location they are best positioned.
- Augments are used in 3 main patterns relative to the position of the acetabular component:
  - Type 1 as a "flying buttress" positioned along the superolateral rim of the acetabulum to enhance peripheral cup support.
  - Type 2 as an "elliptical" construct with the augment placed adjacent to the rim of the cup within an oblong acetabular cavity.
  - Type 3 as a "footing" placed medial to the cup to restore the acetabular floor and create a foundation for cup support and resist medial migration of the component (Figure 26.2).

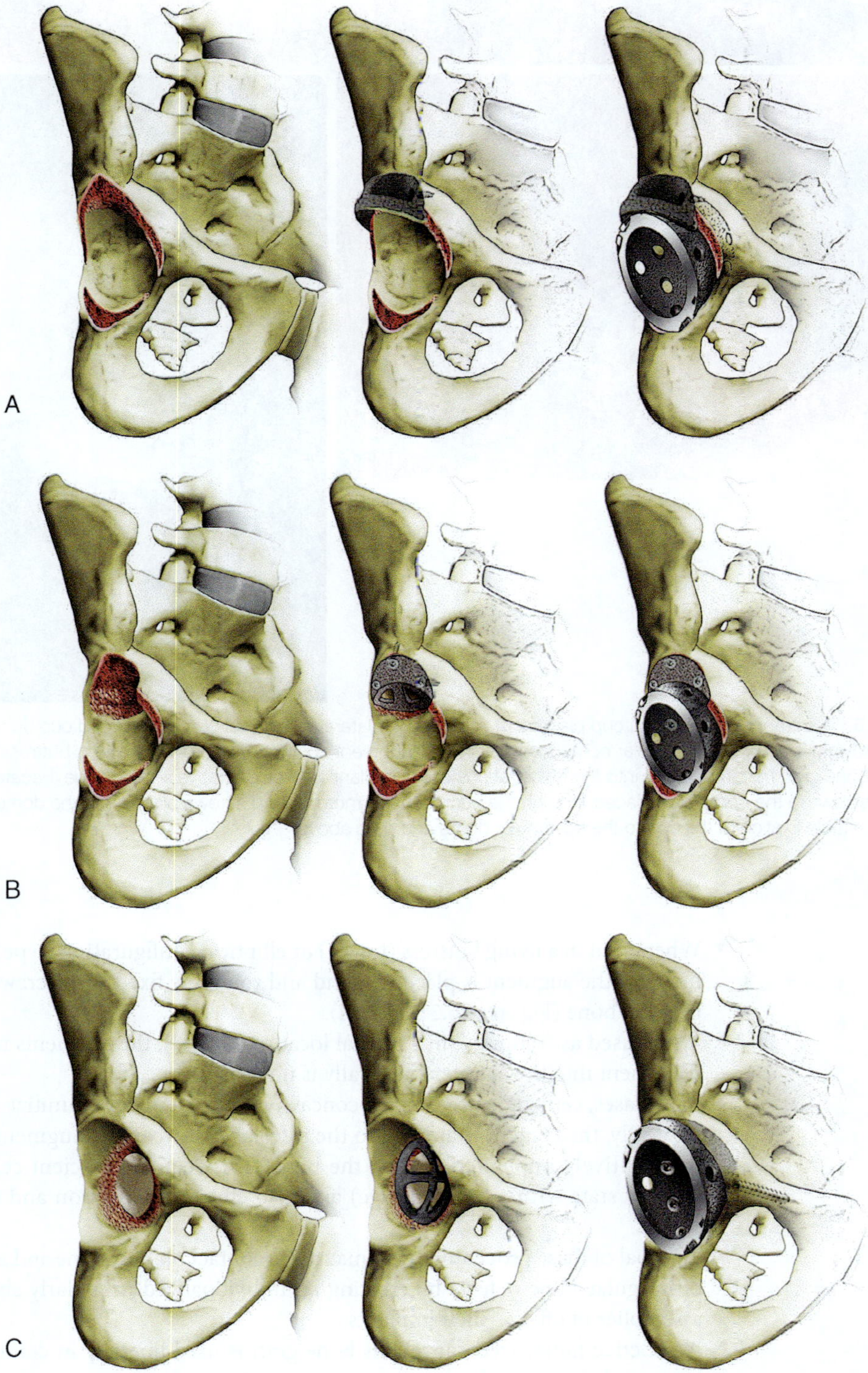

Figure 26.2 | Illustration of the 3 configurations of augment and cup placement used based on the pattern of bone loss encountered: type 1 (flying buttress), type 2 (elliptical), and type 3 (medial footing).

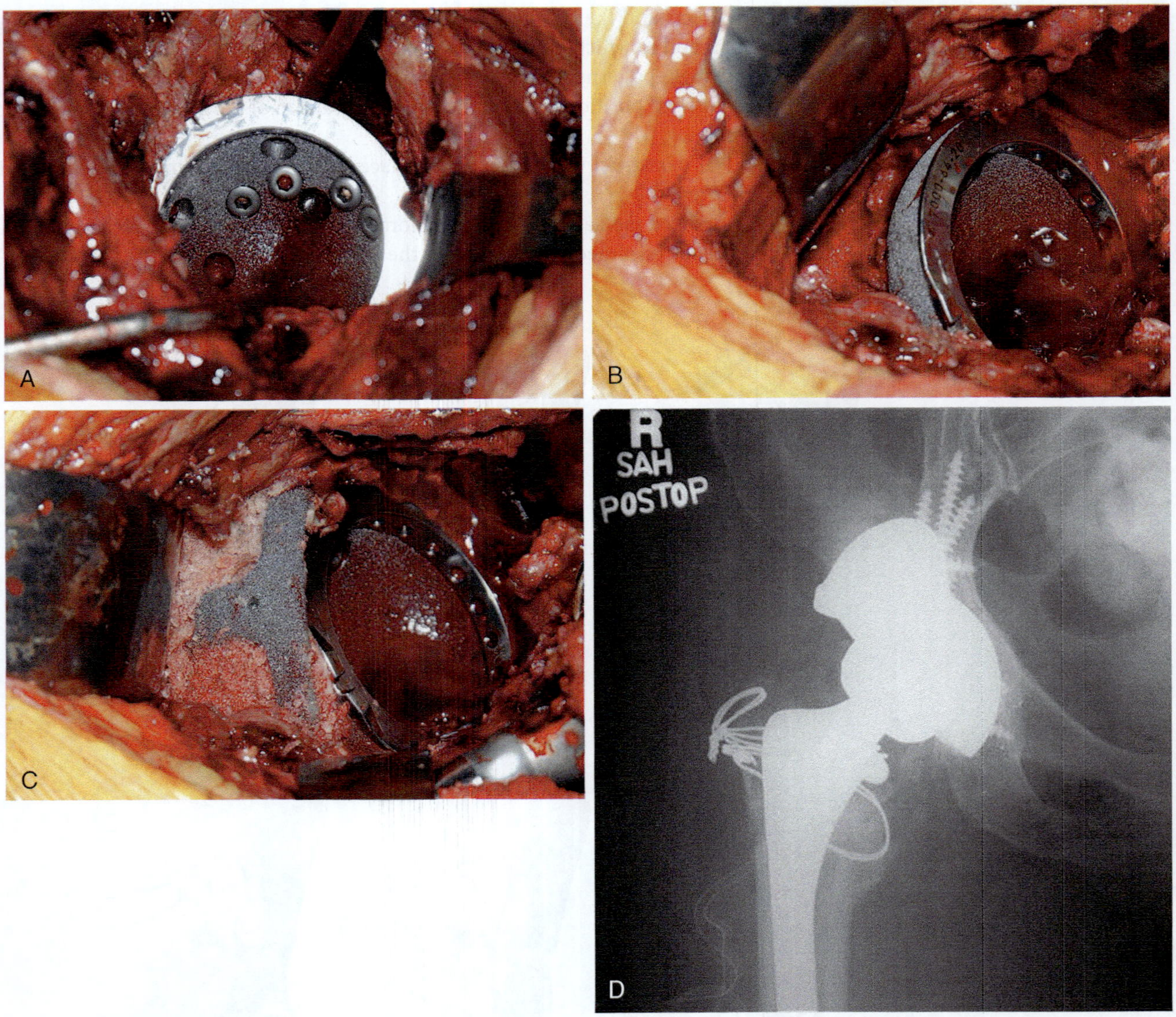

Figure 26.3 | A, Intraoperative view of cup placement with a superolateral segmental bone defect and cup uncoverage. B, Bone defect viewed from the proximal side of the acetabular component. C, Type 1 augment configuration providing "flying buttress" support of the cup with supplemental bone graft material placed into the fenestrations of the implant. D, Postoperative x-ray of type 1 acetabular augment and cup with horizontal screws in the dome area placed through the augment and more vertical screws placed into the dome area of the cup combining to create very stable fixation of the cup to the acetabular dome and ilium above.

- When used in a flying buttress (type 1) or elliptical configuration (type 2), the cup is generally placed first and the augment is placed second and routinely fixed with screws to prioritize cup contact on the host bone (Figures 26.3 and 26.4).
- When used as "footings" in a medial location (type 3), the augments must be placed first and screw placement into the augment generally is not possible.
- In all cases, cement is used on the concavity of the augment to unitize it to the cup (Figure 26.5). Typically, the cement is applied to the interface between the augment and the cup as the augment is definitively implanted against the bone. This requires efficient cement application (usually in a liquid state with a large syringe) and also efficient impaction and fixation of the augment with screws.
- The goal of these procedures is to maximize contact on host bone and aid implant fixation in the face of irregular bone defects by creating an individualized irregularly shaped implant using modular assemblies of off-the-shelf implants.
- Adjunctive morselized cancellous bone graft is used liberally in combination with acetabular augments to help restore bone.

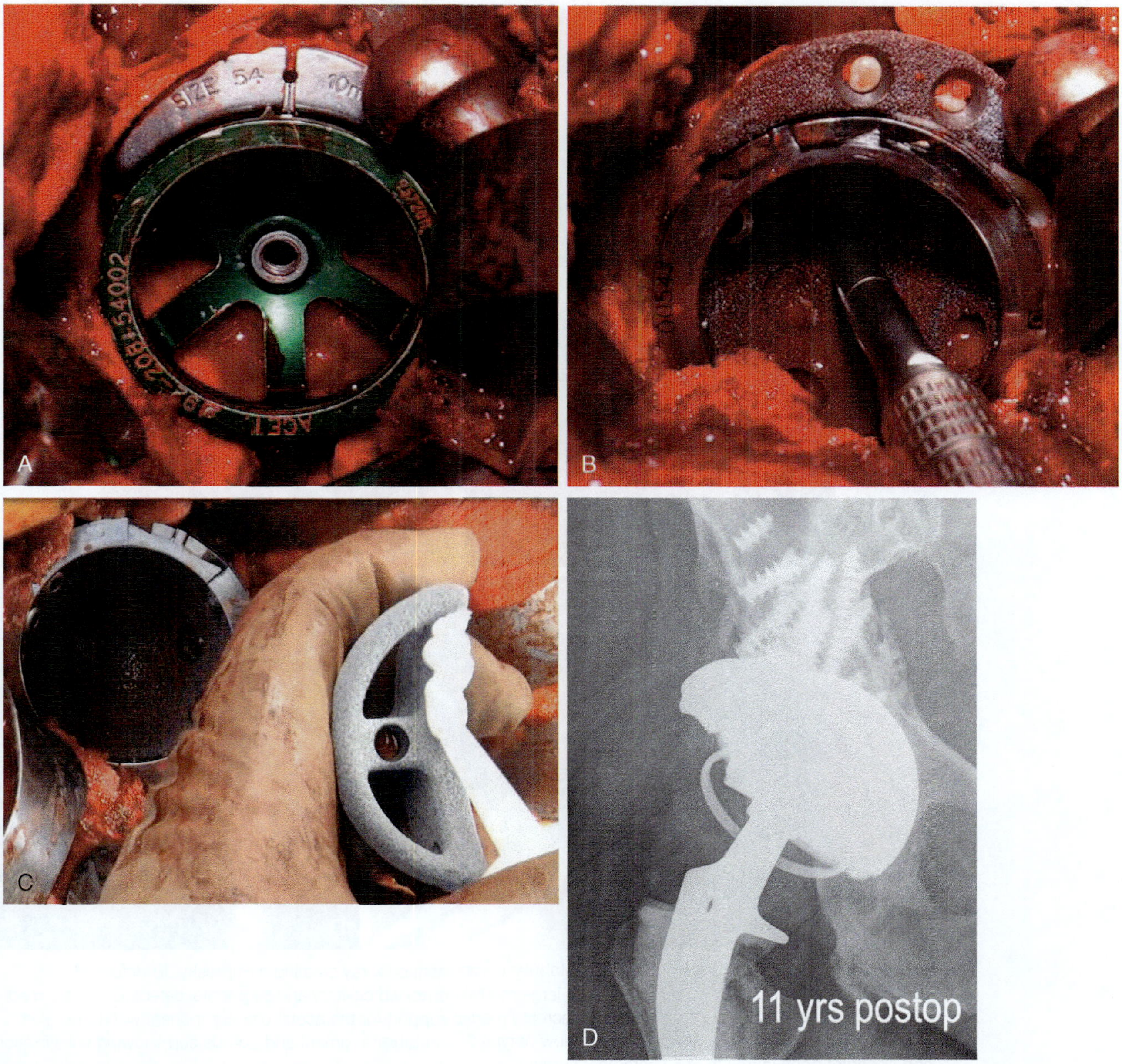

Figure 26.4 | A, Intraoperative view of type 2 construct with provisional acetabular cup and augment trials positioned to fill an elliptical cavity in the acetabulum. B, Cup and augment placement with cement used at the interface of the augment and cup and multiple screws to be placed to fix the combination construct in place. C, Cement placed on the concavity of augment before placement to help unitize augment to cup once the cement has hardened. D, Type 2 augment well fixed along with the acetabular component at 11 years post surgery.

- With successful reconstructions there is an absence of radiolucencies at the implant-bone interfaces.
- Failure to achieve an initially motionless implant-bone interface can result in late migration and failure, especially in the face of pelvic discontinuity whereby additional fixation such as a cup-cage construct may be needed in addition to the uncemented cup and any augments used for defect matching.

Postoperative Care

- Weight bearing is individualized based on assessment of bone defect severity, the resulting implant construct used, and the quality of the fixation achieved (both the femoral and acetabular).
- Any associated fractures (trochanteric vs pelvic discontinuity) and the status of the final soft tissue repair also influence weight-bearing restrictions.
- Most patients, even with sizable defects, who receive acetabular augments are partial weight bearing over the initial 6 to 12 weeks post surgery during healing of the musculature.

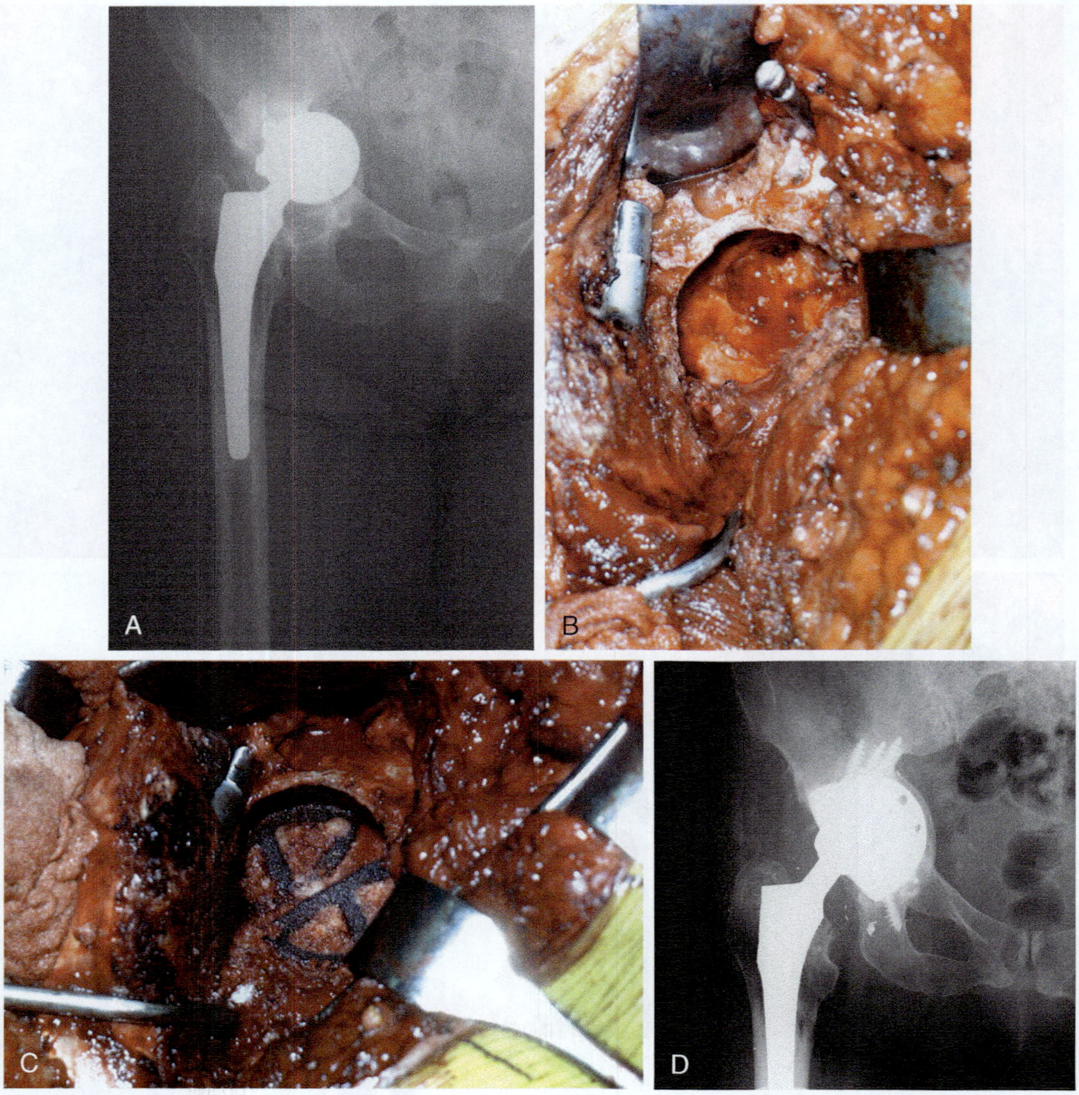

Figure 26.5 | A, Medial migration of loose acetabular component on x-ray creating a Paprosky 3B defect. B, Intraoperative view of intact acetabular rim but large medial combined cavitary and segmental defect. C, Type 3 medially positioned acetabular augments used to recreate medial support for the acetabular component with bone graft material used to fill remaining voids. D, X-ray view of type 3 acetabular augment and porous cup showing solid fixation and apparent bone ingrowth at 5 years post surgery.

- Antibiotics are continued for 10 to 14 days post surgery until final operative culture results are available.
- Abduction hip braces are sometimes used to protect the soft tissue repair and minimize dislocation risk over the first 6 weeks post surgery following revision THA, but use of a brace is unrelated to whether an acetabular augment was used.

Chapter 27
Cup-Cage Constructs

DAVID G. LEWALLEN
ASHTON H. GOLDMAN

Key Concepts

- Major acetabular bone loss may make it difficult or even impossible to achieve stable fixation of a large uncemented porous acetabular component against the remaining host bone.
- Unless a motionless interface between the porous acetabular component and bone is achieved and maintained over the first several months post surgery, bone ingrowth will not occur and the risk of implant migration and failure dramatically increases.
- Chronic pelvic discontinuity is associated with increased failure rates due to cup loosening when standard cup fixation with screws is attempted even when adjunctive augments or posterior column plating is added.
- Charnley zone 3 fixation of the inferior portion of the acetabular component to the posterior column and base of the ischium is important in all acetabular reconstructions but is critical in cases of massive bone loss or pelvic discontinuity.
- The cup-cage technique involves the addition of an antiprotrusio cage over the top of an uncemented acetabular component, which greatly increases the stability of the initial fixation and thereby increases the chances of successful bone ingrowth to the cup over the ensuing weeks post surgery (Figure 27.1).
- When a full cup-cage construct is elected, the ischial flange typically is driven into a bony slot in the ischium. Alternatively, the flange can be placed on the outer surface of the ischium, but this requires additional dissection and can increase the risk of sciatic nerve injury.
- A half cup-cage construct is an alternative in which the ischial flange is removed and the iliac flange is used alone. The half cup-cage technique is technically easier, allows room for screws instead of a flange for fixation into the ischium, and can be used more easily in combination with distraction of any associated pelvic discontinuity.

Sterile Instruments and Implants

- Standard retractors and hip instruments.
- Hemispherical acetabular component instruments and trial and real components in a full range of sizes up to 80 mm.
- Acetabular porous metal augment trials in a variety of sizes and thicknesses to aid in intraoperative assessment, sizing, and planning of final construct.
- Cancellous bone graft to fill any small remaining gaps, defects, or nonunion sites in the acetabulum and to fill the fenestrations of any augments used.
- Antiprotrusio cages in a range of sizes with corresponding malleable trials to aid in bending and fitting of the real component. Fixation screws for the corresponding antiprotrusio cage.

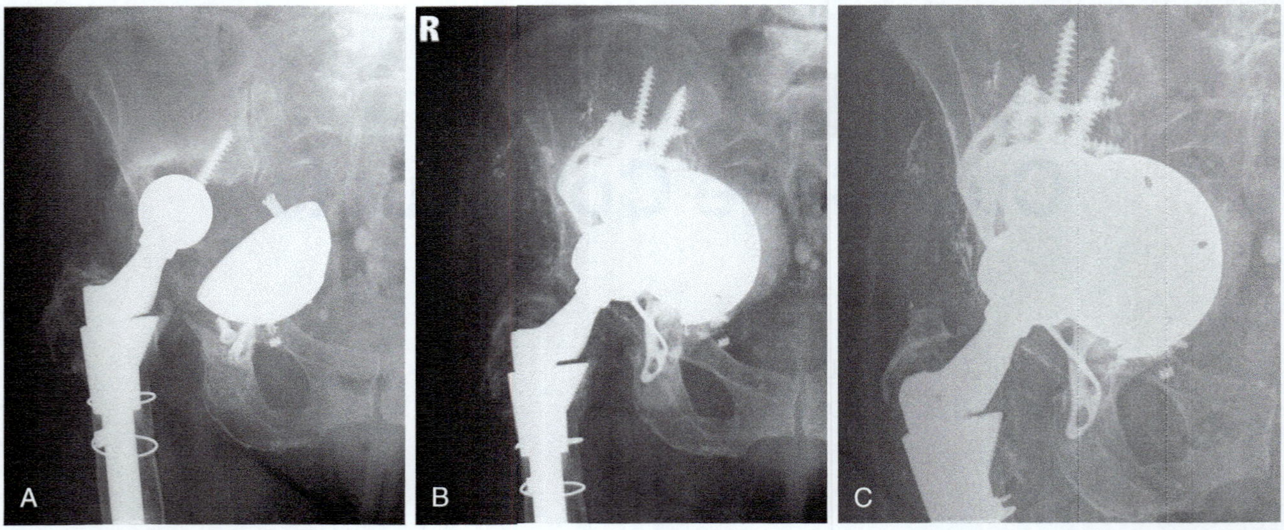

Figure 27.1 I A, Preoperative radiograph of massive Paprosky type 3B bone loss with segmental medial acetabular defect and pelvic discontinuity from migrated cup. B, Postoperative anteroposterior (AP) radiograph of the reconstructed hip showing 2 large medial acetabular augments and bone graft spanning the large medial defect and supporting a jumbo cup fixed with multiple screws and stabilized by a full cage over the top. C, Follow-up radiograph at 6 years post surgery showing solid fixation without implant migration, hardware failure, or radiolucencies.

Surgical Approaches

- Any of the standard potentially extensile surgical approaches can be used per surgeon preference similar to any revision total hip arthroplasty (THA).
- Posterolateral and direct lateral approaches are the most commonly used at our institution, either alone or in combination with an extended trochanteric osteotomy as needed. The exposure is chosen based on exposure requirements on the femoral side and on the acetabular side.
- When a direct lateral approach is used, care must be taken to elevate but not split the gluteus medius too far proximally when exposing the lateral aspect of the ilium above the acetabular cavity to avoid injury to branches of the superior gluteal nerve running to the anterior portion of the muscle.
- When using the posterolateral approach, the superior gluteal nerve is at risk at the sciatic notch at the proximal end of the posterior column, and injury at this level places innervation to the entire gluteus medius at risk.

Preoperative Planning

- An organized assessment of the degree of bone loss on the acetabular side is strongly recommended in cases of major bone loss, and this is ideally based on careful x-ray analysis of key anatomic features.
- The Paprosky classification of acetabular bone defects is helpful in anticipating operative findings and for planning treatment options.
- This classification scheme involves measurement of the amount of cup migration, direction of that migration, status of Kohler line and the tear drop (when medial deficiency and migration of the cup has occurred), and critical assessment of the status of the posterior column as noted on the cross-table lateral radiograph, iliac and obturator oblique (or Judet) views, and occasionally adjunctive computed tomography scanning (Figure 27.2A-C).
- The cup-cage technique is most useful when more severe bone defects as seen in Paprosky type 3A (cup up and out) or 3B defects (cup up and in) make stable fixation of a cementless hemispherical porous cup tenuous despite multiple screws and any adjunctive fixation such as augments.
- Sometimes, decreased residual host bone quality (not just bone deficiency) will play a role in prompting use of a cup-cage to provide more secure fixation of the acetabular component.
- However, the most common current indication for use of a half or full cup-cage is an associated pelvic discontinuity.

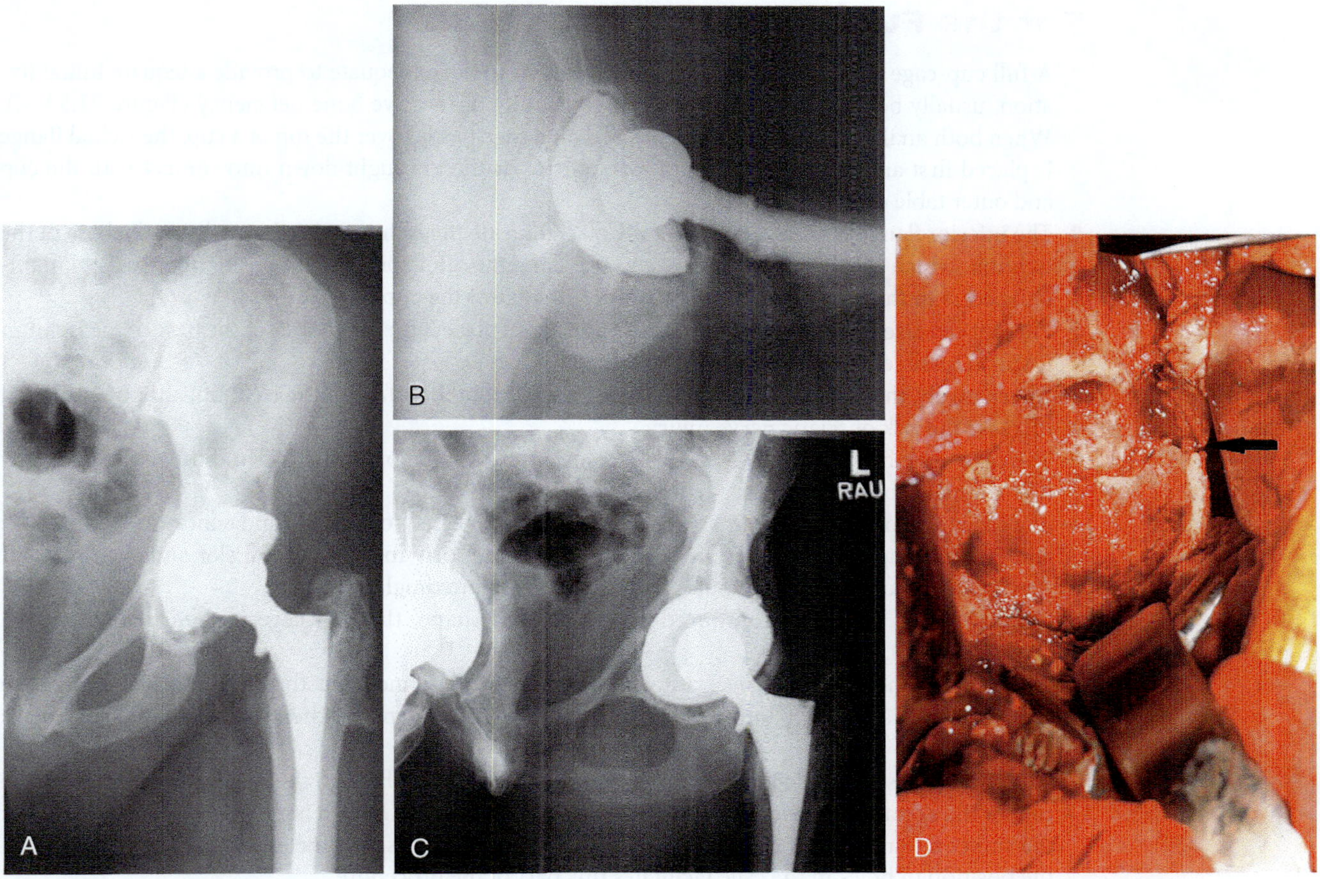

Figure 27.2 | A, Preoperative AP radiograph of the left hip showing radiolucencies at the acetabular implant-bone interface and a bony step off medial to the cup involving the iliopectineal line suggestive of a fracture and possible complete pelvic discontinuity. B, Cross-table lateral view showing the posterior column and a questionable fracture line visible. C, Obturator oblique radiograph more clearly showing the fracture line medially. D, Example of intraoperative appearance of the transverse fracture line of a pelvic discontinuity, which was visible only after removal of the overlying fibrous tissue highlighted here by the arrow where it is exiting the posterior wall of the acetabulum.

- The location and size of the bone defects, size of the patient, and quality of the bone remaining can be difficult to judge despite careful assessment of imaging studies before surgery.
- Thus, planning for more than one potential reconstructive option is important so that a range of implant types and graft materials are readily available after intraoperative assessment makes the precise features of that specific case clear.

Bone, Implant, and Soft Tissue Techniques

- Following exposure and careful removal of the failed implants, the size and location of any acetabular bone defects are assessed. Critical specific details include size of the cavity, shape (elliptical or roughly hemispherical), status of the acetabular dome and posterior superior wall, presence of segmental (versus cavitary) defects, and presence of any fracture lines or actual discontinuity of ilium and ischium.
- Stressing the ilium and ischium separately after wide exposure while looking carefully for any asynchronous motion of the dome versus inferior acetabular cavity is very important because pelvic discontinuity can be occult and difficult to pick up, especially if exposure is suboptimal (Figure 27.2D).
- Presence of pelvic discontinuity is currently our most common indication for use of a cup-cage construct in part due to the increased failure rate previously observed in our hands when a cup alone was used with or without adjunctive augments or posterior column plating.
- Following any bone grafting of the acetabulum, porous cup placement, and initial cup fixation with multiple screws, the decision to add a cage for additional fixation is finalized

For the Full Cup-Cage Technique

- A full cup-cage is used when a cup alone is judged to be inadequate to provide adequate initial fixation, usually because of an associated discontinuity or massive bone deficiency (Figure 27.3A-C). When both an iliac and ischial flange is used on a cage placed over the top of a cup, the ischial flange is placed first and the main cage and iliac portion is then brought down into contact with the cup and outer table of the ilium.
- The inferior flange of the cage is generally placed inside the ischium via a bony slot at the base of the ischium, which is best created before cup placement to allow proper cup positioning so as to maintain access to the bony slot just past the inferior edge of the cup.
- The slot can also be created after the cup is already in place if the target area at the base of the ischium is still accessible past the inferior edge of the cup.
- Alternatively, the ischial flange may be placed on the outer surface of the ischium, although this can increase the risk of sciatic nerve injury.
- The cage must be contoured to fit before placement over the top of the cup and this is facilitated by use of a malleable cage trial as a template.
- The cage trial for the particular size cage selected is subjected to bending and contouring of the iliac and ischial flanges so that the trial can be driven inferiorly into the ischial slot and then brought down and contoured to fit the outer table of the ilium proximal to the cup.
- Once the trial has been contoured to the desired shape, the real cage is then bent to match (Figure 27.3D).
- The ischial flange is then driven into the ischial slot first, and then the cage and iliac flange are brought down superiorly into the cup and onto the outer table of the ilium and fixed into place (Figure 27.3E).
- After the cage is assembled to the cup, a dome screw is placed through the cage and cup and into the roof of the acetabular cavity unitizing the cup-cage construct. Use of a highly porous cup that allows the surgeon to make new screw holes in the cup (with a high-speed metal-cutting burr) that match the position of holes in the cage facilitates this part of the procedure.
- Multiple additional fixation screws are then placed through the iliac flange into the ilium perpendicular to the multiple screws in the dome of the cup.
- When a full cage has been used and the ischial flange has been driven into place inferiorly and the iliac flange secured with screws proximally, it is helpful to check and see if it is possible to place 1 or 2 screws through the shoulder portion of the ischial flange and into the ischium below, although frequently there is not enough room to allow this once the flange is present inside the ischium (Figure 27.3F).
- The desired acetabular insert can then be cemented into the cup-cage, completing the acetabular reconstruction. Cement is simultaneously interdigitated between the cage and the cup to "unitize" the construct.

For the Half Cup-Cage Technique

- The iliac flange may be used alone as a half-cage construct, as this provides excellent added fixation and rotational control for the cup. Insertion of a half cup-cage is technically easier and faster (Figure 27.4A-D).
- When there is major bone deficiency but no actual discontinuity, use of a half cage can also be safer, as it is possible to cause a fracture of a deficient but still intact acetabulum while driving in the ischial flange and inserting a full cage.
- Placement of a half cage over the top of a cup is less traumatic and requires less soft tissue exposure than insertion of a full cup-cage.
- Usually the anatomy of the ischium at the inferior aspect of the acetabulum combined with the frequent small size of the (usually female) patients presenting with pelvic discontinuity requires a choice to be made between a full cage with both an ischial and iliac flange and a half cage with only a single flange onto the ilium above and screws into the ischial base instead (Figure 27.5).
- Cutting away the ischial flange allows room for multiple screws to be used inferiorly through the very periphery of the cup into the base of the ischium out the quadrilateral surface, and this usually results in better fixation than can be achieved with a flange that is press fit into a bony slot in the ischium.

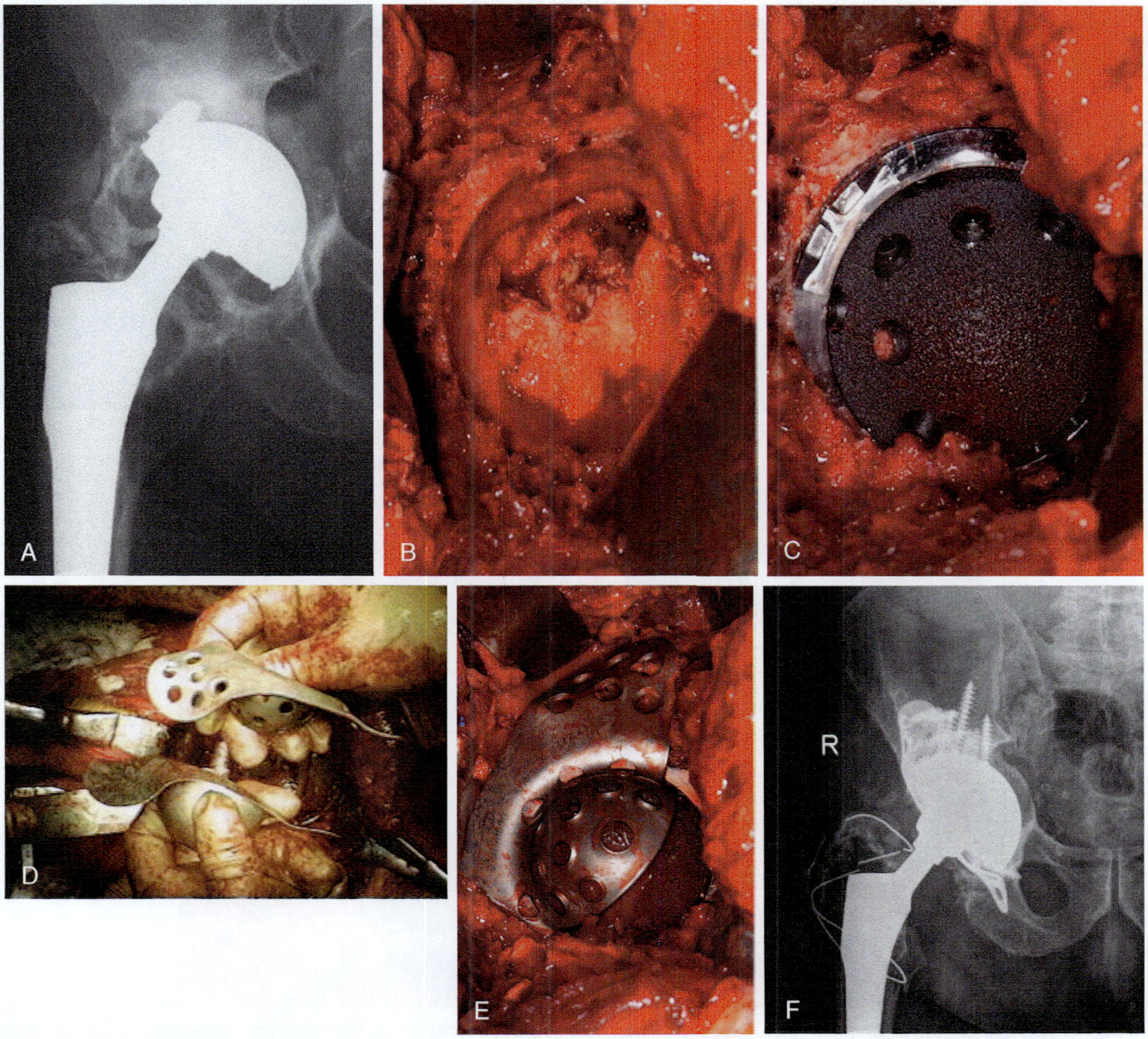

Figure 27.3 | A, Preoperative radiograph of a symptomatic hip with polyethylene wear and medial osteolysis. B, Intraoperative view at surgery during which the posterior column was found to be intact with a thin arc around to the dome. Massive bone loss was present medially and anteriorly, although there was no frank pelvic discontinuity. C, The cup was fixed with 4 screws, but fixation was judged inadequate and the cup was rotationally unstable owing to absent bone and anterior inferior support from the dome distally. D, Cage trial after contouring and insertion into the ischial slot and cup to check fit used to guide bending of the real cage as shown here. E, Real cage inserted into the cup with the ischial flange embedded into the bone at the base of the ischium as seen in the lower left corner. F, AP radiograph 6 years post surgery showing solid fixation without migration or lucencies around the cup or the multiple screws used in the dome of the cup, the iliac flange proximally or the inferior screws placed into the shoulder area of the ischial flange visible at the inferior edge of the cup.

- Another major advantage of the half cage technique is that it is quite easy to combine this method with distraction of an associated pelvic discontinuity.
- Distraction can be accomplished during half cup-cage placement either by impaction of an oversized cup (6-10 mm larger than the resting cavity of the acetabulum) or by impaction of an acetabular augment at the rim of the cup.
- The augment is inserted after placement of an acetabular component that completely fills the resting acetabular cavity and fixation to one side of the discontinuity, opposite the side where the augment will be driven into place.
- The augment size and width are selected to match the cup and the mobility of the proximal and distal segments of the acetabulum so as to allow the augment to be impacted in the manner of a wedge driven between the cup and host bone. The goal is to fully distract and stabilize the discontinuity before final screws are placed through the augment and the cup locking the bone on that side of the

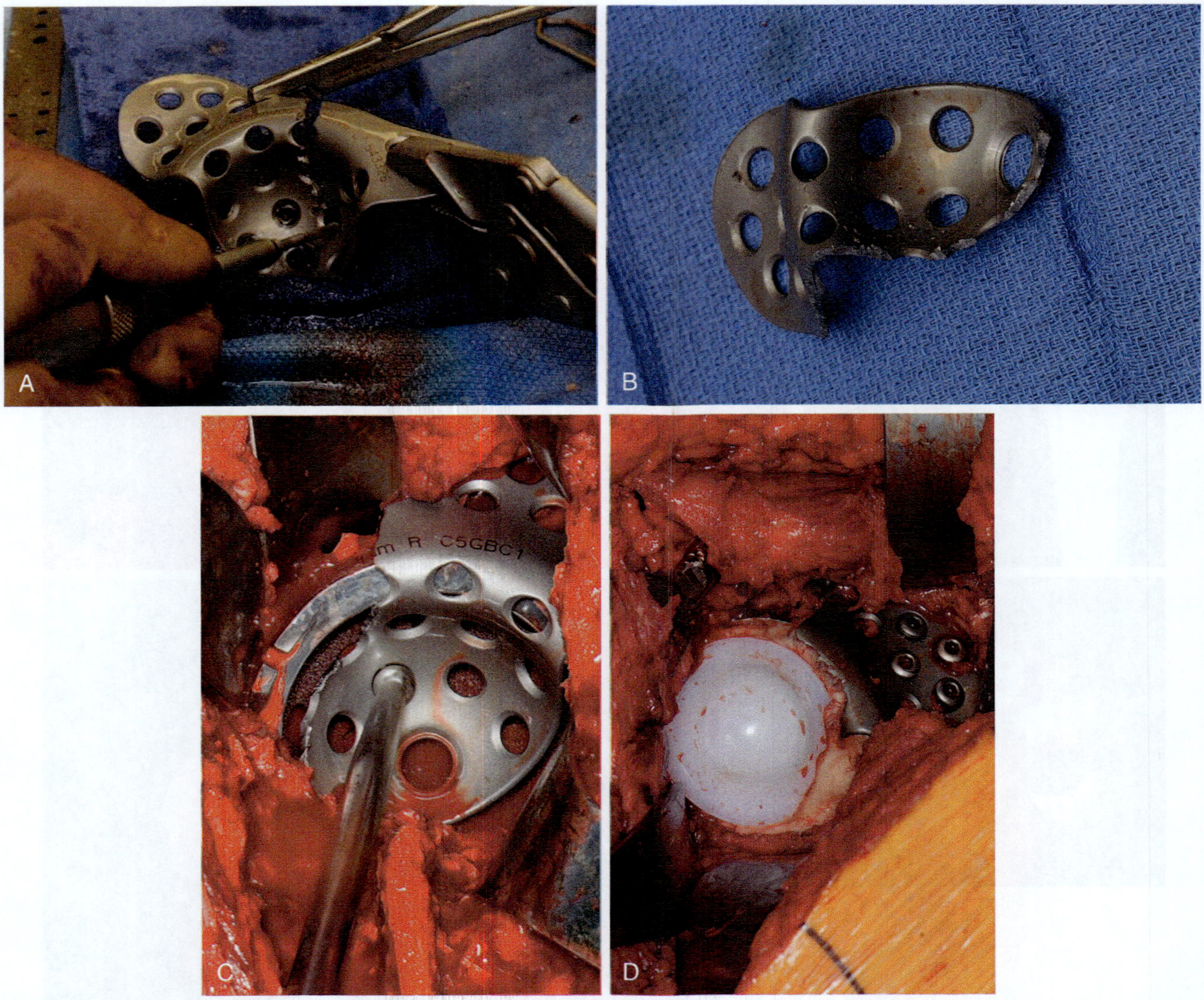

Figure 27.4 | A, Cutting the ischial flange off of a full cage to create a half cup-cage construct. B, Half cage after sectioning. C, The half cage was initially fixed with a screw placed through the cage and cup into the dome of the acetabulum, followed by multiple screws into the iliac flange. D, Completed half cup-cage with iliac screws shown and the polyethylene insert cemented into position with the cement serving to unitize the cage to the cup and create a locking screw effect by enveloping many of the screws used to fix both the cage and the cup to bone.

discontinuity in place. Cement is placed at the junction of the augment and cup to help unitize the reconstruction (Figure 27.6).

- After distraction and completion of cup and augment screw fixation, the half cage can then be placed over the top of the reconstruction and fixed in place, further stabilizing the construct and enhancing overall fixation of the discontinuity. Fixation of the half cage with screws is similar to that described earlier for a full cage.

Postoperative Care

- Weight bearing status is individualized and begun the same or next day following surgery as with any revision THA.
- Patients are protected from full weight bearing for 8 to 12 weeks, depending on surgeon preference and the stability of the initial construct. Moreover. prolonged protection, for at least 3 months, is commonly recommended for pelvic discontinuity cases.

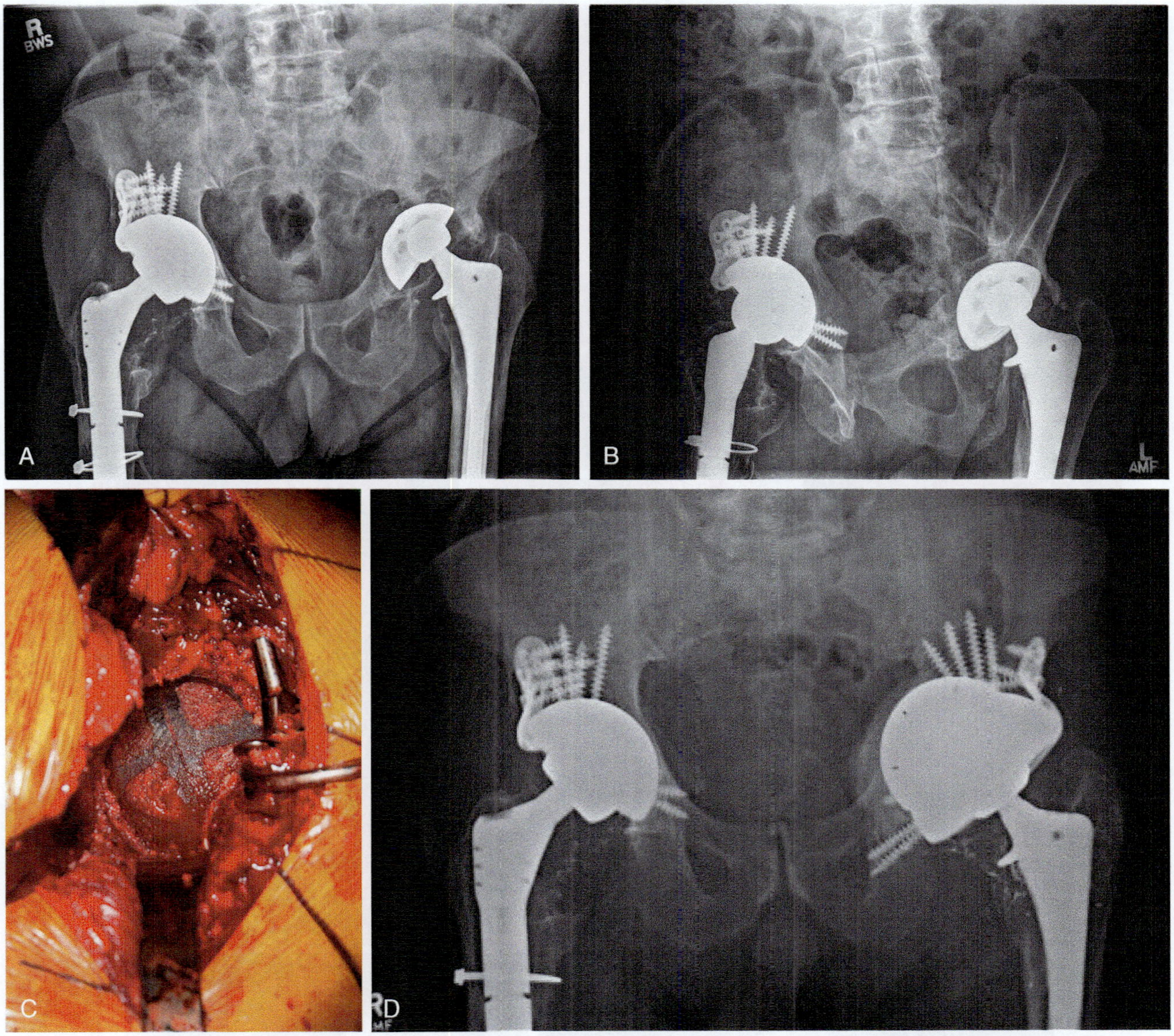

Figure 27.5 | A, Preoperative AP pelvis radiograph of patient with a successful prior half cup-cage on the right side performed as part of a 2-stage reconstruction for infection, now with a symptomatic left hip due to polyethylene wear and aseptic osteolysis resulting in a segmental medial wall defect. B, Obturator oblique radiograph confirming pelvic discontinuity on the left side with a visible defect and a step off due to migration of the inferior half of the acetabulum. C, Intraoperative view of reconstructed medial defect using 2 acetabular augments and morselized cancellous bone graft. D, Radiograph 2 years post surgery on the left with solid fixation, apparent bone healing and bone ingrowth, and no radiographic signs of component loosening or migration. Note the array of screws used in the dome of the cup and the transverse iliac flange screws combining to lock the reconstruction securely to the ilium above. Also, note long screws in an array at the inferior edge of the cup in zone 3 extending into the base of the ischium or quadrilateral surface medially, on both the left and right hips.

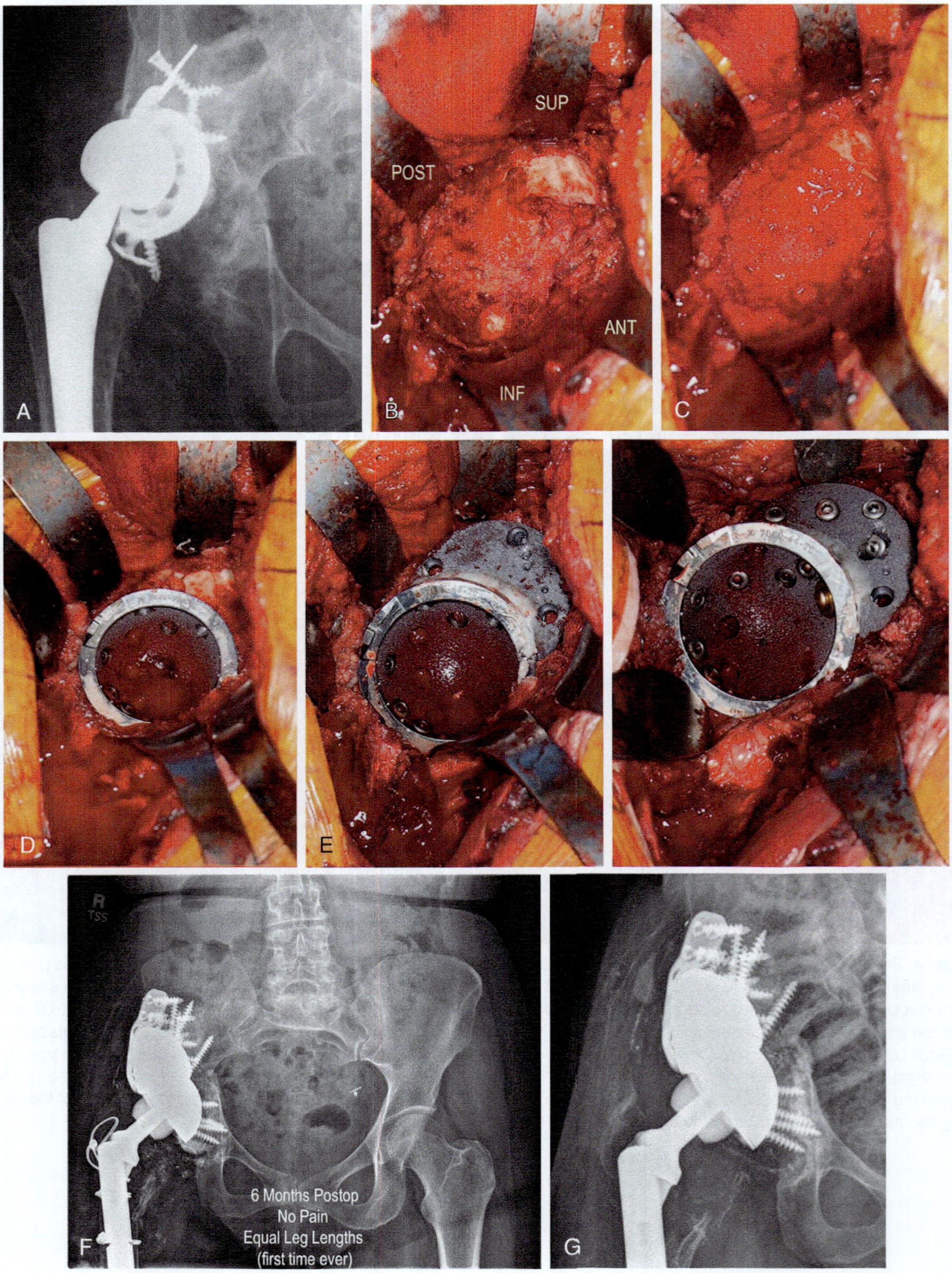

Figure 27.6 | A, Paprosky type 3A defect and an associated pelvic discontinuity in an originally dysplastic patient with reduced superolateral bone stock to begin with and multiple failed reconstructions over the many years before the current failed implant. B, Intraoperative view of long elliptical acetabular defect. C, Same defect after cancellous bone grafting and limited (mostly reverse) reaming down low at the anatomic hip center and up high against the supportive proximal dome and iliac remnants due to a long-standing high hip center. D, As large a cup as possible given AP dimensions of the acetabulum placed low at the correct anatomic level and fixed with multiple screws to the ischium and inferior portion of the posterior column with an approximately 1-cm gap between the upper edge of the cup and the intact "dome" superiorly. E, Oversized acetabular augment driven in as a wedge between the dome and superior edge of the cup causing distraction through the discontinuity of the superior half of the acetabulum proximally and the cup fixed to the inferior half of the acetabulum distally. After impacting as large an augment as possible, in as far as it would go, the augment is fixed in place with transverse screws. Additional multiple long vertical screws are also placed through the cup into the dome of the acetabulum in an array. F, Radiograph of the half cage 6 months after reconstruction with a very long iliac flange placed into the cup, over the top of the augment and fixed with multiple screws to the lateral aspect of the ilium proximally. G, Radiograph at 3 years showing maintenance of solid fixation. The patient was pain free with weight bearing.

Chapter 28
Custom Triflange Implants

MATTHEW W. TETREAULT
MICHAEL J. TAUNTON

Key Concepts

- Custom triflange acetabular components provide a unique solution for bridging large acetabular defects that exceed the limits of defect-matching techniques.
- These implants possess the strength to provide long-term stability without underlying support, the potential for biologic fixation, and the ability to address specific bony defects and pelvic anatomy.
- Collaboration between the surgeon and implant design team is paramount during preoperative planning because intraoperative flexibility is limited.
- A minimum of several weeks is required for implant design and fabrication.

Sterile Instruments and Implants

Instruments

- Routine hip retractors
- A full set of revision total hip arthroplasty (THA) instruments, including:
  - Cup explant system
  - Femoral component explant system
  - High-speed burrs (short and long pencil-tip burrs, 6.5-mm round burr)
  - Osteotomes (straight, curved, flexible)
  - Cement removal set/instruments to clean out intramedullary canal
  - Curettes
  - Cobb elevators
  - Drill, drill bits, threaded drill guides, depth gauge
- In the event of a trochanteric osteotomy:
  - Cabling device/wire passers (also for prophylactic use during femoral component revision)
  - Oscillating saw
- Sterilized models of the hemipelvis and triflange implant

Implants

- Custom triflange acetabular component and liner
- Custom triflange screws
- Femoral heads (with trial heads)
- Revision femoral components (with trial stems)
- Cerclage cables and wires
- Allograft bone chips

Positioning

- Lateral decubitus with hip positioners
- The operative limb should be draped out and sterilely prepared from the iliac crest to the distal thigh.

Surgical Approach

- The authors typically prefer an extensile posterolateral approach, although an extensile anterolateral or transtrochanteric approach may be used.
- A trochanteric osteotomy can facilitate femoral component removal and/or relieve tension when exposure for the iliac flange would risk traction injury to the superior gluteal nerve.

Preoperative Planning

Record Review

- Obtaining the outside operative report and implant stickers is essential.

Laboratory Workup

- Assess for infection preoperatively with inflammatory markers and fluoroscopically guided hip aspiration as indicated.

Imaging

- Preoperative imaging is imperative and includes the following:
  - Anteroposterior (AP) pelvic radiograph
  - AP hip radiograph
  - Cross-table lateral hip radiograph
  - Judet radiographs (obturator and iliac oblique views)
  - Thin-slice computed tomography (CT) scan with 3-dimensional (3D) reconstruction
- The above-mentioned imaging should be used to determine the extent of acetabular bone loss, including the presence and stability of a pelvic discontinuity (separation of the ilium from the ischiopubic segment), as well as the quantity and location of remaining host bone. This imaging also allows for the precise identification of in situ hardware.
- If severe protrusion of the acetabular implant is present, CT angiography may be ordered to assess existing implant proximity to intrapelvic vessels. If vascular structures are at risk, preoperative evaluation by a vascular surgeon (who can be on standby at the time of surgery in the event of vascular compromise) is warranted. Very rarely, a retroperitoneal exposure is indicated to free the intrapelvic structures before implant removal.

Indications

- A custom triflange cup is appropriate for cases of severe acetabular bone loss that exceed the limits of defect-matching techniques whereby the acetabulum can be filled with a larger hemispherical cup or by an augment to achieve stability on host bone (Figure 28.1A-C).
- Indications for a custom triflange cup include selected American Academy of Orthopaedic Surgeons (AAOS) type III combined acetabular defects (or Paprosky 3A or 3B defects[1]) and selected (or in the hands of some surgeon, all) type IV defects (pelvic discontinuities).[2]
- In the setting of a pelvic discontinuity (Figure 28.2A and B), there are 2 simultaneous goals:
  - Long-term acetabular component stability
  - Healing across the bony discontinuity or "unitization" of the pelvis through healing of both the superior and inferior pelvis to the cup construct
- Contemporary reconstruction options for chronic pelvic discontinuities are detailed in Section II-D, Chapter 6. A custom triflange acetabular component is one solution for bridging a large acetabular defect, as the flanges are strong enough for long-term stability without underlying support and also allow for biologic ingrowth on host iliac and ischial bone (Figure 28.3A and B).

Component Design

- For design and production of a custom triflange component, a CT scan of the pelvis with metal subtraction software is needed. Requisite CT specifications should be discussed in advance with the

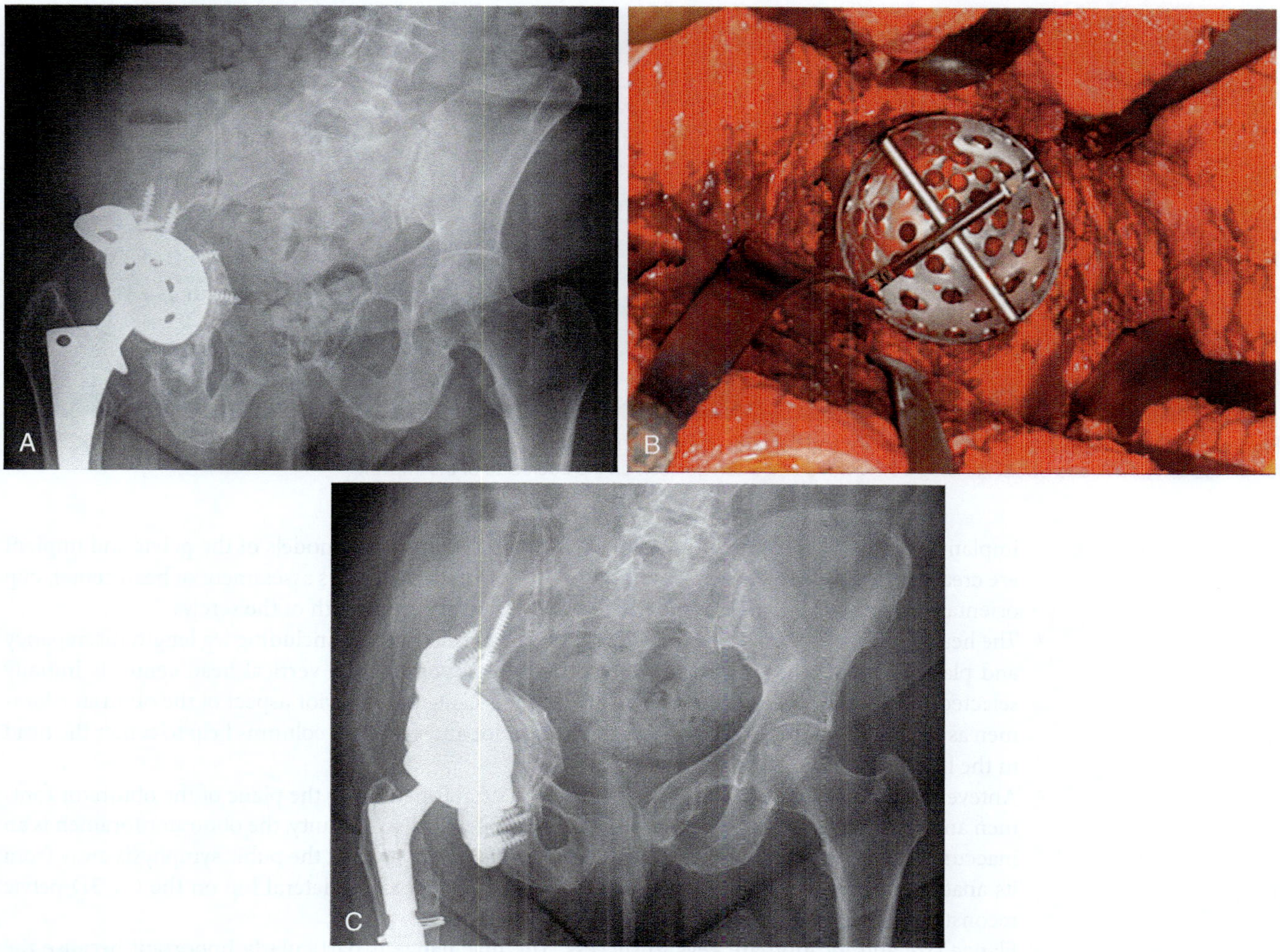

Figure 28.1 | A preoperative AP pelvis radiograph (A) shows a massive right acetabular defect after failed acetabular revision surgery that exceeded the limits of a defect-matching reconstructive technique with a large hemispherical cup. This is illustrated by an intraoperative photograph (B) showing failure of a 70-mm trial reamer to achieve peripheral bony contact when placed in the cavitary defect. The acetabulum was thus reconstructed with a custom triflange component, as seen on 1-year postoperative AP pelvis radiograph (C).

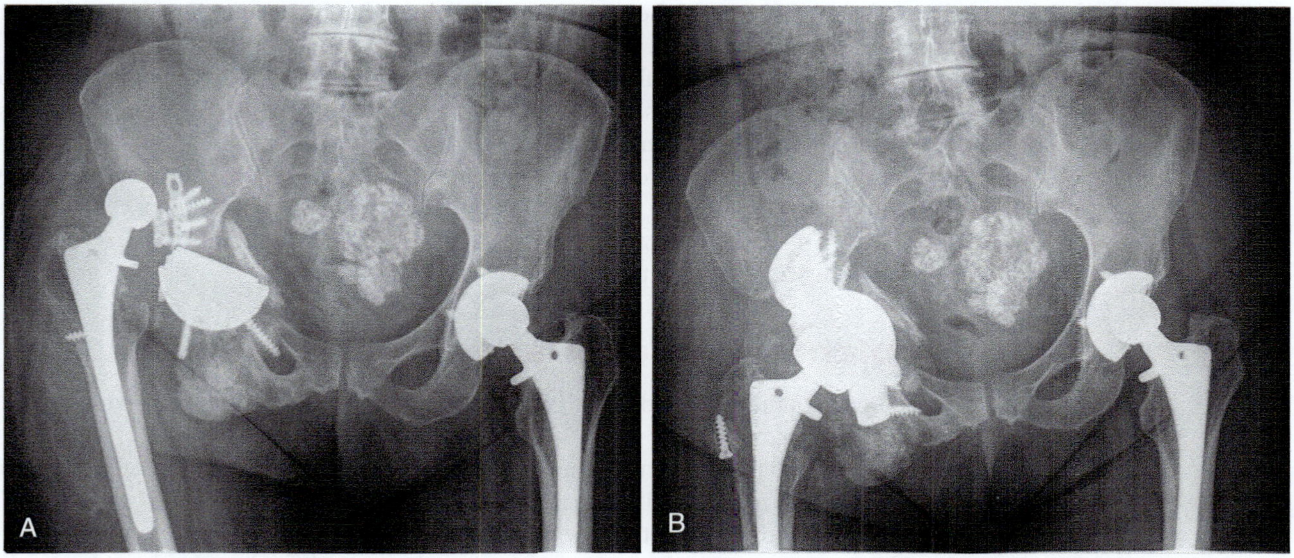

Figure 28.2 | A pelvic discontinuity with associated dislocation of the right hip is demonstrated on preoperative AP pelvis radiograph (A) after failure of an antiprotrusio cage and cemented cup construct placed in the setting of an acetabular periprosthetic fracture. A postoperative AP pelvis radiograph (B) demonstrates reconstruction with a custom triflange acetabular component spanning the discontinuity.

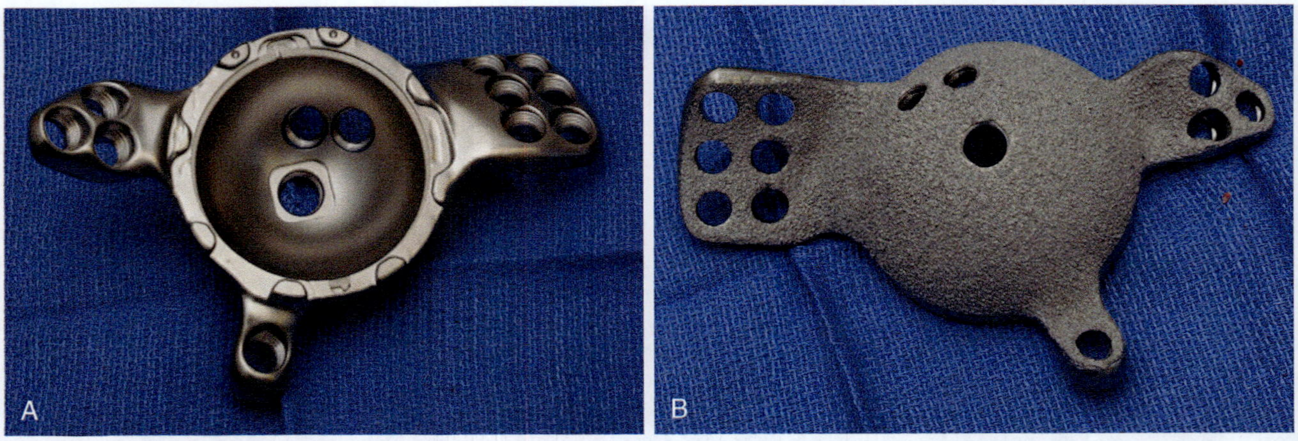

Figure 28.3 | Clinical photographs of the front (A) and back (B) of a custom triflange acetabular component demonstrate the 3 flanges designed for the ischium, ilium, and pubis. A biologic ingrowth surface can be seen on the back side of the implant.

implant manufacturer. Three-dimensional (computer and plastic) models of the pelvis and implant are created for review by the surgeon (Figure 28.4A-C). This includes assessment of head center, cup orientation, size and location of the flanges, and trajectory and length of the screws.

- The head center is chosen based on patient-specific considerations, including leg length discrepancy and planned retention or revision of the femoral component. The vertical head center is initially selected by approximating the anatomic head center using the superior aspect of the obturator foramen as a reference point. The remnants of the anterior and posterior columns help to center the head in the horizontal plane.
- Anteversion and abduction of the cup are initially established using the plane of the obturator foramen and the interteardrop line as guides. In cases of pelvic discontinuity, the obturator foramen is an inaccurate reference point because the inferior pelvis rotates around the pubic symphysis away from its anatomic position. In these cases, the iliac wing and the contralateral hip on the CT 3D pelvic reconstruction are used to determine cup face orientation.
- Flange size and location are keys to success. The iliac flange is particularly important because the best-quality bone and largest surface area for contact is found in the ilium. This flange should be well contoured over the gluteal ridge, and the screw holes should begin at the inferior edge of the remaining structurally sound ilium. The ischial flange sits under the sciatic nerve and should be sufficiently long and broad for screw fixation, and also low profile with rounded edges to avoid irritation of the sciatic nerve. The pubic flange is generally small and triangular in shape and may lack a screw hole. Cup stability on the pelvic model should be assessed. Although the central hemispherical portion does not have to intimately contact the remaining acetabulum, the component should have inherent stability when placed on the model.
- Screw length and trajectory on the flanges should be scrutinized to optimize bony fixation. The authors prefer to use 2 rows of 3 iliac screws (usually 6 total) and a minimum of 3 to 4 ischial screws. Locking screw technology is a key component of modern construct design.
- Typically there are 2 to 3 screws through the dome of the acetabulum. Two of them are usually aimed up the anterior and posterior columns. These screws are usually placed in a compression mode.
- Once the design is finalized, manufacturing typically takes 4 to 6 weeks.

Bone, Implant, and Soft Tissue Techniques

- Perform an approach to the hip based on surgeon preference. We typically utilize an extensile posterior approach.
  - The skin is incised, and the soft tissue planes are reestablished. The tensor fascia is separated from the underlying gluteus medius and vastus lateralis fascia.
  - It is important to identify and protect the sciatic nerve before proceeding with posterior dissection. Significant scar tissue may be present; if surgical planes are difficult to develop, identify the nerve distally (deep to the gluteus maximus insertion or directly over the ischium) and trace it proximally into the sciatic notch. The nerve must be found and mobilized because the ischial

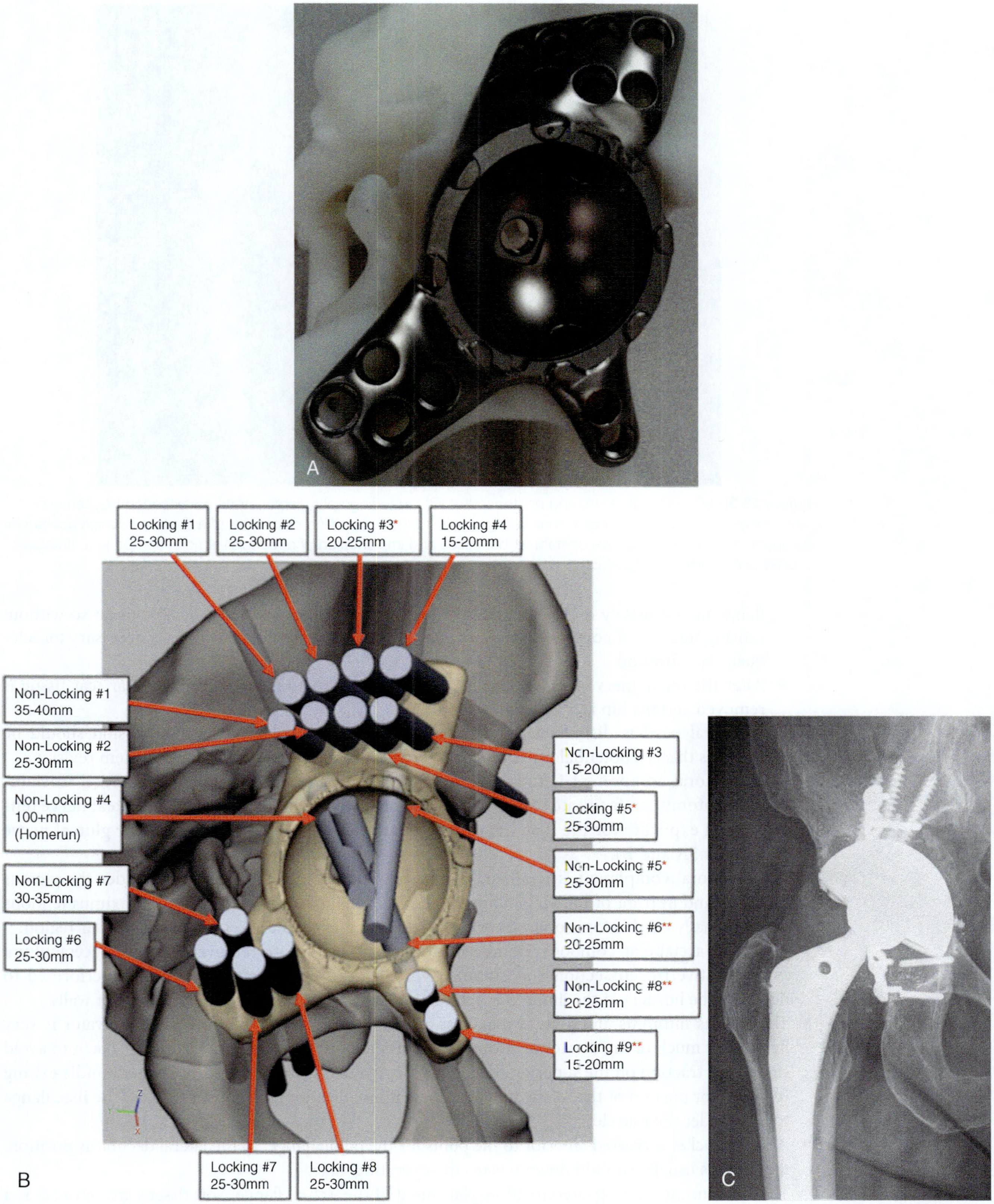

Figure 28.4 | Clinical photograph of implant and hemipelvis models (A) as well as a 3-dimensional CT reconstruction of the patient's hemipelvis with the proposed triflange implant in place (B) for addressing the massive acetabular defect shown on AP hip radiograph (C).

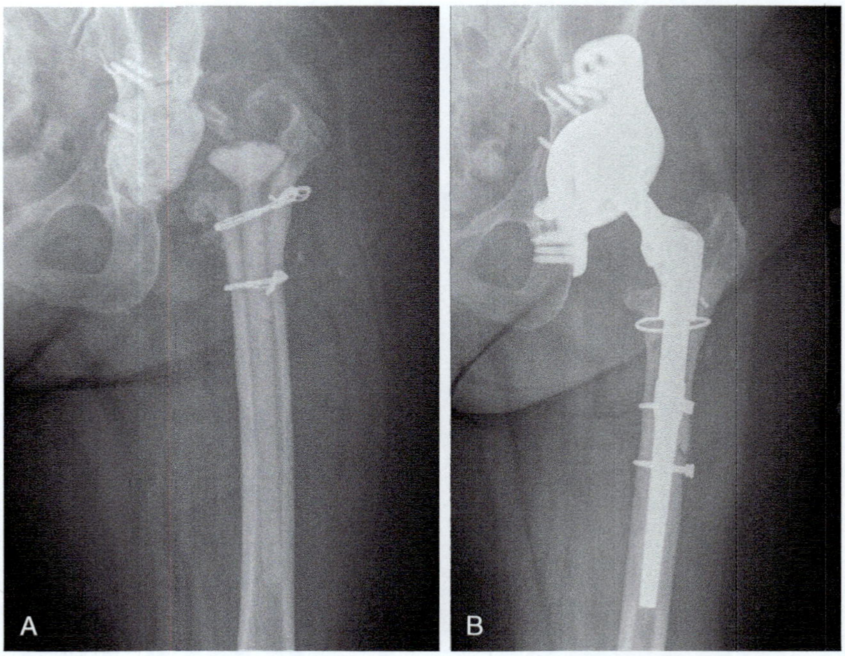

Figure 28.5 | AP preoperative (A) and postoperative (B) hip radiographs demonstrate an extended trochanteric osteotomy utilized to facilitate exposure during revision surgery involving placement of a custom triflange acetabular component to address massive acetabular bone loss and implantation of a modular femoral component. (Images courtesy of Daniel J. Berry, M.D.)

flange fits intimately on the "sciatic" surface of the ischium and must be able to do so without causing traction or compression injury. Occasionally, an external neurolysis is necessary for adequate mobilization.

- After the sciatic nerve is mobilized, a posterior arthrotomy is made. Periarticular scar tissue is removed and the hip is dislocated.

- The femoral head is disimpacted, and the femoral component is inspected. Version should be assessed, as this is a potential cause of intraoperative instability that could warrant stem revision.
- If the femoral component is to be revised, it is extracted at this stage. An extended trochanteric osteotomy can facilitate stem revision and also relieve abductor/superior gluteal nerve tension when exposure for the iliac flange would risk traction injury to the superior gluteal nerve (Figure 28.5A and B).
- If the femoral component is retained, it is mobilized and retracted anteriorly, under the gluteus minimus and in front of the acetabulum. Release of the iliopsoas and/or gluteus maximus tendons is occasionally needed for mobilization of the femur and adequate access to the acetabular region.
- The prior acetabular component and pseudocapsular tissues are removed from the acetabulum. Intraoperative frozen section and cultures typically are sent. Careful dissection is performed to delineate the borders of the ilium, the ischium, the pubis, and the posterior and anterior walls.
- The gluteus minimus and gluteus maximus are elevated off of the ilium. A Cobb elevator is very helpful for much of the dissection around the borders of the acetabulum. Caution is taken to avoid significant traction on the superior gluteal nerve contained within the neurovascular bundle exiting the superior portion of the sciatic notch. Sufficient mobilization must occur to allow the iliac flange to pass under the muscle.
- A small pocket is created anterior to the pubis for the pubic flange. In the lateral decubitus position, the pubis is usually straight down toward the operating table.
- The ischium must be exposed to allow placement of the ischial flange. Soft tissues are elevated as a sleeve off of the residual posterior column, extending from the inferior aspect of the sciatic notch to past the ischium. This may include part of the hamstring origin, particularly in patients with a small pelvis, to facilitate placement of the ischial flange and multiple screws. Keeping the hip in extension and the knee flexed decreases the tension on the sciatic nerve.
- The pelvis is assessed for subtle discontinuity through the application of traction or rotatory torque with ball spike pushers placed on the superior and inferior aspects of the acetabulum. Implantation of the triflange component may differ in the presence of a pelvic discontinuity, as detailed subsequently.

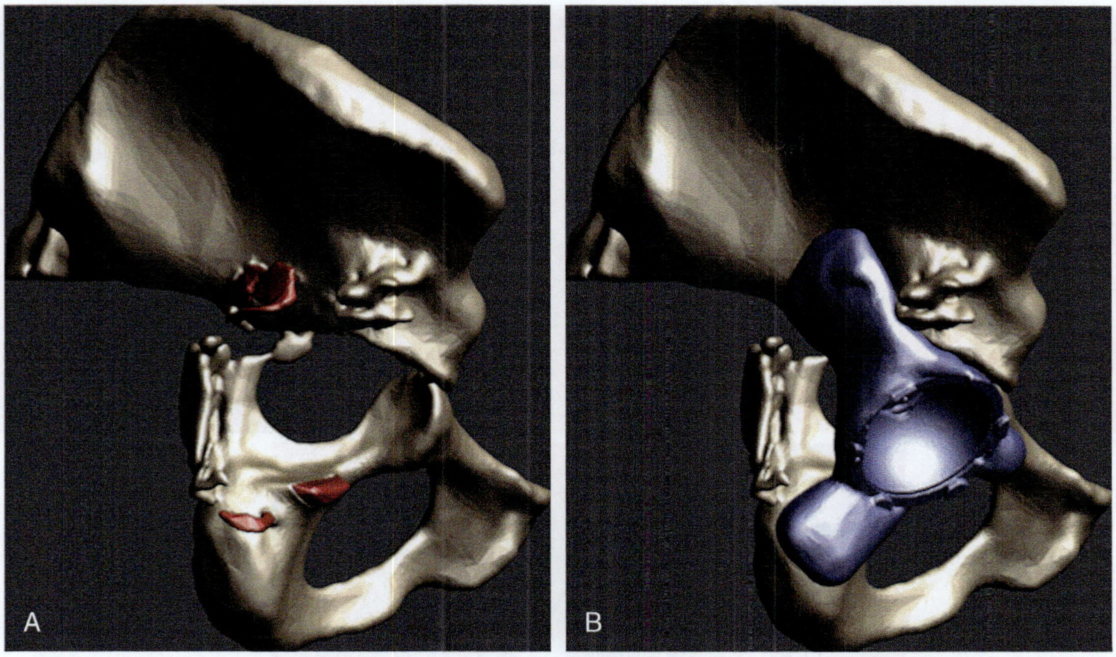

Figure 28.6 | Three-dimensional CT reconstructions of the hemipelvis demonstrate bone to be resected (marked red) (A) to accommodate the planned custom triflange acetabular cup (B). (Images courtesy of Daniel J. Berry, M.D.)

- Small areas of excess bone are removed with a burr in accordance with the preoperative plan to shape the pelvis to accommodate the custom triflange component (Figure 28.6A and B). The acetabular socket may be gently reamed. The sterilized model of the custom triflange is inserted to assess fit and to judge the easiest method of insertion. This iterative process of shaping the pelvis is continued until a good fit of the trial is achieved (Figure 28.7A-C).
  - The surgeon may consider bone grafting at this stage but must be certain that the graft does not force malposition of the component (Figure 28.8A-E). Furthermore, there are often gaps between the component and pelvis where the acetabulum is deficient into which graft can be backfilled after final implant insertion. This graft does not contribute to cup support or fixation but may aid in remodeling of the acetabular defect over time. Antibiotic powder (such as 1 g of vancomycin) may be mixed into the bone graft.
- The real triflange implant is inserted.
  - The iliac flange, which slides between the ilium and gluteus minimus, usually is placed first to minimize tension on the superior gluteal neurovascular pedicle. Placement is facilitated by translating the leg proximally with the hip in a flexed and abducted position to relax the hip abductors.
  - The knee is then flexed and the hip extended to relax the posterior soft tissues and facilitate rotation of the pubic and ischial flanges into place.
  - The ischial flange is critically assessed for overhang to prevent irritation of the sciatic nerve.
  - The triflange cup is gently impacted into its seated position.
  - The model is scrutinized to ensure that fit of the implant and flange location mirror the preoperative plan.
  - The implant is assessed for inherent stability. If placed appropriately, little motion should be observed with moderate stress.
  - If the component does not sit as expected, it may be malrotated, planned bone removal may be insufficient, or morselized bone graft may be preventing the cup from seating.
- Once the implant is seated, screws are placed. A typical screw sequence (in the absence of planned reduction of a pelvic discontinuity) is as follows.
  - One screw is placed in the ischial bone, which is often weakened and osteolytic. The initial ischial screw is generally placed in a nonlocking manner.
  - One screw is placed in the ilium to provide provisional fixation. Because iliac bone is often well preserved, this screw attains reliable purchase. A nonlocking (cancellous) screw is typically used to compress the implant to bone before the placement of locking screws.

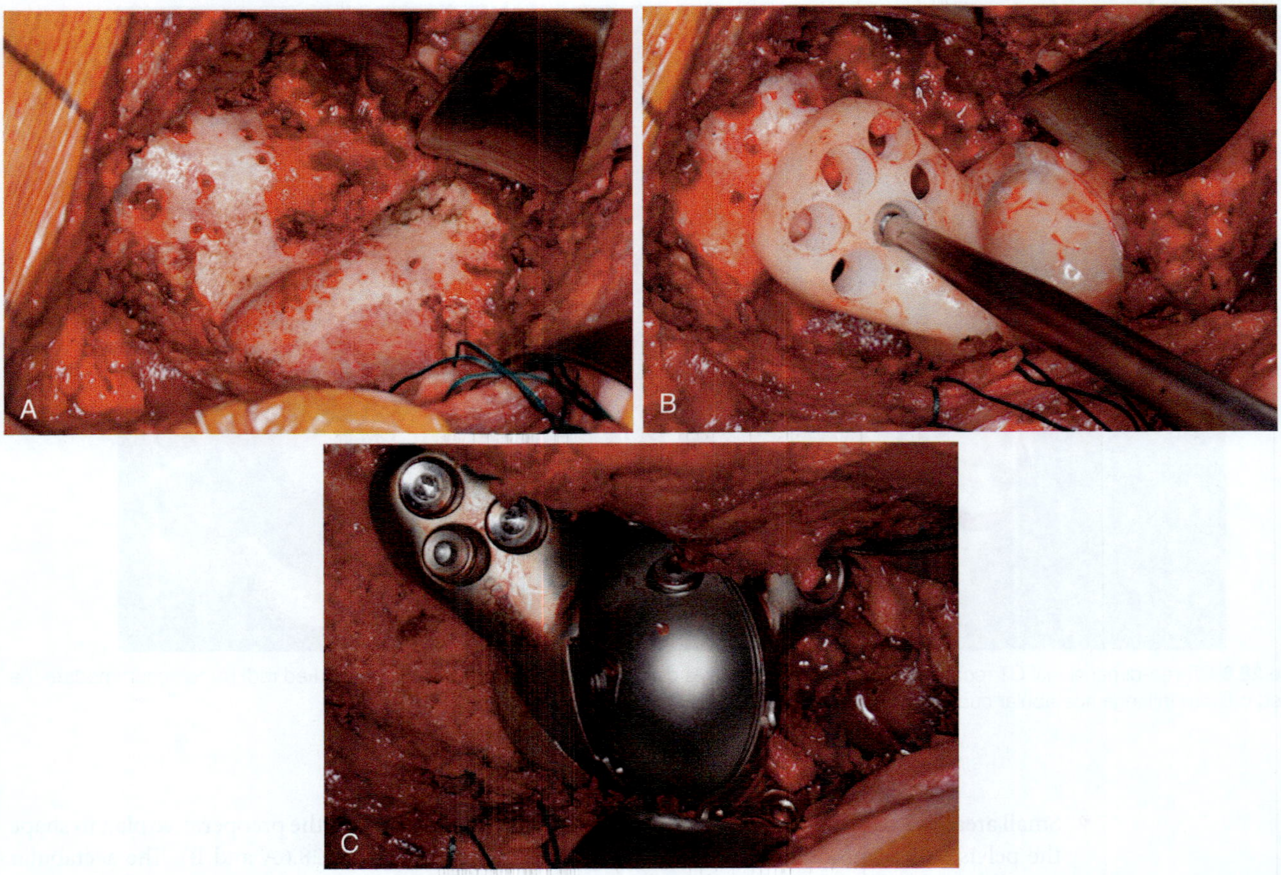

Figure 28.7 | Intraoperative photographs demonstrating a massive acetabular defect (A) that was shaped with a burr to ensure acceptable fit of the custom triflange model (B) before implantation of the real prosthesis (C). (Images courtesy of Matthew P. Abdel, M.D.)

- About 2 to 3 nonlocking screws are placed through the dome of the acetabulum into the anterior and posterior column for maximum compression. The flange nonlocking screws can be retightened at this point.
- Additional screws are inserted to complete fixation.
  - Usually a minimum of 4 ischial locking screws and 4 to 6 iliac screws are placed.
  - During iliac screw insertion, care is needed to avoid traction injury to the superior gluteal nerve. For screws above the distal-most row, drilling and insertion can occur through the gluteus minimus and medius muscles. Palpation rather than direct visualization can be used to verify that the proximal flange is seated.
- In patients with pelvic discontinuity, the custom triflange may be placed with or without a planned reduction of the discontinuity. Reduction of the discontinuity is planned if reduction improves bony support of the custom triflange component and brings the hemipelvis segments into closer contact, increasing the chance of healing the discontinuity. A disadvantage of planned reduction is the risk of being unable to obtain a reduction because of chronic discontinuity. Incomplete reduction results in the inability to properly seat a custom triflange component that was designed to fit with the discontinuity properly reduced.
  - When a reduction is planned, the triflange component is first fixed to the ilium with 1 nonlocking screw. The inferior hemipelvis is then rotated into position against the implant, which reduces the discontinuity, and a screw is placed in the ischium for provisional stabilization. Screw fixation then proceeds according to plan. Bone grafting is considered in patients with residual defects.

- After implantation of the triflange component (and any indicated revision work on the femoral side), trial reduction is performed.
- An intraoperative AP pelvic radiograph is obtained to verify acceptable implant positioning and screw lengths.

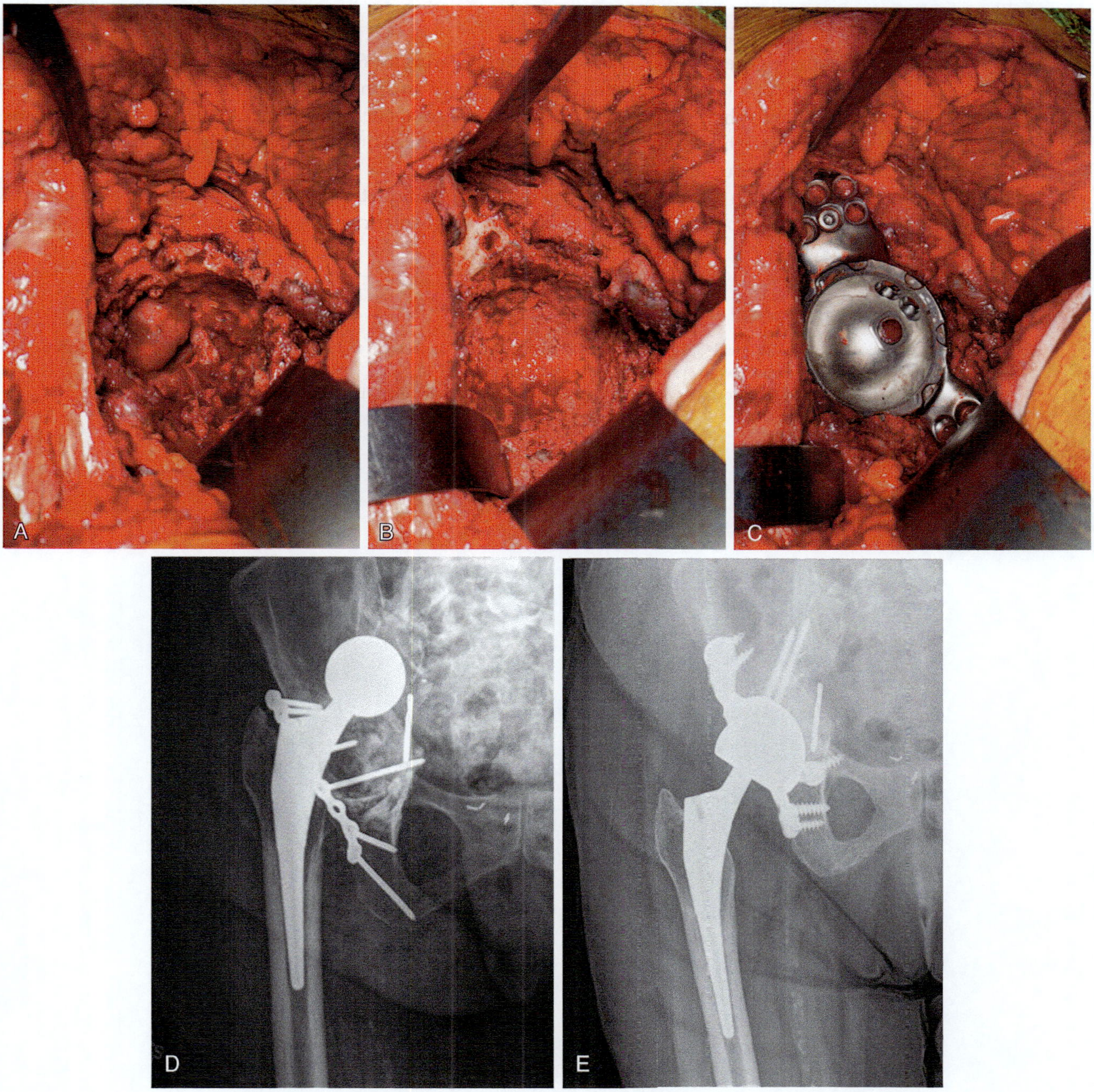

Figure 28.8 | Intraoperative photographs of a massive acetabular defect (A) in which bone grafting with reverse-reamed cancellous allograft chips was performed (B) before placement of a custom triflange acetabular component (C). Preoperative (D) and 2-year postoperative (E) right hip radiographs demonstrate interval acetabular remodeling with stable positioning of the triflange implant.

- Hip stability and leg lengths are assessed.
- The modular insert is placed.
- In patients with poor abductor function (denervation, detachment, or an absent greater trochanter), a constrained liner is used. In other cases, large head-ball diameters are utilized.
- If a trochanteric osteotomy was performed, the fragment is reduced and fixed
- Wound closure proceeds after thorough irrigation. Closure of any remaining posterior capsule structures is attempted. A deep subfascial drain is often placed to avoid postoperative hematoma. Use of vacuum-assisted wound closure may be considered in patients at increased risk of wound complications.

Postoperative Care

- Patients are generally made toe-touch weight bearing for 6 to 8 weeks postoperatively. Weight bearing can be progressively advanced over the next 1 to 2 months based on clinical examination and serial radiographs demonstrating the absence of component subsidence. In patients with pelvic discontinuity, weight-bearing restrictions may be extended until the surgeon appreciates reconstitution of the posterior column.
- A hip abduction brace may be used at the surgeon's discretion for patients believed to be at high risk for dislocation or for protection of a healing trochanteric osteotomy. This is not routinely used in our practice.

References

1. Paprosky WG, Perona PG, Lawrence JM. Acetabular defect classification and surgical reconstruction in revision arthroplasty: a 6-year follow-up evaluation. *J Arthroplasty*. 1994;9:33-44.
2. D'Antonio JA. Periprosthetic bone loss of the acetabulum: classification and management. *Orthop Clin N Am*. 1992;23:279-290.

Chapter 29
Fully Porous Coated Stems

TAD M. MABRY

Key Concepts

- Meticulous preoperative planning and templating are essential to the success of revision femoral reconstruction using fully porous coated stems.
- Liberal use of extended proximal femoral osteotomies will facilitate all aspects of femoral revision surgery and are invaluable in the management of any coexisting femoral deformity.
- Following removal of the existing femoral implant(s), the patient's femur must have at least 4 cm or more of supportive diaphyseal bone to achieve the necessary axial and rotational stability required for bone ingrowth.
  - In the setting of more severe bone loss, alternative methods of reconstruction, such as fluted tapered stems, impaction bone grafting, allograft-prosthetic composites, or megaprostheses, should be considered.

Sterile Instruments and Implants

- Surgical approach-specific hip retractors
- Stem and/or cement extraction tools
- Small saw blades, pencil-tip routers, osteotomes (for extended osteotomy)
- Cerclage wires/cables/instruments (for prophylactic cerclage, osteotomy fixation)
- Instruments and trial implants specific to the selected femoral component

Surgical Approaches

- The surgeon must consider what is needed both to remove the existing implants and to insert the revision fully porous-coated stem, when making the final determination of surgical approach.
- In the absence of significant deformity or the need to access the femur more distally (implant and/or cement removal), both the posterolateral approach and the direct lateral approach may be successfully utilized.
  - In the presence of one or more of these features, the surgeon should have a very low threshold to perform an extended proximal femoral osteotomy.

Preoperative Planning

- The intended hip center is first determined from an analysis of the acetabular side of the hip reconstruction. If the existing acetabular component is to be retained, the hip center will be unchanged; however, if the existing acetabular component is to be revised, the new hip center must be taken into account.
- The existing femoral component planned for revision must then be assessed. If needed for deformity correction or for improved access to the distal femur (implants and/or cement extraction), an extended proximal femoral osteotomy should be planned (Figures 29.1 and 29.2).
  - The length of this osteotomy must be planned to preserve the necessary 4 cm or more of supportive bone in the diaphysis.

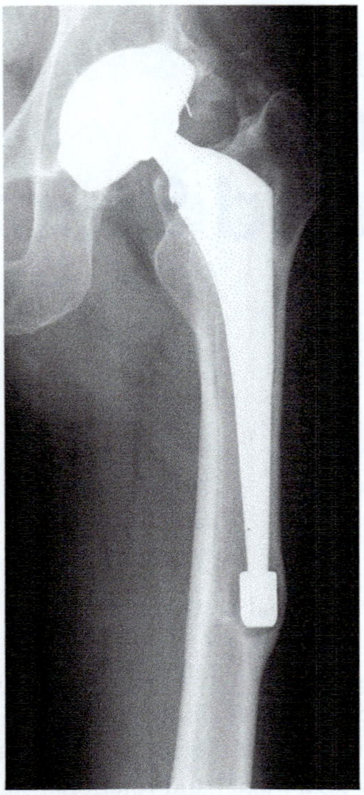

Figure 29.1 | Preoperative anteroposterior (AP) radiograph demonstrating a loose femoral stem with significant varus remodeling of the proximal femur.

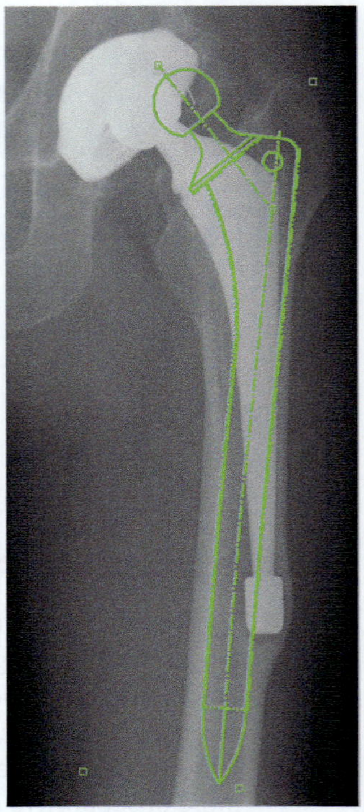

Figure 29.2 | Preoperative AP radiograph with a superimposed template demonstrating the extent of the deformity that will necessitate extended trochanteric osteotomy.

- The stem diameter and stem length are then determined to best achieve diaphyseal contact over ≥4 cm (Figures 29.3-29.5).
  - Most fully porous-coated revision stems are available in several lengths, with the longer devices typically also slightly curved to account for the natural femoral bow.

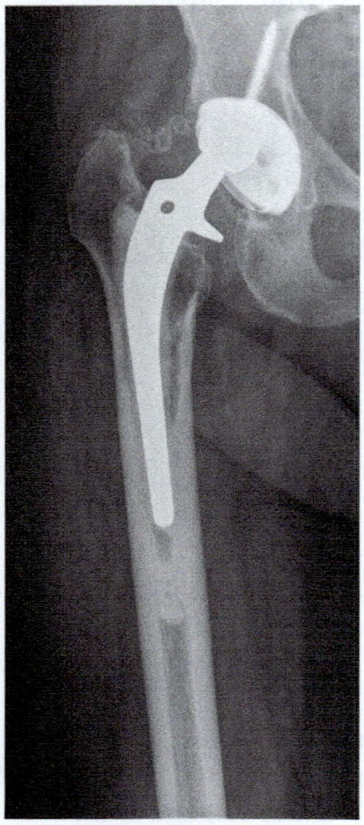

Figure 29.3 | Preoperative AP radiograph of a patient with a debonded cemented stem, polyethylene wear, and progressive femoral osteolysis. Note the well-fixed cement more distally in the femoral canal.

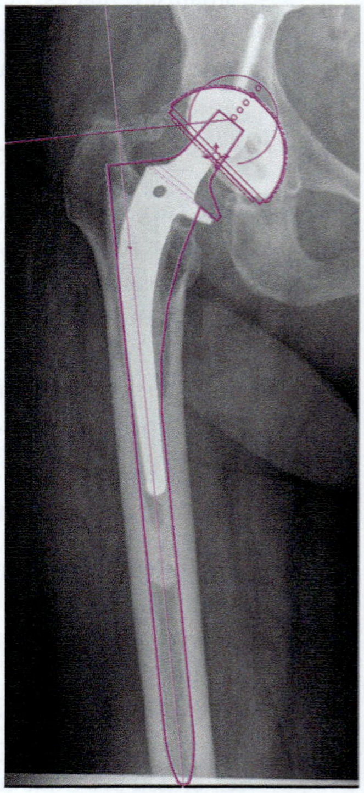

Figure 29.4 | Preoperative templating demonstrates outstanding fit of an 8-inch straight, fully porous-coated revision stem with cortical contact >6 cm.

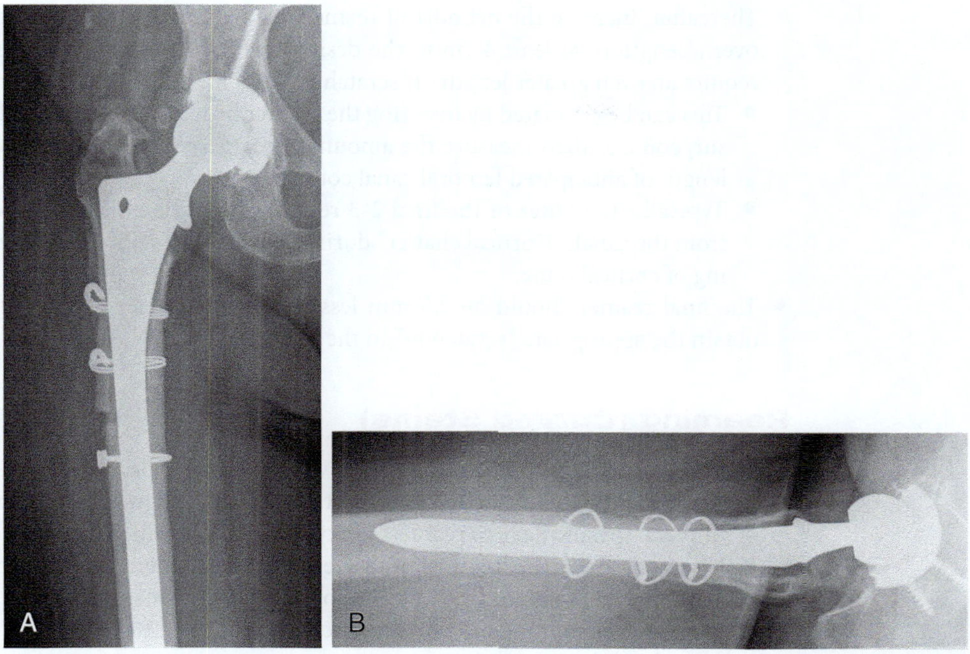

Figure 29.5 | A and B. Final follow-up radiographs demonstrating excellent bony integration of the stem. Note healing of the anteriorly based extended trochanteric osteotomy (needed for distal cement extraction) with a prophylactic cerclage cable distal to the osteotomy site and 2 cerclage wires more proximally for osteotomy fixation.

Bone, Implant, and Soft Tissue Techniques

Exposure and Implant Extraction

- Careful surgical exposure and removal of existing implants, with or without associated cement, is essential to maximize the bone stock remaining for revision femoral reconstruction. Full details of this process are noted in separate chapters.

Prophylactic Cerclage

- Prophylactic cerclage wires or cables should be utilized distal to any cracks that may occur during implant extraction.
- It is also essential to perform prophylactic cerclage distal to the end point of any extended proximal femoral osteotomy.
- In cases of more severe bone loss, the surgeon may wish to reinforce the distal bone stock with both cerclage and an allograft strut.

Reaming (Straight Stems)

- A T-handle starting reamer is often useful to initiate reaming.
  - In the presence of a significant bony pedestal, the surgeon may require a sharp drill with or without fluoroscopic guidance to access the canal more distally. Once the canal is re-established, back-biting instruments can be used to remove the residual pedestal before reaming with rigid reamers (which otherwise may be deflected by the hard bone of the pedestal).
- Begin reaming with cylindrical reamers of the smallest diameter, increasing by 1 mm increments until cortical contact is first achieved.
  - Further expand the starting point, or consider extended trochanteric osteotomy as needed, if the reamer seems to be deflected away from the central axis of the femoral canal by the proximal bone.
  - Control the depth of reaming by reconciling measurements on the reamers with local bony landmarks.
    - The surgeon must prepare for the full length of the stem to avoid underseating of the final implant or femoral fracture, while avoiding unnecessary removal of bone from reaming to an excessive depth.

- Thereafter, increase the cylindrical reamer diameter by 0.5 mm until cortical reaming is achieved over a length of at least 4 cm to the desired depth. Note that smaller-stem diameters are likely to require an even greater length of "scratch fit" to achieve the necessary stability.
  - This can be estimated by inserting the reamer by hand as far as possible with gentle pressure. The surgeon can then measure the amount of reamer still exposed, which would correspond to the length of anticipated femoral canal contact.
  - Typically, the flutes of the final 2-3 reamers should be filled with cortical bone when removed from the canal. "Cortical chatter" during reaming does not always correspond to the actual reaming of cortical bone.
- The final reamer should be 0.5 mm less than the diameter of the anticipated real component to obtain the appropriate "scratch fit" in the femoral canal.

Reaming (Curved Stems)

- The process of canal preparation for curved, extensively porous-coated femoral stems is essentially the same as that noted earlier for straight stems, with 2 significant exceptions:
  - Implant-specific flexible reamers are typically utilized in place of rigid, cylindrical reamers.
  - It is standard practice to ream line to line, rather than underream by 0.5 mm, when using curved stems.
  - Trial and real implants may need to be rotated into position as they are advanced, starting with more anteversion than the final desired anteversion. This allows the curved stem to navigate the curved canal.

Trialing and Radiographs

- Using implant-specific trial stems, the surgeon should assess leg length, soft tissue tension, and hip stability in the standard fashion.
- If there is any bony impingement in the metaphyseal area preventing full seating of the trial stem, the surgeon should remove this bone with a high-speed burr.
- Plain radiographs in 2 planes with the trial stem in place should always be obtained to assess implant size, alignment, and appropriate depth of reaming.
- Before removing the trial stem, the surgeon should note the appropriate stem anteversion needed for stability and, if possible, mark the corresponding stem rotation on the local bone stock. The surgeon should also note the level of seating needed to provide optimal leg length and hip stability. If notable calcar deficiency is present, a calcar replacing implant may be used. The proximal bone may need contouring to fit the calcar build-up on the implant.

Final Implantation

- The diameter of the real stem can be measured very accurately with a hole gauge (Figure 29.6). If the stem size various slightly from the stated size, reamed size may be adjusted by 0.05 mm if needed.
- The real femoral stem is first inserted by hand as far as possible, and in the appropriate amount of anteversion, corresponding to the final determination made during trialing. As noted earlier, the surgeon may need to begin insertion of long curved stems with extra anteversion and gradually rotate the stem into correct anteversion as the stem is advanced.
  - If the stem seems to be excessively proud before impaction, the surgeon should consider removing the stem and line-to-line reaming as needed, until the real stem can be inserted by hand with only 5 to 7 cm remaining for further insertion.

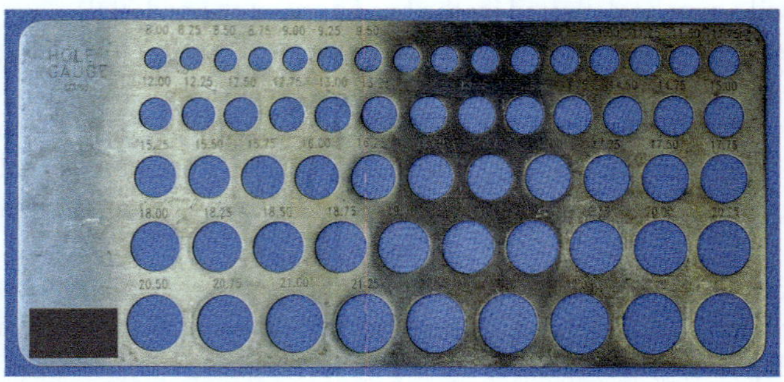

Figure 29.6 | Hole gauge used to accurately measure the diameter of extensively porous coated stems.

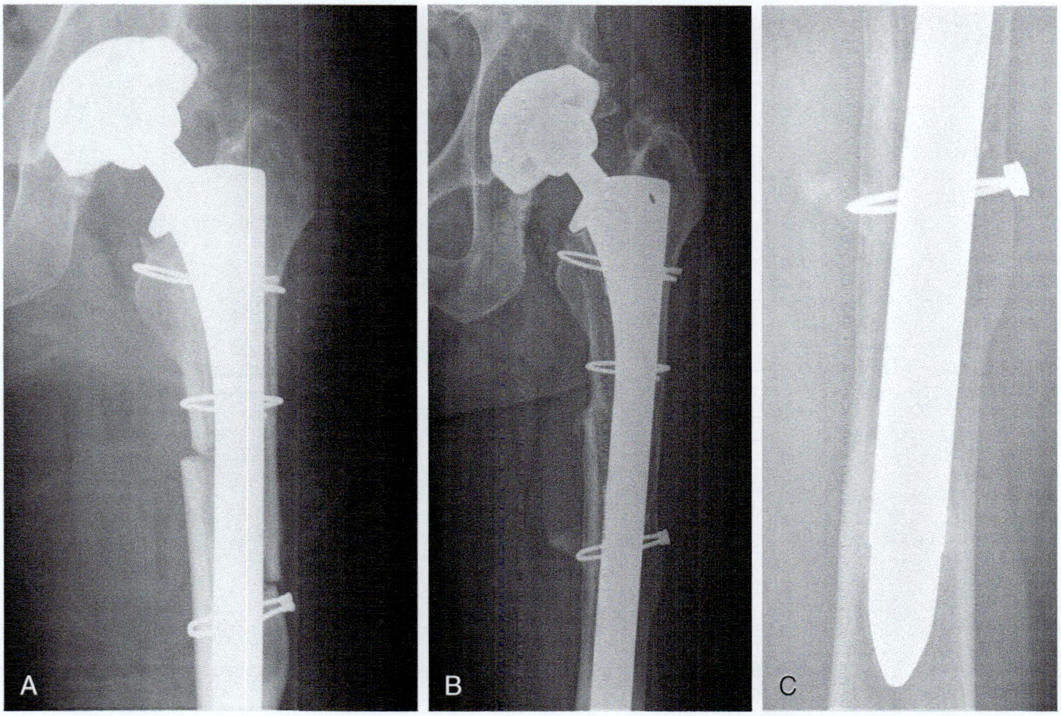

Figure 29.7 I A-C. Initial postoperative and final follow-up radiographs demonstrating excellent bony integration of the stem and complete healing of an extended trochanteric osteotomy requiring a secondary medial osteotomy for complete deformity correction. Note the prophylactic cerclage cable distally and the additional 2 cables proximally for osteotomy fixation.

- The stem is then carefully impacted with repetitive mallet blows. It is critical that the surgeon uses an assistant as needed to control the stem anteversion during the final seating of the implant. Without this control, the stem can rotate into a suboptimal position that cannot be corrected intraoperatively.
    - During final insertion, one should visualize slow and steady progress of the stem. Especially over the last 1 to 2 cm, if it appears that the stem advances an unexpectedly great distance with a single mallet blow, one should assess for a distal fracture with intraoperative radiographs.

Osteotomy Fixation

- Fixation of an extended trochanteric osteotomy varies according to the type of osteotomy and the patient's bone quality and quantity.
- In general, all patients should receive a prophylactic wire or cable distal to the osteotomy site, which is placed before any subsequent femoral preparation or component implantation.
- The osteotomy itself is typically secured with a total of 2-4 wires or cables. Occasionally, a secondary osteotomy is needed to fully correct significant proximal femoral deformity (Figure 29.7A-C).

Postoperative Care

- Immediate postoperative radiographs must include 2 views that capture the entire construct, including the tip of the femoral stem.
    - Consideration should be given to obtaining these radiographs during closure, so that one has the immediate ability to recognize and treat any distal fractures without a secondary return to the operating room.
        - Distal expansion cracks that do not exit the cortex on either view may be treated with protected weight bearing (Figure 29.8). If such a crack is identified intraoperatively, a cerclage cable may be placed for added security.
        - Distal expansion cracks that exit the cortex should be considered less stable and are typically treated with cable cerclage.

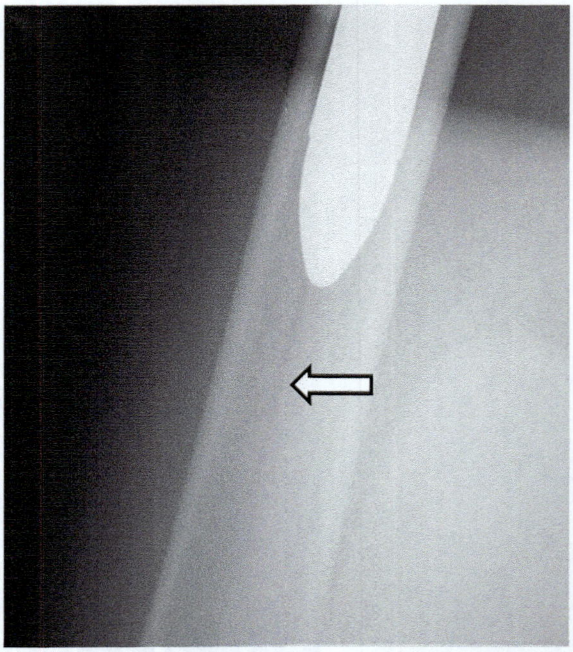

Figure 29.8 | Distal expansion fracture as seen on a postoperative radiograph that does not exit the cortex, treated successfully with protected weight bearing.

- The determination of weight-bearing status immediately following surgery is based on the presence or absence of an osteotomy, the quality of the patient's bone stock, and the perceived immediate fixation of the stem.
  - Typically, no more than partial weight bearing is recommended for the first 6 weeks.
    - In the presence of an osteotomy or more compromised bone stock, toe-touch weight bearing typically is recommended for the first 6 weeks.
- Clinical follow-up with radiographs at 6 weeks is standard to determine the status of early healing and to determine advancement of weight-bearing status.

Chapter 30
Fluted Tapered Modular Stems

NICHOLAS M. HERNANDEZ
MATTHEW P. ABDEL

Key Concepts

- Modular fluted tapered (MFT) stems have become popular in the last decade because of favorable reported results, ease of use, and versatility (Figures 30.1-30.4).
- Preoperative templating is essential for planning the diameter and length of the fluted tapered portion of the stem, as well as the length and offset of the proximal modular components.
- A prophylactic cable around the femoral shaft may be utilized before preparation or implantation of the fluted tapered portion of the stem to minimize risk of failure. Hoop stresses are high during implantation.
- Obtaining immediate axial and rotational stability with the fluted tapered portion is key to success and preventing implant subsidence or loosening.
- The proximal modular portion of the component is used to optimize anteversion, length, femoral offset, and hip stability.
- An extended trochanteric osteotomy (ETO) helps provide good exposure for optimal femoral canal preparation, especially when there is proximal femoral deformity, a large femoral bow, and/or overhanging greater trochanter (please see Section 1-B, Chapter 4). The ETO allows canal preparation under direct vision, creation of a well-reamed supportive cone of bone, and optimal axial and rotational stability of the implant. The goal is for a supportive cone of bone to support the tapered stem, not for the stem to wedge by 3-point fixation (which provides less support against subluxation and less surface area for bone ongrowth).
- Intraoperative radiographs in orthogonal planes should be obtained with trial components in place, particularly to assess for diameter and length of the fluted tapered portion.
- Modular fluted tapered stems can be used for most femoral revisions so long as femoral diaphyseal bone is sufficient to be reamed to a supportive tapered cone of bone that will provide good axial support and rotational stability of the implant (Figures 30.1-30.4).

Sterile Instruments and Implants

Instruments

- Routine hip retractors
- Routine hip instruments to remove preexisting uncemented or cemented femoral components
- Routine instrumentation for the fluted tapered stem
- Small and large oscillating saw if ETO is required
- Pencil-tip burr if ETO is required
- Multiple wide osteotomes if ETO is required
- Cerclage cables (one prophylactic cable and additional cables if ETO is required)

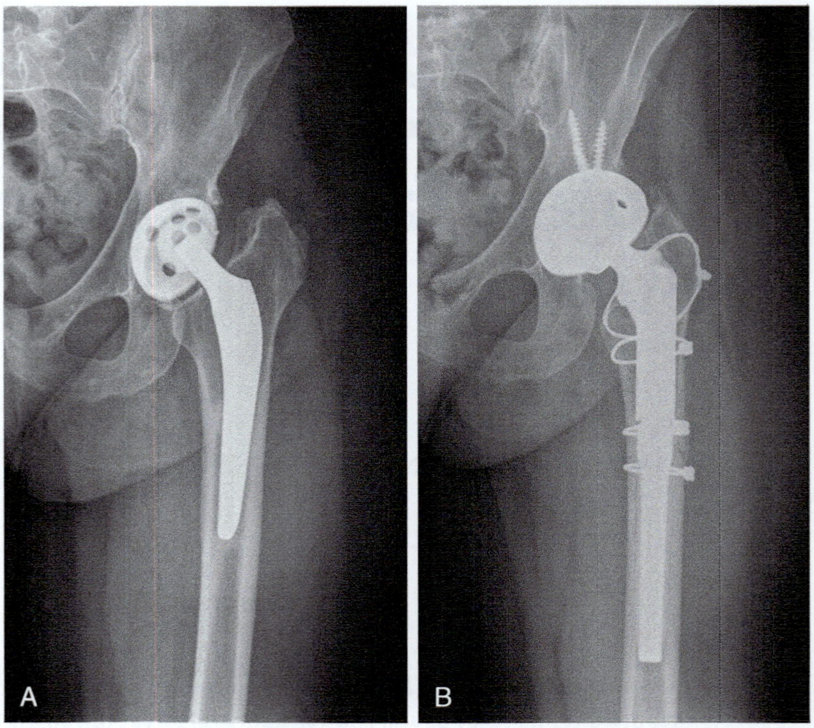

Figure 30.1 | A, Radiograph of hip with loose subsided uncemented stem with good proximal bone. B, Radiograph after revision with mid-length modular fluted tapered stem. (Courtesy of Daniel J. Berry, MD.)

Implants

- Trial and real fluted tapered stems of various diameters and lengths
- Trial and real proximal bodies with various lengths and offsets
- Appropriate femoral heads with the size and composition at the surgeon's discretion
- Dual-mobility implants may be considered in those patients at high-risk for postoperative dislocations

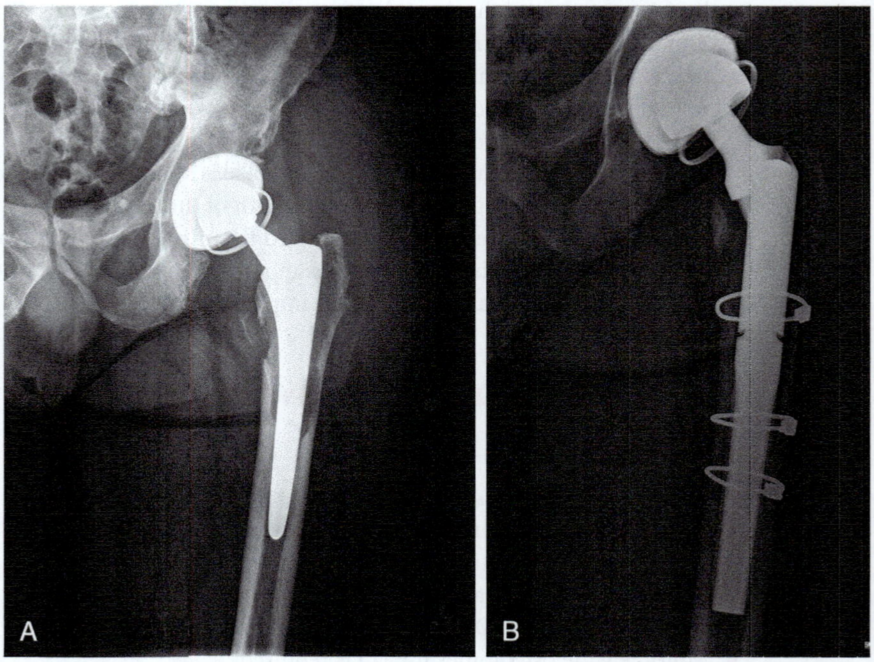

Figure 30.2 | A, Radiograph of hip with well-fixed uncemented dual-modular neck stem and severe lysis due to taper corrosion. B, Radiograph after revision with mid-length modular fluted tapered stem. Note the stem obtained good axial and rotational stability distal to the osteolytic lesions and the ETO. (Courtesy of Daniel J. Berry, MD.)

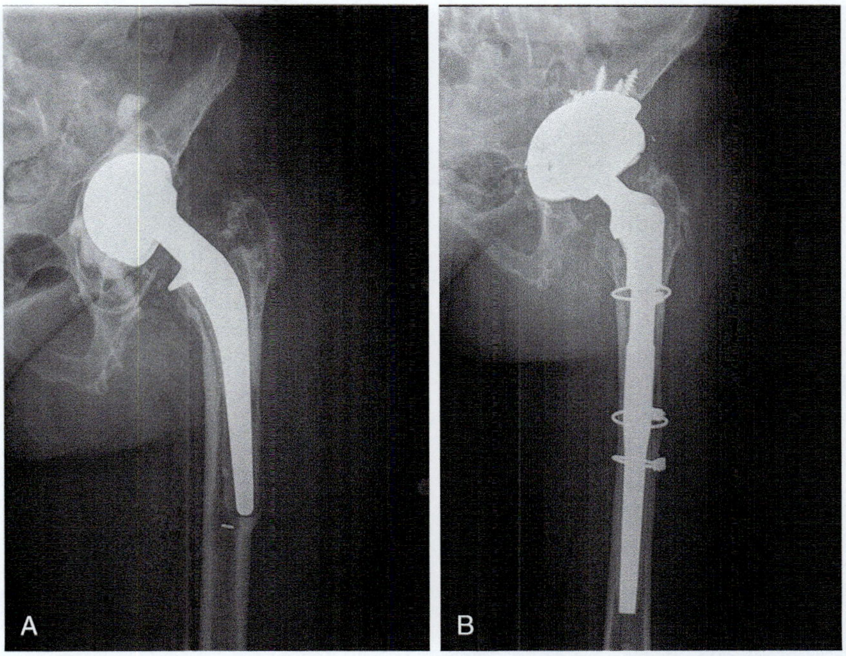

Figure 30.3 | A, Radiograph of hip with loose stem and damaged proximal bone. B, Radiograph after reconstruction with modular fluted tapered stem. (Courtesy of Daniel J. Berry, MD.)

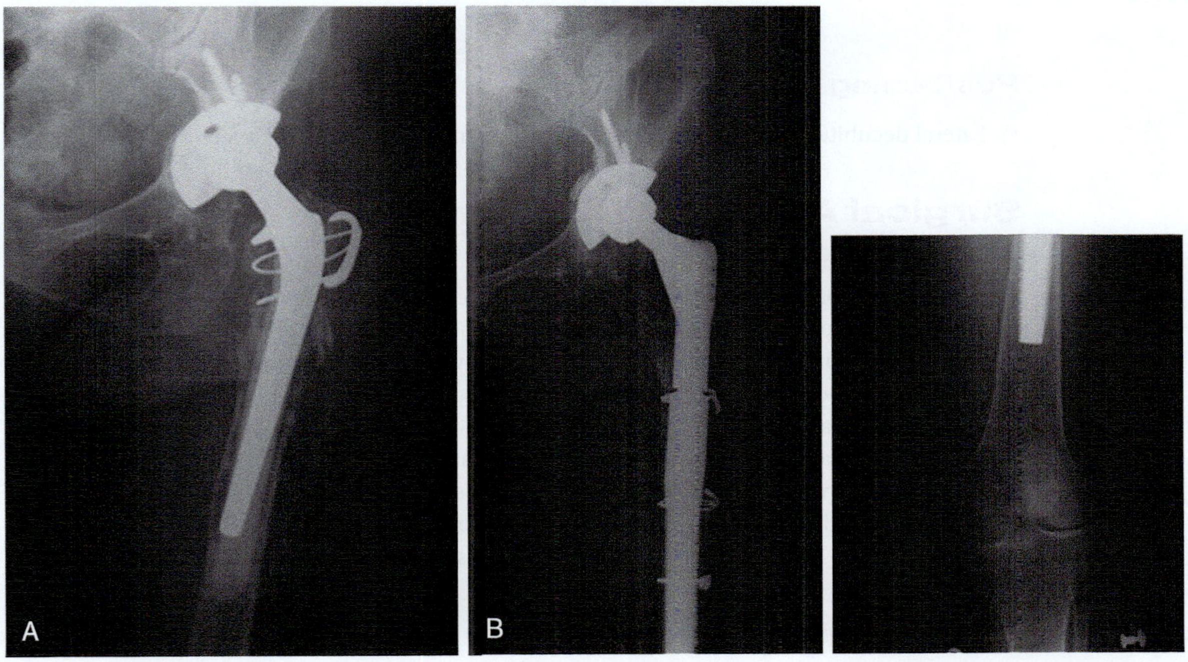

Figure 30.4 | A, Radiograph of hip with loose femoral component and notable proximal bone loss. B, Radiograph after reconstruction with long modular fluted tapered stem. The poor proximal bone has been bypassed, and the prosthetic axial and rotational stability is gained in the mid-diaphysis. (Courtesy of Daniel J. Berry, MD.)

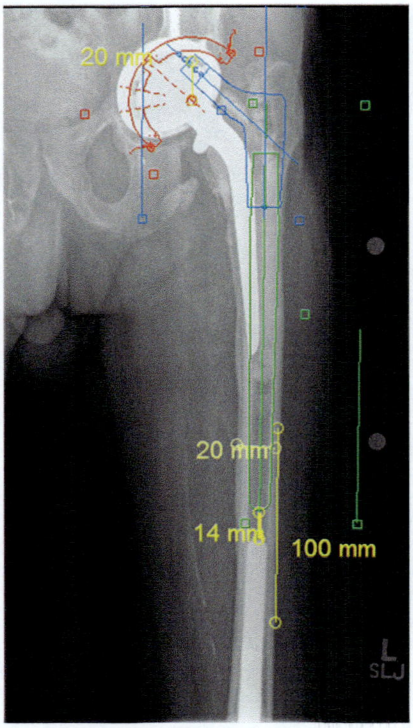

Figure 30.5 | This preoperative template with accurate magnification markers depicts the estimated diameter and length of the proposed fluted tapered portion of the stem and the length and offset of the proximal body.

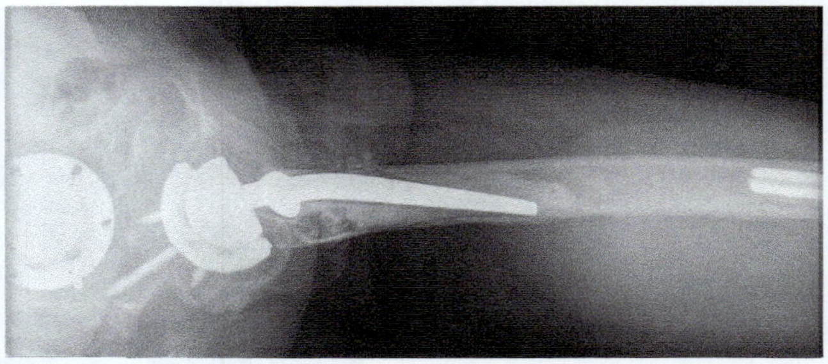

Figure 30.6 | A cross-table lateral radiograph is helpful to evaluate for abnormal or excessive femoral bowing that might lead to anterior cortical perforation.

Positioning

- Lateral decubitus position with access to entire femur and ipsilateral knee

Surgical Approaches

- A posterior approach is preferred as it allows for a laterally based ETO.
- An anteriorly based "Wagner-style" ETO also is acceptable. A Wagner-style ETO is especially useful for placement of very long fluted tapered stems because it helps the surgeon negotiate the anterior femoral bow without distal anterior perforation by the straight portion of the stem.
- An ETO may be performed for the following indications:
  - Removal of a well-fixed uncemented stem
  - Removal of a stem with an extensive cement mantle
  - Proximal femoral deformity or trochanter at risk of fracture
  - To assist with acetabular exposure (if concurrent acetabular revision is being performed)
- In addition, an ETO will allow unobstructed access to the distal femur for canal preparation.

Preoperative Planning

- Determine the limb length inequality and planned center of hip rotation.
- Utilize an anteroposterior (AP) radiograph of the hip with magnification correction to determine the approximate diameter (to provide 2-4 cm of secure isthmic fit) and length (to bypass defects by 2 cortical diameters if possible) of the proposed implants (Figure 30.5).
- Template an appropriately sized proximal femoral body that will restore length and offset (Figure 30.5).
- Plan the length of an ETO (usually 12-16 cm from the tip of the trochanter) that may be needed, but be certain to evaluate remaining bone stock for the MFT stem.
- Evaluate the cross-table lateral radiograph for abnormal or excessive femoral bowing that may increase the risk of anterior cortical perforation (Figure 30.6).

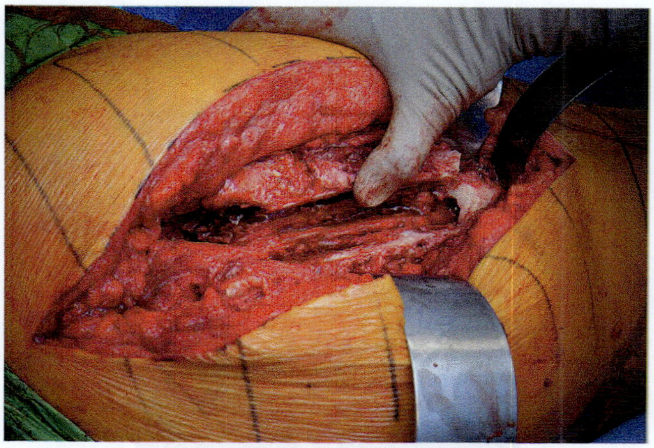

Figure 30.7 | Example of an extended trochanteric osteotomy utilized to garner direct access to the diaphyseal canal for reaming and implantation of the fluted tapered portion in a patient with excessive femoral bow and risk for anterior cortical perforation (as well as 3-point fixation).

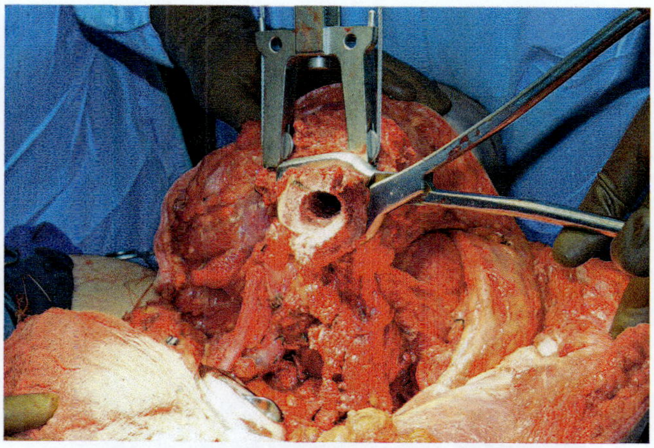

Figure 30.8 | In this intraoperative picture, a prophylactic cerclage cable is placed around the femoral shaft before preparation and implantation of the fluted tapered portion of the stem.

Bone/Implant/Soft Tissue Techniques

- Perform an approach to the hip based on surgeon's preference, but typically a posterolateral approach is preferred.
- Prior implants and any cement are removed with or without the use of an ETO.
- If an ETO is used (Figure 30.7), a prophylactic cerclage cable is placed just below the distal most extent of the osteotomy around the femoral shaft (Figure 30.8). It is tightened, but not secured, as this allows for further tightening throughout the case.
- The femoral diaphysis is then reamed in single-millimeter increments until a supportive cone of bone is achieved. The reamers tend to "self-center" in the femoral canal, but attention to desired alignment in the coronal and sagittal planes is important.
- A trial fluted tapered stem is then impacted carefully and under direct visualization. As the trial stem is advanced, the prophylactic cable is carefully tightened.
- Impaction is discontinued once the trial stem does not advance (i.e., axial stability obtained).
- AP (Figure 30.9) and lateral radiographs are obtained with the trial stem in place. The lateral radiograph is simply obtained by dislocating the hip and rotating the operative limb 90° (Figure 30.10).
- Adjustments to the length and diameter of the fluted tapered portion of the stem are then made if necessary. In addition, if a stem appears to place the anterior cortical bone at risk for cortical perforation, the angle of reaming and subsequent stem insertion are adjusted.
- Next, trial proximal modular bodies are utilized to optimize anteversion, length, femoral offset, and hip stability (Figure 30.11).
- If radiographs are satisfactory, then the trial components are removed and the real fluted tapered portion of the stem is impacted into the femur. It should seat at approximately the same stem depth as the optimized trial component. It is key for the implant to be very stable axially. If its seating level is slightly different from that of the trial, adjustments may be made using the proximal modular portion of the stem. One must be familiar with the specific implant, as some implants have flutes that are not circumferential and require special attention so that they are oriented correctly when implanted.
- The proximal body may be retrialed if necessary. Next, the real modular proximal body is selected and placed in the appropriate version on the fluted tapered portion of the stem. The proximal body is usually secured with a set screw and torque-limiting wrench (Figure 30.12). It is essential to utilize the anti-torque device on the sterile trunnion to minimize the risk of intraoperative torsional fracture distally. Typically, it is easiest to pass cerclage cables for osteotomy fixation at this stage of the procedure, before the hip is reduced, because there is less tension on the soft tissues.

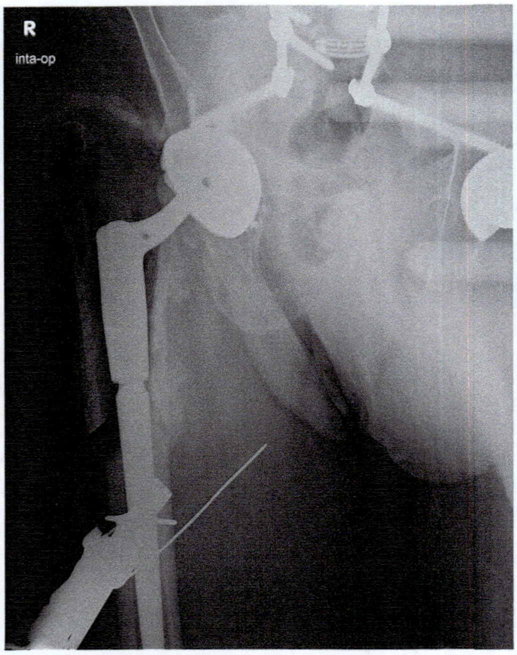

Figure 30.9 | An anteroposterior intraoperative radiograph depicting excellent fit of a trial fluted tapered stem in regards to diameter and length in a patient who required an extended trochanteric osteotomy at the time of reimplantation.

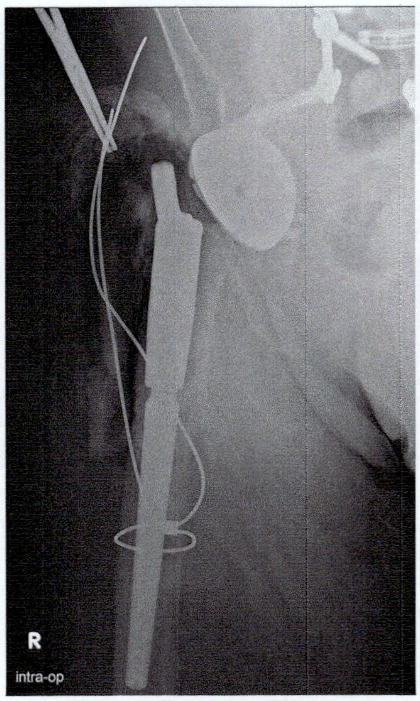

Figure 30.10 | A lateral intraoperative radiograph depicting excellent fit of a trial fluted tapered stem in regards to diameter and length in a patient who required an extended trochanteric osteotomy at the time of reimplantation. Note the central placement of the tip of the stem, which is achieved with the use of an extended trochanteric osteotomy.

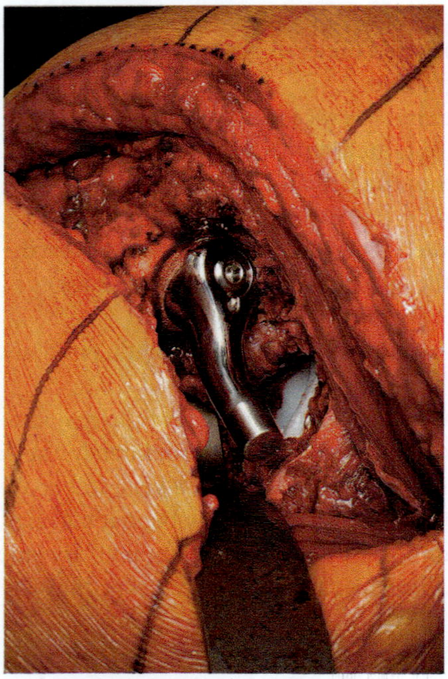

Figure 30.11 | The proximal bodies are modular and allow for refinements in anteversion, limb length, and offset.

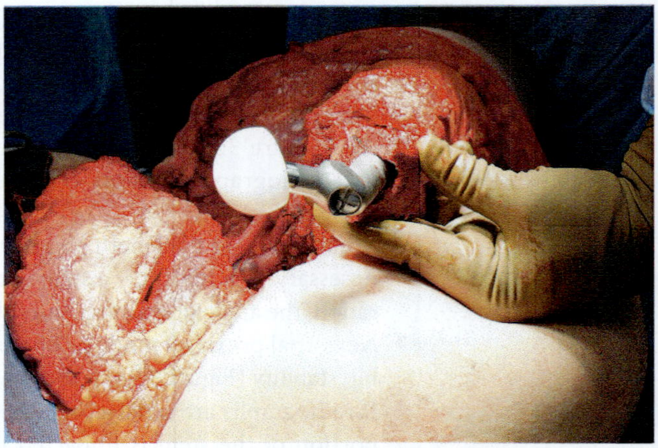

Figure 30.12 | The proximal set screw should be placed with a torque-limiting wrench and counter-torque device on the trunnion before final seating.

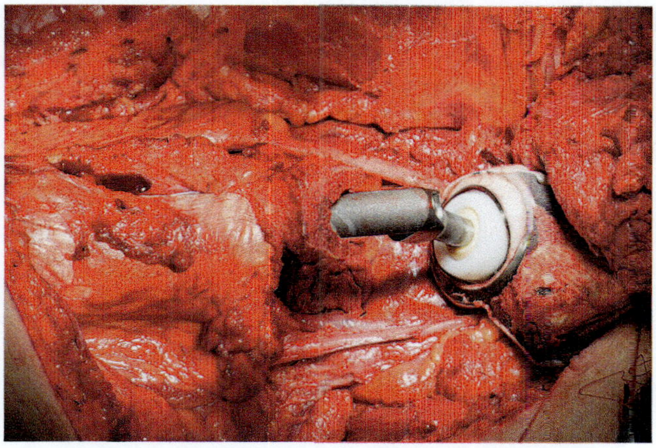

Figure 30.13 | The final construct should then be reduced and evaluated for hip instability. Modular fluted tapered stems can be utilized in the most complex cases, such as this patient treated with internal hemipelvectomy who underwent a subsequent acetabular reconstruction and total hip arthroplasty.

- The hip is then reduced with a trial head, and limb lengths and hip stability are confirmed. The osteotomy can be held over the proximal body to check tension and fit of the osteotomized fragment in its bed.
- A final femoral head is selected and impacted on the sterile trunnion (Figure 30.13), and definitive hip reduction is performed.
- If an ETO was performed, it is closed with cerclage wires and/or cables (Figure 30.14A and B) as per Section 1-B, Chapter 4.

Postoperative Care

- Most patients are made toe-touch weight bearing for 6 to 8 weeks. A hip abduction brace may be used at the discretion of the surgeon.
- Formal physical therapy is not routinely recommended as an outpatient.
- After 6 to 8 weeks, patients may advance to weight bearing as tolerated if the stem appears stable and without subsidence on radiographs.

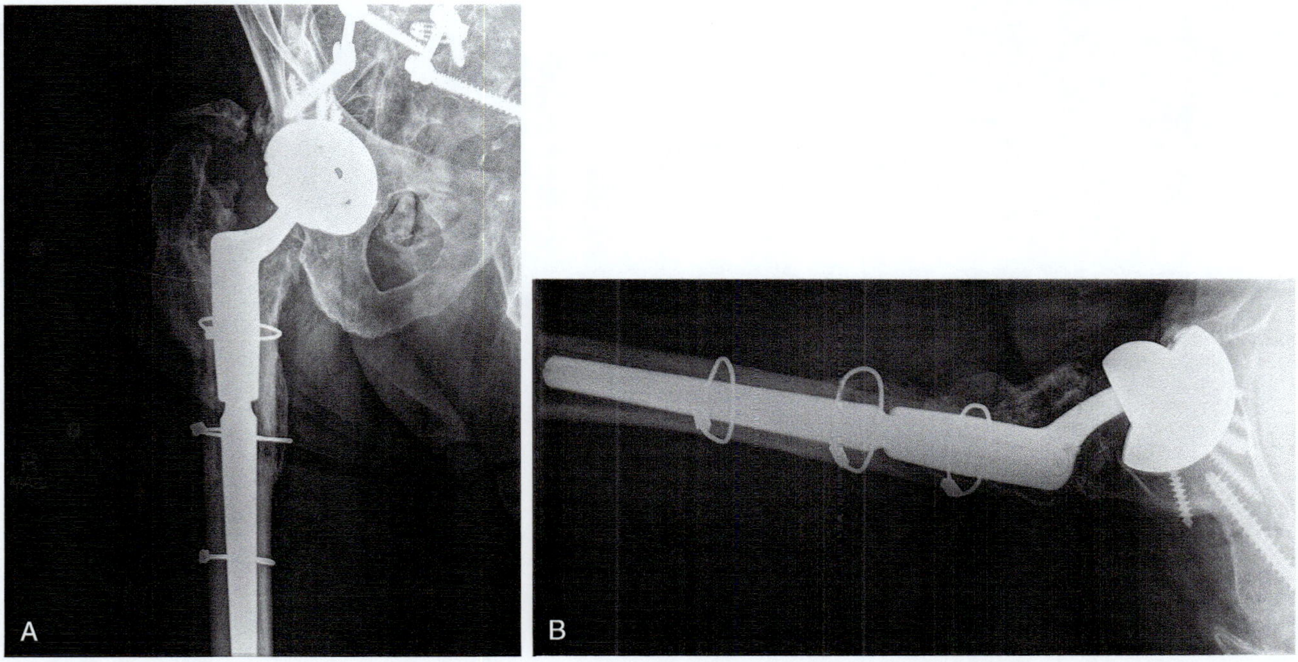

Figure 30.14 | Cables allow the surgeon to close extended trochanteric fragments with compromised proximal bone around a stem with solid diaphyseal fixation as noted in these postoperative anteroposterior (A) and cross-table (B) radiographs at 2 years.

Suggested Reading

1. Abdel MP, Cottino U, Larson DR, Hanssen AD, Lewallen DG, Berry DJ. Modular fluted tapered stems in aseptic revision total hip arthroplasty. *J Bone Joint Surg Am*. 2017;99(10):873-881.

Chapter 31
Cemented Stems

CORY G. COUCH
ROBERT T. TROUSDALE

Key Concepts

- Cement-in-cement revision technique refers to a revision method in which a femoral component is removed from an intact cement mantle and a new femoral component is cemented back into the previous cement mantle.
- The technique is predicated on the old cement mantle being well fixed at the bone-cement interface and the concept that new cement bonds effectively to the old cement.
- The technique is only applicable to a modest number of revision scenarios, typically those in which a stem has debonded from the cement at the implant-cement interface, or situations in which for exposure or biomechanical reasons it is desirable to remove a smooth-surfaced femoral component from a well-fixed cement mantle by deliberately debonding it at the cement-implant interface during revision.
- Reported results of the technique have been mostly favorable.

Indications

- The main indication for cement-in-cement revision is a previously cemented femoral implant that must be removed but in which the cement-bone interface remains intact.
- This technique improves exposure for acetabular revision and is ideal for a broken cemented stem, a monoblock cemented stem with damaged or incompatible head diameter, a stem that is loose at the cement implant interface, a cemented modular stem with damaged or incompatible taper, or component malposition (requiring change of stem offset, stem version or leg length).
- The advantage of cement-in-cement revision is the potential to minimize blood loss, operative time, bone loss, and risk of fracture and femoral perforation. The technique can also improve acetabular exposure and usually allows early full weight bearing (Table 31.1).

Contraindications

- The technique is contraindicated if the bone-cement interface is poor with extensive radiolucencies.

Sterile Instruments and Implants

- Routine hip retractors and system-specific revision hip instrumentation.
- Cemented femoral component extraction system.
- High-speed burr.
- Revision cemented femoral component of choice (polished tapered stems work well for this technique).
- Bone cement

Surgical Approaches

- Positioning: lateral decubitus position.
- Both the posterior and direct lateral approaches may be used. The senior author prefers the posterior approach as it is reproducible and may provide better access and visualization to the femoral canal.
- The senior author reserves the anterolateral approach to patients with severe abductor damage seen at the time of exposure. The cement-in-cement technique is not typically considered compatible with extended greater trochanteric osteotomy.

Radiographic Evaluation—Evaluate Serial Radiographs of the Arthroplasty if Possible

- Component fixation: Evaluate for radiolucencies at the bone-cement interface. Evaluation preoperatively on both anteroposterior and lateral radiographs is important. The cement mantle must be intact and well fixed to bone below the level of the lesser trochanter.
- If the failure of the femoral component has occurred at the cement-bone interface, or if the patient has developed extensive radiolucencies around the cement mantle, then cement-in-cement revision is contraindicated.

Review prior operative reports

- Obtain implant-specific extraction devices as needed and anticipate needs related to the acetabular portion of the revision.

Surgical Procedure

- Perform a routine exposure of the hip joint according to surgeon preference.
- Safe extraction of the existing femoral component begins with removal of cement superior to the lateral shoulder of the implant, usually with a high-speed burr. This allows the cemented stem to be more easily and safely disengaged at the cement-implant interface.
- Collared, matte-finished, or curved stems may be difficult to extract, whereas polished, tapered stems typically are extracted easily with a slap hammer or bone tamp.
- Prevention of greater trochanteric fracture is important and can be facilitated by clearing the path of the femoral component of overhanging greater trochanteric bone or cement before extraction is attempted.
- Resect 2 to 3 mm of calcar bone with a high-speed burr to inspect the bone-cement interface. If the bone-cement interface is compromised with soft tissue interposed, alternative revision methods should be used.
- To optimize bonding of the new cement to the old cement mantle, roughening of the original cement with a burr allows for improved surface area contact and integration with the new cement. While performing this maneuver, the cement mantle also may be burred to optimize position or size of the new implant. Stem anteversion also may be adjusted in this manner.
- A polished collarless stem smaller than the extracted stem is most commonly used for the cement-in-cement revision (Figures 31.1 and 31.2). Be aware that if the stem being removed is relatively short or narrow in diameter, the cement mantle may need to be expanded with a burr or ultrasonic instruments before a new implant can be placed. Alternatively, a relatively small new implant may be used, but in some cases, this will limit prosthetic offset and proximal implant length options.
- Anteversion and depth of insertion of the stem will depend on stability and limb length during trialing of the prosthesis. The trialing process is important to determine how deeply to seat the real implant. If the trial implant seats too deeply, a surgical sponge may be wrapped around the trial implant to hold it temporarily in a "prouder" position.
- Preparation of the cement mantle after roughening includes thorough cleaning with irrigation and drying.

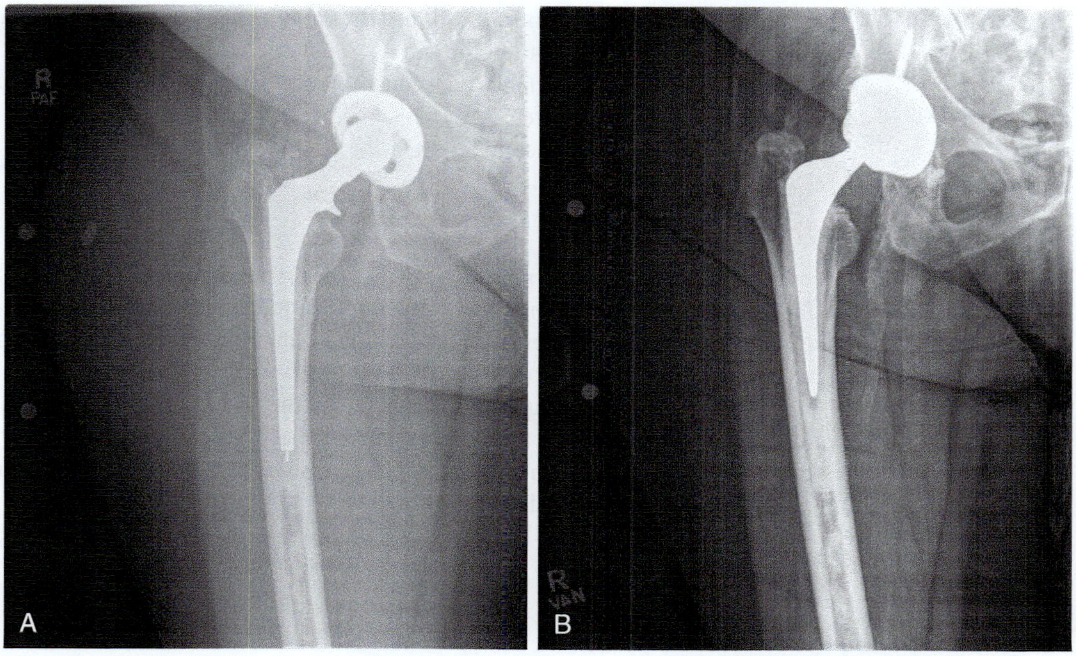

Figure 31.1 | Preoperative (A) and postrevision (B) radiographs of a 21-year-old patient treated with a cement-in-cement revision using a polished tapered femoral component.

- Chemical bonding is optimized if the new cement is injected in the liquid phase from distal to proximal and pressurized.
- Additionally, if desired, liquid monomer can be used to prepare the interface and facilitate chemical bonding before actual cementation.
- After optimal preparation of the femoral canal, cement is injected into the canal in a liquid phase and pressurized.

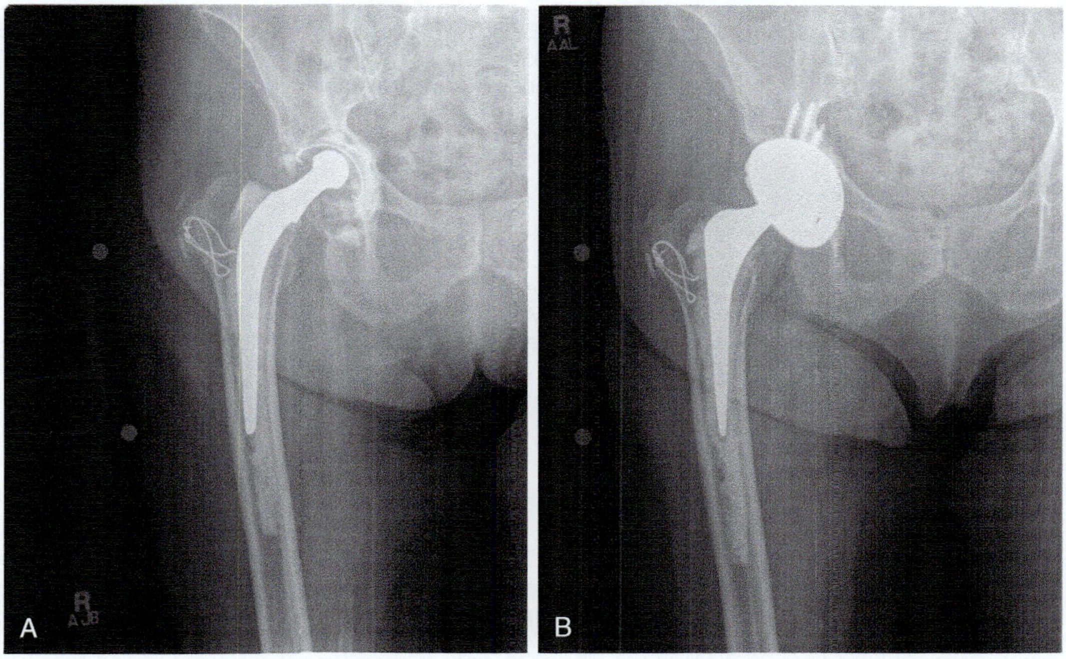

Figure 31.2 | Preoperative (A) and postoperative (B) radiographs of a 41-year-old patient treated with revision THA using cement-in-cement technique and a polished tapered femoral component.

- The new implant is then introduced into the canal and held in place in the appropriate anteversion and at the appropriate depth in the canal.
- After all cement has hardened, trial reductions are performed and the appropriate modular femoral head is chosen and impacted.
- Wound closure is performed in layers.

Special Cases

- In cases of Vancouver B2 periprosthetic fracture around a cemented stem, if the bone cement interface remains intact, the cement-in-cement technique can be utilized for revision after fracture reduction. Leaving the intact cement may facilitate reduction. Appropriate fixation with wires or cables and a long fixation plate construct should be utilized.
- In transverse or short oblique periprosthetic factures near the cemented stem tip, a revision cement-in-cement technique with a longer cemented stem bypassing the fracture by 2 cortical diameters is ideal. This can be performed by using a burr through the distal cement mantle and placing a new cement restrictor or plug distally.

Results

Table 31.1 | Results of Cement-Within-Cement Revisions

Authors (Year)	Number of Hips (Patients)	Implant Type	Reason for Revision	Mean Patient Age in Years (Range)	Mean Follow-up in Years (Range)	Stem Success Rate (%)	Results
Amanatullah et al (2016)	63 (62)	43 Omnifit (Stryker), 20 Exeter V40 (Stryker Howmedica Osteonics)	Aseptic loosening (74%), periprosthetic fracture (14%), instability (8%), implant fracture (6%)	69.2 (14.1 SD)	5.5 (3.8 SD)	98	11 required revision THA, 1 revision for aseptic removal of femoral component, HHS 49.8-68.3
Cnudde et al (2017)	1179	894 Exeter, 285 Lubinus	Aseptic loosening of one or both components (78%), fracture (2%), instability (14%), implant fracture (2%), infection (2%)	74 (10 SD)	4.2 (3.2 SD Exeter), 5.2 (3.5 SD Lubinus)	98	20 re-revisions that were undertaken with a diagnosis of aseptic loosening of one of the components
Stefanovich-Lawbuary et al (2014)	44 (44)	C-Stem AMT (DePuy)	Cup loosening (64%), dislocation (23%), hemiarthroplasty failure (5%), infection (5%), facture (3%)	72 (42-90)	5 (2-12)	95.2	2 revisions (1 for pelvic discontinuity, 1 for infection), no radiographically loose stems, mean scores: OHS, 34; EQ-SD, 0.814; self-administered patient satisfaction scale, 94

HHS, Harris hip score; OHS, Oxford hip score; THA, total hip arthroplasty.

Postoperative Management

The patient is mobilized, and weight bearing is determined based on the details of the entire revision reconstruction. Typically, if just the femoral component has been revised using a cement-in-cement technique, early weight bearing is allowed.

Suggested Reading

1. Amanatullah DF, Pallante GD, Floccari LV, Vasileiadis GI, Trousdale RT. Revision total hip arthroplasty using the cement-in-cement technique. *Orthopedics*. 2017;40(2):e348-e351.
2. Cnudde PH, Kärrholm J, Rolfson O, Timperley AJ, Mohaddes M. Cement-in-cement revision of the femoral stem: analysis of 1179 first-time revisions in the Swedish Hip Arthroplasty Register. *Bone Joint J*. 2017;99-B(4 supple B):27-32.
3. Stefanovich-Lawbuary NS, Parry MC, Whitehouse MR, Blom AW. Cement in cement revision of th efemoral component using a collarless triple taper: a midterm clinical and radiographic assessment. *J Arthroplasty*. 2014 29(10):2002-2006.

Chapter 32
Impaction Bone Grafting With Cemented Stems

ASHTON H. GOLDMAN
RAFAEL J. SIERRA

Key Concepts

- The most common indication for impaction grafting is the stove-pipe Paprosky type IV femur in a younger patient.
- Other indications include an ectatic femur over a distal diaphyseal blockade prohibiting press-fit fixation (a long diaphyseal cement plug, a long stemmed revision total knee arthroplasty component, old fracture deformity, etc.)
- Femoral impaction grafting follows 5 steps: diaphyseal stabilization, diaphyseal grafting, metaphyseal fixation, metaphyseal grafting, and cementation of implant.
- Intraoperative and postoperative femur fractures are not uncommon with this technique. Longer cemented implants may mitigate the risk of postoperative fracture when diaphyseal defects can be bypassed.
- An extended trochanteric osteotomy for implant removal is not a contraindication to femoral impaction grafting.

Sterile Instruments and Implants

- Plates or struts for diaphyseal stabilization
- Wires or cables per surgeon preference
- Wire mesh if desired for metaphyseal stabilization
- Cement restrictor with wire suited for cannulated impactors
- Bone chips of varying sizes (3-8 mm is preferred)
- Femoral impaction system: distal impactors, phantom implants, square-end impactor, half-moon impactor
- Cement
- Polished tapered stem designed for cementation with the taper-slip philosophy

Surgical Approaches

- The posterior approach most commonly is used because of ease of access to femoral canal and extensile nature.
- The anterolateral approach can be used as well.
- Extended trochanteric osteotomy or Wagner-type osteotomy can be performed as well if needed for implant removal. Very secure subsequent fixation of the osteotomy is needed before impaction grafting.

Preoperative Planning

- Templating is important to plan for an implant that (1) recreates appropriate length and offset and (2) bypasses area of bony deficiency.
- Determine whether extended trochanteric osteotomy is likely to be needed for prior stem removal.
- Assess deficiencies to determine whether a plate, strut, or mesh will be required for reconstruction.

Bone, Implant, and Soft Tissue Techniques

- Following implant removal, the femoral canal is debrided of all fibrous material to establish a fresh bone bed for subsequent grafting.
- If diaphyseal defects are present, expose them for reconstruction while maintaining vascularity of the femur.
- The diaphysis is stabilized in the areas of deficiency as needed. If a full-thickness defect is present, an allograft strut or mesh may be used to close the defect (Figure 32.1A). If no defect is present, cerclage wires can be enough to protect the weakened femur from fracture during the impaction process. If a distal defect is present that will not be bypassed adequately by the stem (2 cortical diameters), a plate may be used to protect the femur.
- A central cement restrictor is placed approximately 2 cm below the level of the planned implant. The cement restrictor must fit securely and provide a firm stop against which to impact the bone. Cement restrictors that provide precise sizing and fit are available with some impaction grafting systems.
- The insertion wire is left in the cement restrictor and used as a cannulated guide for allograft impaction.
- A small amount of the smallest bone chips is added, and the distal impactor is used to impact the bone. This step is repeated until an approximately 2 cm of impacted bone plug is resting on top of the cement restrictor (Figures 32.1B and 32.2A).

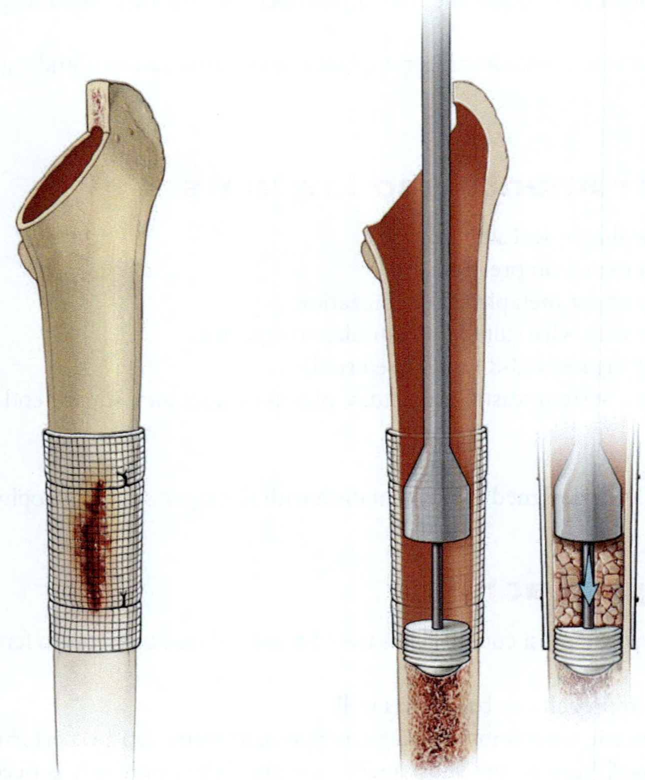
A B

Figure 32.1 | A, Identification of a cortical defect that must be stabilized with a plate, strut, or mesh. If the cortex is intact, simply reinforcing with cerclage wires or cables is appropriate. B, Placement of the distal cement plug with the creation of an impacted distal bone plug resting on top of the cement restrictor by using a cannulated impactor.

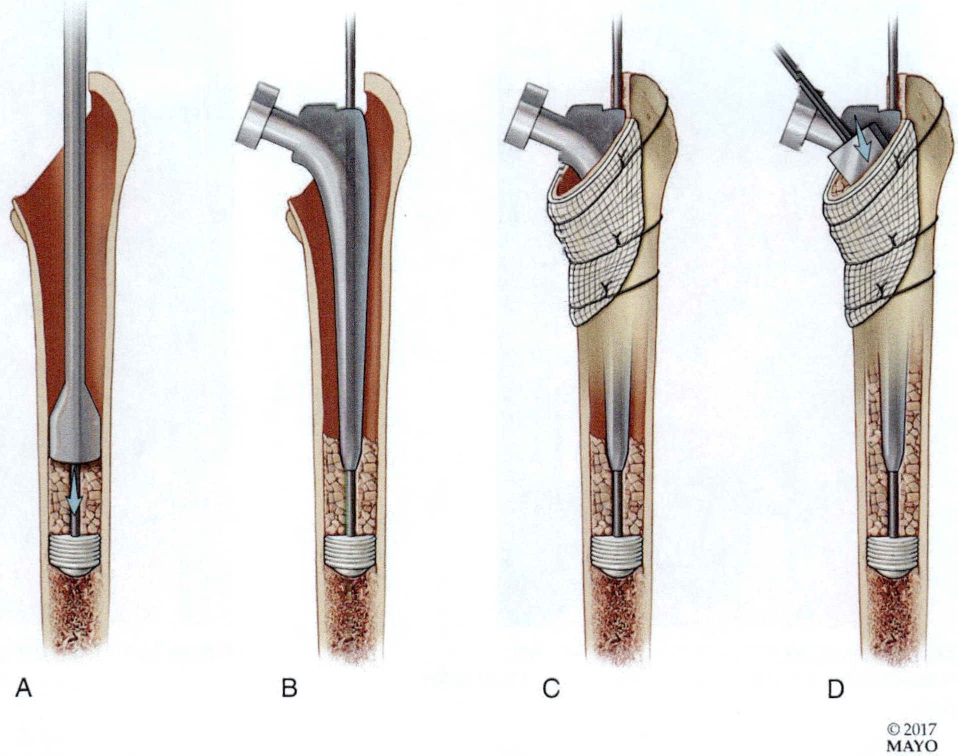

Figure 32.2 | Steps of femoral impaction grafting. A, Distal cement plug with guide wire. Fresh frozen allograft is impacted with a cannulated tamp. B, Further impaction of the diaphyseal allograft with cannulated phantom prosthesis. C, Phantom prosthesis based on the preoperative template used as a guide for reconstruction of the proximal metaphysis. D, Final impaction of the metaphyseal place allograft with a squared tamp. A stem is then cemented into the newly created intramedullary canal (not shown).

- Next, the same process of impaction is continued with phantom implants until the diaphysis is completely filled with bone chips and impacted against the host bone (Figure 32.2B). During the impaction grafting process, very high hoop stresses are created that can lead to femoral fracture. Prophylactic cerclage with wires or cables may reduce the risk of this problem.
- The metaphysis is then recreated with wire mesh if it is deficient or stabilized with cerclage wires if the bone is present (Figure 32.2C).
- Continue impaction with the phantom implant proximally until the metaphysis is filled with allograft. Very dense packing of the allograft chips is a requirement for success of this technique, and this portion of the procedure requires patience and care.
- The square end and half-moon impactors can further impact the most proximal allograft bone in the metaphysis around the phantom implant (Figure 32.2D).
- With the phantom implant removed, an allograft bone tube appearing similar to a normal femur should be seen. The cannulated wire in the cement plug can carefully be removed and the canal suctioned free of fluid (Figure 32.3). A thin suction tube usually is needed to reach the distal aspect of the neomedullary canal without disrupting the allograft chips.
- Vacuum-mixed cement in the early phase of polymerization is added to the newly recreated femur and pressurized in routine fashion. A small-diameter cement nozzle is needed to reach the distal aspect of the neomedullary canal. The small-diameter nozzle only allows cement introduction in an early phase of polymerization.
- While still early in the polymerization process, the prosthesis is introduced. While introducing the implant it is important to start with the correct version and keep a thumb over the calcar to prevent too much cement extravasation. As cement protrudes from the metaphysis, it needs to be removed. Avoid varus placement of the stem.
- An expedient insertion with cement that is still in the liquid phase will allow excess cement to expand out of the top of the metaphysis rather than expand against the placed graft. Furthermore, incorrect version with stem insertion initiation may create mantle defects.

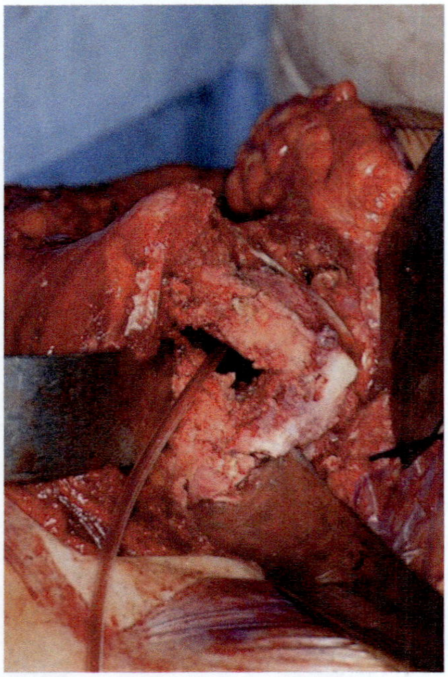

Figure 32.3 I Following recreation of the metaphysis with impacted bone graft, the canal can be suctioned free of fluid before cementation.

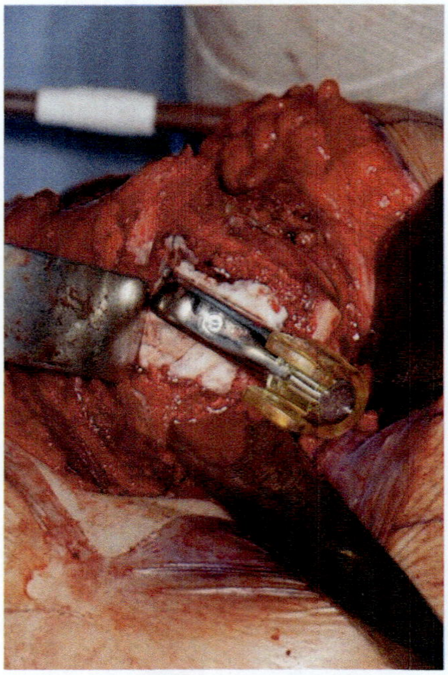

Figure 32.4 I The final implanted prosthesis.

- Advancement of the last few centimeters is done extremely slowly as polymerization is occurring. This further pressurizes the cement against the allograft, causing the allograft to further impact against host bone. However, if one fails to advance the stem completely before final cement hardening, significant leg length may be added by mistake. Be aware that without a collar overinsertion of the stem is possible. Therefore, it is important to identify and rehearse the appropriate level of stem insertion relative to fixed bone landmarks before stem insertion and to reproduce the correct stem depth of insertion during final implantation.
- Figure 32.4 shows the final implanted prosthesis.

Postoperative Care

- Weight bearing is restricted to toe-touch weight bearing for the first 6 weeks and then is gradually advanced to full weight bearing at 3 months.
- Stem subsidence of 3 to 5 mm is expected with this technique owing to the taper-slip geometry of the cemented femoral stem.

Chapter 33
Allograft Prosthetic Composite

DAVID G. LEWALLEN

Key Concepts

- Large segment allograft prosthetic composites (APCs) are used for reconstruction of the femur when other methods of managing femoral bone loss are not possible due to the severity of the defects present.
- *Standard APC reconstructions* involve "end-to-end" contact of the proximal femoral allograft and the more distal host bone which has been resected transversely perpendicular to the long axis of the femur or alternatively the junction can be fashioned into a matching stepcut on both sides for better control of rotation (Figure 33.1)
- As femoral revision techniques have evolved and implant options have increased, massive defects of the proximal half of the femur that may have previously been considered for an APC are currently routinely managed with modular tapered implants using distal fixation into the remaining intact diaphysis and with wrapping of the deficient proximal femoral remnants around the proximal part of the modular stem (Figure 33.2).
- Widespread adoption of modular tapered stems for most cases with severe proximal femoral bone loss has markedly decreased the use of APCs, especially those entailing direct end-to-end or stepcut abutment of allograft to the intact host femur as ability to achieve good distal cortical contact implies sufficient diaphysis for support of a modular stem instead.
- There remain cases of very extensive distal bone loss or vary large capacious damaged femoral canals where adequate support for available tapered fluted implants cannot be achieved and where a special application of allograft prosthetic composites remains useful.
- "Intussusception" *APCs reconstructions* involve the intramedullary placement of the distal portion of the allograft which is driven a substantial distance down inside the intact distal host femur allowing broad contact, reliable union, and excellent proximal support for a very long stem cemented femoral component placed inside the allograft (Figure 33.3).
- With both types of APC reconstructions the trochanteric and proximal femoral host bone remnants are wrapped around the allograft and fixed with cerclage in an effort to achieve bony healing between fragmented host bone fragments and the allograft to aid hip stability and muscle control.
- A competing technique in these extensive bone loss cases is use of a total femoral replacement implant, but this is best reserved for instances where a relatively normal and well-functioning ipsilateral knee joint is no longer present. APC reconstructions have the advantage of allowing preservation of an intact ipsilateral knee joint.

Sterile Instruments and Implants

- Standard hip arthroplasty and revision total hip arthroplasty (THA) instruments and multiple retractors are required.
- A whole femoral allograft of appropriate length and outside diameter is required to allow matching to the host femur dimensions as determined from preoperative templating of x-rays of the entire

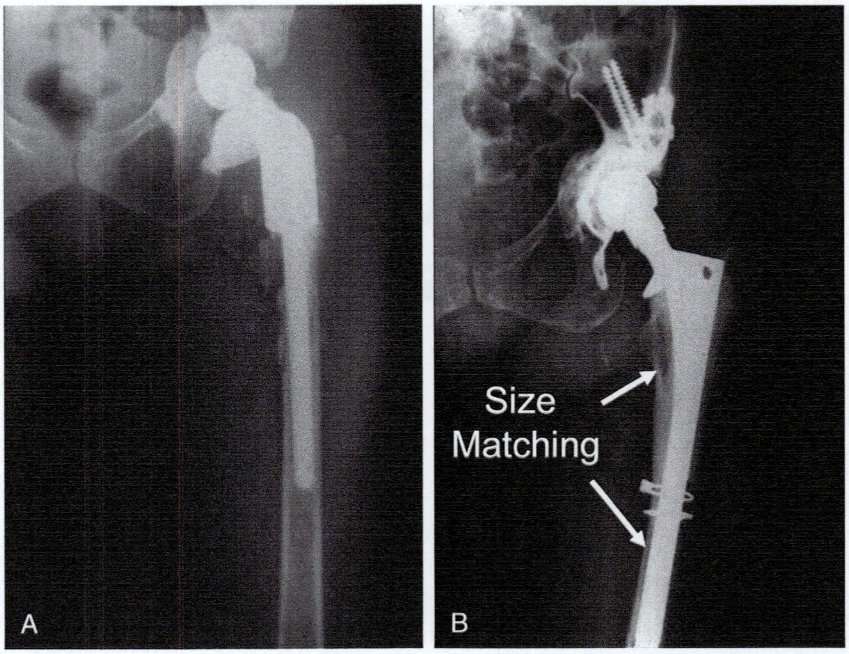

Figure 33.1 | A, Preoperative radiograph of failed loose proximal femoral replacement femoral component and cup. B, Postoperative radiograph showing proximal femoral allograft prosthetic composite with excellent size matching and end-to-end contact.

hip femur and knee of the involved side and of the opposite side for comparison of target anatomic relationships, especially length.

- Calibrated x-rays of any potential femoral allografts are used to find the best match for size and length for the individual patient's hip.

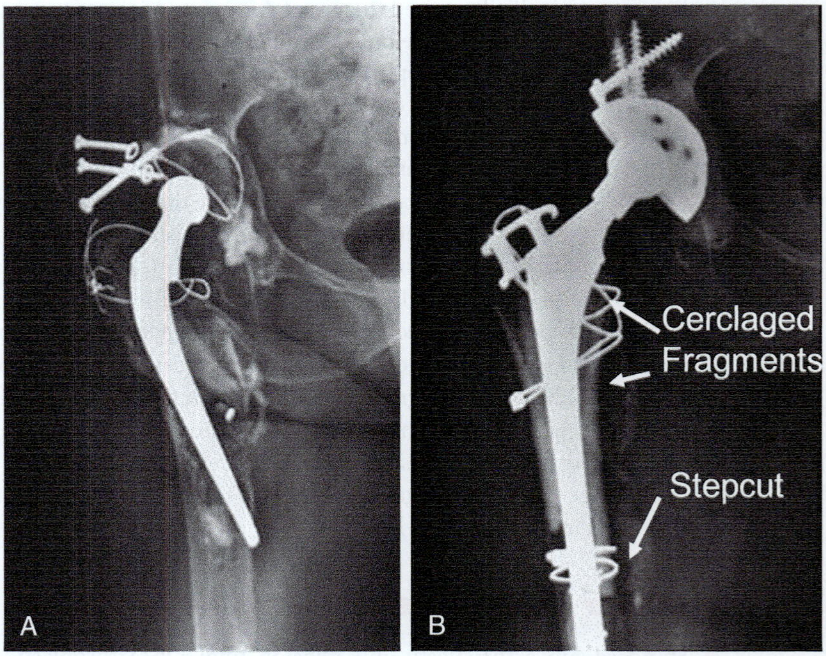

Figure 33.2 | A, Aseptic loosening of a cemented total hip arthroplasty (THA) with massive proximal femoral osteolysis and a Vancouver type B3 periprosthetic femoral fracture. B, Postoperative radiograph of proximal femoral allograft prosthetic composite (APC) using a step cut at the junction between host and allograft. Cerclage fixation of the proximal femoral remnants and associated muscle attachments have been wrapped about the allograft to improve hip stability and function.

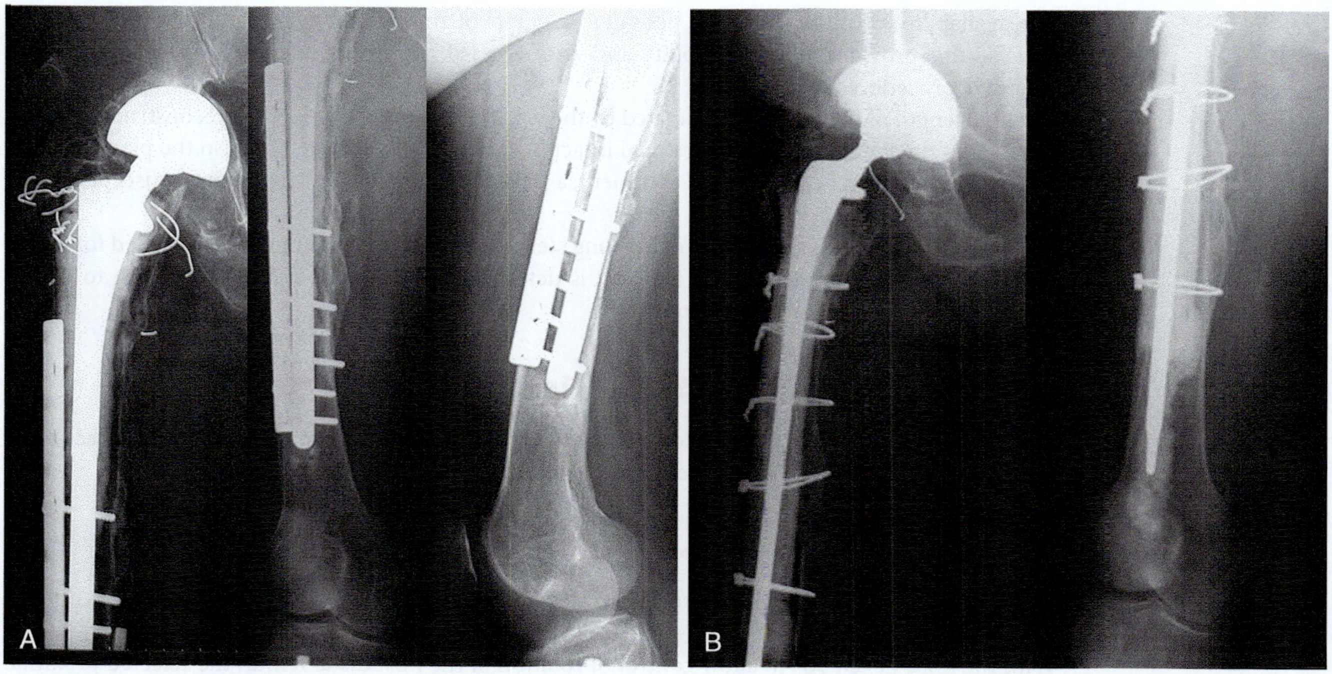

Figure 33.3 | A, Preoperative images showing profound femoral bone loss down to the level of the metaphyseal flare distally due to component loosening and osteolysis. B, Intussusception of a proximal femoral allograft prosthetic composite with the long cemented femoral stem running the length of the allograft which extends well into the distal host femur and shown here to be solidly united and well fixed at 5 years post surgery.

Surgical Approaches

- The procedure is performed in the lateral decubitus position with the entire involved limb draped free and prepared to the level of the knee allowing access to the hip and the entire length of the thigh down to the knee.
- An attempt should be made to incorporate old incisions or approaches when usable, and this will not compromise the ability to perform the needed reconstruction.
- Extensile versions of a posterolateral or direct lateral approach to the hip are generally used proximally at the hip with any of the companion extended osteotomies or existing fracture or nonunion lines used, when expeditious, for intramedullary and more extensile distal exposure of upper portion of the femur.
- In the distal half of the femur the intact segment of the femur is usually exposed as needed by elevating the vastus lateralis along its posterior margin and reflecting it anteriorly.
- To the extent possible, attempts should be made to minimize soft tissue stripping from bone in order to maintain bone blood supply and encourage union especially for comminuted proximal fragments and in the area of the junction between the allograft and host bone.

Preoperative Planning

- Preoperative templating of the failed hip and femur and careful planning of the reconstruction is critical. This allows appropriate arrangements for the required equipment and hip implants and ensures the availability of an appropriate size, length, and type of large segment allograft when an allograft reconstruction is decided upon.
- When a standard allograft reconstruction is planned a proximal femoral allograft is sized in order to mimic the dimensions of the damaged native femur and provide the required length to allow an end-to-end or stepcut abutment of the allograft to the host femur distally.
- When an intramedullary or intussusception type of allograft placement is chosen, a decision must be made about the size and type of allograft needed to achieve a tight fit inside the residual damaged host femur.
- Depending on the inside diameter of the intact distal host femur and the distal extant of the bone loss a long proximal femoral allograft, an inverted long distal femoral allograft (or in smaller patients a humeral allograft) may provide the best fit.

- The availability of more than one potential allograft of the desired type may be a major benefit because this provides added flexibility and an increased margin of safety for these complex and extensive procedures.
- The final length of the allograft is dictated by the original or target length of the reconstructed femur, the level of the junction between residual intact host bone and allograft, and also the planned junction type (which can be end-to-end abutment, a stepcut connection, or a longer intussusception type of reconstruction).
- The estimated length and diameter of the long stem cemented femoral component needed for placement inside the allograft and into the host is determined from preoperative templating to ensure availability of the needed implant inventory.

Bone, Implant, and Soft Tissue Techniques

- After removal of the prior femoral component and any medullary cement, the remaining intact distal femur is exposed, inspected and prepared and sized using intramedullary reamers.

For Standard APC Reconstructions

- The distal femur is cut off transversely or in stepcut fashion at the planned level (generally as proximally as possible).
- With the knee flexed 90° to allow control of rotation of the host distal femur, the selected proximal femoral allograft can be cut as required to match the host bone providing for proper version of the proximal portion of the allograft.
- The proximal femoral allograft is then reamed and prepared on the back table to accept a long stem cemented femoral component that will extend beyond the allograft and well into the host bone distally.
- After cementation of the femoral component into the allograft on the back table using antibiotic impregnated polymethylmethacrylate cement, the APC can be inserted into the host femur with a distal uncemented press fit recommended.
- Adjunctive fixation with strut grafts or cerclage at the junction site between the allograft and host femur and to reattach proximal femoral remnants to the allograft can be used to enhance stability and encourage union.

For *Intussusception* APC Reconstructions

- In order to achieve a tight fit of a cylindrical or gradually tapering segment of allograft well inside the host distal femur, careful planning, allograft selection, and graft preparation are required (Figure 33.3).
- In smaller patients, it may be difficult to find an allograft femur that will actually fit inside the host distal femur, and in these cases, a smaller diameter whole segment allograft humerus can often be used (Figure 33.4).
- Another strategy to allow intramedullary placement of a femoral allograft is to use a whole femoral allograft upside down. Because the normal femur is narrowest at the subtrochanteric level and gradually widens from that point distally, dividing the whole allograft just below the lesser trochanter and flipping it upside down can allow the narrow subtrochanteric section to be driven securely into the distal portion of the host bone with much less machining or modification of the allograft required when compared to the challenge of getting the wide and steadily enlarging distal portion of a femoral allograft inside the similarly gradually widening distal portion of the host femur.
- This upside-down intussusception femoral allograft technique is particularly useful when bone loss extends down to or beyond the junction of the host diaphysis and metaphysis (Figure 33.5).
- While this modification of the technique is quicker and technically easier, it nevertheless requires careful planning, adjustment of the allograft length, and machining of the femoral condylar portions of the allograft which becomes part of the reconstructed proximal femur.
- Proximally one condyle of the inverted femoral allograft is trimmed away to create a calcar-like shape on the medial side, while the other condyle of the allograft can be trimmed to mimic the shape of the greater trochanter in order to provide a site for reattachment of any remnants of the native abductor mechanism or host greater trochanter.

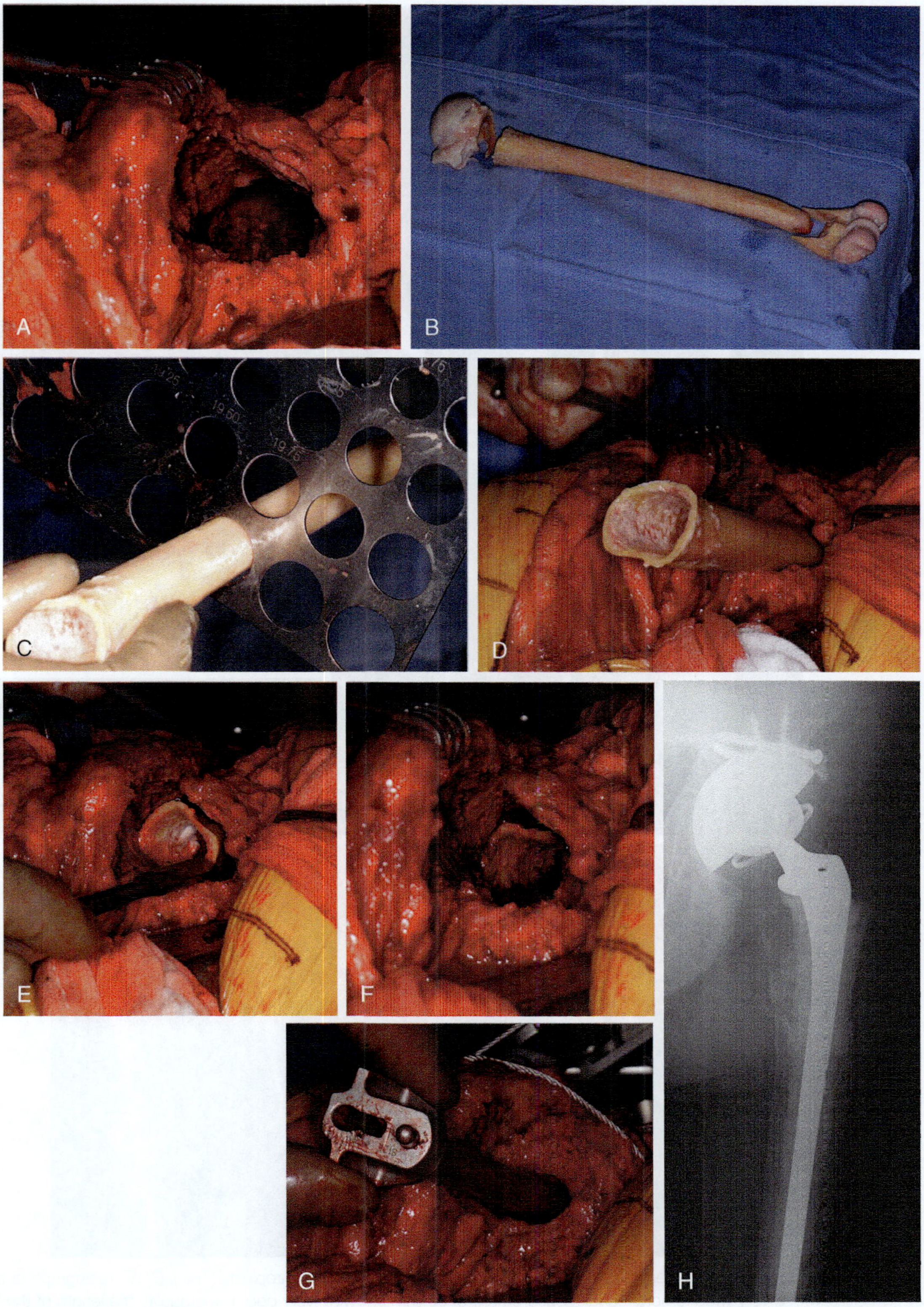

Figure 33.4 | A, Intraoperative view down the inside of a cavitary proximal femur in a patient with a small diameter femur following removal of a prior failed loose component and for whom all available femoral allografts were too large to fit inside the medullary cavity. B, Preparation of a humeral allograft for use as part of an intussusception allograft prosthetic composite (APC). C, Following reaming and sizing of the host femur, a hole or sizing gauge is used to confirm that the allograft has been prepared to the desired matching size using a burr on the outer surface to adjust as needed. D, Insertion of humeral allograft into the host proximal femur. E, Final humeral allograft impaction. F, Allograft reamed and prepared to accept cemented femoral component. G, Trialing femoral component. H, Final radiograph of humeral APC inside host femur.

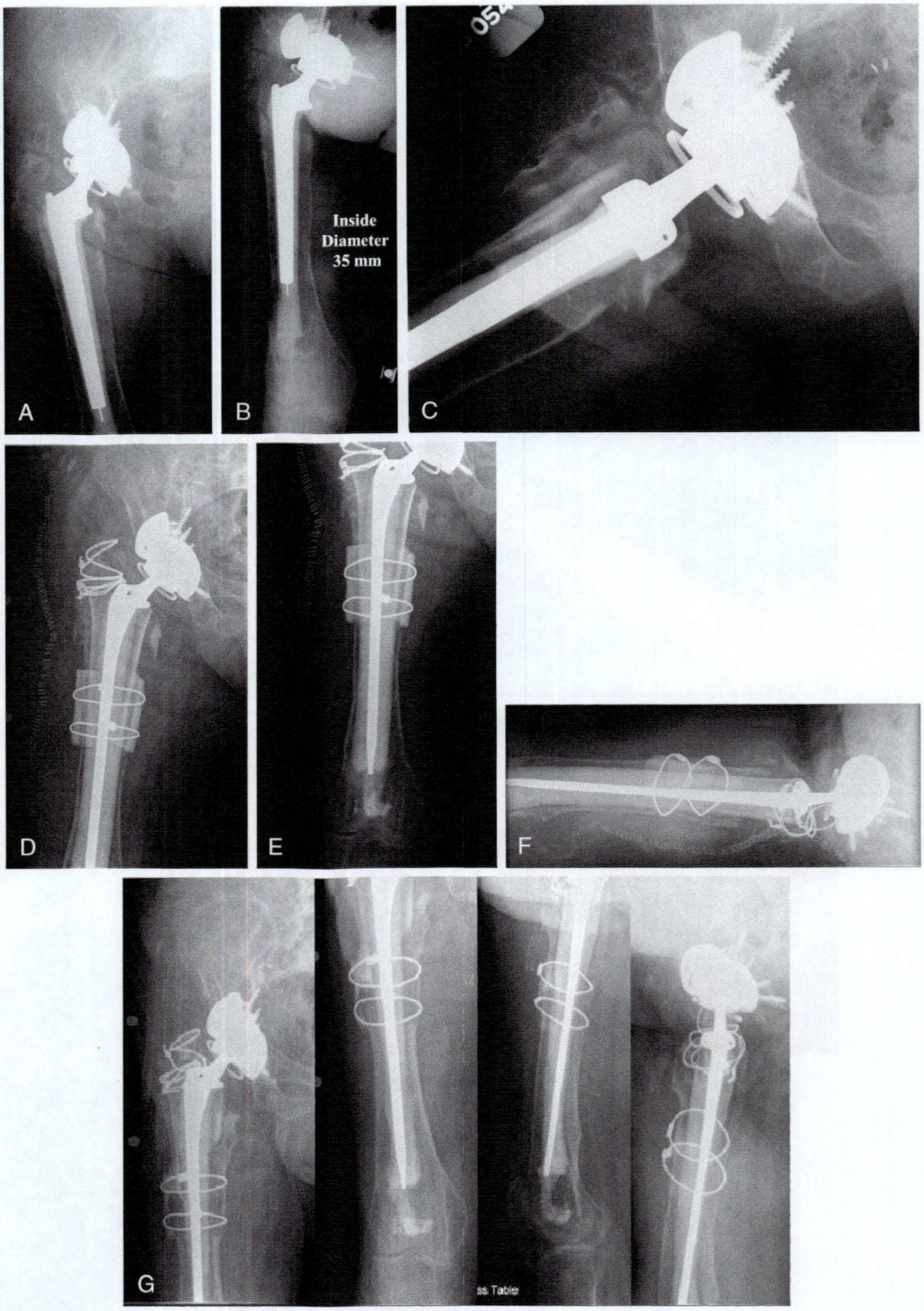

Figure 33.5 I A, Anteroposterior (AP) radiograph of failed total hip arthroplasty (THA). B, AP radiograph of the femur with a very wide femoral canal measurement of 35 mm showing very poor bone quality the length of the bone. C, Lateral radiograph of proximal femur preoperatively showing marked thinning and comminution of bone in the trochanteric region. D, AP radiograph of the hip post surgery with placement of an inverted distal femoral allograft prosthetic composite. E, AP radiograph of the entire femur post surgery showing the flared "distal" portion of the femoral allograft in the proximal portion of the host femur and the tapered subtrochanteric region of the allograft now inside the distal metaphysis of the reconstructed host bone and a cemented femoral component down the inside. F, Lateral radiograph of the femur immediately post surgery. Note the two strut grafts and cerclage used to compress the deficient host femur around the allograft and proximal cerclage fixation of the host trochanter and proximal bone fragments back down to the allograft. G, AP and lateral views at 6 years post surgery showing solid healing of host bone to the allograft and secure fixation of the femoral component.

- In the case of the intussusception allograft technique, it is best to drive the allograft into position first and then cement a long femoral component down the entire length of the allograft or at least well beyond the junctional area after the allograft has been impacted into its final position (because exact seating level of the allograft is difficult to predict until it is driven into the femur).
- If the femoral component is cemented into the allograft on the back table before insertion and then it is driven down the intramedullary portion of the host femur until tight, variation in the actual final level of insertion of the allograft can result in a reconstruction that is either longer or shorter than planned with leg length, hip reduction, or alternatively hip instability issues.

Postoperative Care

- Concerns about healing of the fragmented proximal femoral fragments to the allograft and recovery of the other soft tissues about the hip usually impact weight-bearing status and activity level as much or more as concern about implant fixation and the bony reconstruction.
- Occasionally a hip abduction brace is used to limit abduction and flexion over the initial 6 weeks post surgery as hip instability is more common after such extensive revision procedures.
- Weight-bearing status is individualized but is usually limited to partial weight at most for the initial 6 to 12 weeks post surgery and is advanced once initial bone healing has occurred at around 3 months.
- Antibiotic prophylaxis for dental procedures is recommended for life after major hip revision procedures but especially those involving large structural allografts.

Chapter 34 Proximal Femoral Replacement With Tumor Prosthesis; Total Femur Replacement

KEVIN I. PERRY

Key Concepts

- Massive bone loss of the femur after total hip arthroplasty (THA) can occur secondary to osteolysis, stress shielding, mechanical loosening, infection (Figure 34.1A-D), periprosthetic fracture, tumor resection, and multiple previous reconstructive procedures.
- Salvage of the abductors and reattachment to the prosthesis whenever possible can help with patient function in this difficult cohort of patients.
- Complications following these procedures can be high. Dislocation and infection are two of the most common complications.
- Constrained or dual-mobility acetabular implants should be considered to mitigate the risk of dislocation.
- Patients often ambulate with a significant limp and require some form of gait aid after proximal or total femoral replacement.

Sterile Instruments and Implants

Instruments

- Routine hip and knee (for total femur) retractors, including a Charnley retractor, and assortment of blunt and sharp Hohman retractors
- 2.5- or 3.2-mm drill
- Blunt or sharp bone hook

Implants

- Proximal femoral replacement and/or total femoral replacement systems

Positioning

- Lateral decubitus position for proximal femoral replacement or a sloppy lateral decubitus position on a bean bag for total femoral replacement
- Two hip bolsters
- Operative leg draped free for ease of acetabular and femoral exposure for the hip and for adequate femoral and tibial exposure for the knee

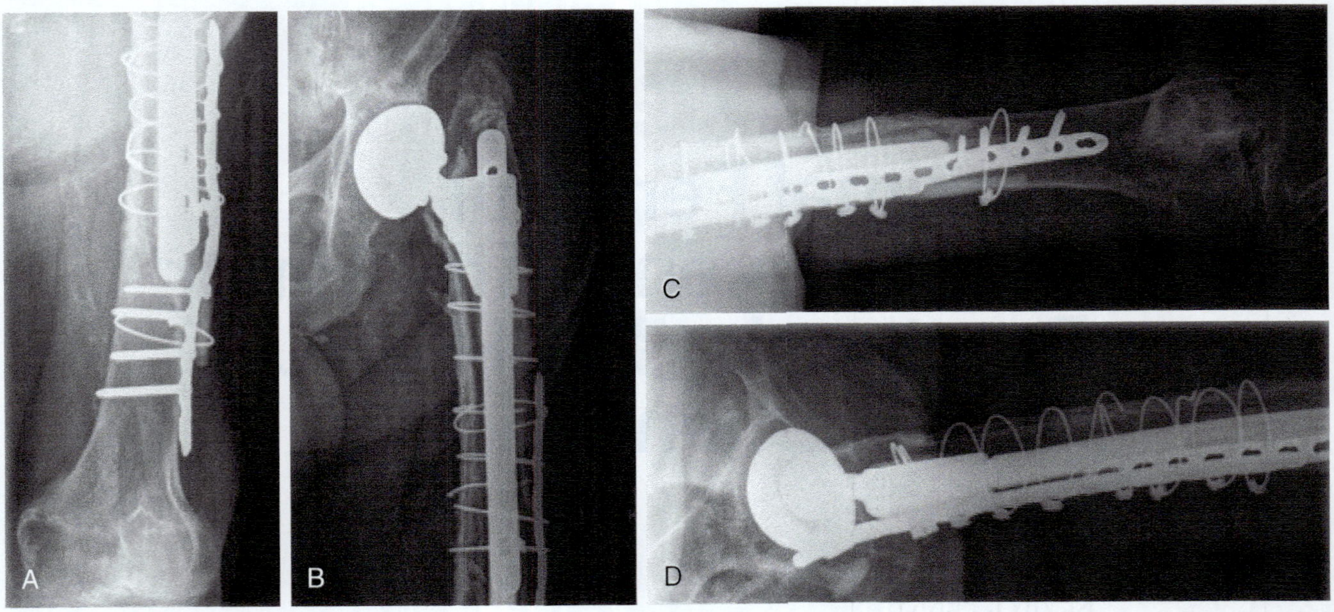

Figure 34.1 | A-D, Preoperative radiographs of an infected total hip with substantial bone loss, infected strut grafts, plates, and cables. Planned proximal femoral resection and antibiotic spacer placement was planned for eventual total femoral replacement.

Surgical Approaches

- Removal of the hip implants can be accomplished from either an anterolateral or posterolateral approach depending on surgeon preference.
- For total femoral replacement, often a combination of a laterally based approach to the hip and an anterior-based approach to the knee is needed. Alternatively, total femoral replacement can be accomplished from an extensive lateral approach to the leg.

Preoperative Planning

- Previous operative reports containing implant information is vital so that the appropriate instrumentation can be available for implant removal.
- Preoperative inflammatory markers (erythrocyte sedimentation rate and C-reactive protein) should be obtained, and the hip should be aspirated preoperatively to rule out infection prior to surgery.
- Preoperative radiographs should be obtained, such as an anteroposterior (AP) of pelvis and an AP and lateral of the femur, which are critical to preoperative planning (Figures 34.2A,B and 34.3A-D). These help determine the level of bone resection (in the setting of a proximal femoral replacement), the diameter of the planned prosthesis, and if there will be any remaining bone stock left in the distal femur. AP and lateral radiographs of the knee should be included if a total femoral prosthesis is planned.
- Consideration of surgical approach, necessity of osteotomy (if removing implants), and understanding the implants in place is imperative to a successful operation

Bone, Implant, and Soft-Tissue Techniques

Proximal Femoral Replacement

- Perform the desired approach to the hip joint.
- If an osteotomy is needed for implant removal, it may be performed during the initial approach.
- Remove the femoral implant (if present) as described in Chapter 24.
- Inspect the acetabular component (if present) and ensure it is in an appropriate position. If the component allows for a constrained or dual-mobility option, these should be considered due to the high risk of dislocation in this difficult patient population.

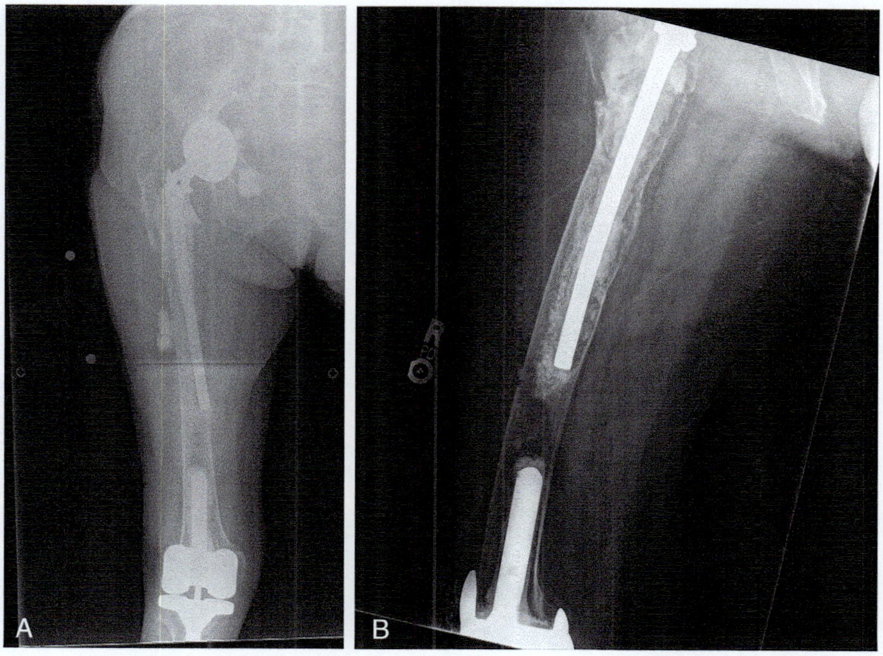

Figure 34.2 | A,B. Preoperative radiographs of a failed long-stemmed cemented femoral component with substantial medial bone loss and total knee arthroplasty (TKA) below necessitating total femoral replacement.

- Resection level of the proximal femur should then be determined. The proximal femur should be sectioned at a level that allows for support of the femoral component distally. The greater trochanter and the abductor attachment should be preserved if possible and reattached once the final implant is in place.
- After the proximal femur has been sectioned, the canal of the remaining femur should be prepared for intramedullary stem of the proximal femoral replacement.
- A trial stem can be assembled on the back table and placed into the femoral canal. The resected specimen can be particularly useful to gauge the length of the prosthesis needed (Figure 34.4A and B).

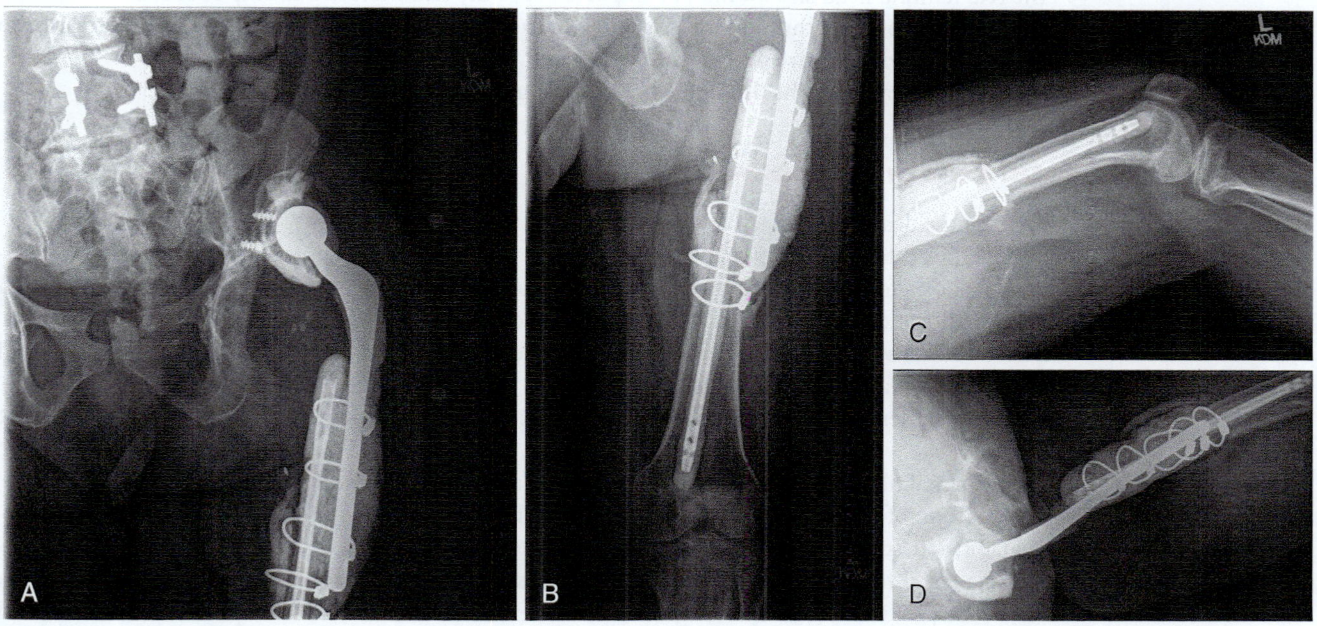

Figure 34.3 | A-D, Preoperative radiographs of an infected, dislocated spacer necessitating proximal femoral replacement.

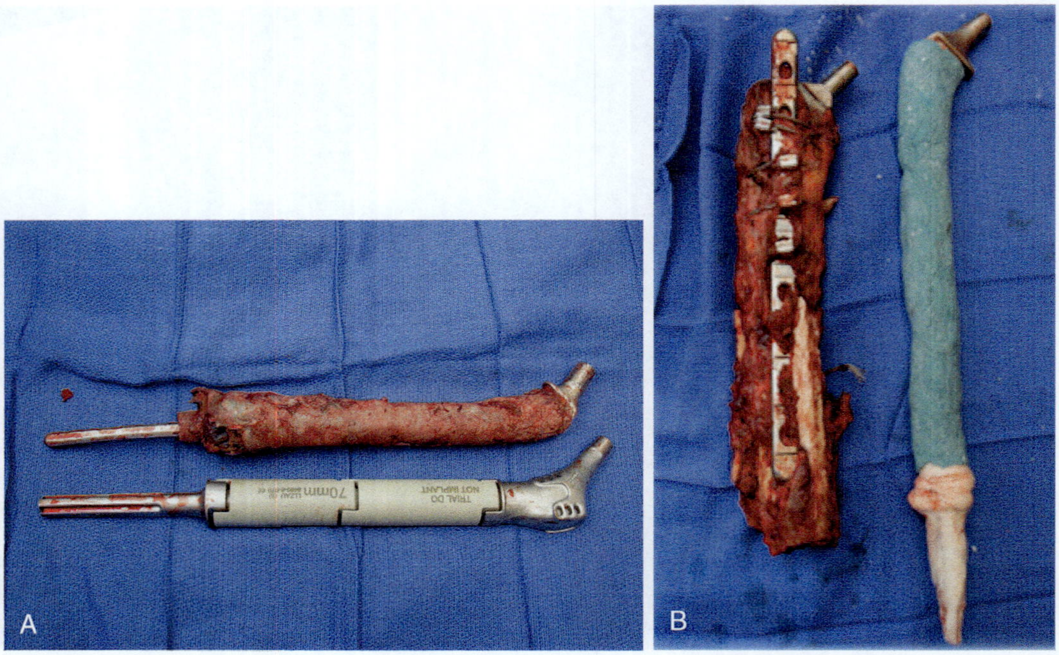

Figure 34.4 | A and B, Intraoperative assessment of prosthesis length based on the resected specimen for a proximal femoral replacement.

Particular attention to stem anteversion is critical as many of the normal landmarks have been removed along with the proximal femur.

- The hip should be reduced and clinical leg lengths and hip stability should be assessed.
- If positioning of the implants is deemed adequate, the remaining femur should be marked so that the femoral component anteversion can be replicated when the real implant is cemented into place.
- A cement restrictor should then be placed at the appropriate level, and the femoral component can be cemented into place.
- A trial reduction should be performed after the cement has hardened to once again assess limb length and hip stability.
- A determination regarding the use of a constrained or dual-mobility implant should be made and implemented as needed.
- The real femoral head should then be impacted onto the trunnion and the hip reduced.
- The wound should be thoroughly irrigated with normal saline and a dilute betadine lavage prior to commencing with closure of the wound in layers.
- Postoperative radiographs should be obtained (Figure 34.5A-D).

Total Femoral Replacement

- Perform the desired approach to the hip.
- Inspect the acetabular component (if present) and ensure it is in an appropriate position. If the component allows for a constrained or dual-mobility option, these should be considered due to the high risk of dislocation in this difficult patient population.
- If a total femur will be utilized, the femoral component can be left in situ and the femur can be removed en bloc from a laterally based incision or through a combined lateral hip and anterior knee incision.
- The resected femoral specimen should be retained to facilitate sizing of the total femoral implant (Figure 34.6).
- The proximal tibial resection can then be made utilizing an extramedullary cutting jig.
- The addition of metaphyseal biologic fixation in the proximal tibia with cones or sleeves is encouraged and is described in Chapter 63.
- The trial total femoral component can then be assembled on the back table and can be placed in a distal to proximal fashion through the midline knee incision if utilized. Special attention should be given to the femoral anteversion such that the native femoral anteversion is replicated as best as possible. The use of a sticky drape over the junctions of the femoral trial is recommended to prevent dissociation of the implant during trialing.

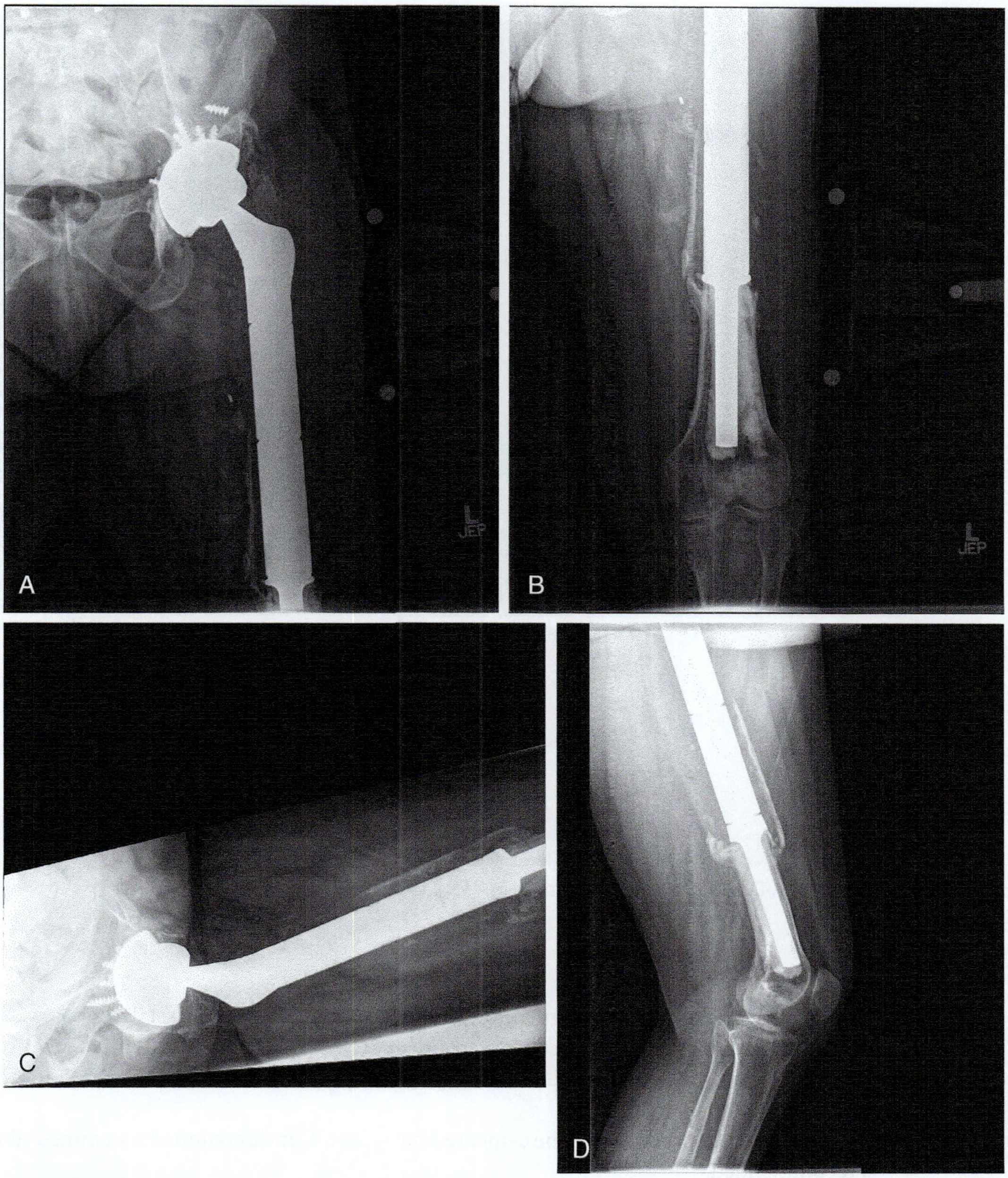

Figure 34.5 | A-D, Postoperative radiographs of a proximal femoral replacement.

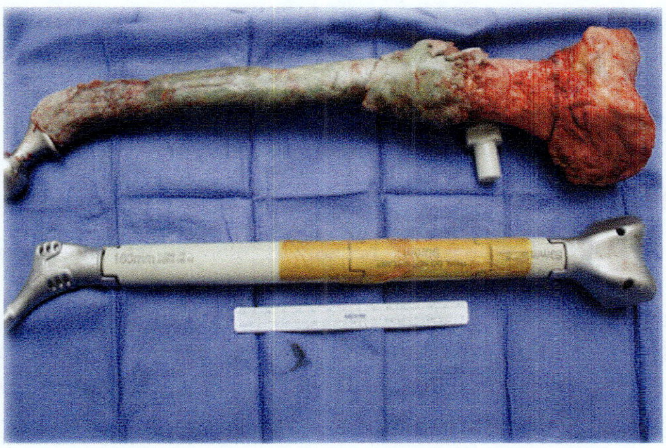

Figure 34.6 | Intraoperative assessment of prosthesis length based on the resected specimen for a total femoral prosthesis.

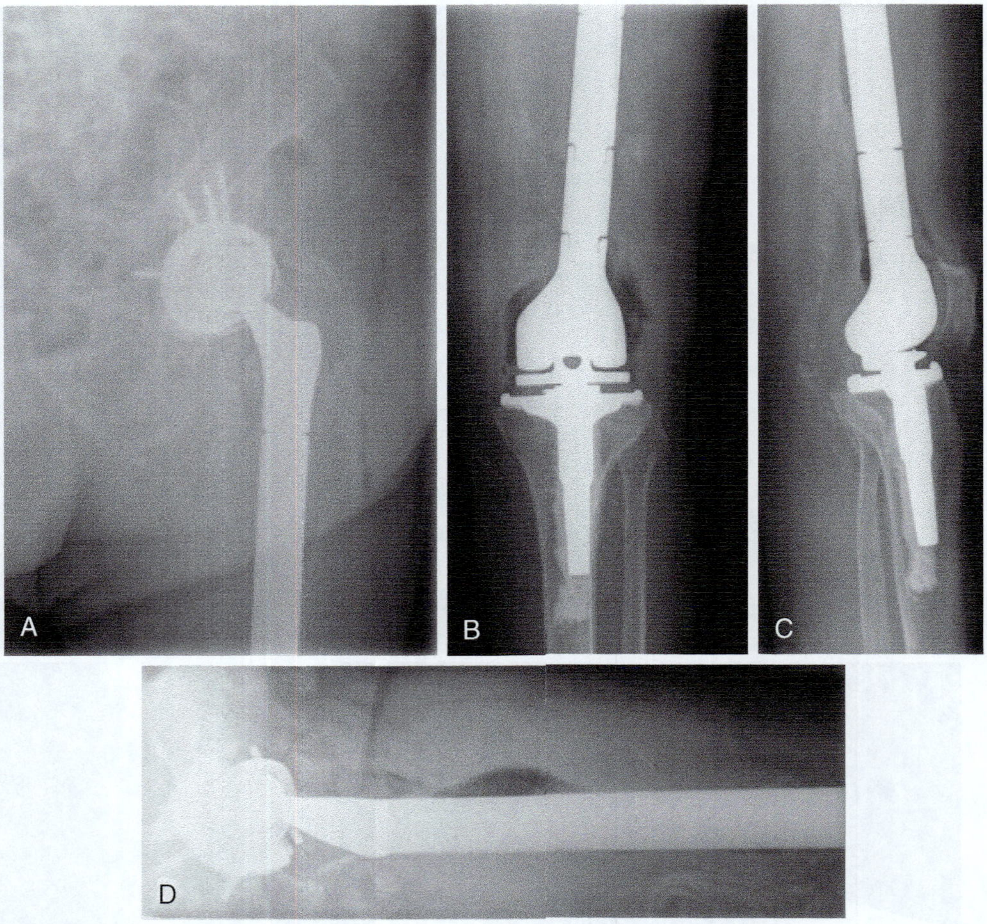

Figure 34.7 | A-D, Postoperative radiographs of a total femoral replacement.

- Careful consideration of the length of the limb should be given and hip stability assessed when trialing. An intraoperative x-ray is useful to ensure appropriate implant positioning.
- When the desired length has been established, final preparation of the tibia can commence and the real implants can be opened.
- The tibial baseplate should then be cemented into place. Consideration of a stemmed tibial baseplate is recommended.
- The real total femoral component can then be opened and should be assembled such that it replicates the final trial implant.
- The real implant can then be inserted in a distal to proximal fashion. The hinged portion of the knee should be assembled, and femoral head neck lengths can be trialed.
- The real femoral head should then be impacted onto the trunnion, and the constrained mechanism, assembled or the dual-mobility liner, reduced.
- The wound should be irrigated with normal saline and a dilute betadine lavage and the wounds can be closed in layers.
- Postoperative radiographs should be obtained (Figure 34.7A-D).

Postoperative Care

- Patients are typically allowed to be weight bearing as tolerated with the use of crutches or a walker after surgery.
- The abductor attachment is often severely compromised or completely absent and therefore patients should be placed on strict THA precautions to minimize the risk of hip dislocation. Postoperative immobilization in a hip abduction brace can also help to prevent postoperative hip dislocation.

- A course of oral antibiotics is recommended until intraoperative cultures come back at 14 days given the magnitude of the surgery and devastating implications of infection in this group of patients.
- Most patients will need permanent use of a gait aid during ambulation due to the severe soft-tissue compromise associated with proximal femoral and total femoral replacement.

Chapter 35
Cortical Strut Bone Grafts

DAVID G. LEWALLEN

Key Concepts

- Cortical strut grafting of the femur during revision total hip arthroplasty (THA) can help reconstruct bone defects and restore bone stock, eliminate stress risers which might cause later fracture, provide stable fixation of periprosthetic fractures, and can reduce pain from mechanical mismatch of the bone and implant at the tip of some femoral components.
- Disadvantages include expense, increased associated infection risk, need for greater exposure, and chance of devascularization of the host bone, irritation of overlying soft tissues, possible graft resorption, and occasionally adjacent joint stiffness from scarring of the soft tissues.
- Strut grafts may be applied as needed along one cortex or double strut grafts may be applied either medial and lateral or at 90° to one another (usually on the anterior and lateral cortices) (Figure 35.1).
- Strut graft union rates to the host bone are high as long as contouring and host bone contact are good and reasonable efforts are made to respect and preserve remaining soft tissues attachments to the underlying femur as much as possible.
- Excessive stripping of soft tissues from the host bone can prevent healing of any fractures of the host bone and can impair allograft incorporation.

Sterile Instruments and Implants

- Standard revision hip instruments and retractors are needed to facilitate extended femoral side exposure.
- A large segment cortical strut allograft (usually from the femur) of adequate length and size to complete the reconstructive plan and provide distal extension well on to the intact portion of the host bone is needed.
- A saw and high-speed burr are both needed to allow strut graft preparation and contouring.
- Fixation of the strut graft is accomplished by cerclage wires, cables, or plastic loops with instrumentation for insertion of the planned cerclage type a requirement.
- It is important to have many more cerclage devices available on hand than would likely be needed in the event the initial fixation of bone or strut grafts is suboptimal and must be redone.

Surgical Approaches

- Any surgical approach used for revision THA including the posterolateral, direct lateral, and extended trochanteric version of these approaches can be adapted to allow strut grafting as needed.
- Often struts are placed onto areas exposed distally along the diaphysis of the host bone by either longitudinal splitting or reflection of the vastus lateralis anterior-ward.
- A concerted effort must be made to limit the extent of soft tissue stripping off of the femur to that required for strut graft contact on host bone—and no more—in order to avoid devascularization of the femur.

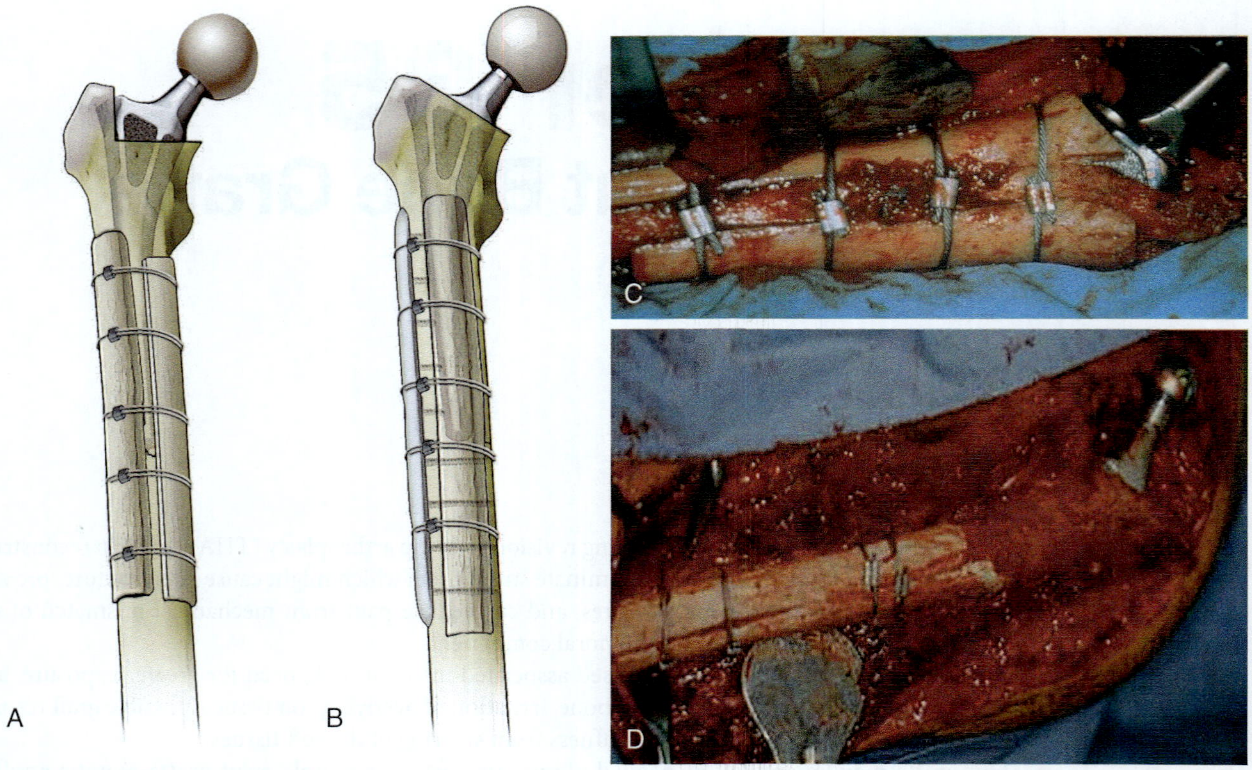

Figure 35.1 | Illustration and corresponding intraoperative photographs of double strut allografts applied during revision total hip arthroplasty (THA) with strut placement on opposing medial and lateral surfaces (A and C) and at 90° to each other on the anterior and lateral surfaces of the femur (B and D).

Preoperative Planning

- Planning for potential strut graft use is reasonable when there are major segmental or cavitary femoral bone defects that compromise or threaten the integrity of the proximal femur and associated muscular attachment sites like the trochanter.
- Strut grafts are a useful tool for spanning stress risers due to boney defects or stress risers created by the tip of the femoral implant. The strut grafts can help reduce the risk of subsequent fracture especially in patients with impaired bone quality (Figure 35.2).
- Fixation of periprosthetic femoral fractures and femoral osteotomies can be greatly enhanced by the use of strut grafts, as they can span areas of missing bone or gaps between remaining bone fragments. Used judiciously strut grafts also can compensate for associated poor host bone quality while enhancing both initial implant stability and longer term bone stock (Figure 35.3).
- The optimal length and size of the strut should be estimated from calibrated preoperative radiographs. Arrangements should be made to ensure the availability of an appropriate allograft.
- Useful allograft types for femoral side applications that are commercially available include already precut cortical struts, whole femoral allografts, whole distal femoral, and hemicondylar distal femoral allografts.
- Whole distal femur or hemicondylar distal femoral allografts with both a metaphyseal and diaphyseal segment can allow harvest of the cancellous bone from the condylar portion of the allograft while still providing the desired long cortical strut graft from the same allograft specimen (Figure 35.4).
- Cerclage fixation of strut grafts requires planning for the availability of cerclage wires, double-looped wires or cables, and the instrumentation needed to insert and tighten them.

Bone, Implant, and Soft Tissue Techniques

- Strut grafting of the femur usually is performed after reconstruction of the femoral side with insertion of the real femoral component, though occasionally it may help in achieving an intact femoral tube for insertion of trials or the real stem and can be done before implant placement as well.

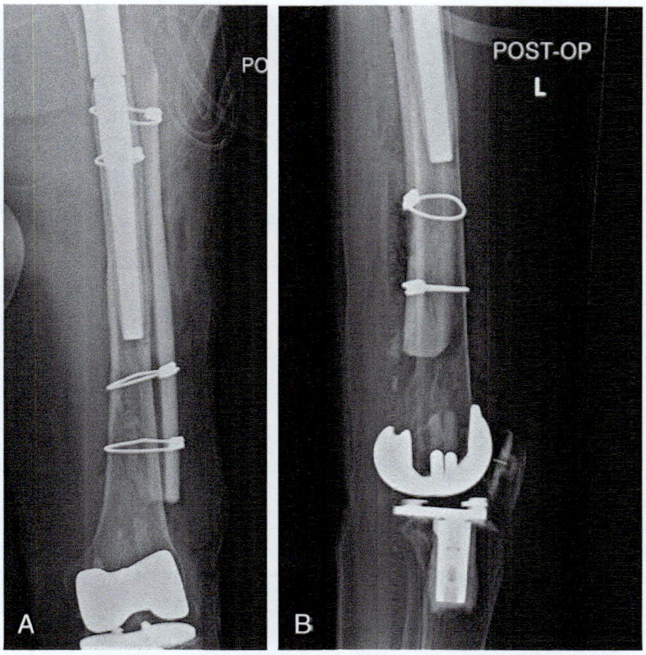

Figure 35.2 | A and B, Postoperative radiographs of a revision total hip arthroplasty (THA) with a long distal femoral strut allograft performed for a loose femoral component and associated comminuted proximal femoral fracture in an osteoporotic rheumatoid patient on prednisone.

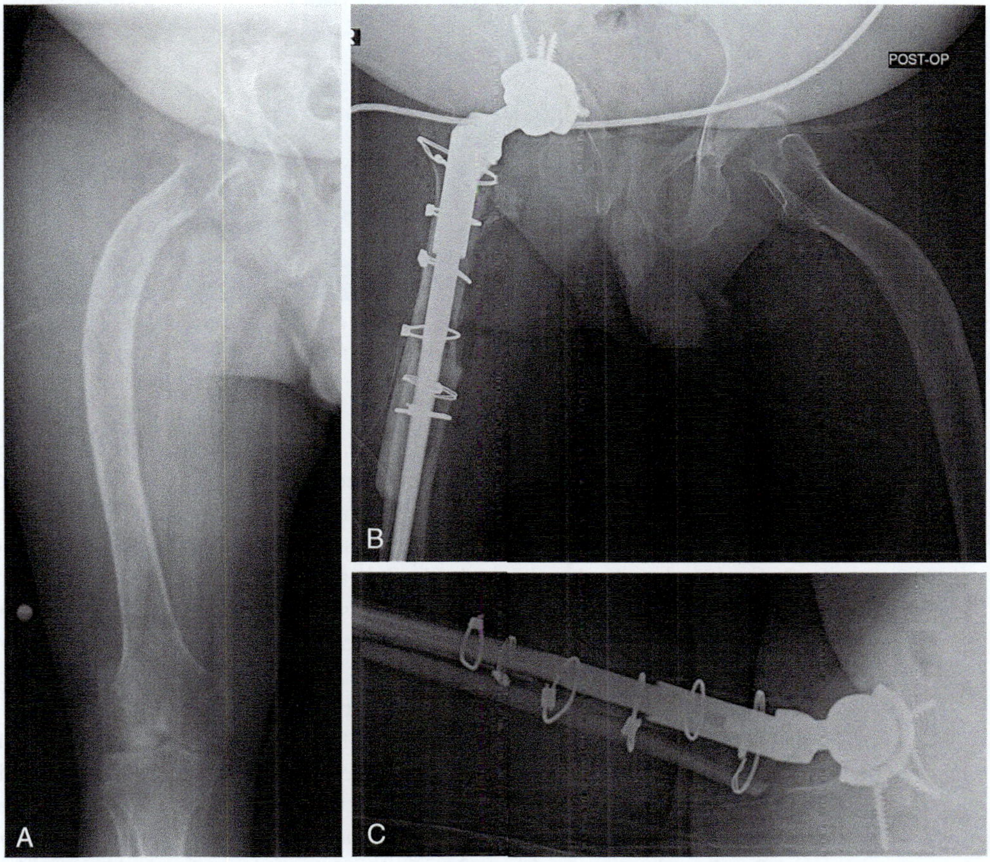

Figure 35.3 | Preoperative radiograph of patient with osteogenesis imperfecta and a painful femoral neck nonunion complicated by marked varus and apex anterior bowing of the the proximal femur due to multiple prior malunited femoral fractures (A). Postoperative radiographs following complex combined osteotomies of the femur showing a long onlay strut graft used to help fix the osteotomy and improve overall bone stock and future bone quality (B and C).

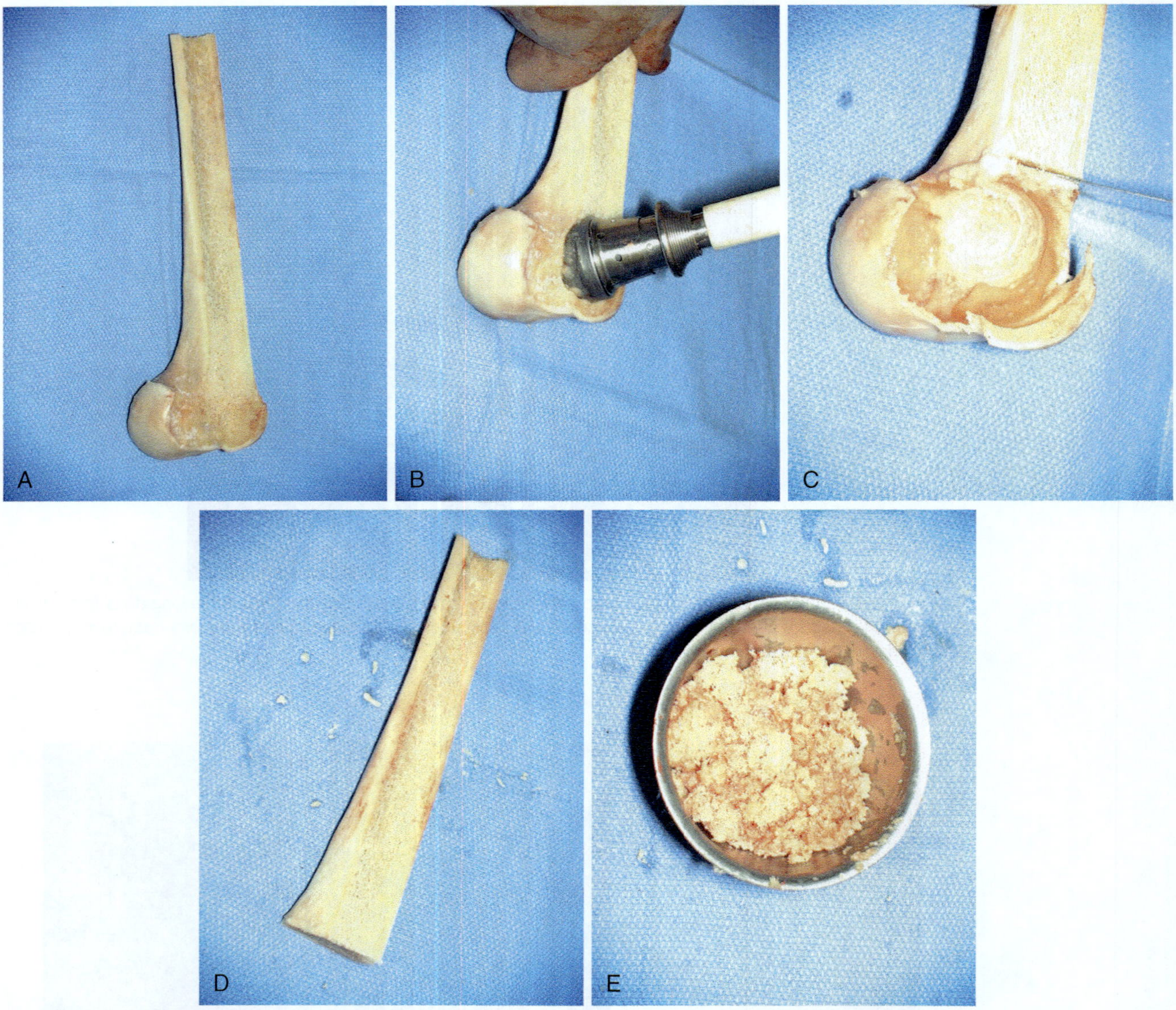

Figure 35.4 I Hemicondylar distal femoral allograft (A) prepared by reaming the condyle with small acetabular reamers (B) followed by cutting the strut with a saw in order to remove the condylar portion (C). Final strut graft and cancellous bone harvested from the same hemicondylar allograft (D and E).

- In some cases of periprosthetic fracture, it is best to use a limited number of cables or wires directly around the host bone to securely hold the reduction of the fracture first, followed by placement of the strut over the bone and cerclage and fixation of the strut graft with additional wires of cables which can be passed through the same soft tissue windows as the initial cerclage.
- Care is taken, as already emphasized, to avoid excessive soft tissue stripping of the bone, but it is optimal to have direct strut contact with host femur along as much of the length of the strut as possible.
- Direct and intimate strut allograft contact with bone is achieved by three main methods: (1) Choosing a strut graft that fits the surface of the underlying host. When a cortical strut graft is cut from a full-circumference large-segment allograft, choosing the bone with the best contour is important. Typically about one-third of the circumference of a whole segment allograft is used. (2) Contouring the undersurface of the graft to optimize host bone contact. This usually involves making the undersurface of the graft a larger diameter circumference that intimately fits the outer circumference of the host femur. This contouring can be done most effectively with a high-speed acorn-shaped burr. (3) Bending the strut graft to a final intimate fit with the femur. Tight cable fixation can help with this, but most grafts bend only a modest amount.
- A minimum of two cerclage wires or cables are needed for each strut, but fixation is improved by additional cerclage, though the price paid is added soft tissue stripping and devascularization of the host bone. Most commonly two cables are used proximal and two cables are used distal to the area being protected by the strut graft.

- Cable fixation is much stronger than wire and can be used to actually reduce bone fragments into position before final tightening, while wire is merely capable of holding reduced bone and strut grafts in place.
- One cost-saving and -effective method is to use gradual tightening of a cable to reduce fragments into the desired position and before crimping or tightening the cable, to pass a wire in the same area and tighten the wire first.
- Once the wire has been tightened the companion cable can be removed before it is crimped or locked into position. Once removed, the cable can be reused elsewhere for the same purpose or left in at another location where cable fixation is desired.
- This technique is very useful when multiple areas of cerclage are needed along an extensive section of the femur and especially if a mix of both cerclage wire and cables is desired.
- An intraoperative X-ray can be obtained with the cables provisionally tightened but not yet crimped to ensure a satisfactory reduction of bone fragments and strut graft placement before final tightening.
- Once in final position and tightened cable ends are cut short and wire ends bent over and tucked into bony recesses as much as possible to try and minimize the irritation of any overlying soft tissues.
- It is very important to be careful working around the cut ends of any wires and especially cut off cables as the sharp ends can perforate gloves, injure surgical team members and increase the risk of bacterial contamination and postoperative infection.
- Any small gaps between strut and host at the end of the procedure are filled with available cancellous graft to encourage union.

Postoperative Care

- Routine revision THA weight bearing and management protocols may be used, though generally with more major bone defects, stress fracture cases, or periprosthetic fracture patients are restricted from full weight bearing until 3 months post surgery to allow initial bone healing (Figure 35.5).
- After more extensive revision procedures extending distally along the femur, knee range of motion should be a focus of the postoperative rehabilitation program to avoid knee contracture, loss of motion, or stiffness symptoms.

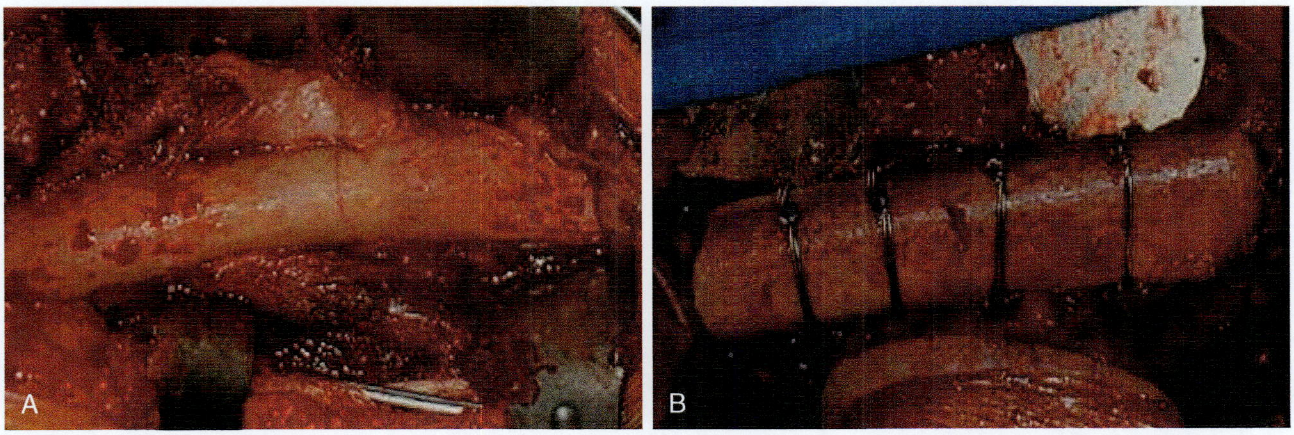

Figure 35.5 | Intraoperative photograph of an incomplete femoral stress fracture near the tip of a femoral component (A) treated with an onlay cortical strut allograft (B) and prolonged protected weight bearing post surgery until bony healing.

Chapter 36
Periprosthetic Osteolysis

CORY G. COUCH
MICHAEL J. TAUNTON

Key Concepts

- Osteolysis can have a number of etiologies including infection, tumors, and inflammatory reactions related to particulate debris. In joint replacement, non–infection-related osteolysis is most commonly caused by reactions to polyethylene debris, cement debris, or metal debris or metal ions.
- Osteolysis may be asymptomatic or may lead to pain and decreased function (typically due to the associated particle generated synovitis), loosening of the femoral and/or acetabular component, and periprosthetic fracture.
- In many cases, periprosthetic acetabular osteolysis can be treated with component retention in the case of a well-fixed acetabular shell with the benefit of reduced surgical time, blood loss, cost, and avoidance of additional bone loss.
- Surgical treatment of osteolysis is recommended when there is imminent wear-through of the acetabular polyethylene, progressive expansile lesions that may cause implant loosening, or periprosthetic fracture.
- Prior imaging, over the lifetime of the arthroplasty, is helpful for comparative purposes to evaluate for changes in osteolysis and radiolucent or reactive lines.

Basic Science of Osteolysis

- The formation of particulate debris or corrosion products from total hip implants leads to an inflammatory response and macrophage activation that leads to osteolysis.
- The particulate debris can be formed from any type of wear of the total hip arthroplasty (THA) implants. Particulate debris can be formed from polyethylene (particularly non-cross-linked polyethylene), either at the bearing surface or on the back side of the polyethylene. Cement debris may be created from a loosened cemented implant (due to abrasion of the cement by implant or bone). Metal wear particles may be created from metal-on-metal bearings. Additionally, modular metal junctions maybe subject to taper corrosion in which mechanically assisted crevice corrosion leads to release of cobalt and chromium ions that lead to osteolysis and tissue necrosis through other pathways.
- It is important to first rule out infection in the setting of osteolysis as both may have similar presenting clinical pictures in regard to bone loss. This can be done with laboratory workup of erythrocyte sedimentation rate, C-reactive protein, and aspiration if warranted and intraoperative cultures.

Sterile Instruments and Implants

Instruments

- Routine hip retractors
- Revision instruments
  - Cup explant system
  - Femoral component explant system instruments and tools
  - High-speed burrs (short and long pencil-tip burrs, 6.5-mm round burr)
  - Osteotomes (straight, curved, flexible)

- Cement removal instruments if cement is present
- Ultrasonic cement removal device if available and if cement is present in femur
- Curettes
- Cobb elevators
- Drill, drill bits, threaded drill guides, depth gauge

Implants

- Highly porous revision acetabular components
- Various acetabular liner options: standard, dual mobility, constrained
- Acetabular screws
- Porous metal augments
- Acetabular cages
- Revision femoral components (with trial stems)
- Femoral heads (with trial heads)
- Cerclage cables and wires
- Allograft bone chips

Positioning

- Lateral decubitus position
  - Typical position for most procedures
  - The operative limb should be sterilely prepared from the iliac crest to the foot and draped out to the distal thigh
    - Allows for intraoperative assessment of distal blood flow in emergency
    - Allows for management of distal femoral fracture intraoperatively

Surgical Approaches

- The operative approach is at the discretion of the surgeon and may be chosen based on the location of the osteolysis and the planned operative intervention.
- For many cases the authors prefer the posterior approach as it may easily be made extensile if needed. Additionally, posterior column osteolysis is more readily approached posteriorly.
- The senior author reserves the anterolateral approach in those with severe abductor damage seen at time of exposure or for cases in which cup retention is planned and there is relatively less prosthetic cup anteversion present.
- The direct anterior approach, in expert hands, is useful for a minority of revision hip arthroplasties, but extensile exposure is more difficult.

Preoperative Planning

Record Review

- The size, manufacturer, and brand of the femoral and acetabular implants should be identified for proper planning of removal. If some modular components will be retained, having compatible modular implants such as femoral heads or polyethylene inserts is essential and advance planning is necessary to ensure their availability at surgery.
- Prior operative reports for determining the type of articulation and for determining the implant-specific (especially the polyethylene bearing) track record.
- Implant stickers are essential.
- Identifying features of the implant such as an extraction hole or threaded insertion for an extractor may aid in stem removal with a universal or stem-specific extraction device.

Laboratory Workup

- Assess for infection preoperatively with inflammatory markers and fluoroscopically guided hip aspiration as indicated.
- If metal corrosion or wear is thought to be the etiology, obtain serum cobalt and chromium levels.

Evaluation and Treatment of Acetabular Osteolysis

- Periodic screening of all patients with THA is recommended; more frequent screening is appropriate for patients who are young and active or have components known to be poor performers. This should be performed with anteroposterior (AP) pelvis, AP and lateral hip, and potentially Judet view radiographs.
- Plain radiographs may inadequately detect the extent of osteolysis; however, there is increased sensitivity with computed tomography (CT) (and sometimes magnetic resonance imaging [MRI]). These modalities may be recommended in cases in which there is progressive wear and/or symptoms with little radiographic evidence of lysis. However, advanced imaging is not cost-effective for screening. Additionally, in settings of massive osteolysis or if pelvic discontinuity is suspected, CT may help the surgeon further investigate and perhaps plan further surgical intervention.
- CT is more effective in assessing bone loss in the pelvis; however, MRI is particularly useful in assessing soft tissue reactions especially in situations of osteolysis in conjunction with metal reaction and soft tissue mass.
- It is an important exercise to classify osteolytic bone loss in the setting of revision THA, as the classification systems may help guide treatment.

Paprosky Classification for Acetabular Bone Loss

- Type 1: Completely supportive rim without significant bone loss or migration
- Type 2:
  - 2A: Global cavitation of the acetabulum with direct superior hip center migration; sufficiently intact superior dome and teardrop prevent concomitant lateral or medial displacement.
  - 2B: Deficient superior dome, allowing for superior and lateral component migration owing to the lack of a lateral stabilizing buttress.
  - 2C: Deficient medial wall causing direct medial migration of the hip center.
- Type 3:
  - 3A: Acetabular rim is deficient from the 10- to 2-o'clock position, moderate to severe destruction of the acetabular walls and posterior column.
  - 3B: Acetabular rim is deficient from the 9- to 5-o'clock position, destruction of all acetabular supporting structures including both walls and both columns, causing the hip center to migrate in a superior-medial direction.

Radiographic Signs of Fixed Acetabular Component (Figure 36.1A-C)

- No radiolucent lines
- Superolateral buttress
- Inferomedial buttress
- Medial stress shielding
- Radial trabeculae

Radiographic Signs of Loose Acetabular Component (Figure 36.4A and B)

- Appearance/progression of radiolucent lines >2 years postoperatively
- Continuous radiolucent line in all 3 DeLee and Charnley zones
- Radiolucent line >2 mm in any DeLee and Charnley zones
- Component migration >2 mm, lack of osseous integration is indicated by motion of the acetabular component

Surgical Treatment

- The decision to proceed with surgical treatment often is a longitudinal one. Frequently, some patients may be followed for years with known modest polyethylene wear, modest osteolysis, and maybe some mild symptoms.

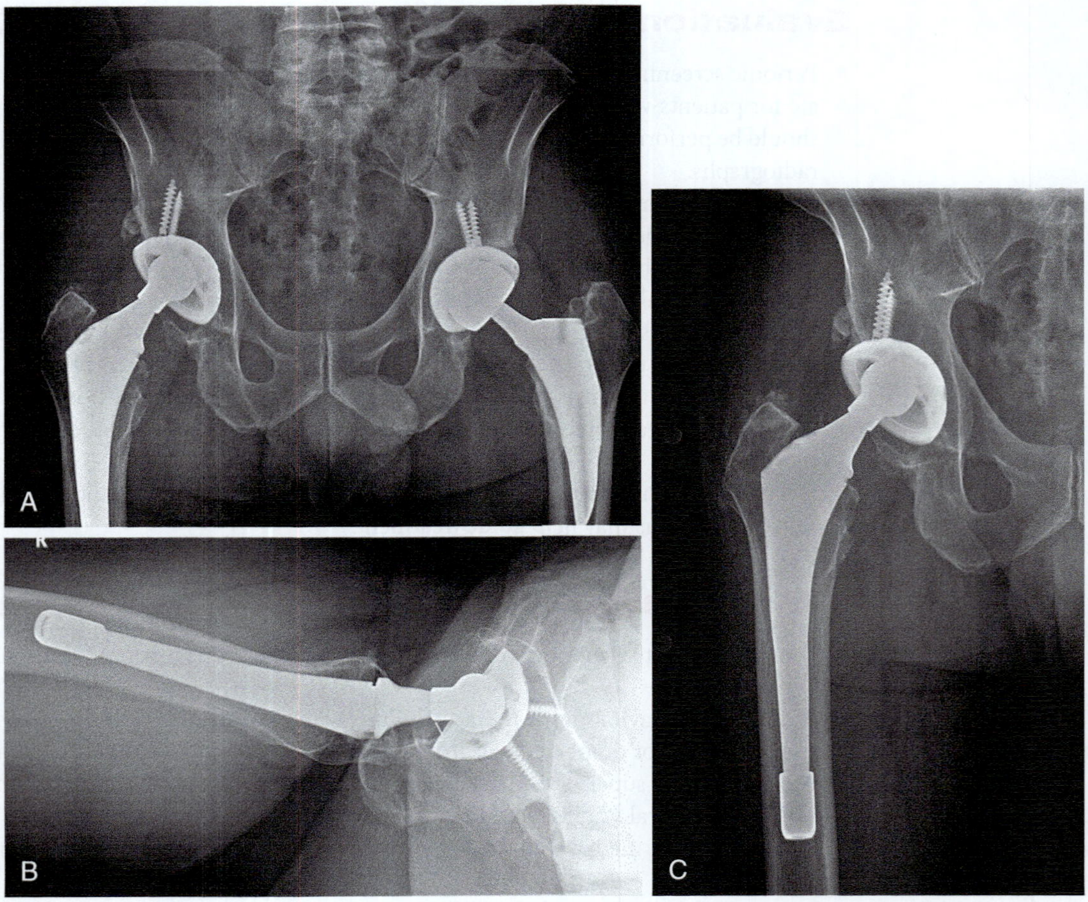

Figure 36.1 | AP pelvis (A) radiograph demonstrating significant periprosthetic osteolysis of the acetabulum, the greater trochanter, and the medial calcar area in the right total hip of a 62-year-old man. The cross-table lateral (B) radiograph reveals 2 large osteolytic defects behind the acetabular component, but there is no pelvic discontinuity. The AP femur radiograph (C) further demonstrates that there are spot-welds at the margins of the cup and more distally on the femoral component suggesting the implants are still well fixed. Despite the significant polyethylene wear and osteolysis, the patient was only mildly symptomatic.

- However, surgical treatment typically is recommended in reasonably healthy patients when there is development of persistent symptoms, imminent wear-through of the polyethylene, or progressive expansile lesions leading to potentially unstable implants or periprosthetic fracture.
- The specific acetabular component's track record and the type of polyethylene (especially cross-linked versus conventional) should be considered.

Retaining the Acetabular Component

- The benefits of retaining a well-fixed acetabular shell include reduced surgical time, less blood loss, lower cost, and avoidance of additional bone loss.
- There are a number of drawbacks to acetabular component retention.
  - There will be an incomplete access to retroacetabular lesions for complete debridement of the osteolytic lesion and bone grafting.
  - The surgeon is unable to change the component position. Some cups have a thick shell and therefore in smaller sizes can accept only a smaller head diameter, which can lead to an increased risk of hip instability.
  - Additionally, there are typically fewer off-the-shelf options for newer bearing surfaces when the cup is retained, but in many cases a cross-linked polyethylene implant may be cemented into a retained shell if other options are not available.

Bone, Implant, and Soft Tissue Techniques Acetabulum

Surgical Technique: Retaining the Acetabular Component

- The surgical approach to the hip is usually dictated by the surgeon's preference. However, in cases of osteolysis, the usual approach may need to be varied to allow for appropriate visualization, access, or even protection of certain osteolytic areas. For instance, if there is a large posterior column defect, it may be much easier to gain access from a posterior approach. Hip instability is one of the most frequent complications of this procedure. Anterolateral approaches have a lower risk of instability and deserve particular consideration if retention of a relatively less anteverted cup is planned (because a posterior approach in this circumstance may destabilize the hip).
- The pseudocapsular tissues are removed as usual, and the femur is inspected. If the femur is to be revised, it is much easier to remove it before treating the pelvic bone loss, whether the cup is being revised or not. The osteolytic areas are noted, and retractors are placed appropriately. The worn liner is removed. The cup is then assessed for gross stability. If it is grossly loose, then one would proceed to immediate revision. If the cup is found to be apparently well fixed, the screws should be removed, and an area of tissue should be removed from the cup-bone interface (exposing the component-bone interface with a high-speed bur is recommended), to ensure bony ingrowth is truly present. The mechanical stability of the cup should be reassessed, if possible, by attaching the cup-specific inserter/extractor to the cup and rigorously assessing rotational mechanical stability. After the cup has been found to be well fixed, bone grafting may proceed.
- The techniques and extent of bone grafting needed in the situation of retained acetabular component are varied and debated. Most agree that if there is easy access to lesions, it makes sense to debride the lesions and pack with bone graft.
- If the defect is central, and the center cup hole is large, grafting may proceed at least partially through that hole. The surgeon may use multiple screw holes to access the osteolytic lesions. Or alternatively, if there is a plan to cement in a new liner, a triangle may be cut between 3 holes and treatment of the lesion may be performed through that portal (Figure 36.2A-C). If there is a plan to snap in a new liner with the existing locking mechanism, it may not be advisable to compromise the structural integrity of the acetabular component.
- Frozen allograft cancellous bone graft is impacted into the osteolytic lesions with bone tamps of various sizes and shapes. The author has no experience with bone graft substitutes or other synthetic bone void fillers.
- If the lesion is peripheral and/or not completely accessible through the center of the cup, a trap door may be made through the ilium to allow for access for grafting superiorly, or down into the anterior and posterior aspects of the cup. If a trap door is made, care should be taken not to go through remaining strong "pseudopods" of bone that stabilize the cup. The ischium typically can be grafted through a lytic space between the ischium and the cup.
- After grafting is complete, screws that were removed may be replaced. If there are screw holes that are appropriately positioned for screws, one may consider putting new screws in those holes.
- In most cases a new polyethylene liner is implanted into the retained shell. The surgeon should use a cross-linked polyethylene if possible. Off-the-shelf cross-linked liners may be available for newer cup designs. For older cup designs a cross-linked polyethylene insert from a new cup design may be cemented into the retained shell. Trial components are used to choose a liner that will fit all the way into the shell and rest securely on the cup rim if possible. The real liner is then prepared for cementation by creating a "spider web" pattern of grooves on the back surface with a 4-mm burr to provide cement interdigitation to secure the liner. Cement is introduced into the retained shell in a liquid phase to allow full seating of the liner. Avoid seating the liner notably "proud" of the shell (Figure 36.3A and B).

Revising the Acetabular Component

- There are a number of benefits of revising the acetabular component in the setting of osteolysis. There is improved access to the osteolytic lesions, and the ability to graft the defect is improved. A new component may be optimally repositioned and may have better options for bearing surfaces.
- There are also many drawbacks to cup revision in the setting of osteolysis. First, if the cup is well fixed, there is always a chance that the new acetabular component will fail to achieve stable bony

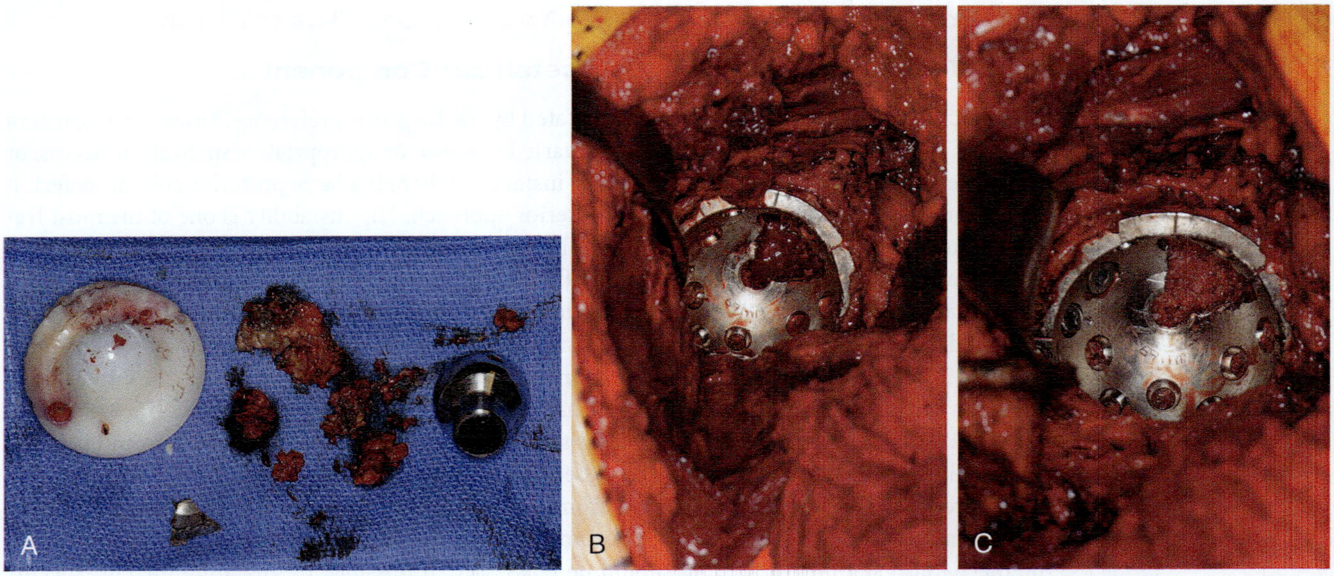

Figure 36.2 | Intraoperative photographs demonstrating revision THA for severe polyethylene wear. The removed polyethylene liner has severe wear. (A) After the liner was removed, the screws were removed. A pencil tip burr was utilized to expose the bone-cup interface, and the stability of the cup was tested and the cup was found to be secure. As per the preoperative radiographs, there was osteolysis in the dome, and a helicoidal cutting burr was utilized to cut a triangle between 3 screw holes to access behind the cup (B). A curette was used to remove the osteolytic tissue behind the cup, and morselized cancellous bone from the bone bank was then impacted into the osteolytic cavity. Two screws were placed in the remaining screw holes with good bony fixation (C).

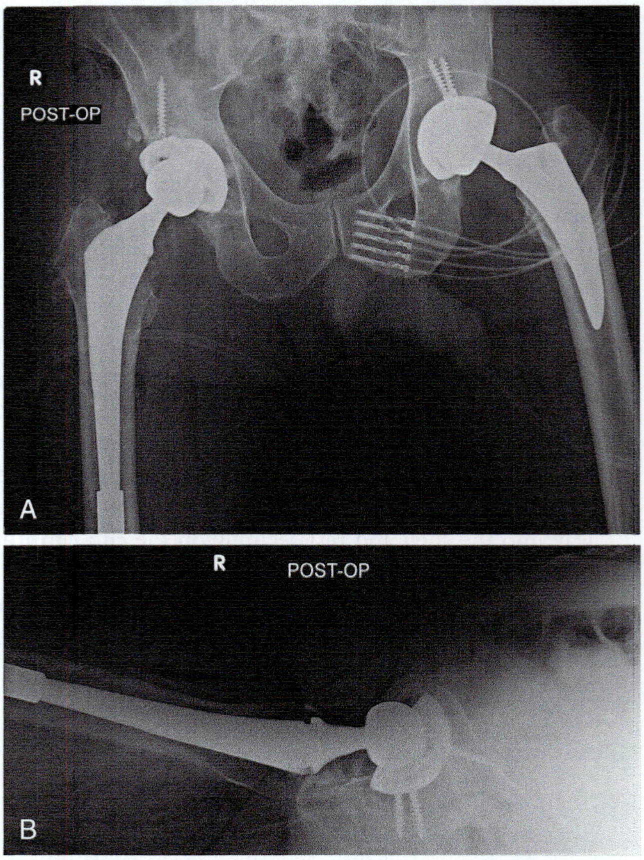

Figure 36.3 | Postoperative AP pelvis and cross-table lateral radiographs (A, B) demonstrating a new acetabular insert that was cemented into the existing metal acetabular component. The femoral component was well fixed; bone grafting was performed of the trochanteric area working from above along the lateral shoulder of the femoral component, packing allograft cancellous bone into the cavitated trochanter.

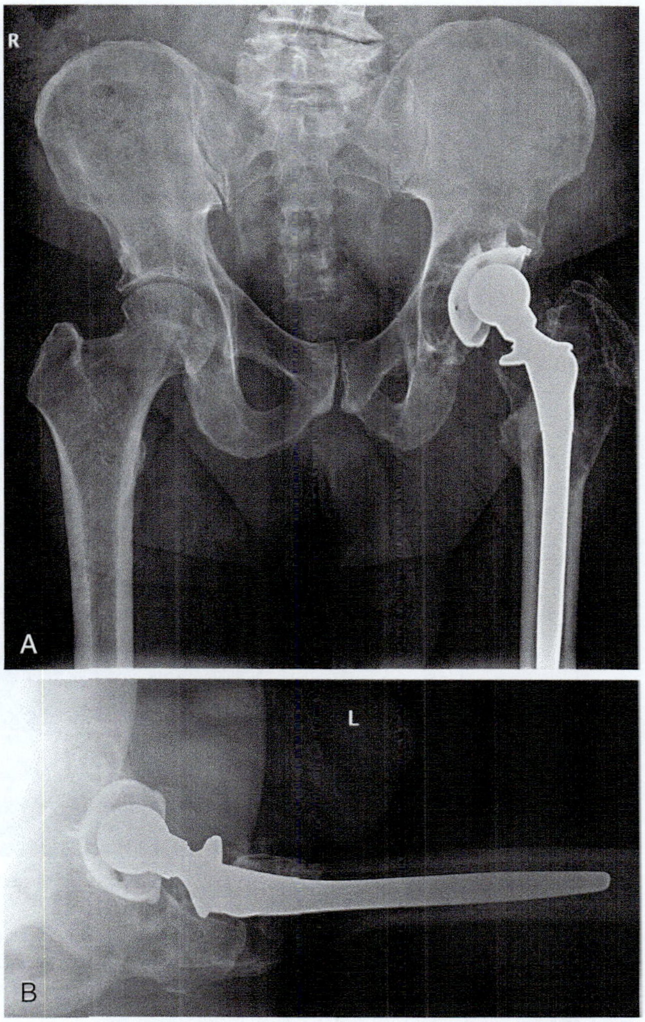

Figure 36.4 | AP pelvis (A) radiograph demonstrating significant periacetabular osteolysis with migration of the acetabular component and loosening. Additionally, there is ballooning osteolysis of the greater trochanter with expansion of the trochanter and impending fracture. Cross-table lateral (B) radiograph demonstrating massive posterior column osteolysis and ischial osteolysis at risk for pelvic discontinuity at the time of revision. (Courtesy of Daniel J. Berry, MD.)

ingrowth. Second, there is a chance during removal or during preparation of the acetabulum that a more severe bone loss pattern is created, making reconstruction less predictable. Additionally, revision of the component typically leads to increased operative time, prolonged recovery through limited weight bearing, bone loss, and cost.

- If the cup is to be removed and it is well fixed, extreme care should be exercised in freeing the cup from the bone. Curved, size-specific self-centering osteotomes for the purpose of cup removal are recommended. The surgeon should be prepared for a larger defect behind the cup than was anticipated (Figure 36.5A and B).
- The lesions are debrided, and cancellous bone graft is then packed into the defects, usually with a reverse reaming technique. If a hemispherical shell cannot be made stable, then the surgeon may employ the use of augments, cage, or custom implants discussed in other chapters in this book.

Evaluation and Treatment of Femoral Osteolysis

- Periodic screening of all patients is recommended, more frequent screening of patients who are young and active or have implants with a poor track record. Dual modular neck implants with a tendency for corrosion-related osteolysis would be one such example. This should be performed with AP pelvis, AP and lateral hip, and potentially Judet views.
- Plain radiographs may inadequately detect the extent of osteolysis. There is increased sensitivity with CT and MRI advanced imaging. CT is more effective in assessing bone loss in the femur. However,

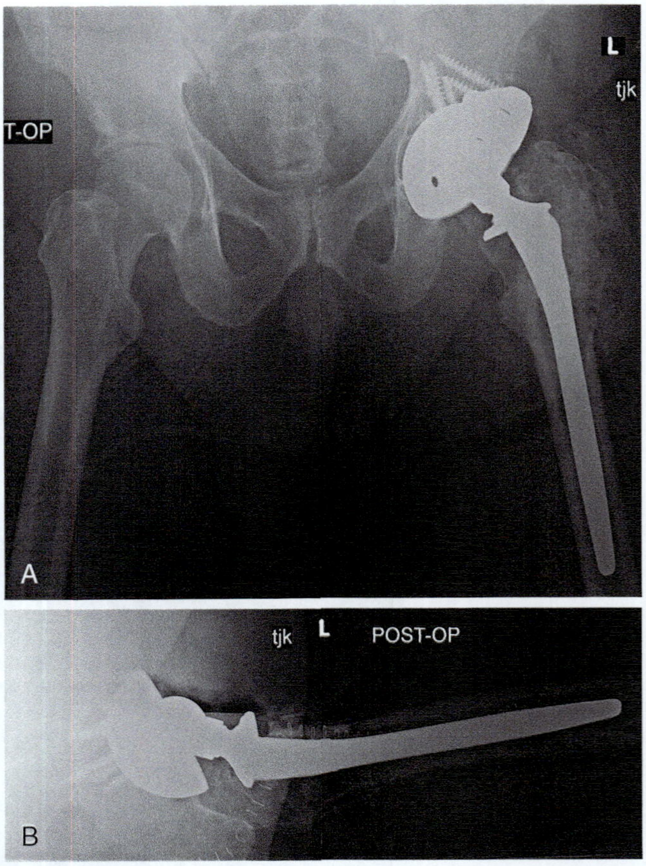

Figure 36.5 | AP pelvis and cross-table lateral (A, B) radiographs demonstrating an acetabular component revision with a hemispherical highly porous component with a superior lateral augment. Severe greater trochanteric osteolysis was addressed by debridement of the osteolytic lesions and bone grafting with a large amount of particulate allograft bone. The well-fixed femoral component was retained. (Courtesy of Daniel J. Berry, MD.)

MRI is particularly useful in assessing soft tissue reactions especially in situation of osteolysis in conjunction with metal reaction and soft tissue mass.

- It is an important exercise to classify osteolytic bone loss in the setting of revision THA, as the classification systems may help guide treatment.

Paprosky Classification for Femoral Bone Loss

- Type 1: Metaphyseal and diaphyseal bone preserved
- Type 2: Metaphyseal bone is compromised, diaphyseal bone intact
- Type 3:
  - 3A: Extensive metadiaphyseal bone loss, defect with at least 4 cm of intact femoral isthmus
  - 3B: Extensive metadiaphyseal bone loss, defect with less than 4 cm of intact isthmus
- Type 4: Extensive metadiaphyseal bone loss without supportive diaphysis

Diagnostic Evaluation of Femoral Osteolysis

Imaging workup should include an AP radiograph of the pelvis and AP and lateral radiographs of the femur. Prior imaging, specifically immediate postoperative radiographs, is helpful for comparative purposes to evaluate for change in stem position and radiolucent or reactive lines.

- Cemented stems: indications of loosening:
  - Presence of progressive radiolucent lines at the cement implant or cement bone interface
  - Subsidence of the femoral implant
  - Fracture of the stem or cement
- Uncemented stems: indications of loosening:
  - Presence of progressive radiolucent lines adjacent to the porous coating
  - Varus or valgus tilting

- Implant migration with subsidence
- Late shedding of femoral porous coating

Treatment of a Well-Fixed Stem in the Setting of Osteolysis

- Evaluation of stem at the time revision is performed by using a high-speed burr to expose the cement-bone interface or bone-implant interface followed by vigorous mechanical testing of the implant to determine if micro motion is present.
- In patients who have a well-positioned femoral implant that is not infected, it is generally preferred to leave the implant in place at the time of acetabular revision for osteolysis.
- In the setting of a large lytic lesion of the greater trochanter with impending trochanteric fracture, retaining the femoral component with bone grafting of the trochanteric defects is a reasonable option.
- If the well-fixed stem does not allow modularity to restore limb length and soft tissue tension, revision may be considered.
- If the well-fixed stem is cemented, a cement-in-cement technique may be considered if the cement mantle is intact. However, if notable osteolysis is present around the implant, this technique usually would not be indicated.

Treatment of a Loose Femoral Component in the Setting of Osteolysis

- The size, manufacturer, and brand of the femoral implant should be identified for proper planning of removal. Identifying features of the implant such as an extraction hole or threaded insertion for an extractor may aid in stem removal with a universal or stem-specific extraction device.
- If the stem is cemented, the evaluation of the cement mantle quality and the length of distal cement are important in planning revision.
- If the stem is uncemented, the surgeon should pay particular attention to the design of the implant, the geometry, and the extent of the porous coating.

Bone, Implant, and Soft Tissue Techniques Femur

Surgical Technique for Femoral Revision

- The operative approach to the hip usually is dictated by the surgeon's preference. However, in cases of femoral osteolysis, just as in the case of pelvis osteolysis, the usual approach may need to be varied to allow for appropriate visualization, access, or even protection of certain osteolytic areas.
- If there is known extensive proximal femoral osteolysis that encompasses the entire proximal femur, a Wagner-type osteotomy that bivalves the proximal femur may be the best option to allow for efficient revision, and then allow for the 2 fragments to be "wrapped" around the revision implant.
- In more typical situations, after a posterior or anterolateral approach, excision of the reactive pseudocapsule allows for greater exposure and mobility of the femur and reduced risk of greater trochanteric fracture, as well as improved visualization of the acetabulum.
- Release of the gluteus maximus insertion on the femur may allow for greater femoral mobilization and reduce the risk of intraoperative fracture.
- An osteotomy can be utilized to facilitate exposure; osteotomy configurations include Wagner anterior extended osteotomy, lateral extended trochanteric osteotomy (ETO), standard trochanteric osteotomy, and trochanteric slide osteotomy.
- In many cases of osteolysis there may be remodeling of the proximal femur. If there is varus remodeling of the proximal femur, the femoral implant may be removed without an osteotomy, but preparation and placement of a new implant may be impossible. Therefore, an ETO performed at the time of the approach may be a more judicious decision. An ETO often is required to safely remove extensively porous-coated and double tapered noncemented stems.
- As with femoral revision in any situation, implant extraction can be facilitated with flexible osteotomes and high-speed burrs. Cement removal after cemented implant extraction can be facilitated with ultrasonic devices.
- The most commonly used category of implants for most revisions of Paprosky 2-3b and some type 4 femurs is the fluted-tapered stem. These are either modular or nonmodular and are utilized according to surgeon's preference.

- Osteolysis is one particular diagnosis for which there is a possibility the surgeon may need to use an atypical technique. If proximal bone deficiency extends beyond the isthmus of the femur, a cemented proximal femoral replacement (for elderly patients) or an allograft-prosthetic composite (APC) (for young or more active patients) may be options.
- In a capacious type IV femur, the APC may again be an option, but impaction bone grafting may also be an option. The meticulous impaction of allograft bone into the medullary canal rebuilds bone stock, and a long polished tapered cemented stem is implanted into this newly created cancellous support.

General Revision Bone, Implant, and Soft Tissue Techniques

- After implantation of the femoral and acetabular components a trial reduction is performed.
- An intraoperative AP pelvic radiograph is obtained to verify acceptable implants positioning and acetabular screw lengths and positions.
- Hip stability and leg lengths are assessed.
- The modular insert is placed.
- In patients with poor abductor function (denervation, detachment, or an absent greater trochanter), a constrained or dual mobility liner may be used. In other cases, large femoral head diameters are utilized.
- If a trochanteric osteotomy was done, the fragment is reduced and fixed with cables below the level of the lesser trochanter, and, if needed, Luque wires above the level of the lesser trochanter.
- Wound closure in layers is performed after thorough wound irrigation. Closure of any remaining capsular structures is attempted. Muscle is reapproximated if elevated from bone. A deep subfascial drain often is placed to avoid postoperative hematoma. Use of vacuum-assisted wound closure may be considered in patients at increased risk of wound complications.

Postoperative Care

- Patients generally are made toe-touch weight bearing for 6 to 8 weeks postoperatively and particularly if an osteotomy has been performed, a complex acetabular revision has been performed, or if bony or soft tissue fixation is in any was tenuous. Weight bearing can be progressively advanced over the next 1 to 2 months based on clinical examination and serial radiographs demonstrating the absence of component migration. In patients with pelvic discontinuity, weight-bearing restrictions may be extended until the surgeon appreciates reconstitution of the posterior column.
- A hip abduction brace can be used at the surgeon's discretion for patients believed to be at high risk for dislocation or for protection of a healing trochanteric osteotomy. This is not routinely used in our practice.

Suggested Readings

1. Paprosky WG, Perona PG, Lawrence JM. Acetabular defect classification and surgical reconstruction in revision arthroplasty: a 6-year follow-up evaluation. *J Arthroplast*. 1994;9:33-44.
2. Valle CJ, Paprosky WG. Classification and algorithmic approach to the reconstruction of femoral deficiency in revision total hip arthroplasty. *J Bone Joint Surg Am*. 2003;85-A(suppl 4):1-6. PMID: 14652388.
3. Maloney WJ, Herzwurm P, Paprosky W, Rubash HE, Engh CA. Treatment of pelvic osteolysis associated with a stable acetabular component inserted without cement as part of a total hip replacement. *J Bone Joint Surg Am*. 1997;79(11):1628-1634. PMID: 9384421

Chapter 37
Metal Wear or Corrosion

ADAM HART
MICHAEL J. TAUNTON

Key Concepts

- Metal ions leading to an adverse local tissue reaction (ALTR) as exemplified in Figure 37.1 may be generated from any implanted metallic part:
  - Metal-on-metal (MoM) hip resurfacings (Figure 37.2A)—Metal ions are generated from wear of the bearing and are most problematic with smaller acetabular component inside diameters (and therefore females > males), vertically positioned acetabular components, and select implants with a poor track record.
  - MoM total hip replacements (Figure 37.2B)—Metal ions may be generated from the bearing surface or, more commonly, the taper at the head-neck junction. Many designs of these implants generally have had high failure rates.
  - Taper corrosion—Metal ions generated from corrosion at the head-neck junction (Figure 37.2C). Although the etiology is likely multifactorial, both galvanic corrosion (the result of contact between dissimilar metals) and mechanically assisted crevice corrosion (partly the result of micromotion) appear to be predominantly responsible.
  - Modular junctions—Analogous to taper corrosion of the head-neck junction, metal ions may be generated from any modular interface (such as modular revision stems, double modular neck implants (Figure 37.2D), or the junction between a screw and the acetabular component). Ions and/or metal debris are generated at the interface between 2 metal implants by mechanical processes and/or electrochemical processes.
  - Impingement—Unintentional wear of any metal component (such as impingement of the neck on the acetabular component) may generate metal debris.
- Goals of surgery include:
  - Debulking of the inflammatory ALTR—Excision of the membrane, drainage of the cystic collections, and extensive debridement of necrotic muscle, capsule, tendon, and bone. In situations in which the ALTR tracks into the retroperitoneal space, it is generally acceptable to perform an incomplete resection unless there is significant compression of noble structures such as the femoral nerve or artery, in which case an additional intrapelvic approach may be needed.
  - Remove the source of metal ions—Revision of components to eliminate the source of metal debris.
  - Reconstruction of the hip—Accounting for the potentially deficient bone and soft tissues.
  - Avoiding complications—Chiefly infection and instability.

Sterile Instruments and Implants

- Perioperative—Intraoperative blood salvage and tranexamic acid, Foley catheterization, intraoperative fluoroscopy or radiographs.
- Implants—Depend on the source generating metal ions:
  - Hip resurfacing—Replacement of the femoral component with a primary titanium implant (such as a single-taper, double-taper, or cylindrical stem depending on surgeon's preference) and a ceramic on polyethylene bearing. If the acetabular component is well fixed, adequately positioned, and of an even size, it may be retained and a dual-mobility head/liner can be placed (off-label use) (Figure 37.3). Otherwise, the acetabular component should be removed and revised to a nonmetal bearing.

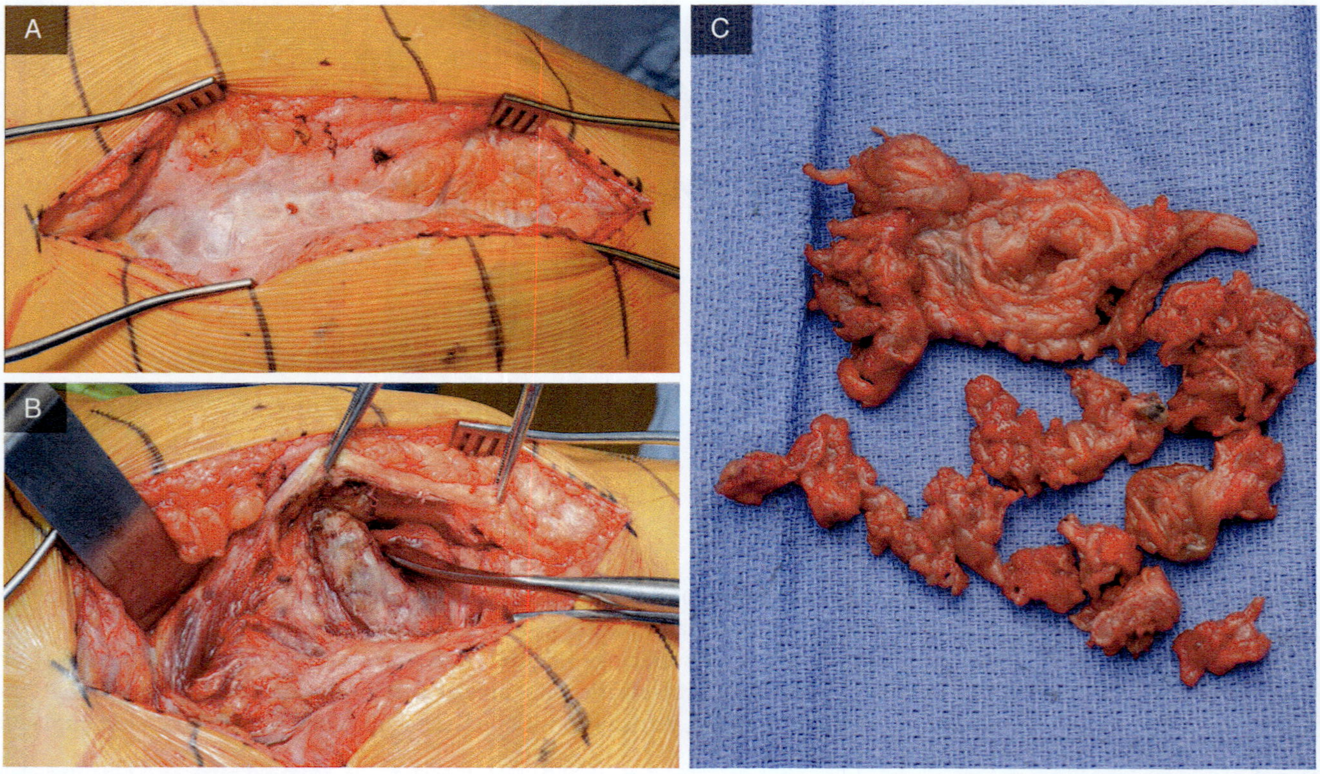

Figure 37.1 | Example of a patient with a MoM total hip replacement and large ALTR involving the gluteus medius and minimus as seen during the exposure (A, B) and excised tissue following debulking of the pseudotumor (C).

- Modular head-neck taper corrosion—If the stem is well fixed and the trunion is not significantly damaged (Figure 37.4A and B), a ceramic head may be placed (against manufacturer recommendations) or a ceramic head with titanium sleeve adaptor (preferred) may be implanted. If the stem is loose or malpositioned or the trunnion is badly damaged (Figure 37.4C), the component should be revised to a revision stem, typically one not made of Co-Cr.
- MoM total hip—The metal debris and active ions typically are generated from both the trunnion and the metal-metal bearing surface and can be treated as described earlier. The acetabular component management depends on whether or not the bearing is modular. Modular implants may be treated with revision to a highly cross-linked polyethylene bearing. Nonmodular implants may be treated as described for hip resurfacing implants.

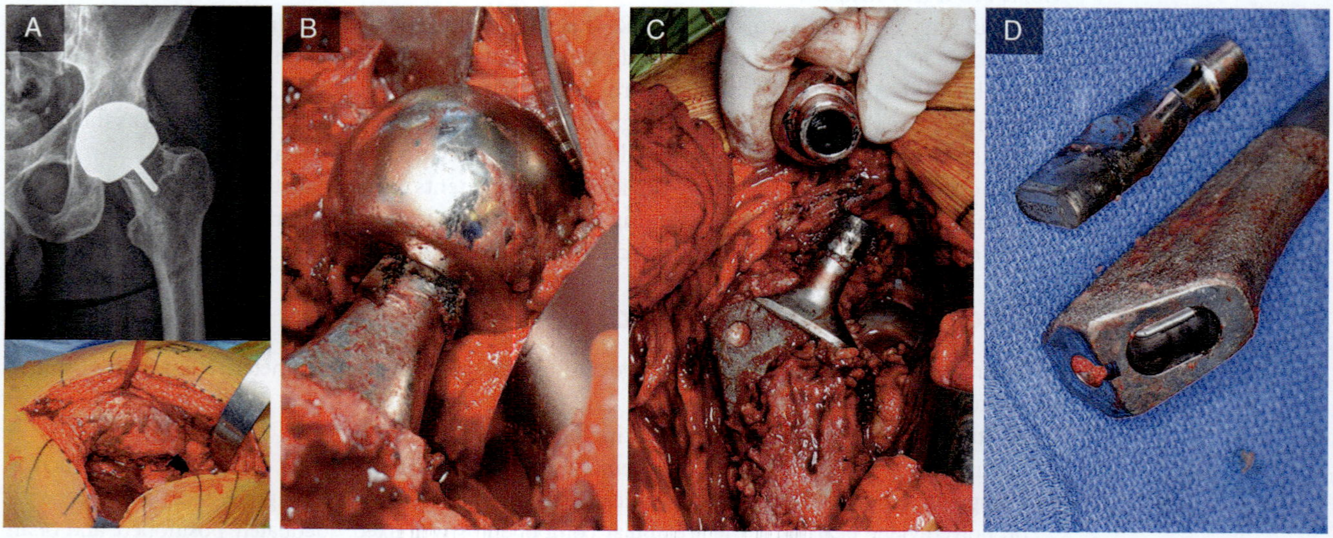

Figure 37.2 | Sources of metallosis include the bearing of a hip resurfacing (A), trunnion of a MoM total hip replacement (B), trunnionosis of a metal-on-polyethylene total hip replacement (C), and double modular neck stem (D).

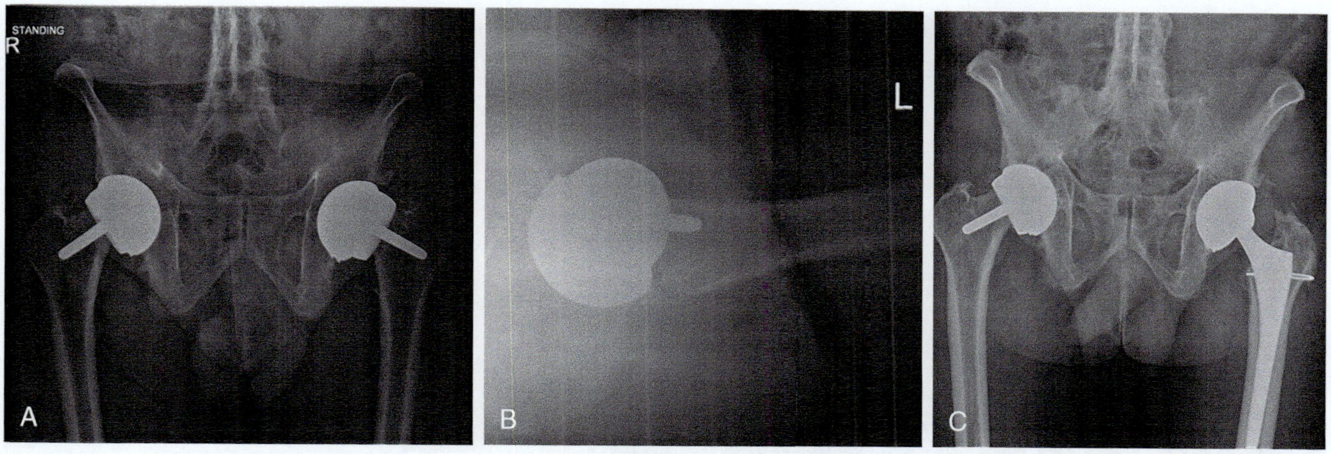

Figure 37.3 I Radiographs of a 45-year-old man with ankylosing spondylitis and bilateral hip resurfacings with elevated metal ion levels and bilateral hip pain (A, B) and revision of the left hip to a cementless titanium double taper stem, retention of the acetabular component, and insertion of a dual mobility bearing (C).

- Double-modular neck implants—These stems, even if well fixed, should be revised to a titanium revision stem with a ceramic on cross-linked polyethylene bearing.
- Extras—Consider the need for a high-speed burr, cables or wires, acetabular component explant, curettes, pulse lavage, drains.

Surgical Approaches

- Anterolateral or posterolateral based on surgeon preference. In cases with significant ALTR affecting the abductors, the anterolateral approach is favored as it can facilitate an abductor repair and has a lower risk of postoperative instability.

Preoperative Planning

- Detailed history and physical examination—In particular, compressive signs and symptoms related to a pseudotumor abutting the femoral nerve or artery or retroperitoneal structures may merit vascular or general surgery preoperative consultations. Signs and symptoms of systemic metal toxicity should be sought, including mental alterations, thyroid, and cardiac dysfunction. Furthermore, history of instability and signs of abductor deficiency are important considerations for the reconstruction.

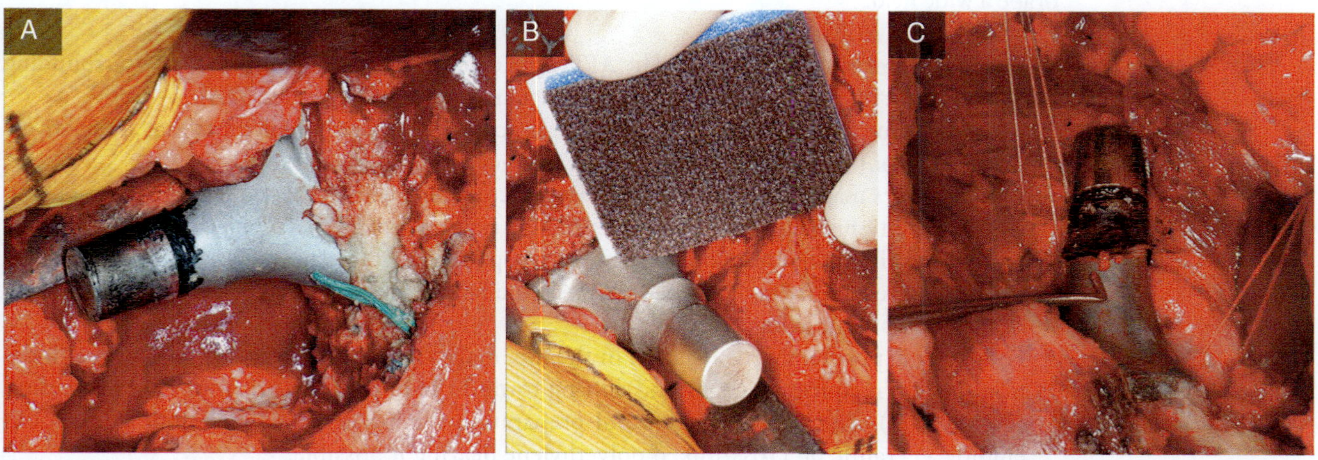

Figure 37.4 I Intraoperative photographs demonstrating trunnionosis of a titanium stem and cobalt chrome head that resulted in an ALTR (A), cleaning of the trunnion using a cautery scratch pad and retention of the stem (note that a scratch pad is no longer recommended and a clean damp sponge should be used), and comparison with another case of trunnionosis with a severely damaged stem and notching of the neck (C) (this stem cannot be retained).

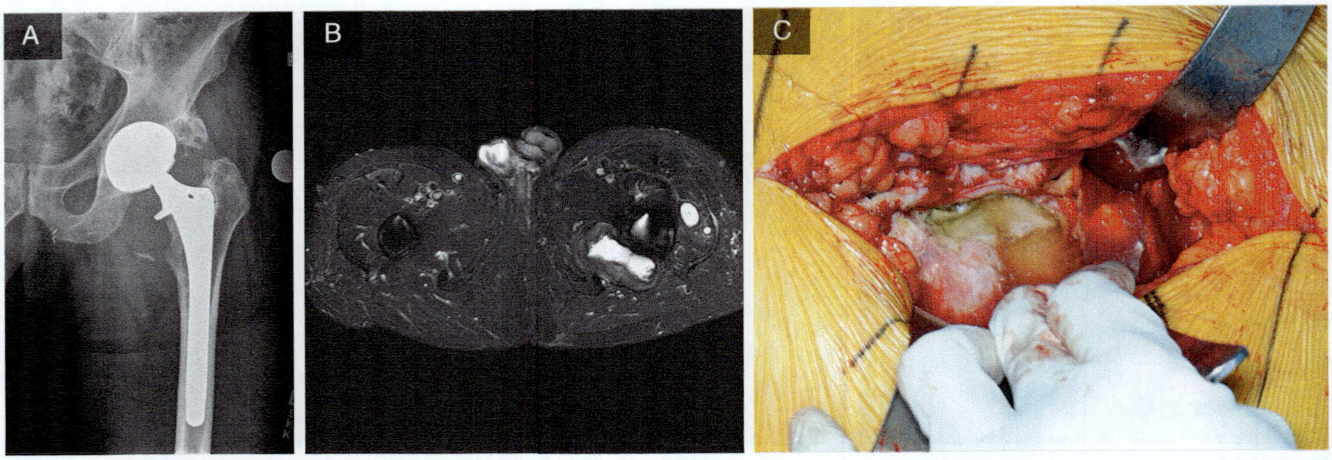

Figure 37.5 | Radiograph (A), MARS MRI axial image (B), and intraoperative photograph (C) of a pseudotumor from trunnionosis in a patient with a primary metal-on-polyethylene hip replacement with a CoCr stem and head.

- Obtain prior operative reports—Review what approach was used and specifics of the implanted components. For example, some dual-modular neck stems have specific removal tools that will greatly facilitate explantation. In cases in which the stem can be retained, availability of a ceramic head with titanium sleeve must be assessed preoperatively.
- Metal ion levels (Co, Cr, Ti)—Note the absolute levels, trend of levels over time, and ratio of Co to Cr (a high Co to Cr ratio suggests taper corrosion). Creatinine and kidney function should also be evaluated, as this may affect clearance of metal ions.
- Infection workup (C-reactive protein, erythrocyte sedimentation rate, and hip aspiration with manual differential)—Noting the high incidence of concomitant infections with ALTR and diagnostic challenge of differentiating these 2 entities.
- Radiographic evaluation and templating—To assess the position, stability, and presence of osteolysis around the existing components (Figure 37.5A). Careful templating of appropriate implants depending on the situation.
- Ultrasound or metal artifact reduction sequence MRI—To assess the presence, location, and extent of soft tissue damage resulting from the ALTR (Figure 37.5B and C). Cross-sectional images allow for assessment of the abductors for damage and fatty atrophy.

Bone, Implant, and Soft Tissue Techniques

- Place the patient in the lateral decubitus position with solid pelvic supports (ideally radiolucent) and drape a wide field.
- Debridement of ALTR:
  - Wide exposure of the area involved by ALTR and debulking of its capsule, fluid, and surrounding damaged soft tissues using electrocautery, rongeurs, and curettes (Figure 37.6).
  - Remove as much of the ALTR as possible. It is acceptable to leave small parts that are relatively inaccessible or that track to inaccessible areas inside the pelvis.
  - Pseudotumors may surround neurovascular structures and should therefore be approached with sufficient caution. Additional approaches and the assistance of a general or vascular surgeon may be required and should be anticipated in the preoperative assessment.
  - Intraoperative cultures and histopathology should be sent routinely.
- Revision of a hip resurfacing:
  - Following exposure and dislocation of the hip, make the femoral neck cut in the usual location using a reciprocating saw and cutting toward the implant's stem from either direction (Figure 37.7). The rest of the femoral preparation follows ordinary technique and should employ a ceramic on cross-linked polyethylene bearing if possible.
  - Retention of the acetabular component and insertion of a dual mobility liner:
    - Ensure that the shell is well fixed by exposing the bone-implant interface circumferentially, and apply axial force to the rim of the component using a round impactor to ensure no motion at the interface.

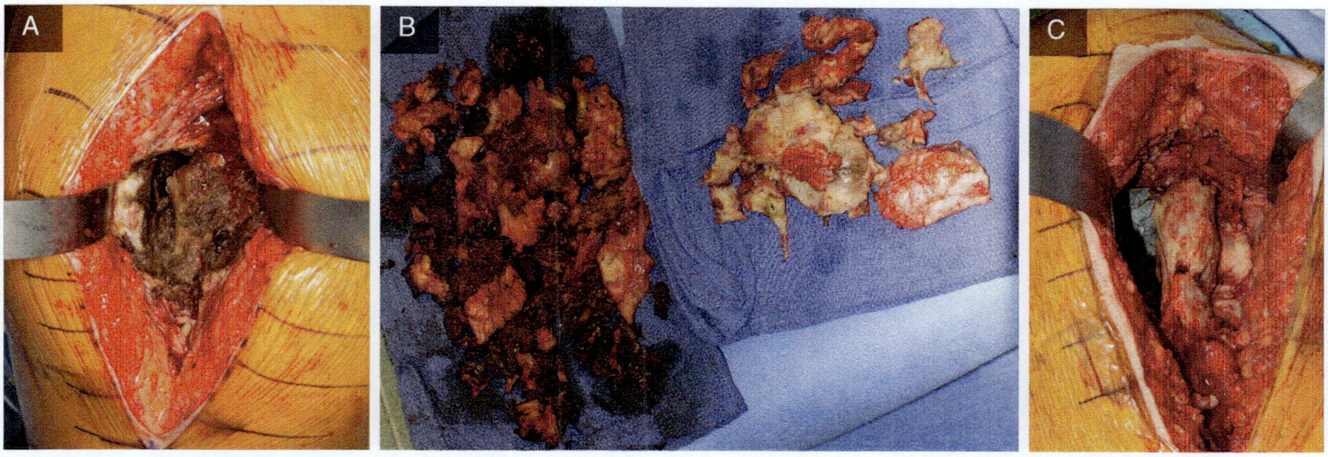

Figure 37.6 | Intraoperative photographs of an infected pseudotumor in a metal-on-metal hip replacement with significant involvement of the abductors (A), debulking of pseudotumour and necrotic periarticular soft tissues (B), and resulting soft tissue deficiency following debridement and placement of a static antibiotic spacer (C).

        - Retention of a 1-piece acetabular component is considered more often in well-positioned implants, able to accept a dual-mobility head, and has a good track record. It is especially advantageous in cases of small pelvic anatomy or medialized implants where bone stock may be very deficient after removal of the acetabular component.
    - Revision of the acetabular component
        - Remove the implant using the self-centering size-specific curved osteotomes.
        - Assess resulting bone deficiency and address with cancellous grafting or porous metal augments as needed.
        - Reconstruct using a revision acetabular component with multiple screws for secure fixation. Larger defects may require a cup-cage construct.
- Revision for head-neck taper corrosion:
    - Remove the femoral head and examine the trunnion for damage. Once metal debris is removed using a damp sponge, evaluate for notching or significant damage of the taper (Figure 37.8). If the trunnion is in acceptable condition, a ceramic head with a titanium sleeve adaptor may be used to replace the metal head. Note that occasionally a custom adaptor sleeve may be needed for this purpose and will have to be ordered ahead of time (Figure 37.9). On the other hand, irretrievably damaged stems will require revision with a non–Co-Cr stem according to the bone loss and surgeon's preference.

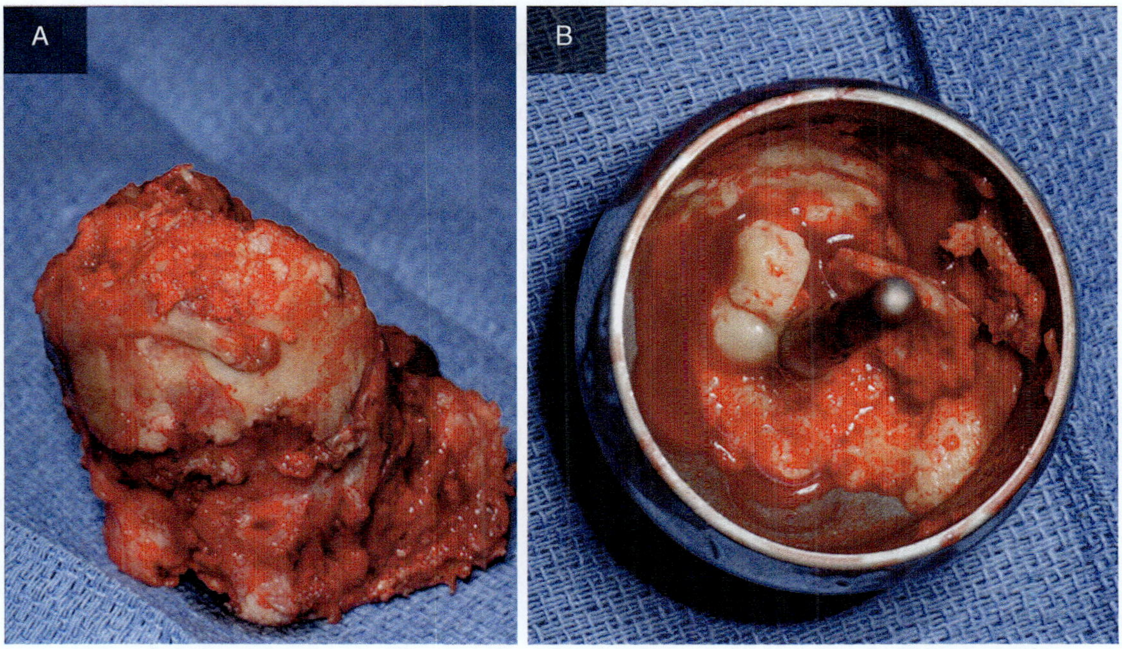

Figure 37.7 | Revision of a hip resurfacing by performing a standard neck cut using a reciprocating saw and photographs of the resected head (A) and femoral implant (B), which had debonded from the head after removal.

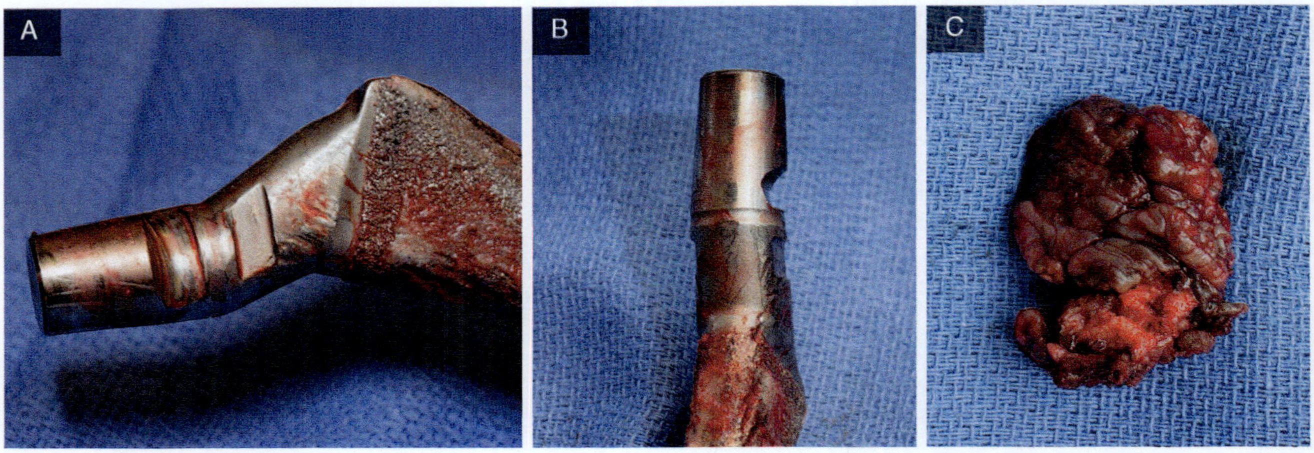

Figure 37.8 | Intraoperative photographs of a titanium stem with severe notching (A,B) and excised ALTR from Ti debris (C).

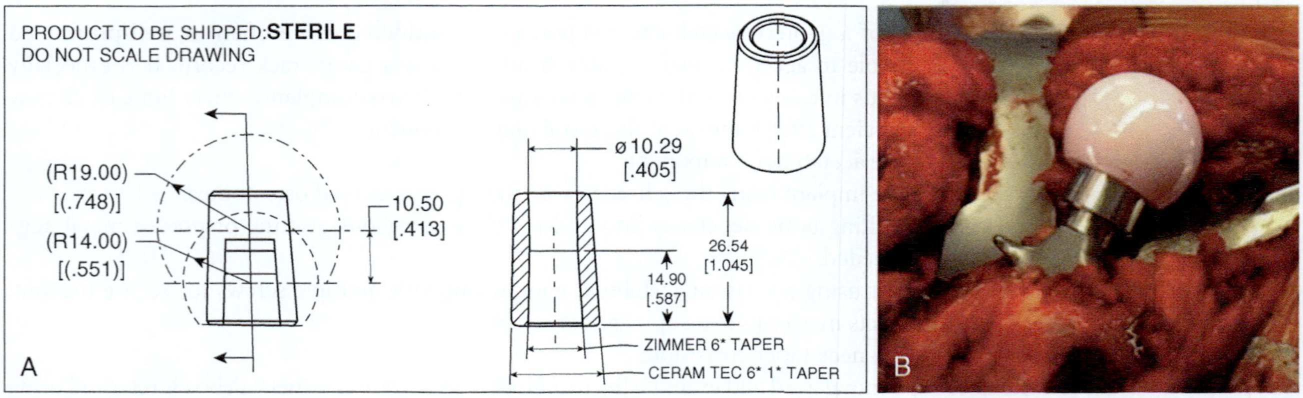

Figure 37.9 | Technical drawings (A) and intraoperative photo (B) of a custom sleeve adaptor for a well-fixed Harris-Galante stem following revision for taper corrosion.

- Revision for metallosis at other modular implant connections—This includes double-modular necks and modular stems. Generally, these components will require removal and should be replaced by a titanium revision stem with a ceramic head.
- Revision for an MoM total hip combines the principles outlined earlier to address the CoCr acetabular component and taper corrosion of the femoral component.
- Abductor damage—Following an extensive debridement of the pseudotumor, there may be significant soft tissue deficits involving the abductors (Figure 37.6C). Several options should be considered to reduce the risk of hip instability.
  - Abductor repair, re-enforcement with Achilles allograft technique, or gluteus maximus muscle transfer as described in Chapter 43 (Abductor Muscle Repair/Reconstruction).
  - Increase stability of the construct using a large-diameter femoral head, dual-mobility components, or a constrained liner (reserved as a last resort).

Postoperative Care

- Depending on the procedure performed, we typically restrict our patients to toe-touch weight bearing for 8 weeks. An abduction brace may be considered if the abductors were repaired/reconstructed or if stability is of concern.
- We routinely keep our patients on oral antibiotics until final culture results are negative at 14 days following surgery.

Chapter 38
Periprosthetic Femur Fracture

BRIAN P. CHALMERS
MATTHEW P. ABDEL

Key Concepts

- The key to fracture management is accurately determining if the femoral component is well-fixed or loose because most well-fixed implants are treated with internal fixation and most loose implants are treated with revision.
- Careful analysis of preinjury and injury radiographs to assess for femoral component fixation helps with accurate classification of the fracture.
- Open reduction and internal fixation (ORIF) of periprosthetic femoral fractures with stable femoral components (Vancouver B_1 and C fractures) should be performed using rigid constructs that include locking plates/screws and cables/wires.
- Revision total hip arthroplasty (THA) of periprosthetic fractures with loose femoral components (Vancouver B_2 and B_3) usually is accomplished with modular fluted tapered femoral stems bypassing the fracture and 2 to 3 cerclage wires proximally to wrap the remaining fracture fragments around the revision femoral component in a biologically friendly manner.
- The focus of this chapter will be on Vancouver B and C fractures.

Sterile Instruments and Implants

Instruments

ORIF

- Pointed reduction clamps
- Lobster claw reduction clamps
- Two ball spikes
- Intraoperative fluoroscopy or imaging
- Revision THA instrumentation available (not open) if conversion needed

Revision THA

- Routine revision hip retractors
- Sagittal and reciprocating saws
- Short and long pencil-tip burrs
- 6.5-mm round burr
- Multiple wide osteotomes
- Intraoperative fluoroscopy or imaging readily available

Implants

ORIF

- Variable-angle locking plates with a radius of curvature similar to that of the femur
- Locking and nonlocking screws

- Cerclage cables and/or Luque wires

Revision THA

- Uncemented modular fluted tapered stem and corresponding instrumentation
- Cerclage cables and/or Luque wires
- Consider femoral head and polyethylene liner exchange if the femoral head diameter can be increased to minimize the risk of instability—in these circumstances have available compatible polyethylene liners and modular femoral heads.

Positioning

ORIF

- We prefer a lateral decubitus position to access the entire femur on a flat radiolucent table with fluoroscopy access to the lower limb; this facilitates fracture reduction, stabilization, and imaging and allows ease of conversion to a revision THA if required intraoperatively.

Revision THA

- Lateral decubitus position to access the entire femur as necessary for fracture fixation and access for fluoroscopy.

Surgical Approaches

ORIF

- In noncomminuted fractures, rigid internal fixation and direct bone healing is the goal.
  - Therefore, a lateral exposure of the femur and direct visualization and reduction of the fracture is needed on a fracture table.
  - Take care not to strip the soft tissues and periosteum circumferentially.
  - A lateral exposure at the knee is required for insertion of the lateral distal femoral locking plate.
  - Screws and cables are placed proximally via a percutaneous approach.
- In comminuted fractures, the goal is to bridge and stabilize the fracture in appropriate alignment.
  - Therefore, indirect reduction techniques with minimal soft-tissue stripping and minimal exposure at the fracture site are ideal.
  - A lateral exposure at the knee is required for insertion of the lateral distal femoral locking plate.
  - Screws and cables are placed proximally via a percutaneous approach.

Revision THA

- In revision THAs, a lateral incision directly over the lateral proximal femur is required.
  - Oftentimes, an extended trochanteric osteotomy (ETO) or transfemoral osteotomy is used to minimize soft-tissue stripping of the proximal fracture fragments.

Preoperative Planning

- For both ORIF and revision THA, the most important factor in treating periprosthetic femur fractures is the stability and fixation of the femoral component. As such, a thorough history and radiographic evaluation are essential.

Careful Clinical History

- Timing of the injury with respect to the primary THA
  - Implants should be considered loose if the fracture occurs within 6 to 8 weeks of the index primary THA.
- Antecedent hip/thigh pain
  - If there is significant prior groin or thigh pain, procurement of preinjury radiographs to assess for subsidence, progressive radiolucent lines, and/or component migration is helpful.

Radiographic Evaluation

- Careful analysis of orthogonal injury radiographs (anteroposterior [AP] and lateral) to assess the location and nature of the fracture is essential.

- Evaluation of the stability of the implant is key. In particular, the surgeon should evaluate for:
  - Subsidence
  - Radiolucent lines around the implant
  - Change in implant positioning
  - Fractured cement mantle
- Comparison with preinjury radiographs is imperative if there is any uncertainty about implant stability.
- Computerized tomography (CT) scans are warranted in highly comminuted fractures, distal spiral femoral fractures where the distal extent of the fracture is not clear, and in situations in which the femoral component stability is in question.

Fracture Classification

- Fractures should be classified via the Vancouver classification given the fact that it guides treatment decisions:
  - Vancouver A_G (Figure 38.1A and B): A fracture of the greater trochanter
  - Vancouver A_L (Figure 38.2A and B): A fracture of the lesser trochanter
    - Uncommon fracture pattern, most often related to osteolysis from one source or another.
    - Consider a CT scan to assess for occult spiral fractures around the femoral component or oncologic lesions.
  - Vancouver B_1: Periprosthetic femur fracture near the stem tip of a well-fixed femoral component (Figure 38.3A and B)
  - Vancouver B_2: Periprosthetic femur fracture around a loose femoral component (Figure 38.4A and B)
  - Vancouver B_3: Periprosthetic femur fracture around a loose femoral component with significant bone loss or extremely poor bone quality (Figure 38.5A and B)
  - Vancouver C: Periprosthetic femur fracture far distal to a well-fixed femoral component (Figure 38.6A and B)
- In general, loose femoral components (Vancouver B_2 and B_3) are best treated with revision THA, whereas well-fixed femoral components (Vancouver B_1 and C) are best treated with ORIF.

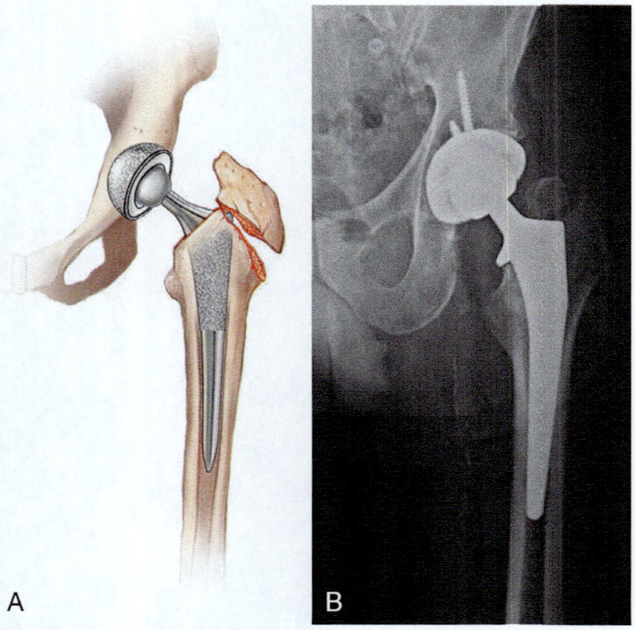

Figure 38.1 | Illustration (A) and AP radiograph (B) of a Vancouver A_G periprosthetic femur fracture. (Used with permission of Mayo Foundation for Medical Education and Research. All rights reserved.)

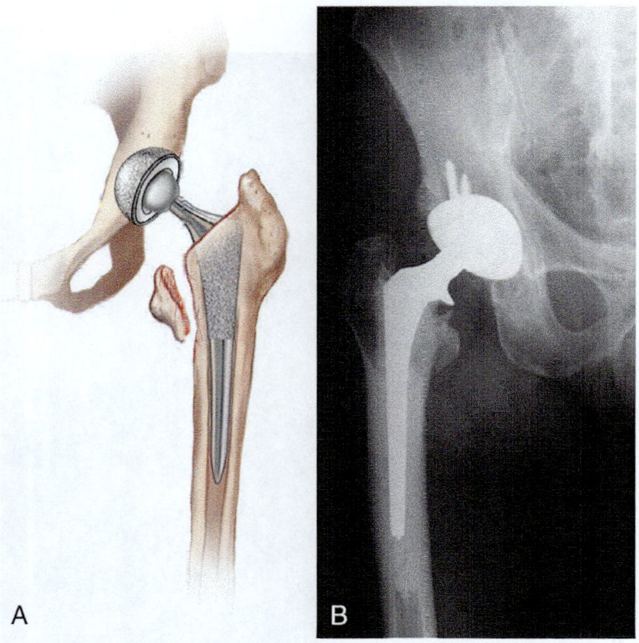

Figure 38.2 | Illustration (A) and AP radiograph (B) of a Vancouver A_L periprosthetic femur fracture. (Used with permission of Mayo Foundation for Medical Education and Research. All rights reserved.)

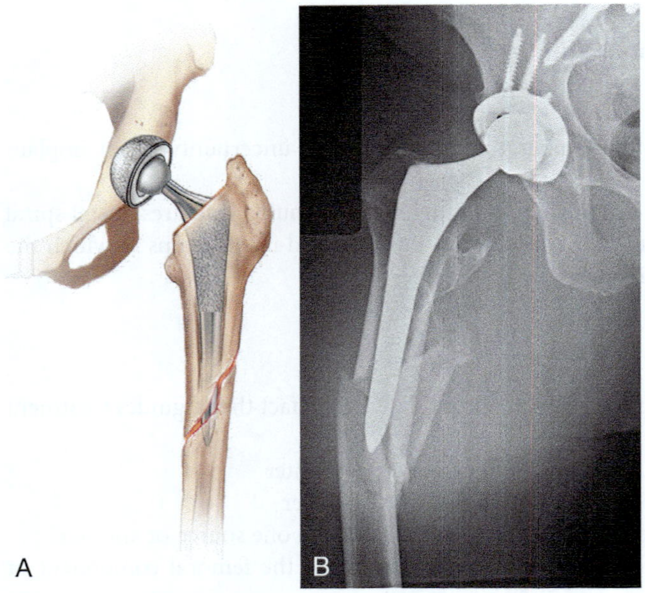

Figure 38.3 | Illustration (A) and AP radiograph (B) of a Vancouver B_1 periprosthetic femur fracture. (Used with permission of Mayo Foundation for Medical Education and Research. All rights reserved.)

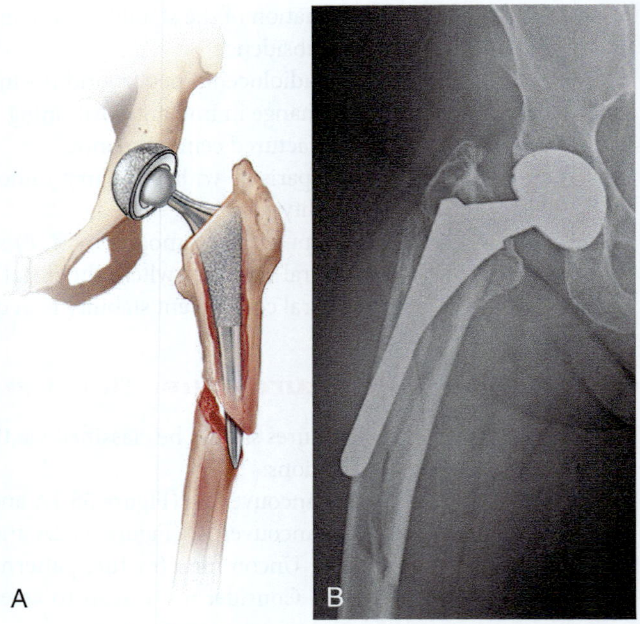

Figure 38.4 | Illustration (A) and AP radiograph (B) of a Vancouver B_2 periprosthetic femur fracture. (Used with permission of Mayo Foundation for Medical Education and Research. All rights reserved.)

Operative Planning and Templating

For both ORIF and revision THA, every effort should be made to obtain the operative report and implant records of the primary THA, with particular emphasis on prior surgical approach and in situ implants.

ORIF

- On full femoral radiographs, tentatively plan the approximate length of the desired plate to ensure the appropriate equipment and implants will be available.
- Note any femoral deformities (e.g., increased anterior bow, varus or vagus deformities) in case special implants need to be acquired.

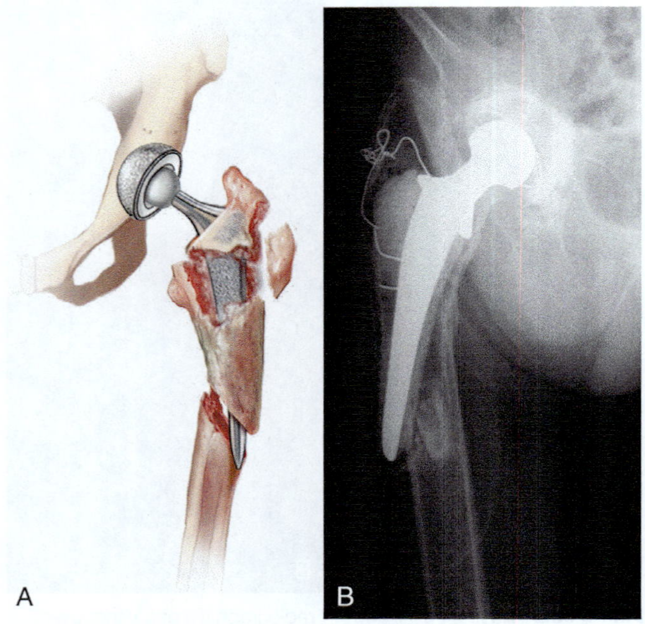

Figure 38.5 | Illustration (A) and AP radiograph (B) of a Vancouver B_3 periprosthetic femur fracture. (Used with permission of Mayo Foundation for Medical Education and Research. All rights reserved.)

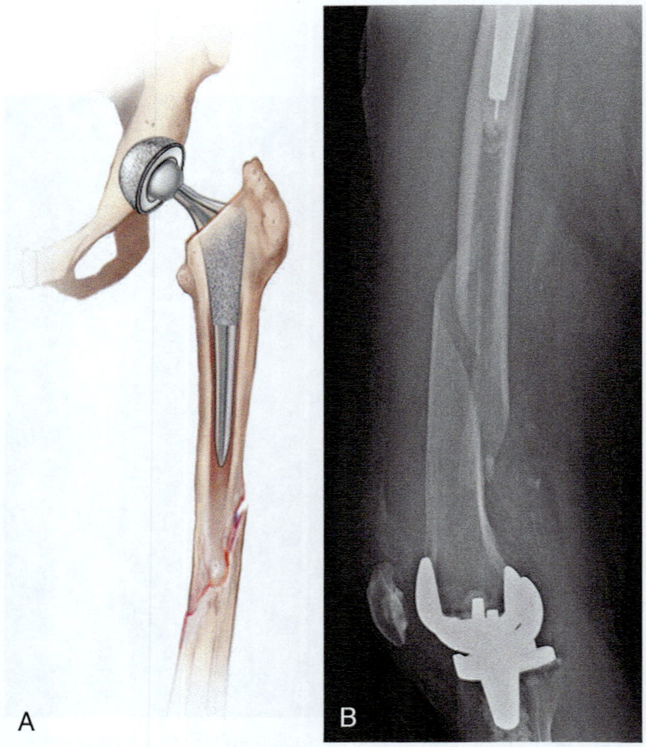

Figure 38.6 | Illustration (A) and AP radiograph (B) of a Vancouver C periprosthetic femur fracture. (Used with permission of Mayo Foundation for Medical Education and Research. All rights reserved.)

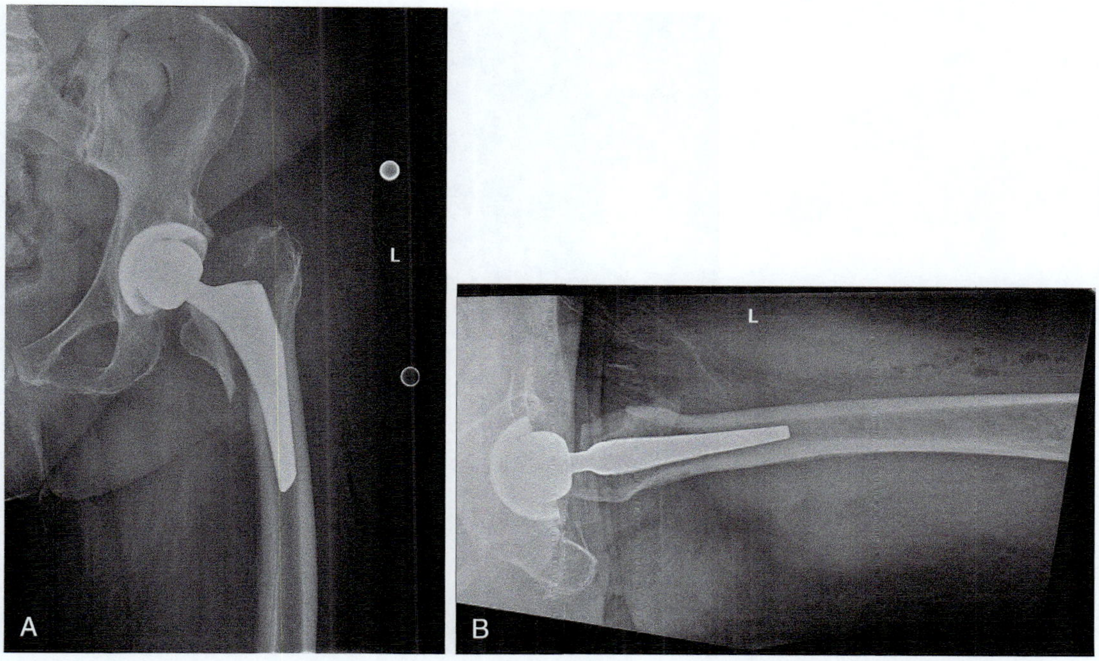

Figure 38.7 | Anteroposterior (A) and lateral (B) radiographs of a Vancouver B_2 periprosthetic femur fracture with a loose femoral component mandating a modular fluted tapered stem at the time of revision total hip arthroplasty in a 79-year-old woman.

Revision THA

- If planning for a modular fluted tapered stem (Figure 38.7A and B), templating should follow the recommendations enumerated in Section II-C, Chapter 6.
- Be prepared to change the initial treatment strategy based on intraoperative findings and revise the femoral and acetabular components if necessary (e.g., femoral component loose, intraoperative instability after revision THA).

Bone, Implant, and Soft Tissue Techniques

Open Reduction and Internal Fixation (Vancouver B_1 and C Fractures)

- For fractures around or distal to a well-fixed femoral stem (Figure 38.8A and B), the goal should be open reduction and internal fixation with direct exposure and reduction of the fracture.
- The fracture site is first accessed directly and provisionally reduced with pointed reduction clamps or lobster claw clamps.
- Provisional fixation can be completed with low-profile Luque wires to allow a lateral plate to be placed directly on top (Figure 38.9A and B).
- If the fracture is amenable, compression of the fracture fragments with lag screws (by technique rather than by design) should be performed.
- Exposure through a direct lateral approach to the distal femur is then performed to place the distal femoral locking plate up the femur in a retrograde fashion.
- Select a lateral distal femoral locking plate that appears to be of appropriate length, usually to the vastus ridge or top of the greater trochanter (Figure 38.10A and B).
- In a retrograde fashion, slide the distal femoral locking plate from the distal incision at the knee directly on bone to the proximal femur.
- Obtain AP and lateral fluoroscopic images proximally and distally to ensure that the plate is the appropriate length and positioned appropriately in the sagittal plane (Figure 38.10A).
- Once satisfied with the plate length and position, it should be secured with K-wires proximally and distally (Figure 38.11A and B).
- Place 2 to 3 distal screws through the plate to secure the plate to the bone distally.
- Then place at least 1 screw or cable proximally to secure the plate to the bone.

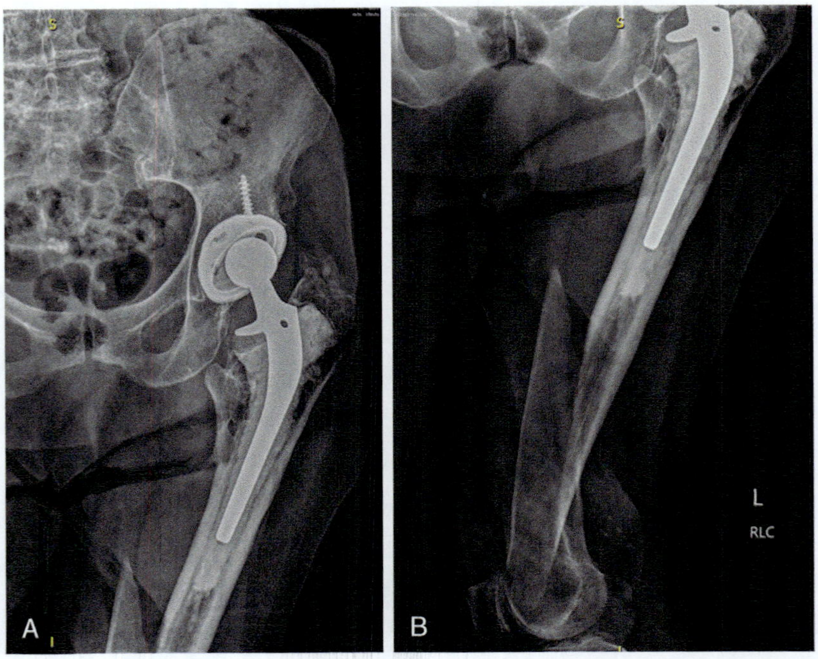

Figure 38.8 | Anteroposterior (A) and lateral (B) radiographs of a 95-year-old woman who sustained a Vancouver C distal spiral periprosthetic femur fracture below a well-fixed hybrid THA. (Images courtesy of Brandon J. Yuan, MD.)

- The first screws should be nonlocking cortical screws; never place a nonlocking cortical screw after placing a locking cortical screw.
- Thereafter, place the rest of the locking screws in the distal portion of the plate.
- The goal for proximal fixation is bicortical nonlocking screws. This is typically done with a small lateral incision more proximally and is achievable if the femoral component is small and there is adequate bone anterior or posterior to the implant. Bicortical fixation through a cement mantle will further enhance fixation (Figure 38.12A-C).
- With larger, uncemented femoral components, bicortical screw fixation is challenging. As such, one bicortical screw into the lesser trochanter and a combination of unicortical locking screws and cables can be used.

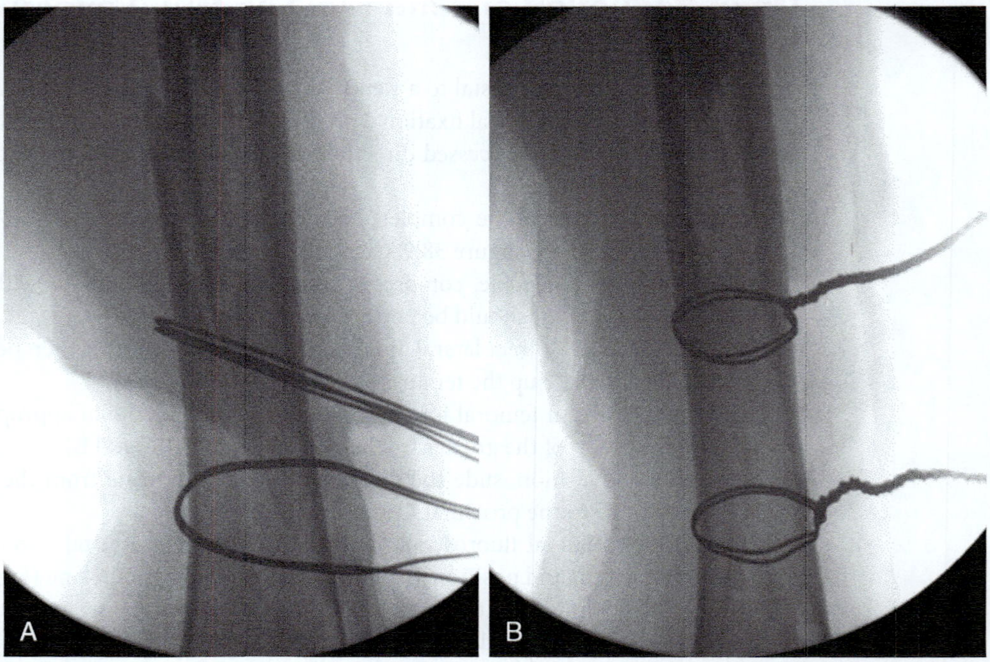

Figure 38.9 | Intraoperative fluoroscopic images (A, B) of the patient from Figure 38.8 with adequate exposure and provisional fixation of the oblique spiral fracture with Luque wires. (Images courtesy of Brandon J. Yuan, MD.)

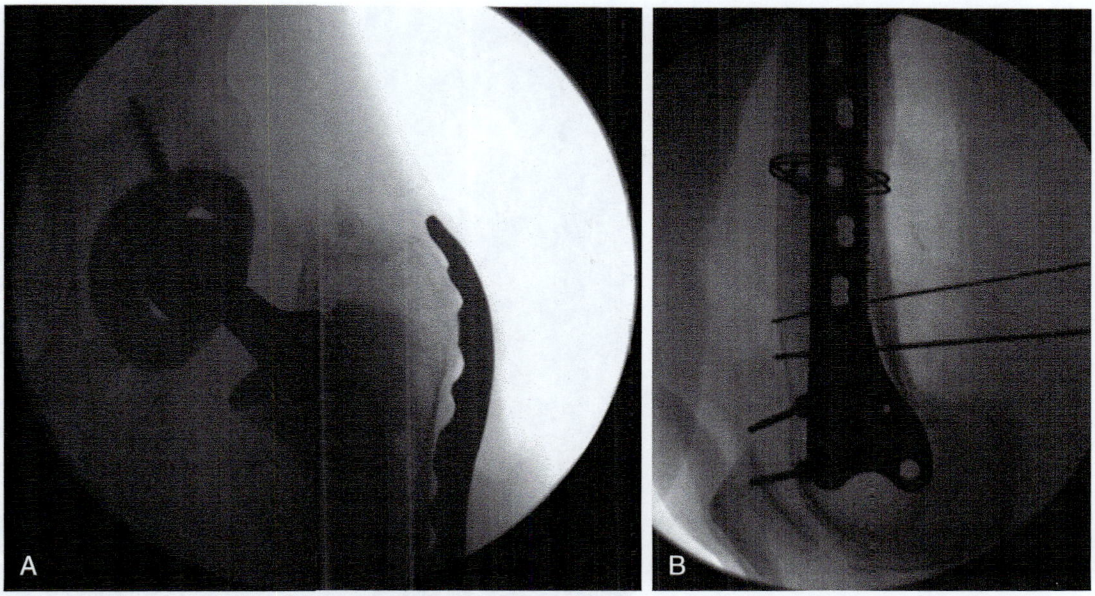

Figure 38.10 | Intraoperative fluoroscopic images depicting adequate plate length from the greater trochanter (A) to the lateral condyle (B) in the patient from Figure 38.8. (Images courtesy of Brandon J. Yuan, MD.)

- If direct reduction and compression of the fracture is obtained, the plate is acting as a neutralization construct. As such, place 2 to 3 nonlocking screws in the femoral shaft between the knee and the femoral component. Every screw hole does not need to be utilized (Figure 38.12A-C). These screws can often be placed through the exposure needed for fracture reduction. Otherwise, they should be placed percutaneously.
- If indirect reduction of a comminuted fracture is performed, the plate is acting as a bridge plate. As such, allowing some strain by spacing the locking screw fixation will induce secondary bone healing.

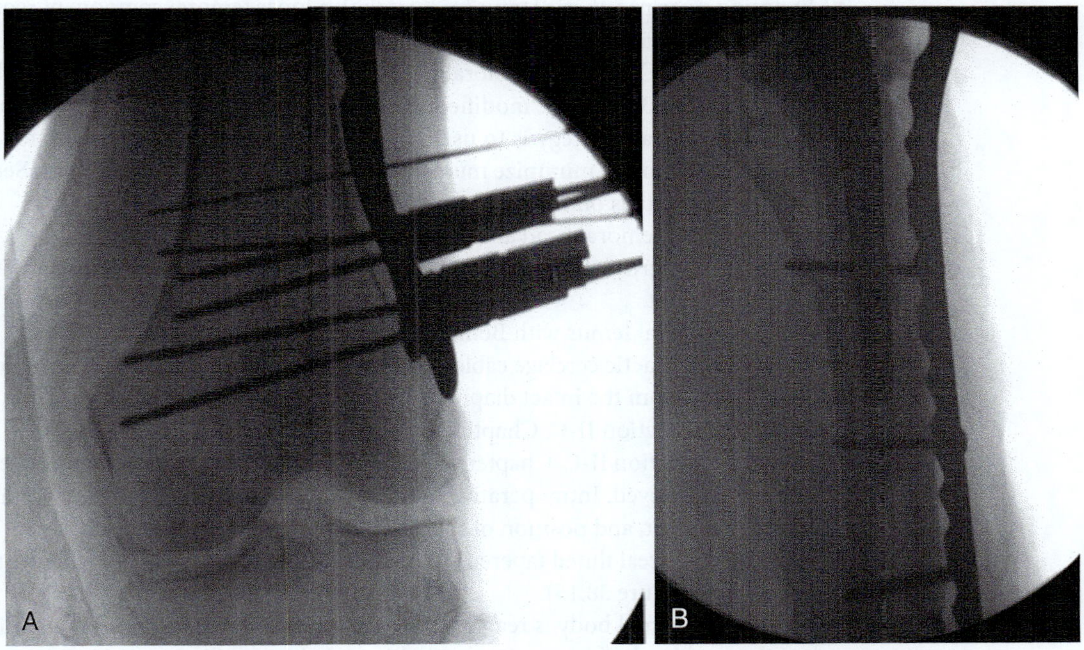

Figure 38.11 | Intraoperative fluoroscopic images revealing drilling and measurement of distal screws (A) and placement of multiple bicortical screws proximally (B) in the patient from Figure 38.8. (Images courtesy of Brandon J. Yuan, MD.)

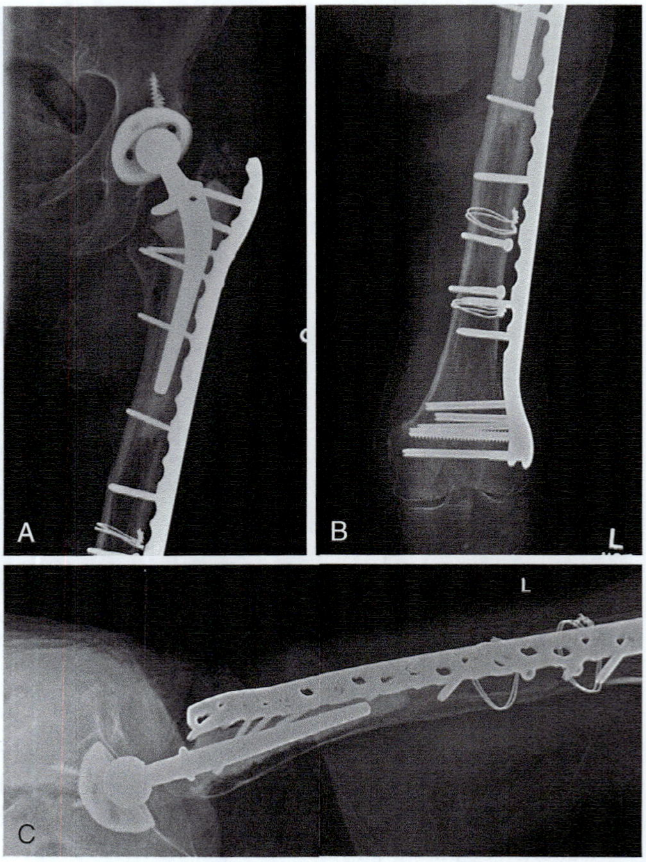

Figure 38.12 I Postoperative anteroposterior (A, B) and lateral (C) radiographs of the patient from Figure 38.8 revealing direct compression across a distal femoral spiral fracture with Luque wires and compression screws and proximal bicortical screw fixation around the cemented femoral component. (Images courtesy of Brandon J. Yuan, MD.)

Revision Total Hip Arthroplasty (Vancouver B_2/B_3)

- Exposing a periprosthetic femur fracture with a loose femoral component requires access not only to the fracture but also to the intramedullary femoral canal and acetabulum.
- A modified ETO or a transfemoral exposure through the fracture site typically is possible and very helpful (Figure 38.13). The modified ETO often involves splitting the proximal femur in mid coronal plane. The overall strategy is to use fracture lines or limited osteotomies for access to the joint and femoral canal and to minimize muscle stripping from any bone fragments. See Section II-B, Chapter 2 for further details on revision exposure.
- Disimpact the femoral head and remove the loose femoral component.
- Check the integrity of the polyethylene bearing surface and the fixation and position of the acetabular component.
- Expose the distal femur with Bennet retractors on each side.
- Place a prophylactic cerclage cable on the nonfractured, viable, diaphyseal bone (Figure 38.14).
- Sequentially ream the intact diaphysis with fluted tapered reamers until there is a supportive cone as described in Section II-C, Chapter 6.
- As noted in Section II-C, Chapter 6, the fluted tapered stem is trialed to ensure that axial and rotation stability is achieved. Intraoperative radiographs in orthogonal planes are obtained to ensure that the length, diameter, and position of the fluted tapered stem are optimal.
- Thereafter, the real fluted tapered stem is gently impacted while sequentially tightening the prophylactic cable (Figure 38.15).
- Next, the proximal body is reamed and trial modular proximal bodies are utilized to optimize limb length, combined offset, version, and ultimately hip stability.
- At this point, the hip is abducted and pointed reduction clamps and ball spike are used to reduce the osteotomy and fracture fragments.

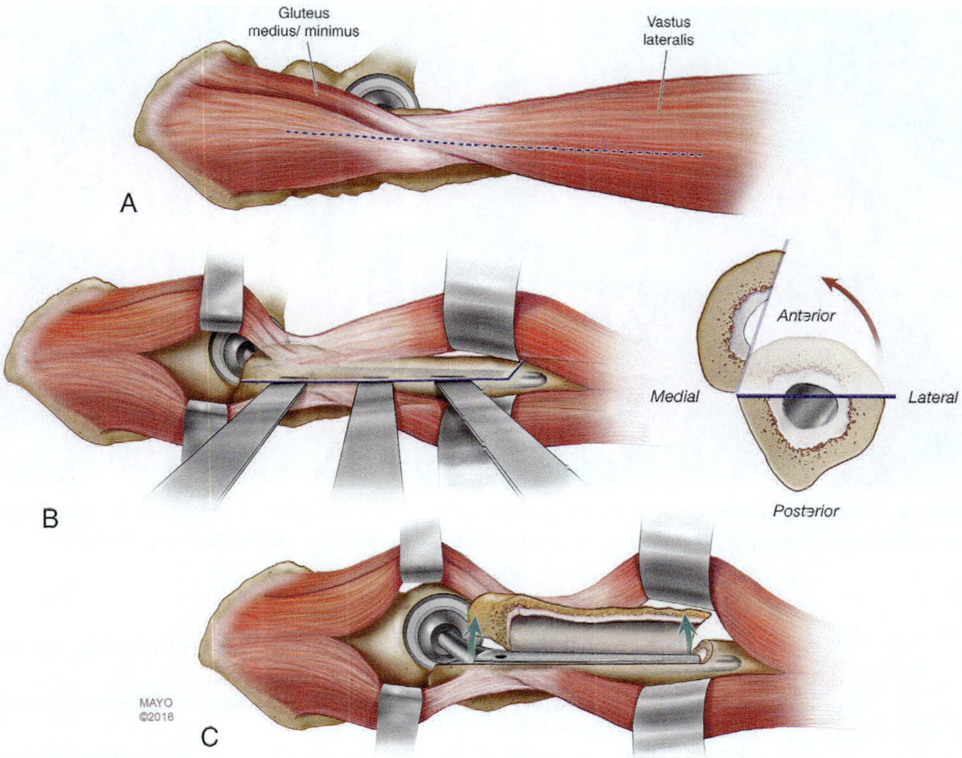

Figure 38.13 | Illustration depicting an anteriorly based extended trochanteric osteotomy to exposure the femur. The soft tissues are first separated along the lateral axis of the femur to access the bone (A). The lateral cortex of the femur is split with a saw and burr and the medial cortex is perforated in order to create a stress riser; wide osteotomes are then utilized to gently elevate and complete the osteotomy (B). The anterior portion of the proximal femur can then be elevated as a sleeve to access the femoral component (C). (Used with permission of Mayo Foundation for Medical Education and Research. All rights reserved.)

- Finally, 2 to 3 cerclage cables or wires are placed in a biologically friendly manner around the proximal osteotomy and fracture fragments around the proximal aspect of the stem (Figure 38.16A).
- Occasionally a burr will be needed to remove sclerotic bone from the inner surface of the trochanter and remaining osteotomy fragment to ensure enclosure around the proximal aspect of the stem (Figure 38.16B).

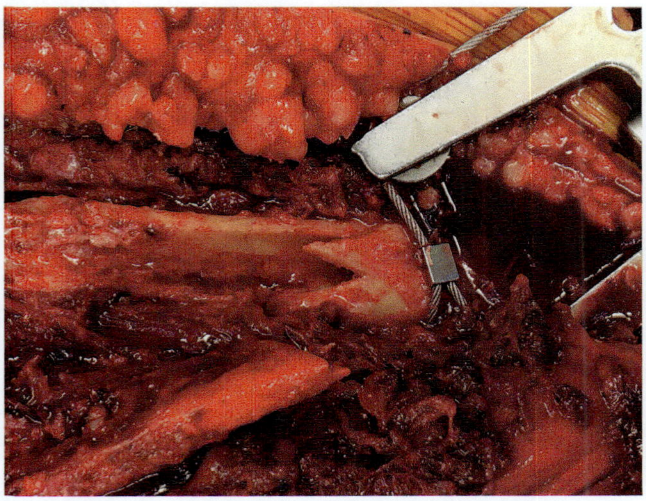

Figure 38.14 | Intraoperative photograph of a prophylactic cerclage cable placed distal to the distal extent of a Vancouver B_3 periprosthetic femur fracture in a 69-year-old woman.

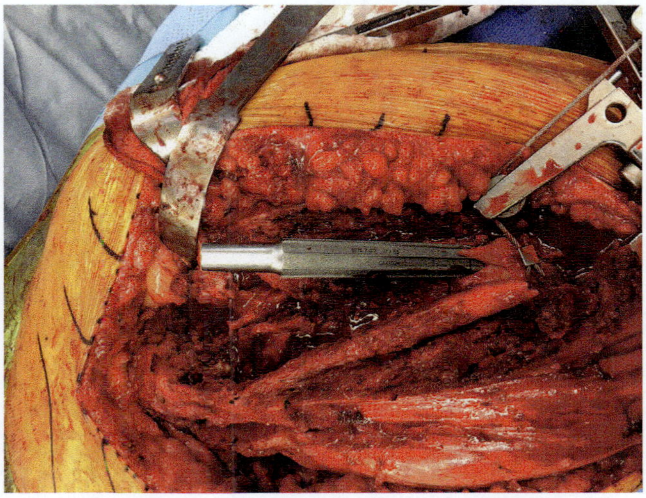

Figure 38.15 | Intraoperative photographs of the real fluted tapered portion of the stem impacted until axial and rotation stability was achieved in the patient from Figure 38.14.

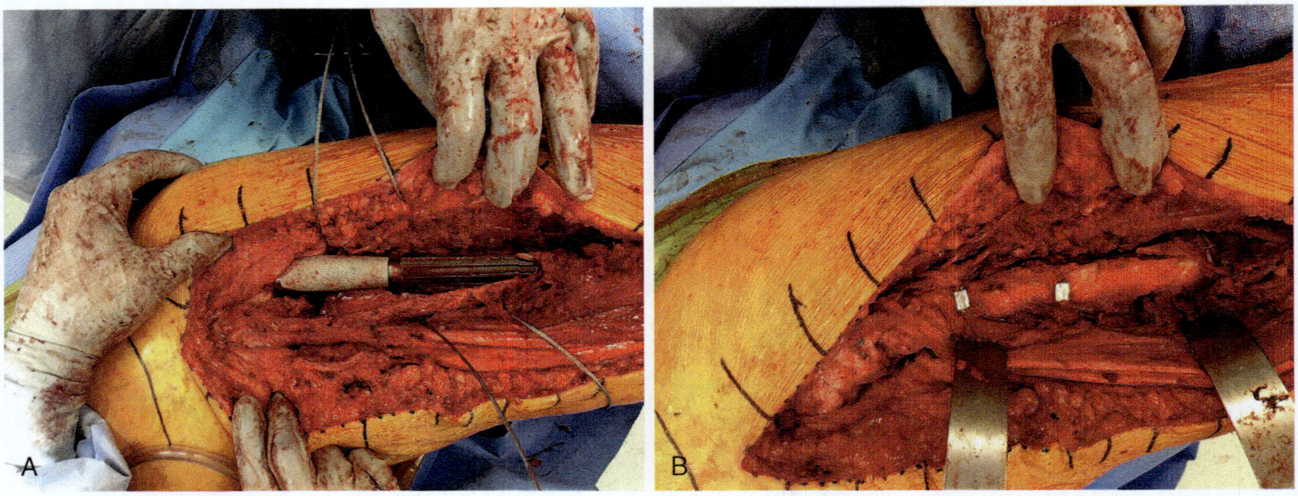

Figure 38.16 | Intraoperative photographs of the patient from Figure 38.14 with 2 cerclage cables placed in a biologically friendly manner to minimize soft-tissue stripping (A) and also adequate to close the osteotomy and fracture fragments (B).

Suggested Readings

1. Abdel MP, Cottino U, Larson DR, Hanssen AD, Lewallen DG, Berry DJ. Modular fluted tapered stems in aseptic revision total hip arthroplasty. *J Bone Joint Surg Am*. 2017;99(10):873-881.
2. Abdel MP, Lewallen DG, Berry DJ. Periprosthetic femur fractures treated with modular fluted, tapered stems. *Clin Orthop Relat Res*. 2014;472(2):599-603.
3. Abdel MP, Watts CD, Houdek MT, Lewallen DG, Berry DJ. Epidemiology of periprosthetic fracture of the femur in 32 644 primary total hip arthroplasties: a 40-year experience. *Bone Joint Lett J*. 2016;98-B(4):461-467.

Chapter 39
Hip Instability

BRIAN P. CHALMERS
ROBERT T. TROUSDALE

Key Concepts

- Careful patient evaluation is important to identify clinical and physical risk factors that place a patient at risk for instability. These include lumbar spine pathology, abductor mechanism dysfunction, underlying neuromuscular disorders, and cognitive disorders.
- Careful radiographic evaluation of the lumbar spine, implants, component fixation, component position, hip offset, and hip length is paramount.
- Address instability in revision total hip arthroplasty in a step-wise fashion:
  - Fixed bearing.
    - Address component malposition, soft tissue and bony impingement.
    - Restore soft tissue tension with hip length and offset.
    - Utilizing a large-diameter fixed-bearing femoral head increases jump distance and range of motion free of impingement, thereby increasing hip stability.
  - Dual mobility construct.
    - Increases the effective femoral head diameter and the arc of motion before prosthetic impingement and may be preferred in high-risk patients.
  - Constrained liners.
    - Reserved for severe abductor and soft tissue insufficiency and/or failure of the above-mentioned approaches.

Sterile Instruments and Implants

- Basic hip retractors and instrumentation.
- Acetabular explant system.
- Acetabular component position tester.
- Implant-specific femoral heads and modular polyethylene liners, including lateralized, lipped, and face-changing liners.
- Revision uncemented acetabular components of choice (with instrumentation), including large-diameter femoral head articulations.
- Revision uncemented femoral component of choice.
- Dual mobility construct of choice (with instrumentation).
- Constrained liner of choice (with instrumentation).

Surgical Approaches

- Positioning—lateral decubitus position.
- Both the posterior and anterolateral approaches may be used as they may be made extensile, allowing for wide exposure, if needed. as it is reproducible and extensile.
- The direct anterior approach, in expert hands, is useful for a minority of revision hip arthroplasties, but extensile exposure is more difficult.
- The senior author reserves the anterolateral approach in those with severe abductor damage seen at the time of exposure.

Preoperative Planning

Analysis of Patient Clinical Risk Factors

- Analyze patient demographics—elderly patients and women are more prone to dislocation (Figure 39.1).
- Consider comorbid conditions:
  - Neurologic conditions, e.g., Parkinson disease, Charcot arthropathy, cerebral palsy, post poliomyelitis.
  - Lumbar spine fusion/stiffness, especially extending to the pelvis.
- Recognize the indication for primary total hip arthroplasty—posttraumatic (e.g., prior femoral neck fracture) and avascular necrosis have higher risk for postoperative dislocation.

Analysis of Physical Examination Risk Factors

- Abductor strength/abductor lurch.
- Limb length, both actual and perceived, discrepancy.
- Stiffness of the lumbar spine.

Radiographic Evaluation—Compare Preoperative and Current Radiographs

- Polyethylene wear/osteolysis.
- Component fixation.
- Acetabular component position (Figure 39.1).
  - Ideal acetabular inclination = 40° (Figure 39.2).
  - Ideal acetabular anteversion = 15° to 20° (Figure 39.2).
    - Should be analyzed on a true/direct lateral radiograph of the hip.
- Cup position may vary based on lumbar disease.
- Hip length and offset (Figure 39.3).

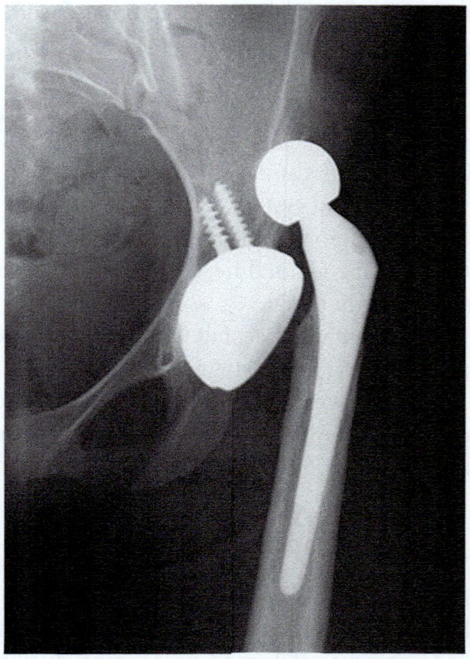

Figure 39.1 | A patient with a posterior-superior total hip dislocation with an overly abducted acetabular component.

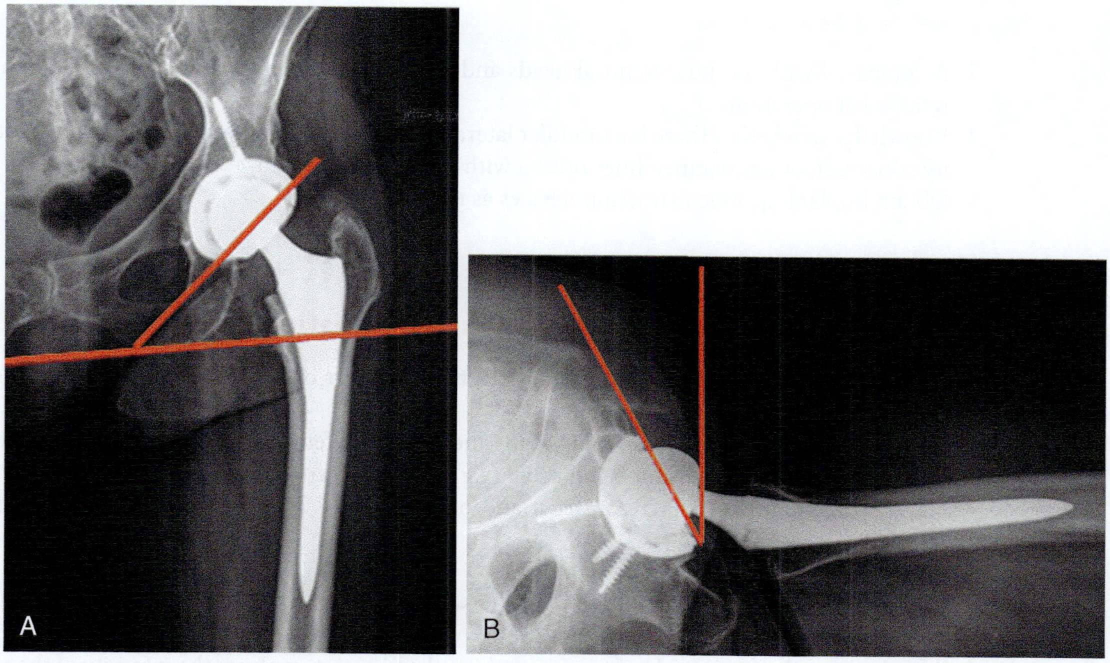

Figure 39.2 | Radiographs showing important measurements to assess component position and restoration of hip offset and length. The ideal acetabular inclination is 40° (A). The ideal acetabular anteversion is 15° to 20° (B).

Prior Operative Reports

Prior Surgical Approach

- Guides surgical planning and better understanding of instability mechanism, along with knowledge of the *direction* of recurrent dislocations.
  - For example, if a primary total hip arthroplasty was done via a posterior approach but is dislocating anteriorly, close evaluation of acetabular and femoral anteversion should be completed.

Type of Articulation

- Metal-on-metal articulations or concern for taper corrosion should prompt evaluation of metal ion levels and evaluation of the abductor mechanism (by physical examination and magnetic resonance imaging with neutral artifact reduction sequences).

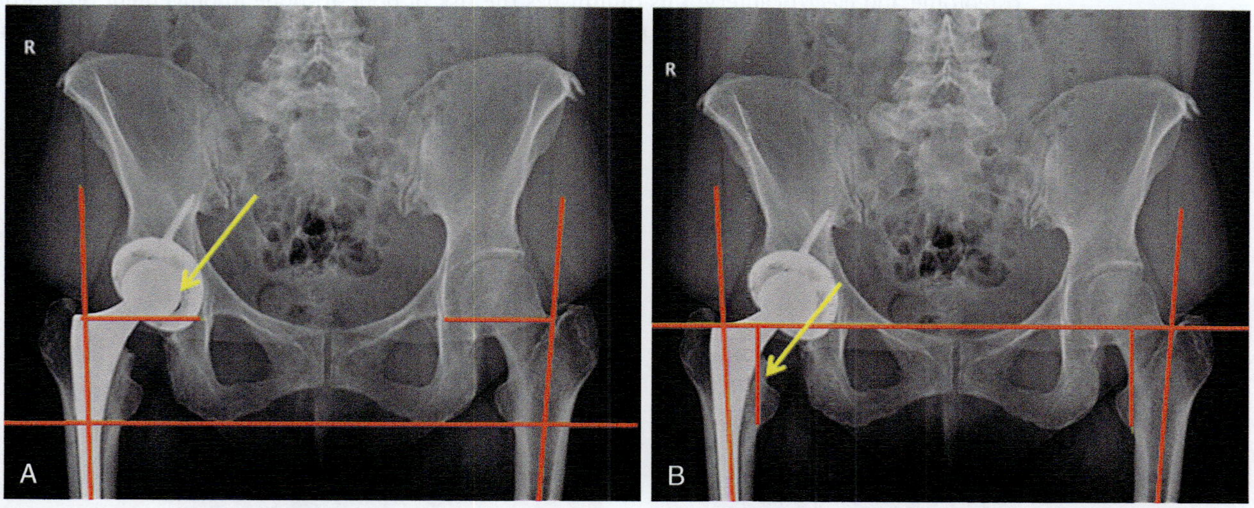

Figure 39.3 | Restoration of both hip offset (arrow, A) and hip length (arrow, B) compared with preoperative radiographs and the contralateral hip is also important to assess.

Implant Records

- Be prepared with modular femoral heads and polyethylene liners that match implants that may be retained at operation.
- Knowledge of whether there is a modular lateralized or face-changing polyethylene liner, dual mobility construct, or constrained liner option with the implant system.
- Obtain implant-specific extraction devices as needed.

Surgical Preparation

Be Prepared With Surgical Multiple Options

- Obtain the modular femoral heads and polyethylene liners of current implants if plan to obtain the original components.
- Template a revision acetabular component and a revision femoral component and have them available before surgery if revision is indicated (e.g., loosening, component malposition,).
- Have available dual mobility construct and/or constrained liner of choice if additional stability is needed.

Bone, Implant, and Soft Tissue Techniques

- After incising the fascia and before approaching the hip joint, evaluate the integrity of the soft tissues.
  - Note any posterior capsular deficiency (especially if a prior posterior approach was utilized) (Figure 39.4).
  - Note the integrity and quality of the abductor mechanism (especially if a prior lateral or anterolateral approach was utilized) (Figure 39.5).
- Dislocate the hip anteriorly or posteriorly depending on the surgical approach utilized with a bone hook.
- Remove the femoral head with a square tip impactor (do not impact directly on the trunnion) (Figure 39.6).
- Test the stability/fixation of the femoral component manually.
- Evaluate the femoral component position.
  - Ideally there should be approximately 15° of femoral anteversion (for a combined anteversion of 30° to 40° with the acetabular component).
  - Expose the acetabular component circumferentially with retractors per surgeon's routine; Hohmann retractors or bent Hohmann retractors are the senior authors' preferred retractors (Figure 39.7).
- Remove any osteophytes and/or bone that is prominent to the acetabular component with a curved osteotome and electrocautery; this diminishes the risk of bone-to-bone impingement on a prominent acetabular rim or osteophytes that may push the femoral head out of the acetabular component (Figure 39.8).

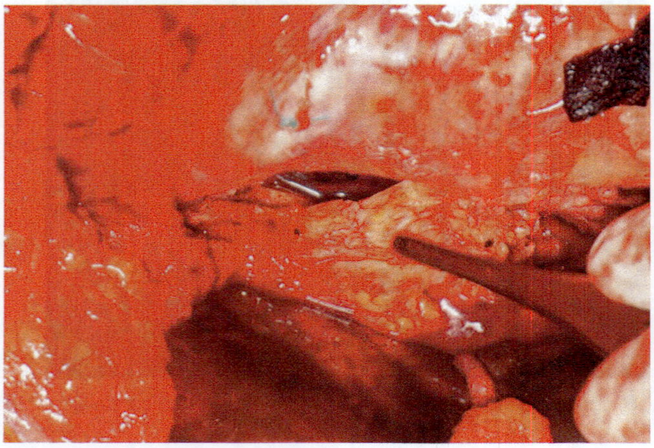

Figure 39.4 | Photograph of posterior capsular deficiency encountered on revision total hip arthroplasty from a prior posterior approach.

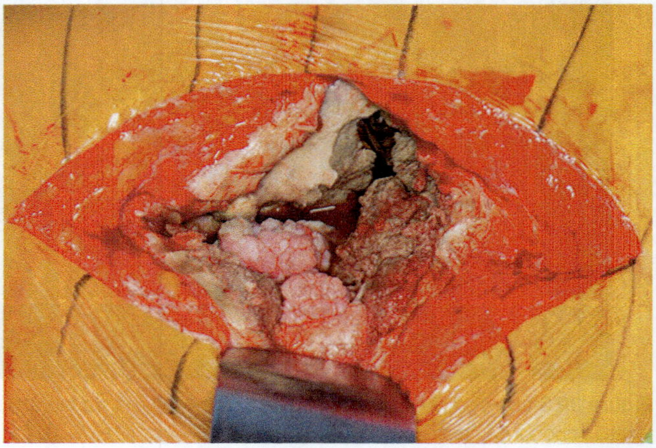

Figure 39.5 | Photograph of a severely deficiency abductor mechanism.

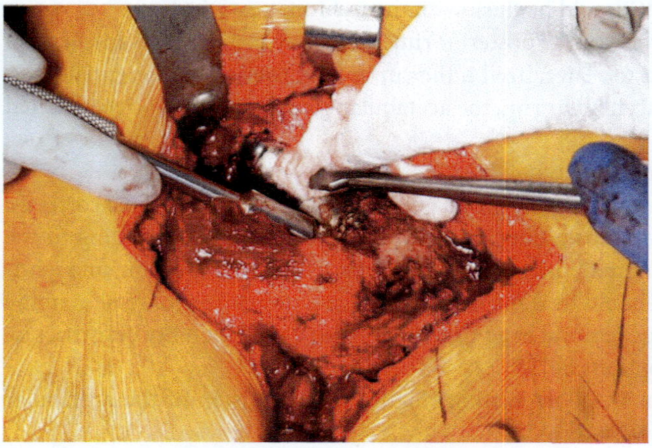

Figure 39.6 | A total hip dislocated and the femoral head disimpacted from the trunnion with a square tip impactor and a sponge protecting the trunnion integrity.

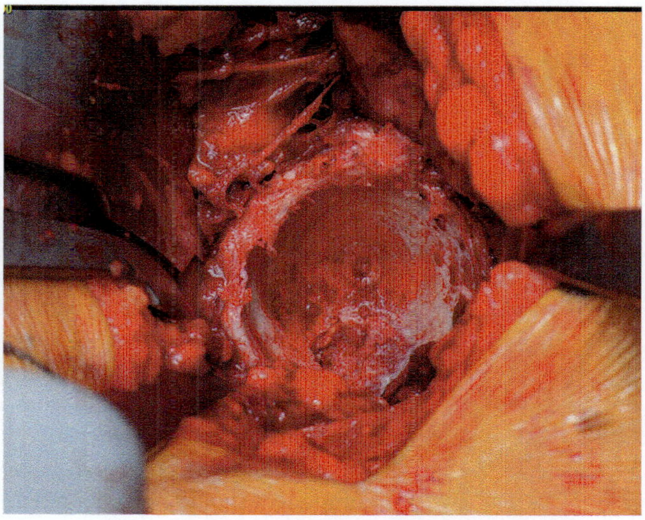

Figure 39.7 | Photograph of circumferential acetabular exposure with Hohmann retractors to properly evaluate the position and fixation of the acetabulum and/or acetabular component.

- Remove the polyethylene liner from the acetabular component; many acetabular components have a company-specific removal device; however, stacked osteotomes at the interface of the cup and polyethylene liner or placement of a 4.5-mm screw (from the acetabular screw set) into the cup are also proven techniques for removing polyethylene liners; if these fail, reaming the polyethylene liner is a last option.
- Remove the screws (if any) from the acetabular component.
- Test the stability of the acetabular component manually with the implant-specific insertion/extraction device if available. Alternatively, place a square-tip impactor on the rim and lightly tap it, looking for micromotion. With a small instrument, inspect the circumferential interface of the acetabular component to assess for bony ingrowth.

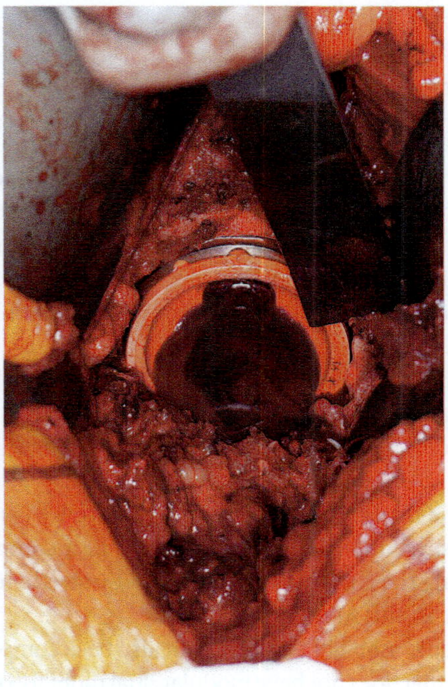

Figure 39.8 | Photograph of the technique of removing osteophytes around the acetabular component with a curved osteotome.

- Evaluate the position of the acetabular component; our preferred technique is to utilize a suction cup holder with a trial acetabular insert, anatomic landmarks, and preoperative radiographs.
  - In general, the acetabular component should be flush with the ischium posteriorly.
    - If the acetabular component is proud of the posterior rim, there may be too much anteversion (or the acetabular component was too lateralized if the cup is too proud circumferentially).
    - If there is a prominent posterior acetabular rim, the acetabular component may be retroverted or underanteverted.
  - The goal acetabular inclination should be about 40°.
    - The acetabular component typically sits slightly proud of the superior rim if positioned correctly.

Note: The key principle in addressing hip instability is to solve the problem that is leading to the recurrent instability; issues with component malposition, bony and soft tissue impingement, and inadequate restoration of leg length and offset should be done first. We utilize a step-wise progression in the articulation to increase stability from a large femoral head fixed bearing to a dual mobility construct to, rarely, a constrained liner when all other options fail.

- If the acetabular component is loose or in poor position (Figure 39.9), revision of the acetabular component should be undertaken.
  - Remove the acetabular component with minimal bone loss with an acetabular explant system; starting with the smaller blade, pass the blade circumferentially around the acetabular component right along the cup; retractors may need to be removed or shifted positions to release 360°; once completed, move onto the larger blade and repeat the process, making sure the blade buries as deeply as possible; the acetabular component often becomes loose and remains attached to the explant system once all bone ingrowth is detached.
  - Clean the acetabulum and assess remaining bone stock.
  - Sequentially ream with larger reamers until excellent rim fit is achieved; we prefer to utilize a revision acetabular component.
  - Impact the real acetabular component into place, taking care to place it in proper abduction and anteversion.
  - We routinely place multiple acetabular screws through the acetabular component to ensure adequate fixation in the revision setting.
- If the acetabular component is well fixed and in good position, trial of lateralized or face-changing acetabular liners and modular femoral heads to increase hip offset and length should be attempted to improve hip stability (Figure 39.10).
- Increased femoral head diameter also augments hip stability (Figure 39.10).

Note: Although an isolated head/liner exchange is possible, it is infrequent that it will solve recurrent instability issues except in the simplest of cases; we avoid the temptation to use simple modular femoral head/polyethylene liner exchange in more complex patients status post multiple revision total hip arthroplasties.

Dual Mobility Constructs

- Dual mobility constructs allow for a larger effective femoral head diameter, increase the prosthetic jump distance, and allow for a greater arc of motion before prosthetic impingement.
- Dual mobility constructs are our preferred approach to addressing hip instability in many high-risk patients, including patients with conversion total hip arthroplasty from a hemiarthroplasty (Figure 39.11), patients with extensive lumbar spine fusions (Figure 39.12), patients with neuromuscular conditions, and in selected patients undergoing complex acetabular reconstructions in which constraint should be avoided.
- Dual mobility constructs can be placed either at the time of acetabular revision (if the component is loose or malpositioned) or during modular exchange into a compatible acetabular component, or a dual mobility compatible liner designed for cement may be cemented into a well-fixed, well-positioned acetabular component.
- Revision acetabular component with a dual mobility construct (Figure 39.11): we recommend revision acetabular component per the surgeon's routine with the use of a component that has a dual mobility option; we suggest assembling the femoral head and larger polyethylene articulation on the back table as it is difficult to assemble in situ in most systems.
- Cementation of a cement-compatible dual mobility construct can also be accomplished into a well-fixed, well-positioned acetabular component that does not have modular dual mobility options (Figure 39.13A).

- After confirmation of ideal component position and stability, trial the dual mobility component, utilizing one that is 2 to 4 mm smaller than the inner diameter of the revision acetabular component to allow for a cement mantle.
    - Open the real dual mobility acetabular cup; we prefer a component with a porous or roughened surface that will interdigitate with cement better than a polished surface (Figure 39.13B).

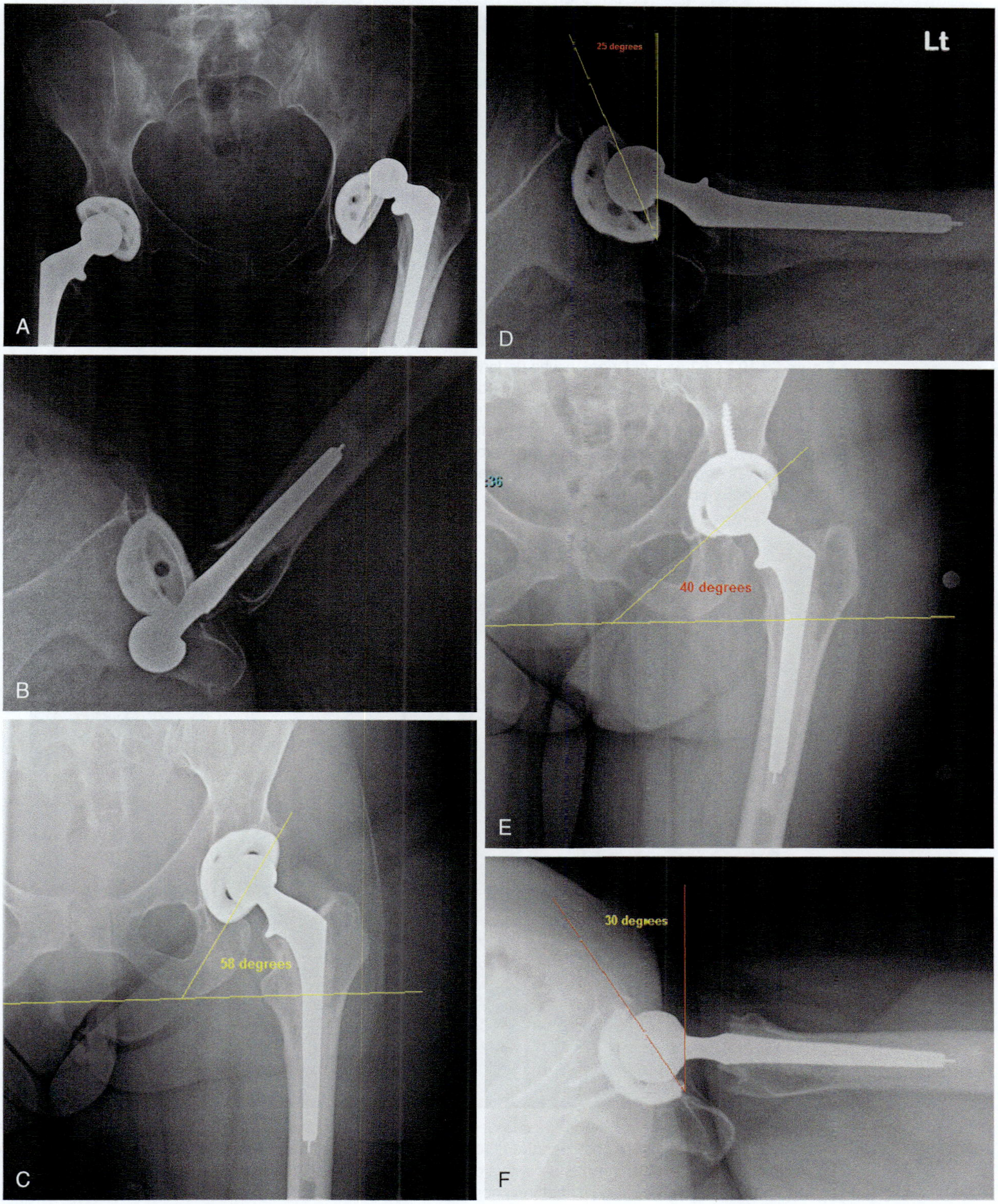

Figure 39.9. | A 62-year-old woman who underwent a bilateral total hip arthroplasty 12 years ago via posterior approaches was referred to us for recurrent posterior-superior prosthetic dislocations (A and B). Her left acetabular component had increased acetabular inclination at nearly 60° (C). She underwent an acetabular component revision to a more ideal acetabular component position (E and F) and an upsizing of the femoral head to 36 mm. She remained stable without recurrent dislocation at 3 years' follow-up.

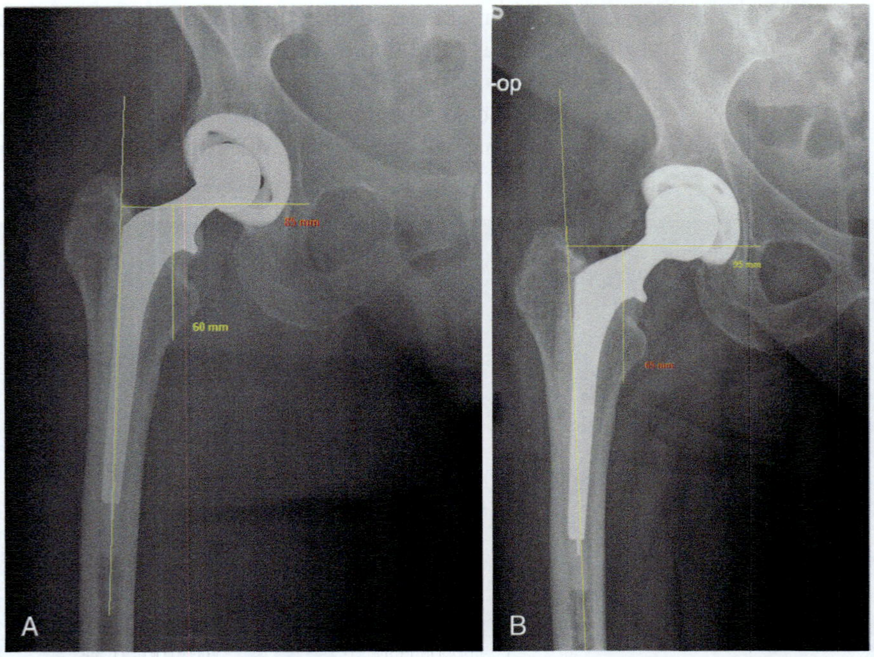

Figure 39.10 | A 62-year-old woman who underwent a bilateral total hip arthroplasty 12 years ago via posterior approaches for acetabular dysplasia was referred to us for recurrent hip dislocations. Her right acetabular component was in good position. She underwent a revision right total hip arthroplasty with implantation of a 4-mm lateralized, 10° face-changing liner with the build-up placed posterosuperior and a modular femoral head exchange to increase her length and offset. Overall, offset and length were increased 10 and 5 mm, respectively (A and B), from preoperatively. She was also upsized to a 36-mm fixed-bearing femoral head. She remained stable without recurrent dislocation at 3 years' follow-up.

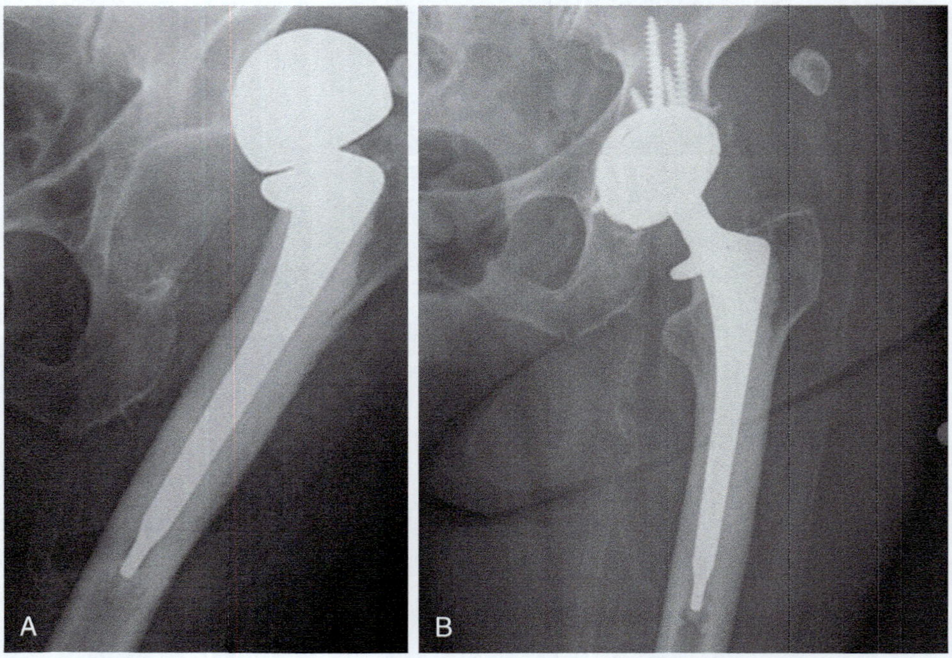

Figure 39.11 | An 86-year-old woman who underwent a cemented hemiarthroplasty for an intracapsular femoral neck fracture experienced recurrent postoperative dislocation (A) and was referred to us for management. She underwent implantation of an acetabular component with a dual mobility construct (B) given her prior dislocations and multiple risk factors for recurrent instability (prior fracture, prior large femoral head, elderly, and female).

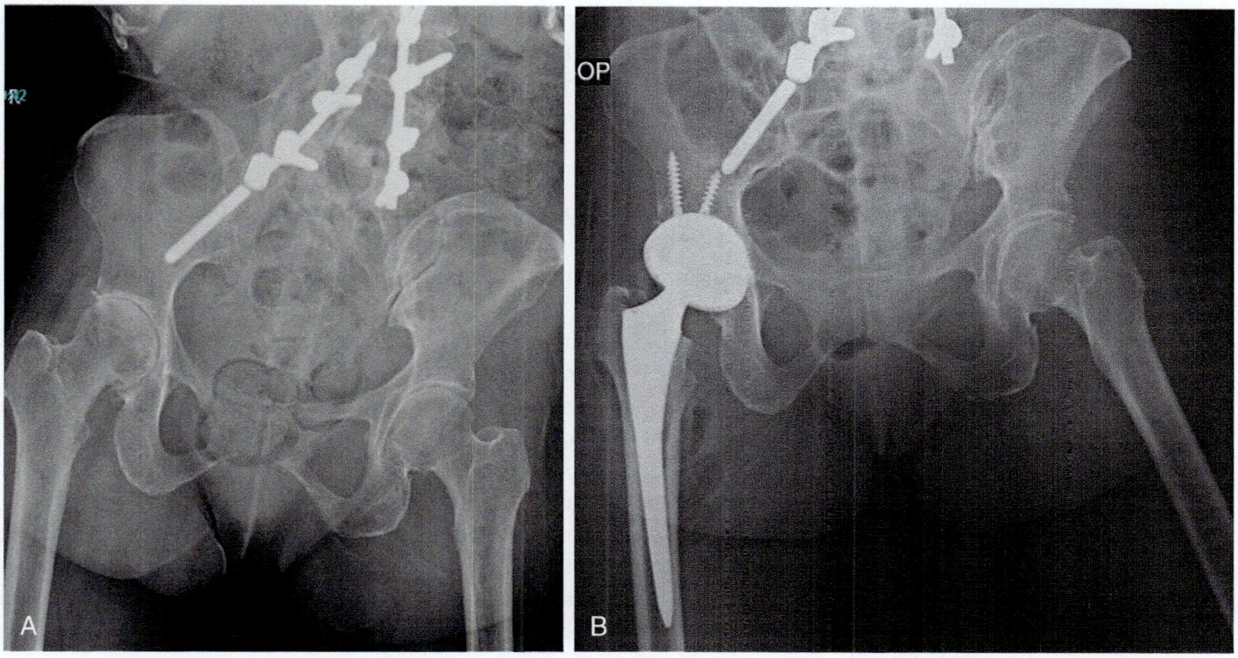

Figure 39.12 | Preoperative (A) and postoperative (B) radiographs of a patient with extensive spinal deformity that is fused down to the pelvis who underwent primary total arthroplasty with a dual mobility construct.

- Score the inner surface of the acetabular component (if needed) with a metal cutting burr; copiously irrigate to dispose of any metal debris.
- Mix one batch of cement with 1.2 g of gentamicin on the back table; finger pack this into the acetabular cup while it is still in a doughy state.
- Utilize a polyethylene impactor to insert the dual mobility acetabular component into the cement, making sure that it is seated evenly and fully in the revision cup.
- Remove excess cement and maintain even circumferential pressure on the cemented cup with the polyethylene inserter.

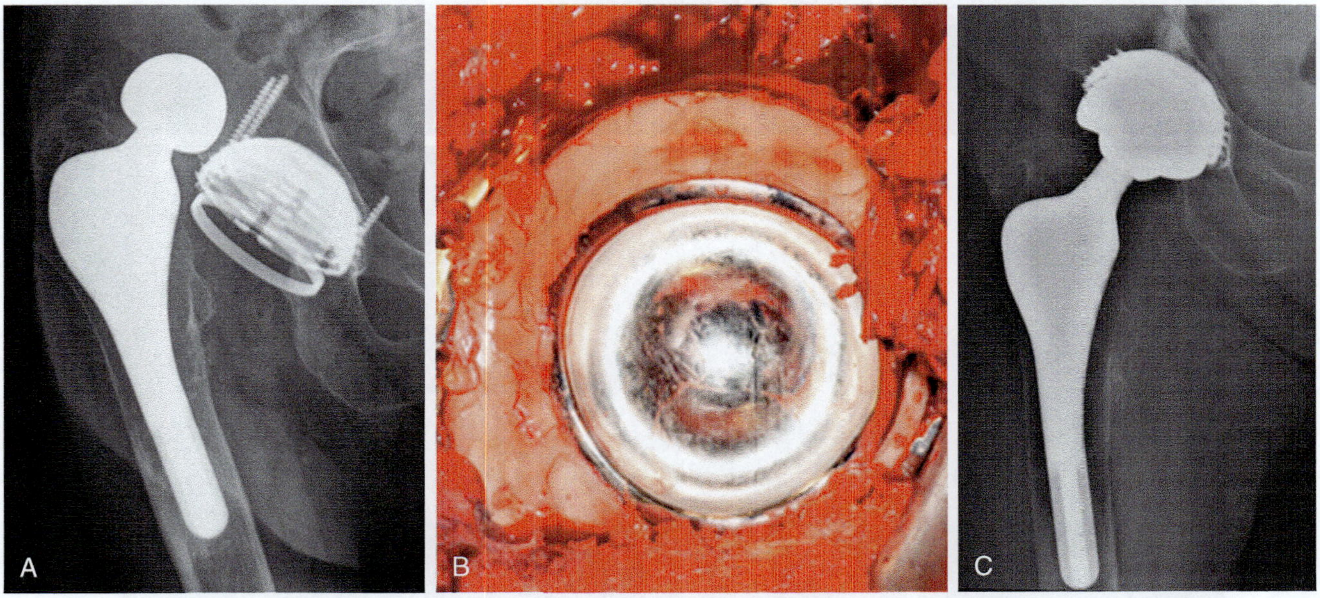

Figure 39.13 | A 53-year-old woman with rheumatoid arthritis who underwent implantation of a constrained liner at an outside hospital for recurrent dislocation. She was referred to us for management of her dislocated hip (A). To avoid massive bone loss during revision of her threaded acetabular component, a dual mobility construct was cemented in place (B and C). She remained stable at 4 years post operation.

- Assemble the femoral head and larger polyethylene articulation on the back table as outlined earlier.
- Impact the dual articulation onto the femoral trunnion and relocate the hip (Figure 39.13C).
- Test the stability of the hip intraoperatively.

Constrained Liners

- Constrained liners prevent dislocation by holding the hip in the acetabular component, compensating for deficient soft tissues.
- The main indications for the utilization of constrained liners in the recurrently dislocating total hip arthroplasty are:
  - Severely deficient abductor mechanism and/or periarticular soft tissue (Figures 39.14 and 39.15).
  - Recurrently dislocating dual mobility constructs.
- Our preference in patients with reasonable soft tissues and abductor mechanism is to utilize a dual mobility construct because of several key factors:
  - Constrained liners nearly always require operative intervention in the event of a recurrent dislocation.
  - Constrained liners increase prosthetic impingement.
  - Constrained liners increase acetabular component-bone stresses, which is especially problematic in complex acetabular reconstructions with bone graft, augments, and/or cup-cage constructs.
- As outlined earlier in the dual mobility revision section, constrained liners can be placed into compatible implant-specific acetabular components or cemented into place; the surgical technique follows that of the above-mentioned techniques for dual mobility constructs.
- Once the final implants are selected, assembly order follows from the type of constrained implant chosen.

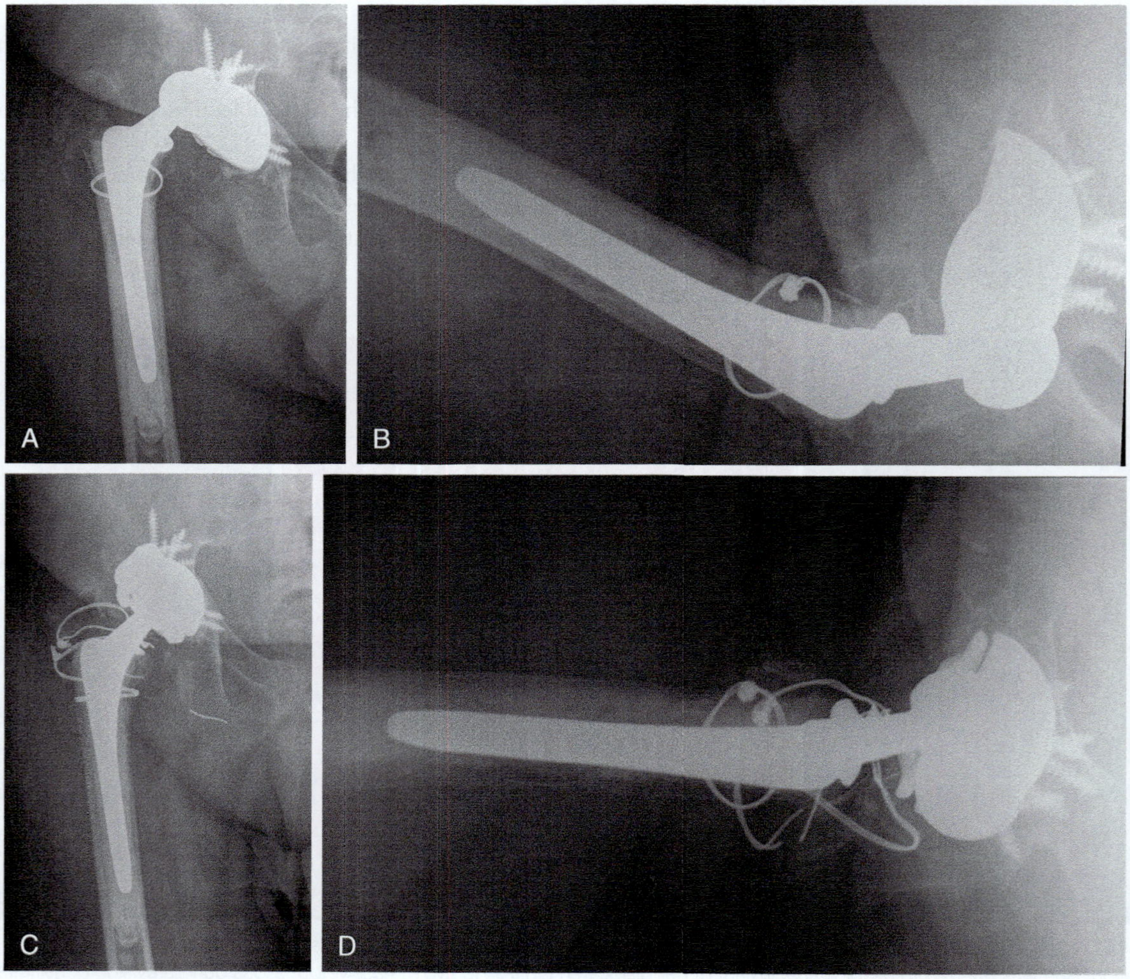

Figure 39.14 I A 52-year-old man who is status post complex revision acetabular reconstruction with a tantalum revision acetabular component and modular augments experienced recurrent posterior-superior dislocations (A and B). Note the trochanteric fracture and escape (A). The patient was over 1 year from acetabular revision and the acetabular component was in good position and had excellent bony ingrowth. He was revised to a cemented constrained liner given the poor abductor mechanism (C and D).

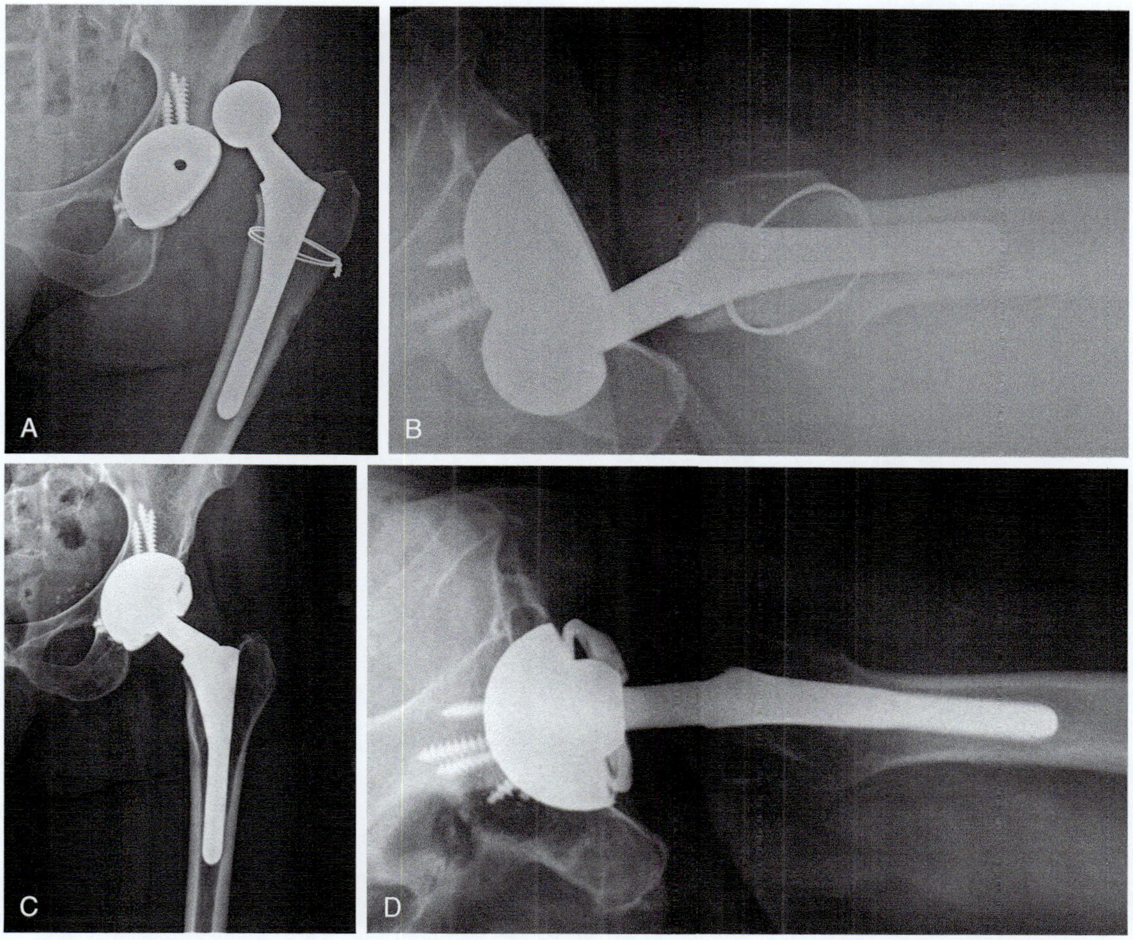

Figure 39.15 | A 63-year-old woman status post revision total hip arthroplasty for a failed metal-on-metal resurfacing with extensive pseudotumor and abductor destruction presented with recurrent superior and posterior dislocations (A and B). The patient's acetabular component was well fixed and in good position. The patient was revised to a cemented constrained liner (C and D) and remained stable at final follow-up.

Postoperative Care

- A hip abduction orthosis for 6 to 8 weeks to allow soft tissue healing can be utilized; the senior author prefers to use these braces only after implantation of a constrained liner to prevent increased range of motion and prosthetic impingement.
- Weight bearing is allowed based on details of the rest of the revision procedure such as whether the acetabular component was revised.

Chapter 40
Infection: Two-Stage Techniques

TIMOTHY S. BROWN
KEVIN I. PERRY

Key Concepts

- Two-stage exchange for chronic periprosthetic joint infection (PJI) of the hip is the gold standard treatment in North America.
- The first stage entails removal of all of the hip implants and cement, a thorough debridement of the necrotic and infected materials, a thorough irrigation of the wound, followed (usually) by placement of an antibiotic loaded spacer.
- Three distinct types of antibiotic spacers exist: a nonarticulating antibiotic spacer, a prefabricated articulated antibiotic spacer, and an articulated spacer fabricated at the time of surgery.
- Prefabricated spacers (Figure 40.1) contain low-dose antibiotics and need to be supplemented with high-dose antibiotic cement if they are to be used.
- Spacers fabricated at the time of surgery (Figure 40.2) allow the surgeon to control the type of antibiotic and dosage used in the spacer.
- Dislocation of antibiotic spacer is not uncommon and is probably underreported (Figure 40.3).
- Postoperatively, the patient should receive a course of intravenous antibiotics targeted at the offending microorganism guided by an infectious disease specialist.
- After completion of the antibiotics, the patient should undergo a period of time off of antibiotics to ensure the infection has been cleared before proceeding with hip reimplantation.
- During hip reimplantation, multiple cultures should be obtained and intraoperative pathology should be sent to ensure the infection has been cleared.

Sterile Instruments and Implants

Resection and Spacer Insertion

- Routine hip retractors
- Large oscillating saw (if performing an osteotomy)
- Pencil-tipped burr (short and long)
- Thin osteotomes for removal of uncemented implants
- Ultrasonic cement removal devices if removing a cemented stem

Implants

- Antibiotic spacer molds (if fabricating spacer at the time of surgery)
- Cement gun for antibiotic dowel fabrication (if utilizing nonarticulating spacer)
- Luque wires

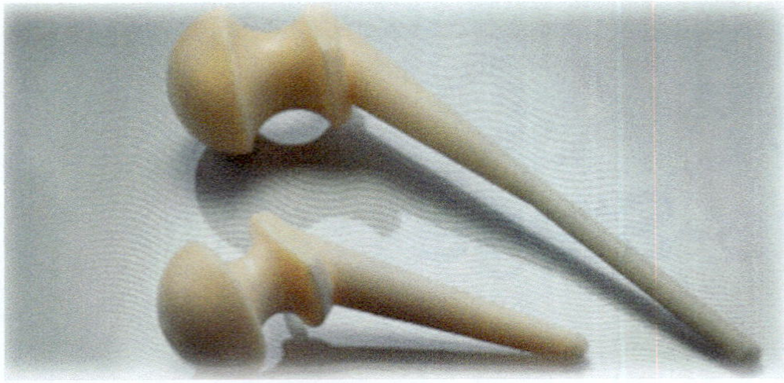

Figure 40.1 | Example of a prefabricated antibiotic spacer.

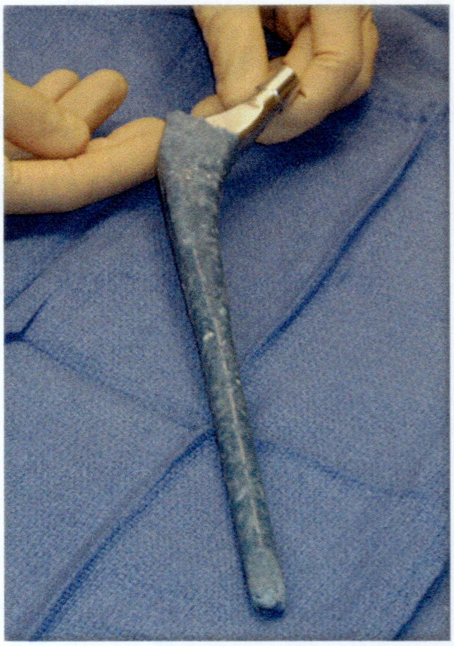

Figure 40.2 | Intraoperative photo demonstrating an antibiotic spacer fabricated with high-dose antibiotics at the time of surgery.

Reimplantation

- Osteotomes and rongeurs to remove cement
- High-speed burrs and curettes to remove cement
- Wire cutters if cerclage wires are in place
- Routine hip retractors
- Revision total hip arthroplasty acetabular and femoral revision implants
- Consider high-stability bearings

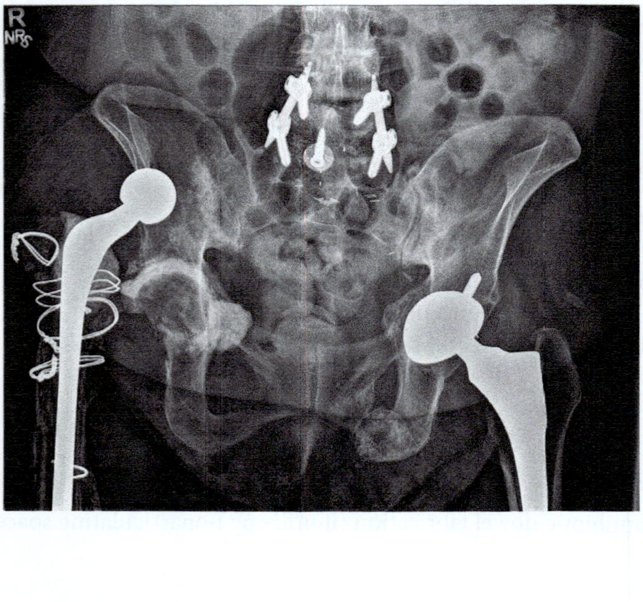

Figure 40.3 | AP pelvis demonstrating dislocation of an articulating antibiotic spacer.

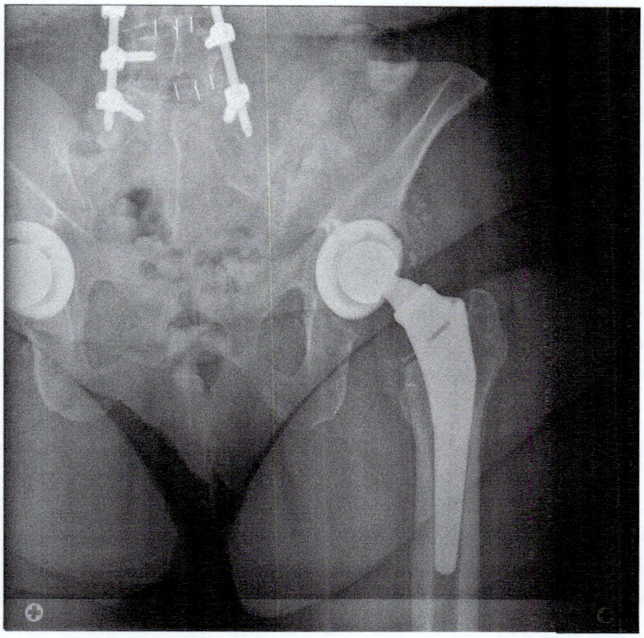

Figure 40.4 I AP raciograph of infected total hip arthroplasty.

Positioning

- Lateral decubitus position or supine position based on surgeon's preference.

Surgical Approaches

- Removal of the hip implants can be accomplished from either an anterolateral or posterolateral approach depending on surgeon preference.
- If an extended trochanteric osteotomy will be utilized for femoral implant removal, the posterolateral approach to the hip is preferred.

Preoperative Planning

- Previous operative reports containing implant information is vital so that the appropriate instrumentation can be available for implant removal.
- Preoperative radiographs should be obtained, including an anteroposterior (AP) pelvis, a lateral of the affected hip, and an AP view of the affected hip (Figure 40.4).
- Consideration of surgical approach, necessity of osteotomy, and understanding the implants in place is imperative.
- A plan regarding the use of a nonarticulating versus an articulating antibiotic spacer is useful preoperatively so that the appropriate instrumentation may be readily available.
  - No spacer (resection alone)
    - Used rarely
    - Predominately for patients who are very sick or immunocompromised or those who have already failed treatment with antibiotic spacers
  - Nonarticulating spacer
    - Used in some cases, especially when extensive bone loss or soft tissue deficiency precludes the use of an articulating spacer
    - Advantages of nonarticulating spacer:
      - No risk of spacer dislocation
      - Little risk of bone erosion
    - Disadvantages of nonarticulating spacer:
      - Poorer patient function during resection interval
      - More difficult exposure at second stage

- Articulating spacer
  - Used in most patients
  - Good soft tissue envelope reduces risk of spacer dislocation
  - Advantages of articulating spacers:
    - Better patient function during resection interval
    - Easier exposure during reimplantation
    - The patient needs to be compliant to minimize risk of spacer dislocation and to sufficiently protect construct to minimize risk of femur fracture or bone erosion
  - Disadvantages of articulating spacers:
    - Risk of articular spacer dislocation
    - Increased risk of bone erosion due to spacer loading
    - Increased risk of periprosthetic fracture around spacers

Bone, Implant, and Soft Tissue Techniques

- Perform the desired approach to the hip joint.
- If an osteotomy is to be performed, this may be performed during the initial approach.
- Remove the implants as described in Chapter 24.
- Once the implants have been removed, a thorough debridement of all infected and necrotic tissues should be performed.
- Make sure all cement and cement restrictors (which usually are radiolucent) are removed.
- Multiple cultures and an intraoperative pathology specimen should be sent to identify the offending microorganism and confirm the presence of PJI.
- Once the debridement has been completed, the wound should be thoroughly irrigated.
  - Irrigation is performed using the following solutions in sequence:
    - 3 L normal saline, pulse lavage
    - 15 mL sterile povidone-iodine in 500 mL normal saline
    - 3 L normal saline, pulse lavage
    - 500 mL Dakin solution, H_2O_2, or Hibiclens
    - 3 L normal saline, pulse lavage
- If no spacer is being placed, the wound can then be closed in layers according to surgeon preference.
- If utilizing a nonarticulating spacer, a dowel should be created to place into the femoral canal utilizing high-dose antibiotic cement.
  - High-dose antibiotic cement recipe:
    - One batch cement
    - 3 g vancomycin
    - 3.6 g tobramycin
    - 150 mg amphotericin B (if there is a possibility of fungal/yeast infection)
    - 1 to 2 drops sterile methylene blue
    - Mix the cement monomer and polymer together first until they react and create a liquid
    - Add the 2 drops of sterile methylene blue
    - Slowly mix in the powdered antibiotics until the cement becomes doughy
  - Creating the dowel:
    - One batch high-dose antibiotic cement, mixed and placed into cement gun.
    - Push cement to tip of gun and unscrew the barrel. Push cement in the cup of the barrel away from threads of the barrel.
    - Allow the cement to harden completely until cool (otherwise it will be difficult to remove), then remove the dowel from the barrel. If the dowel gets stuck, use a sagittal saw to disrupt the plastic at one end and then remove with a rongeur.
    - Create one dowel for implantation into the femur.
    - Place the dowel into the femoral canal (Figure 40.5).
- If utilizing an articulating antibiotic spacer fabricated at the time of surgery, the antibiotic spacer should be made at this time utilizing the mold in the set (Figure 40.6) with the high-dose antibiotic recipe listed earlier.
- The polyethylene acetabular portion of the antibiotic spacer can be burred on its backside to facilitate better cement interdigitation and fixation (Figure 40.7).

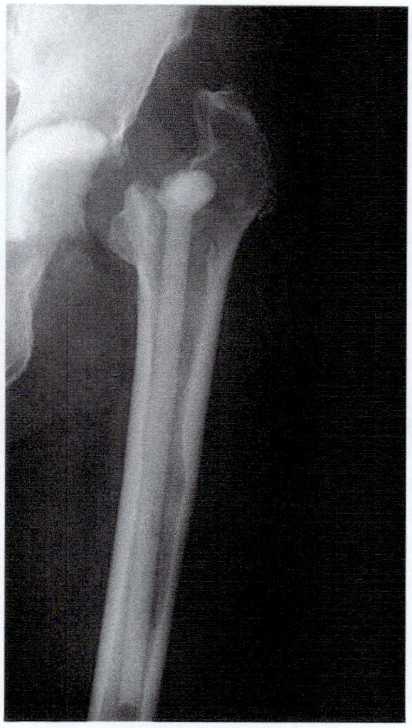

Figure 40.5 | AP radiograph of nonarticulating antibiotic spacer.

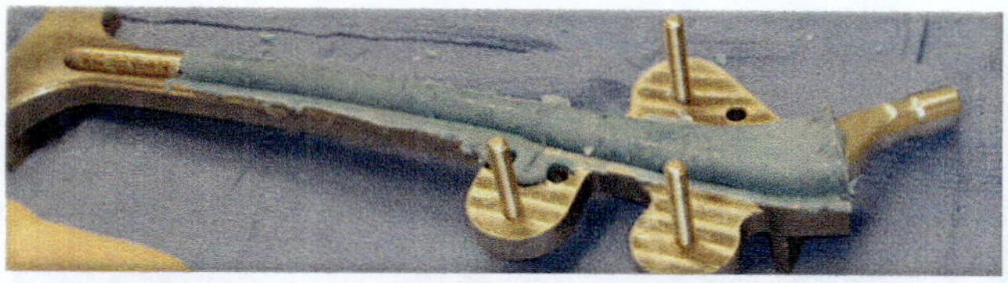

Figure 40.6 | Mold for the antibiotic spacer with the spacer in situ.

- The acetabular portion of the spacer can be cemented into place (Figure 40.8) utilizing the high-dose antibiotic recipe noted earlier.
- When mixing antibiotic cement, it is helpful to mix the cement first and then slowly incorporate each batch of antibiotics so that nice, doughy cement can be achieved (Figure 40.9).
- If the acetabular bed is particularly bloody and cement interdigitation is difficult, one can consider making 3 small burr holes in the socket to allow for better component fixation.
- The femoral portion of the antibiotic spacer may then be cemented into place with the same antibiotic ratio. Typically, 1-2 batches of methylmethacrylate are required. The implant should be cemented in judiciously, balancing the desire to fix the spacer sufficiently for function with the anticipated need

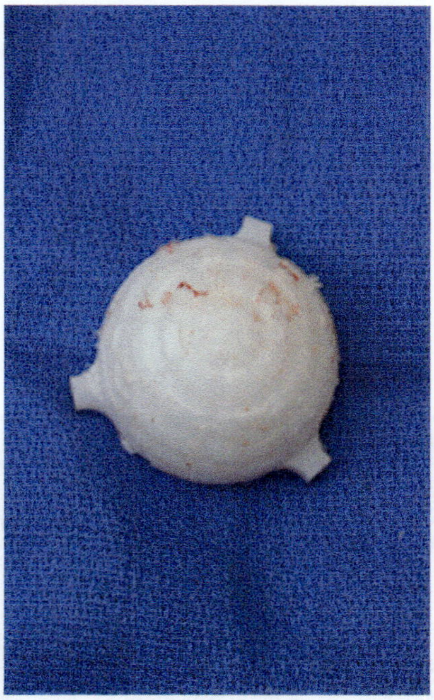

Figure 40.7 | Intraoperative photo demonstrating the back of the acetabular component that has been burred to facilitate cement interdigitation.

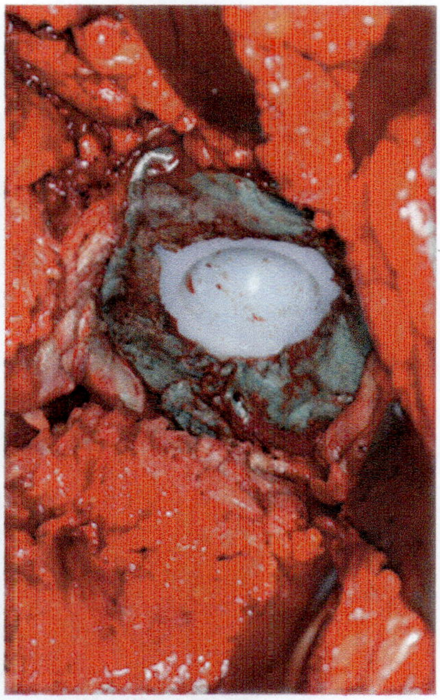

Figure 40.8 | Intraoperative photo demonstrating the acetabular component that has been cemented into place. Note the excess antibiotic cement at the periphery of the implant that facilitates antibiotic elution.

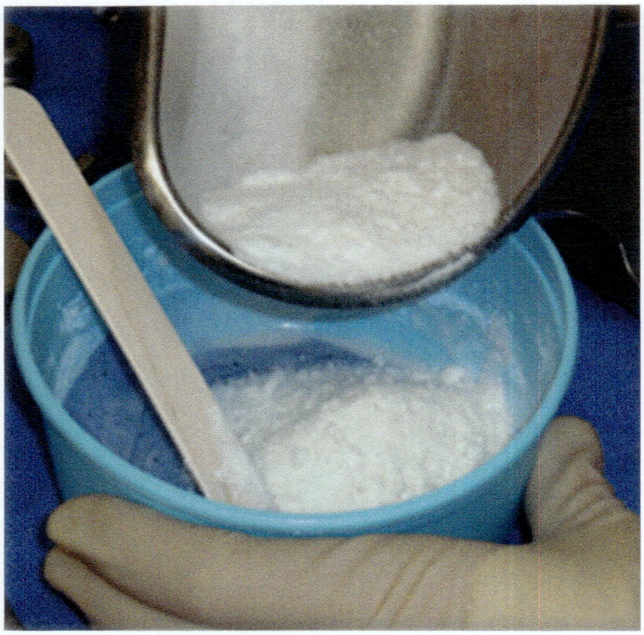

Figure 40.9 | Intraoperative photo demonstrating antibiotics being mixed into the cement.

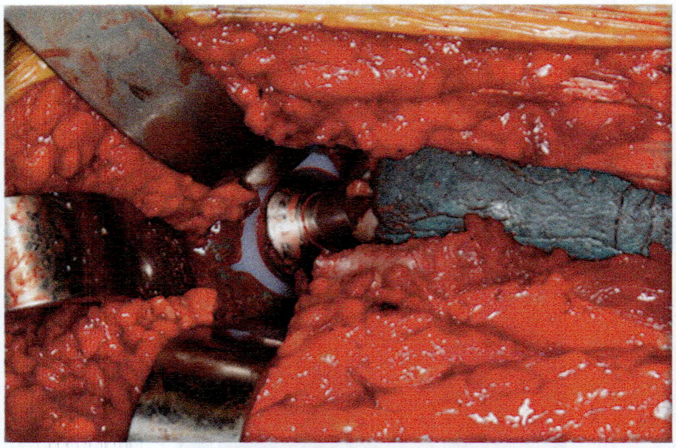

Figure 40.10 | Intraoperative photo of the reduced antibiotic spacer after final cementation.

to remove the spacer in a few months without excessive bone loss. (Note: If an osteotomy has been performed, it may be reduced and fixated with monofilament wires before cementation of the femoral component.)

- After the cement has hardened, the hip should be reduced (Figure 40.10) and taken through a range of motion to ensure stability of the hip. If a captured polyethylene cup is used, sometimes a tight seal and air pressure will prevent reduction. This problem can be solved with a small drill hole in from the rim into the cup or a small nick on the inner rim of the cup.
- The wound should then be closed in layers according to surgeon protocol and a postoperative radiograph obtained (Figure 40.11A and B). If an ETO has been used, it should be closed with monofilament wires, not with polyfilament cable owing to infection risk.

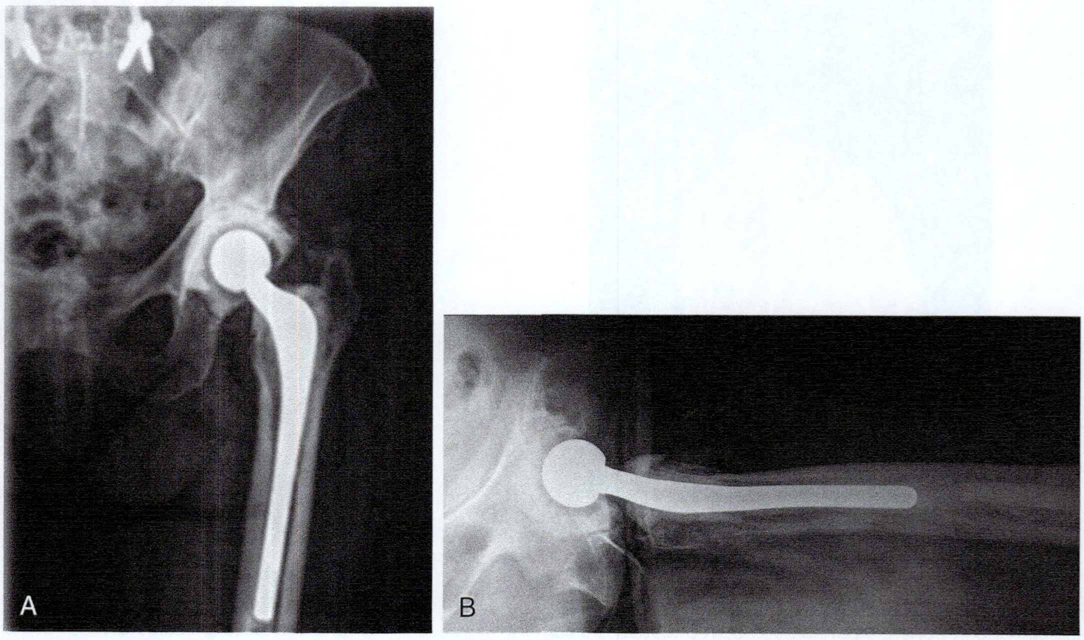

Figure 40.11 | AP (A) and lateral (B) radiographs of the final antibiotic spacer.

Postoperative Care

- Postoperatively, patients should be made toe-touch weight bearing if an osteotomy was performed for femoral component removal. Otherwise, patients are typically made partial weight bearing with the use of crutches or a walker for at least 6 weeks and usually for the duration of the resection interval.

Management of the Patient During the Resection Interval

- Placement of a long-term intravenous (IV) access line is required for antibiotic administration after the first stage of the 2-stage approach.
- A course of IV antibiotics should be administered directed at the specific offending microorganism.
- After completion of the antibiotics, a 4- to 6-week antibiotic-free period should commence and inflammatory markers monitored.
- If the inflammatory markers and clinical picture suggest clearance of the infection, reimplantation of the hip can be considered (at least a 12-week window between the first and second stages of the operation is preferred). This interval allows the patient to recover metabolically, the soft tissues to heal, and the surgeon to observe for clearing of the infection.
- A decision is made to proceed with reimplantation once laboratory test results have normalized and the clinical examination is consistent with clearance of the infection.
- We do not hesitate to extend the period with an antibiotic spacer in place if there is any question as to whether the infection has been cleared.
- On occasion the patient may need to be returned to the operating room for a repeat irrigation and debridement with spacer exchange if the examination and serum laboratory test results are not consistent with clearing of the infection.

Reimplantation

- We usually attempt to excise the previous scar during reimplantation.
- An extensile exposure to the hip is again made, using an extended trochanteric osteotomy if needed. If previous cerclage wires were placed on the femur, they should be removed.
- The spacer is carefully removed using techniques described in Chapter 24.
- Multiple cultures are sent.

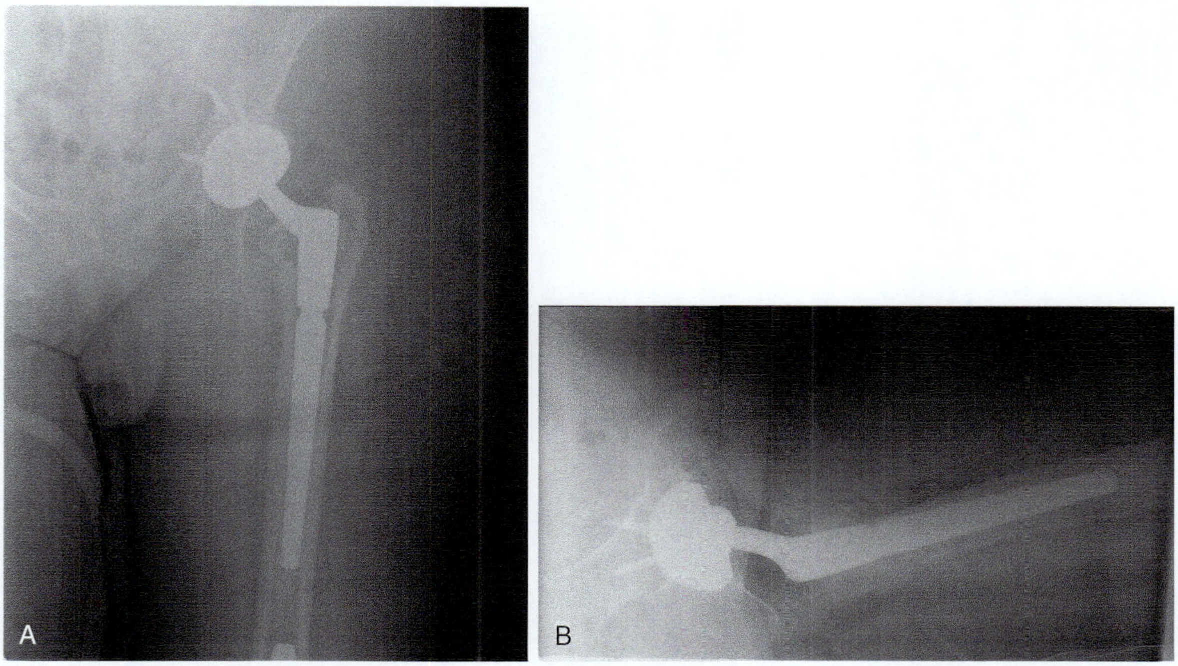

Figure 40.12 | AP (A) and lateral (B) radiographs of the hip after final reimplantation.

- The femoral canal is thoroughly debrided, ensuring that all aspects of the spacer are removed.
- The acetabulum is exposed and thoroughly debrided.
- The acetabular reconstruction depends on bone loss but typically utilizes a highly porous component with multiple screws. Patients are at high risk for dislocation, and the use of large-diameter femoral heads or dual mobility components is effective in reducing this complication.
- The femoral component used depends on anatomy and bone loss, but the most commonly used in our practice is a modular fluted tapered stem. The distal diaphysis is occasionally prophylactically wired to prevent fracture while reaming. Particularly in the case of previous infection, where recurrent infection risk is 5 to 20%, avoid using a longer stem than needed to prevent more severe bone loss should later extraction be required.
- Trial components are utilized to confirm a stable implant, and an intraoperative radiograph is obtained to ensure appropriate positioning.
- The real femoral component is then inserted as described in Chapter 30.
- The wound should then be thoroughly irrigated and closure can commence.
- Postoperative radiographs should be obtained including an AP pelvis and lateral of the hip (Figure 40.12A and B).
- The patient is kept on oral antibiotics directed against the prior organism for at least 14 days postoperatively. The role of extended antibiotic treatment for selected patients is under study at this time.

Chapter 41

Pelvic Discontinuity

MATTHEW P. ABDEL

Key Concepts

- Pelvic discontinuity is a separation of the ilium superiorly from the ischiopubic segment inferiorly (Figure 41.1).
- When performing a revision total hip arthroplasty (THA) in such a cohort, there are 2 simultaneous goals:
  1. Gaining long-term acetabular component stability.
  2. Healing across the bony discontinuity *or* "unitization" of the pelvis by healing of the superior pelvis to the superior aspect of the cup-construct and the inferior pelvis to the inferior aspect of the cup-construct.
- Preoperative imaging is essential and includes the following:
  1. Anteroposterior (AP) pelvic radiograph
  2. AP hip radiograph
  3. Cross-table hip radiograph
  4. False profile hip radiograph
  5. Judet radiographs including obturator oblique and iliac oblique views
  6. ± Computerized tomography (CT) scan with 3-dimensional (3D) reconstruction
- Contemporary management options for chronic pelvic discontinuities include:
  1. Hemispherical acetabular component placement and open reduction and internal fixation (ORIF) with pelvic plating (Figure 41.2). This method works best for acute pelvic discontinuities and has a lower healing rate for chronic discontinuities with severe bone loss and is not commonly used currently.
  2. Cup-cage construct (Figure 41.3).
  3. Distraction method (Figure 41.4). This method "unitizes" the pelvis but usually does not lead to healing of the actual discontinuity fracture lines.
  4. Custom triflange implant (Figure 41.5). This method requires several weeks' lead time for implant fabrication.

Sterile Instruments and Implants

Instruments

- Routine revision hip retractors.
- Routine hip instruments to remove preexisting uncemented or cemented acetabular components.
- Two ball spikes.
- Two vice grips.
- Intraoperative fluoroscopy or imaging.

Implants

Cup-Cage Construct (Author's Preferred Technique)

- Highly porous acetabular components of various diameters (particularly sizes 60 mm or greater)
- Highly porous acetabular augments (of various sizes)

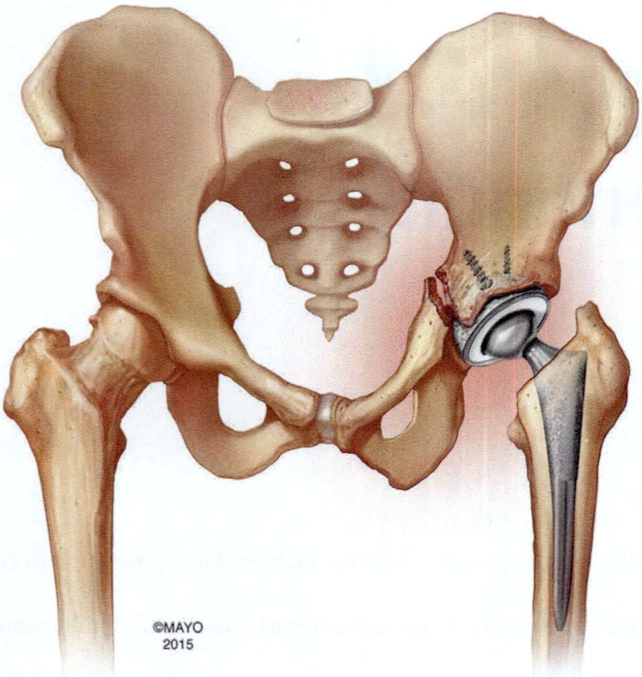

Figure 41.1 I Illustration of an AP view of the pelvis showing a left pelvic discontinuity where the ilium superiorly is separated from the ischium inferiorly. Of note, there are several indicators of a pelvic discontinuity, including the visible fracture line, obturator ring asymmetry, and medial migration of the inferior hemipelvis with disruption of Kohler line. (Used with permission of Mayo Foundation for Medical Education and Research. All rights reserved.)

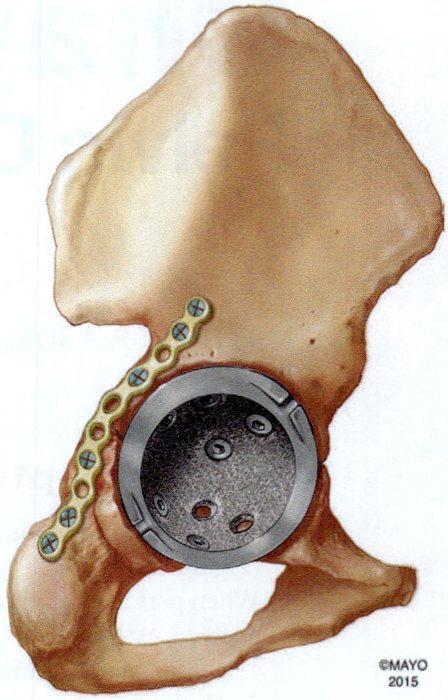

Figure 41.2 I Illustration of a hemispherical acetabular component with posterior column compression plating, typically reserved for acute pelvic discontinuities with adequate bone quality and quantity. (Used with permission of Mayo Foundation for Medical Education and Research. All rights reserved.)

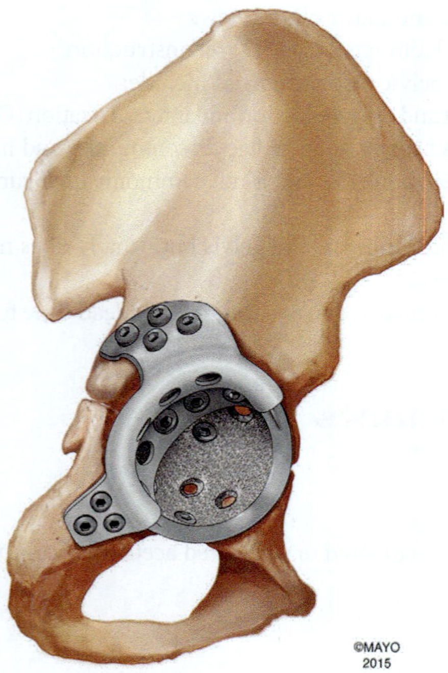

Figure 41.3 I Illustration of a cup-cage construct where the highly porous acetabular component is placed on host bone, supplemental screws are placed superiorly and inferiorly, and a supplemental cage is placed on top of the acetabular component spanning the ilium to the ischium. (Used with permission of Mayo Foundation for Medical Education and Research. All rights reserved.)

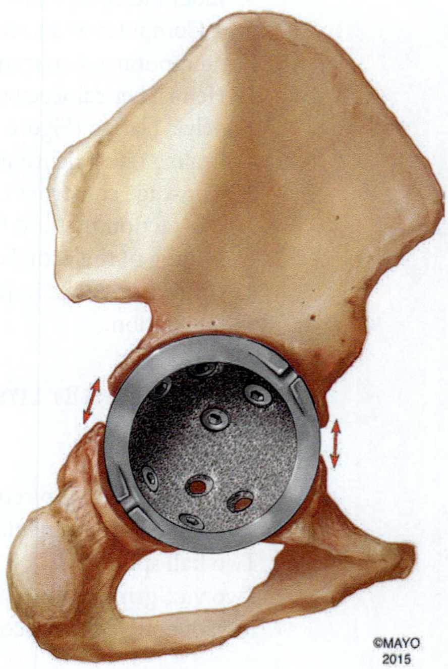

Figure 41.4 I Illustration of the distraction method where an acetabular component that is 6 to 8 mm larger than the last reamer is inserted, allowing the elastic recoil of the pelvis to provide a rigid initial capture. (Used with permission of Mayo Foundation for Medical Education and Research. All rights reserved.)

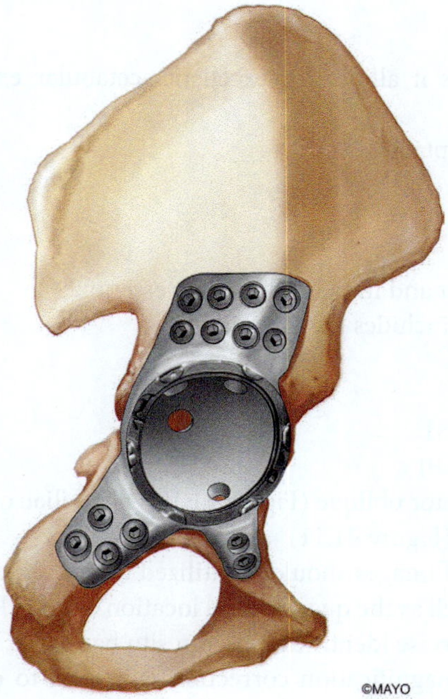

Figure 41.5 | Illustration of a custom triflange, including iliac, ischial, and pubic flanges. (Used with permission of Mayo Foundation for Medical Education and Research. All rights reserved.)

- Supplemental screws
- Supplemental full-cage or half-cage
- Metal-cutting burr
- Allograft bone chips

Distraction Method

- Highly porous acetabular components of various diameters (particularly sizes 60 mm or greater)
- Highly porous acetabular augments (of various sizes)
- Supplemental screws
- Supplemental full or half cage
- Metal-cutting burr
- Allograft bone chips

Custom Triflange

- Custom triflange trial (provided by manufacturer)
- Real custom triflange component (provided by manufacturer)
- Custom triflange screws (provided by manufacturer)

Hemispherical Acetabular Component and ORIF With Plating

- Highly porous acetabular components of various diameters (particularly sizes 60 mm or greater)
- 3.5-mm reconstruction plate with 2 plate benders and compatible drill bits and screws
- Large pointed bone reduction forceps

Positioning

- Lateral decubitus position with access to entire femur in case an osteotomy is required for acetabular exposure.

Surgical Approaches

- A posterior approach is preferred as it allows for excellent acetabular exposure (including the posterior column and ilium).
- An anterolateral approach is also acceptable.

Preoperative Planning

- Obtaining the outside operative report and implant stickers is essential.
- Preoperative imaging is essential and includes the following:
  1. AP pelvic radiograph (Figure 41.6)
  2. AP hip radiograph (Figure 41.7)
  3. Cross-table radiograph (Figure 41.8)
  4. False profile radiograph (Figure 41.9)
  5. Judet radiographs including obturator oblique (Figure 41.10A) and iliac oblique (Figure 41.10B)
  6. ±CT scan with 3D reconstruction (Figure 41.11)
- The above-mentioned constellation of images should be utilized to determine the pattern and relative stability of the discontinuity, as well as the quantity and location of bone loss and remaining host bone. Such imaging also allows for precise identification of in situ hardware.
- An AP radiograph of the hip with magnification correction is helpful to determine the targeted hip center of rotation based on where the ilioischial line should be if pelvic discontinuity were not present, as well as the estimated acetabular component diameter. In addition, templating allows the surgeon to evaluate the current hip offset and limb length discrepancy, as well as the targeted hip offset and limb length corrections.
- If custom triflange component will be utilized, the patient will require a CT scan with metal subtraction software preoperatively. The exact CT specifications should be discussed in advance with the proposed implant manufacturer. Thereafter, a 3D model can be created and reviewed by the surgeon. This includes assessing the head center, cup orientation, size and location of flanges, and trajectory and length of screws.

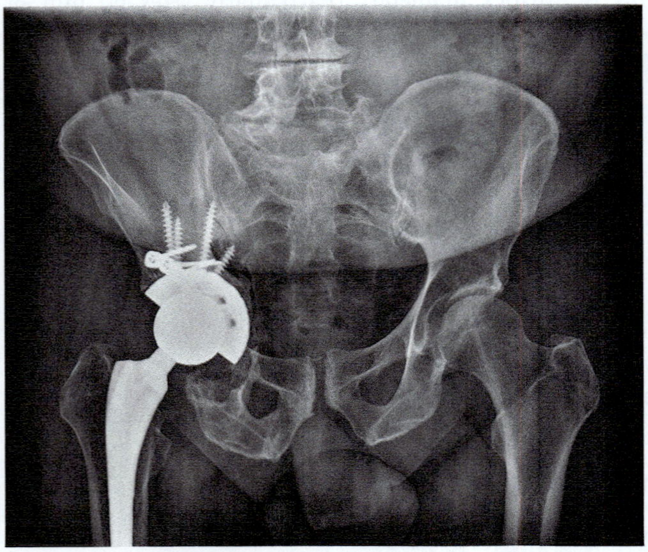

Figure 41.6 | AP pelvis radiograph of a 71-year-old man depicting a failed attempt at treating a pelvic discontinuity with a hemispherical acetabular component and plating completed at an outside institution. Radiographic findings concerning for pelvic discontinuity include a visible fracture line through the anterior and posterior columns, medial translation of the inferior aspect of the hemipelvis relative to the superior aspect (seen as a break in Kohler line), and rotation of the inferior aspect of the hemipelvis relative to the superior aspect (seen as asymmetry of the obturator rings).

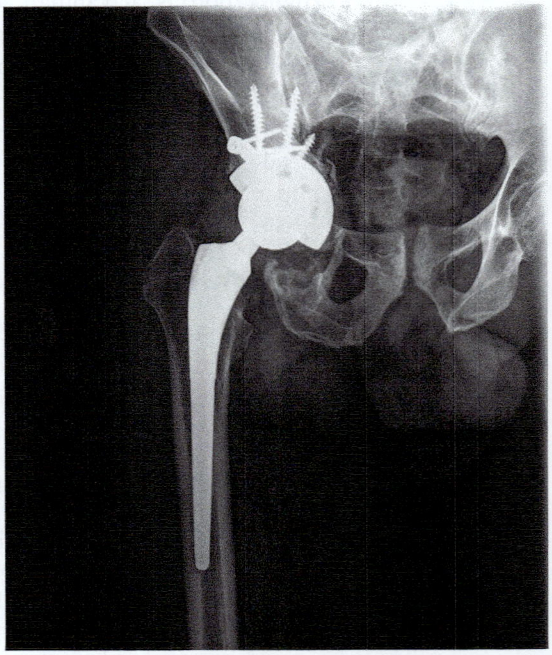

Figure 41.7 | The AP hip radiograph of the same patient also allows for full evaluation of the femoral component.

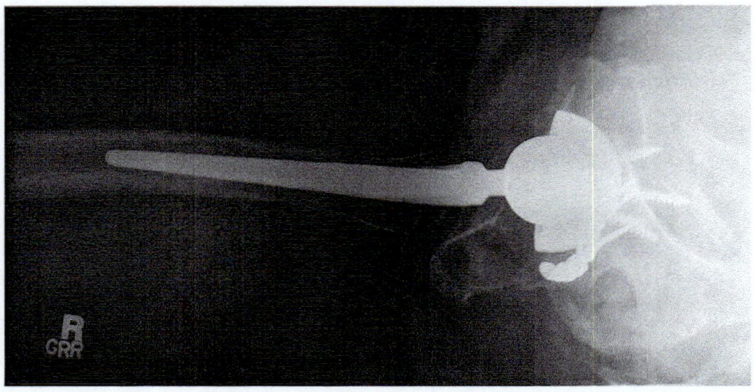

Figure 41.8 | A true cross-table lateral allows for evaluation of the posterior column. It also provides valuable information in regards to the version of the acetabular component, location of in situ screws, and remaining bone stock.

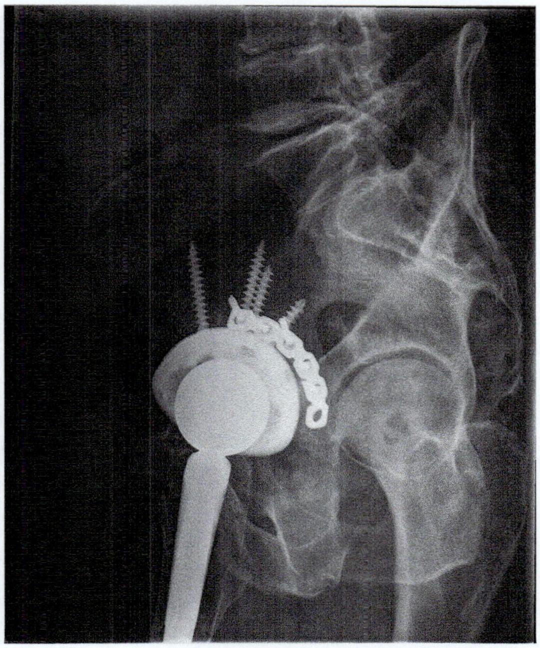

Figure 41.9 | The false profile radiograph is a 65° oblique radiograph that reveals the posterior column en bloc.

Bone/Implant/Soft Tissue Techniques

- Perform an approach to the hip based on surgeon's preference, but typically a posterior approach is used.
- Carefully identify and protect the sciatic nerve if possible. It is uniquely at risk during these procedures because of motion through the discontinuity and, in some cases, posterior column instrumentation.
- Remove the prior acetabular implants.
- Debride the remaining soft tissue and debris from the acetabular fossa until only bony surfaces are exposed.
- Assess the bone loss and remaining bone quality.
- Evaluate the pelvis with the use of 2 ball spikes, with one superior and one inferior to confirm if a discontinuity is present, looking for motion across the fracture site.
- Evaluate the degree of mobility of the discontinuity.

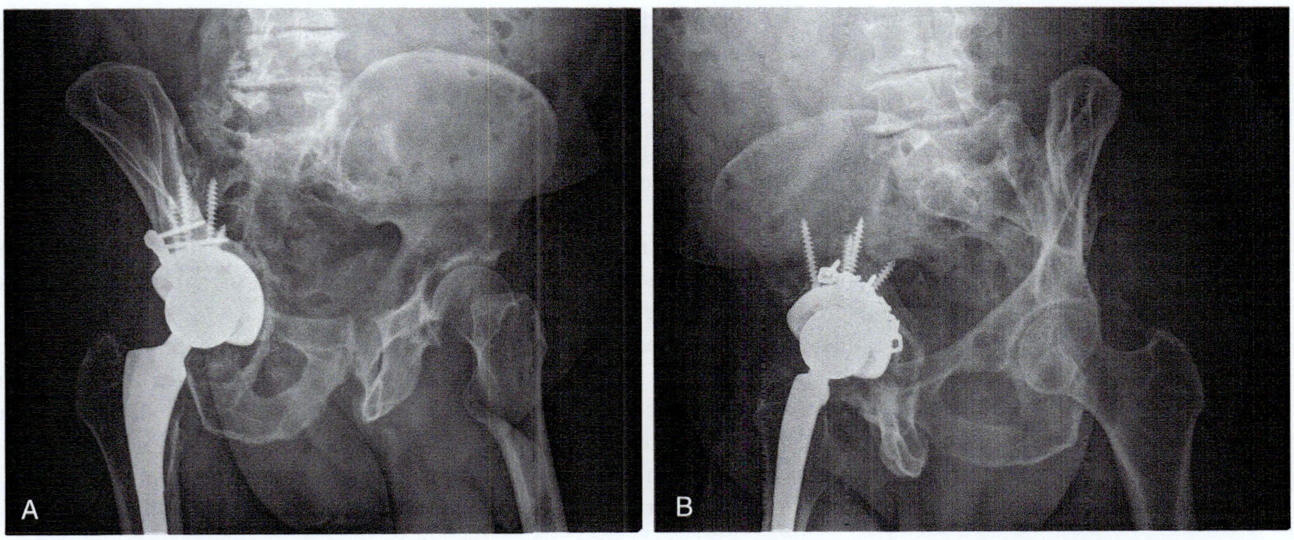

Figure 41.10 | Judet radiographs include an (A) obturator oblique (which evaluates the anterior column) and an (B) iliac oblique (which evaluates the posterior column).

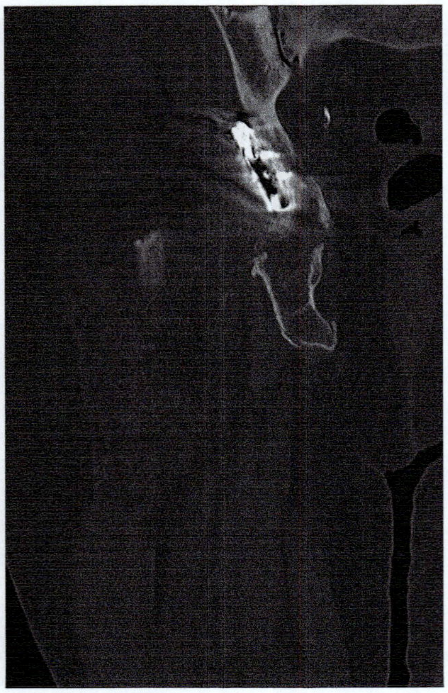

Figure 41.11 I Occasionally, a CT scan with 3D reconstructions can be beneficial in not only diagnosing a pelvic discontinuity but also determining the remaining bone quantity and quality (as well as positioning of in situ prostheses and hardware).

Cup-Cage Construct

- Gently ream the remaining acetabular bone in 2-mm increments until there is contact between the remaining superior and inferior bone.
- Antibiotic-loaded bone graft is then placed in the discontinuity and gently impacted.
- A trial highly porous acetabular component is then placed in the appropriate orientation with a targeted acetabular inclination of 40° and anteversion of 20°.
- If the diameter is correct, then a real highly porous acetabular component is impacted until there is capture, typically between the anterior-superior and posterior-inferior bone.
- Multiple supplemental screws are placed superiorly into the ilium and inferiorly into the ischium and/or pelvis (Figure 41.12). This allows the acetabular component to serve as an "internal plate." Be very cautious to avoid plunging into the soft tissues (and thereby risking neurovascular injury) when placing screws outside the traditional "safe zone."
- A supplemental cage is then placed over the acetabular component spanning the ilium to ischium if supplemental screw fixation inferiorly through the acetabular component is poor (Figure 41.3).
- If supplemental screw fixation inferiorly through the acetabular component was good, then the author's preference is to utilize a half cage (Figure 41.13), where the ischial flange is removed with a metal-cutting burr.
- The cage is then constructed in situ to mate to the acetabular component and remaining iliac bone.
- To place the cage, one iliac screw may be removed, and that screw is now placed through the hole in the cage, through the acetabular component, and back into the ilium (Figure 41.14).
- Typically, 3-4 screws can be placed through the ilium flange of the cage roughly perpendicular to the acetabular cup dome screws in a trajectory that goes from lateral to medial. Using a straight nonflexible drill bit is preferred for these screws.
- A polyethylene liner (with a textured back surface) is then cemented into place with antibiotic-impregnated cement (Figure 41.15). This allows for slight adjustments in the effective acetabular inclination and version of the overall construct (Figure 41.16A and B). If available, an all-polyethylene acetabular component designed for cement may be used. If not, a modular polyethylene liner for an uncemented cup should be used; if this method is chosen the back of the liner should be scored in a "spiderweb" pattern with a 4-mm burr to enhance cement fixation.

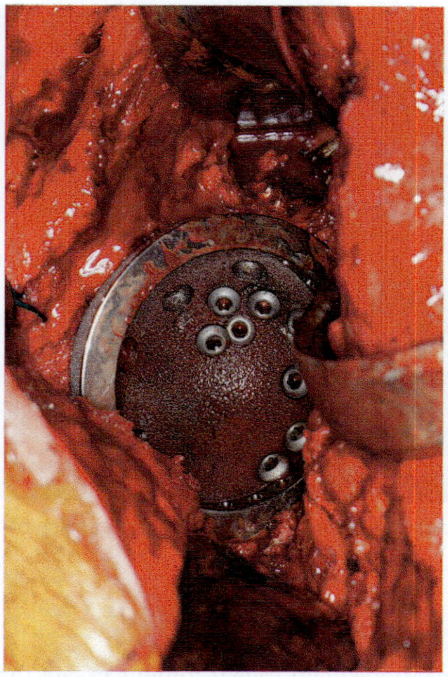

Figure 41.12 | Intraoperative photograph of the above-mentioned 71-year-old male patient at the time of re-revision THA whereby a highly porous acetabular component has been impacted with multiple supplemental screws placed superiorly into the ilium and inferiorly in the ischium. A diamond-cutting burr was utilized to place multiple additional screw holes through the acetabular component.

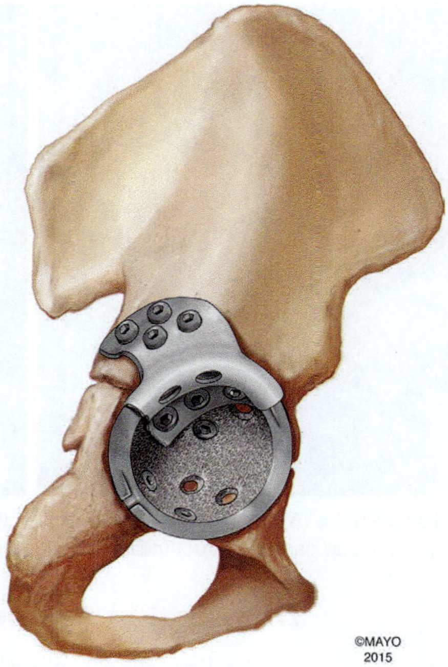

Figure 41.13 | Illustration of a half cup-cage construct where the highly porous acetabular component is placed on host bone, supplemental screws are placed superiorly and inferiorly, and a supplemental half-cage is placed on top of the acetabular component with the ischial flange removed. (Used with permission of Mayo Foundation for Medical Education and Research. All rights reserved.)

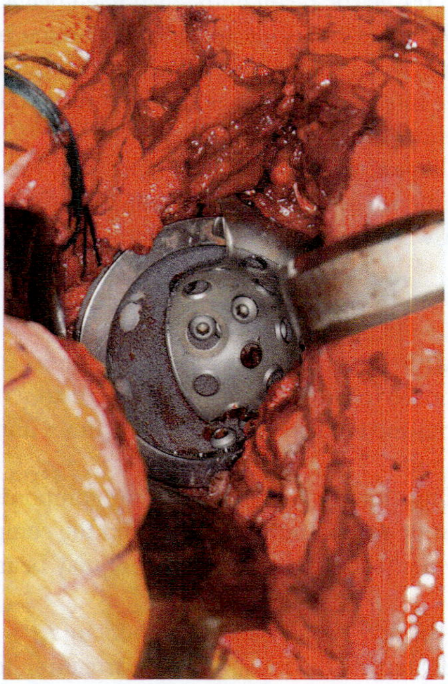

Figure 41.14 | Intraoperative photograph of the 71-year-old male patient mentioned earlier at the time of re-revision THA whereby 1 iliac screw was removed and that screw was placed through the hole in the cage, through the acetabular component, and back into the ilium. An additional 3-4 screws are placed through the iliac flange of the cage and into host bone.

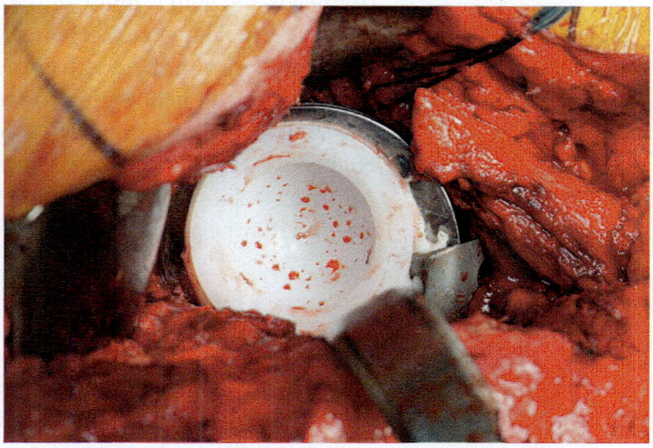

Figure 41.15 | A polyethylene liner is then cemented into place unitizing the half cup-cage construct.

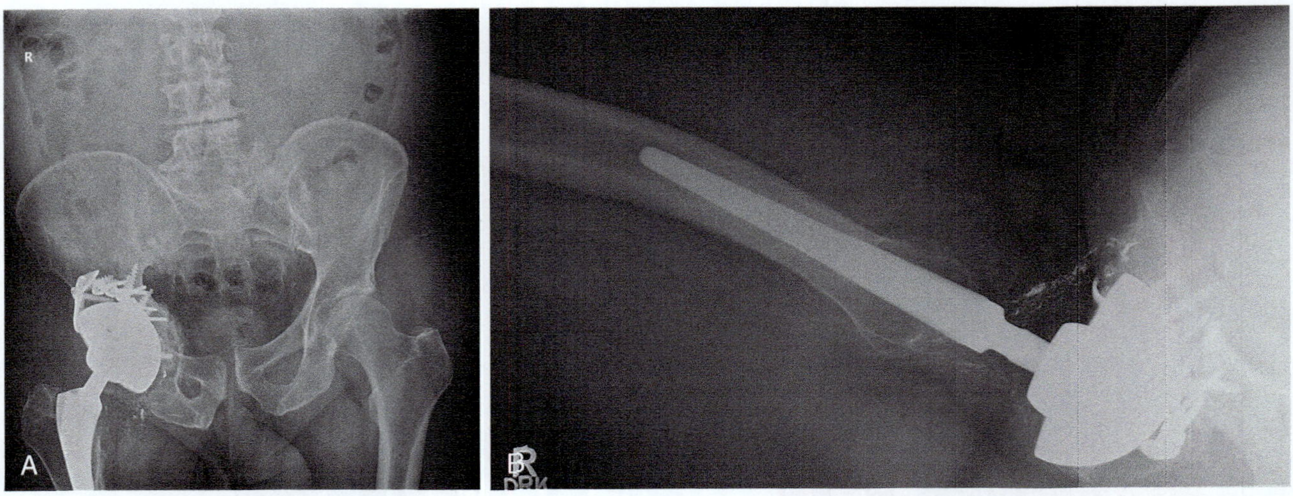

Figure 41.16 I AP pelvis (A) and cross-table lateral (B) of the above-mentioned 71-year-old male patient 3 months after re-revision of his pelvic discontinuity with a cup-cage construct utilizing a half-cage.

Distraction Method

- The distraction method is similar to the above-mentioned cup-cage technique except that sequentially larger reamers are used until the anterior-superior and posterior-inferior margins of the acetabulum are engaged.
- After those acetabular margins are engaged, the discontinuity is distracted by an additional 6 to 8 mm through the use of larger trial components.
- Cancellous bone graft (autograft or allograft) is packed in the discontinuity and remaining bone defects.
- The real highly porous acetabular component, oversized by 6 to 8 mm compared with the reamed size, is then placed again in the remaining ischium and brought into the desired position, allowing the distraction to create an initial press fit. The goal of oversizing is to distract the inferior and superior pelvis and gain stability of the construct from the elastic recoil of the distracted pelvis.
- Multiple supplemental screws are placed superiorly and inferiorly into the remaining host bone. Good fixation with these screws is the key to success of this procedure. Remember the goal is for the superior bone to heal to the superior cup and the inferior bone to heal to the inferior cup thereby unitizing the pelvis even if the discontinuity fracture line itself does not heal.
- Highly porous metal augments may be used to fill large acetabular defects (Figure 41.17) and improve construct stability with respect to the superior or inferior aspect of the hemipelvis. In such cases, distraction may be achieved using a pelvic distractor with screws in the ileum and ischium.

Custom Triflange

- After the failed acetabular component is removed, the preoperative plan and 3D model is reviewed to identify prominences of bone that must be removed to allow optimal fit of the custom triflange.
- Oftentimes, this is an iterative step in which the trial and burr are utilized several times until the trial component fits nicely on the ilium, ischium, and pubis.
- Thereafter, the acetabular socket is gently reamed to allow for a smooth fit of the component.
- The surgeon may consider bone grafting but must be certain not to malposition the component by placement of excessive bone graft. Antibiotic powder (such as vancomycin, 1 g) may be mixed into the bone graft.
- The custom triflange implant is then rotated into the pelvis underneath the abductors.
    - The first row of iliac flange screw holes typically targets the most inferior, structural bone of the ilium.
    - The ischial flange normally has 3-7 screw holes to accommodate 6.5-mm acetabular screws and typically rests on the posterior surface of the ischial tuberosity.
    - The pubic flange is generally the smallest and often does not have screw holes.
- The triflange component is fixed to the ilium with 1 nonlocking cancellous screw, the discontinuity is reduced, and then 1 screw is placed in the ischium for initial stabilization of the inferior hemipelvis.
- Initially, cancellous screws are utilized to compress the implant to the bone.
- Thereafter, locking screws are placed in the remaining holes.
- Usually, 9-13 screws are utilized (Figure 41.18A and B).

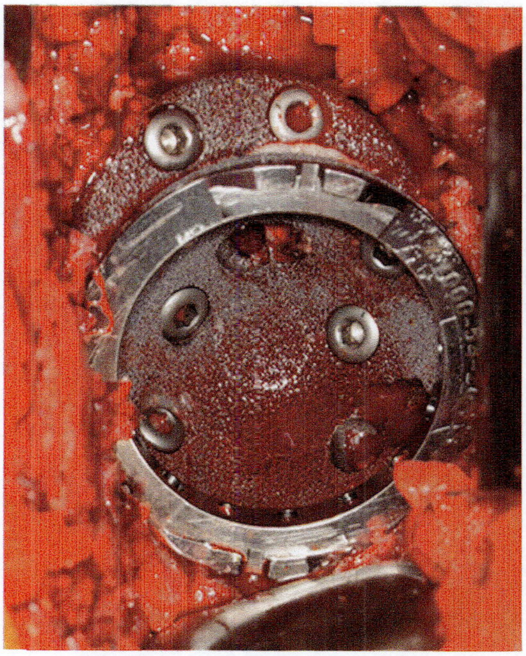

Figure 41.17 | An intraoperative picture of a highly porous augment utilized superior to the acetabular component.

Hemispherical Acetabular Component With ORIF With Compression Plating

- This technique is not discussed in this chapter as it is now rarely used in chronic discontinuity cases. In acute discontinuity cases the posterior column may be plated with a pelvic reconstruction plate and an uncemented hemispherical cup, fixed with screws, implanted.

Postoperative Care

- Generally, patients are made toe-touch weight bearing for 6 to 8 weeks and a hip guide abduction brace may be used at the discretion of the surgeon.
- Formal physical therapy is not routinely recommended as an outpatient.
- At 6 to 8 weeks, patients may advance to weight bearing as tolerated if the revision components appear stable on radiographs.

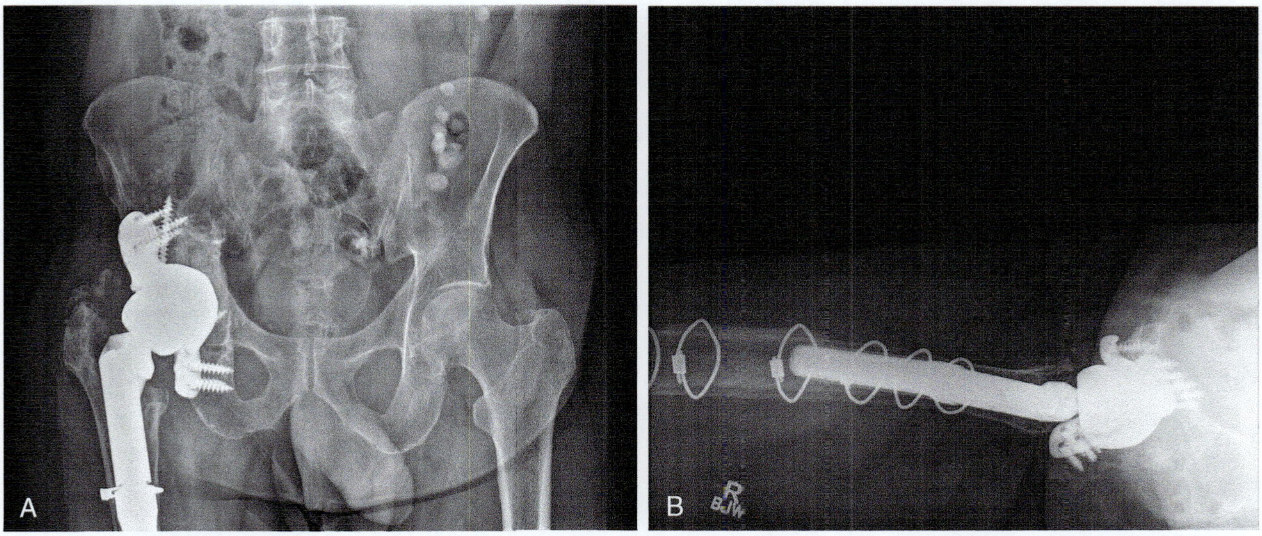

Figure 41.18 | Postoperative AP pelvis (A) and cross-table lateral (B) radiographs of a 64-year-old man with a pathologic pelvic discontinuity secondary to metastatic acinic cell carcinoma treated with a custom triflange at 1 year postoperatively.

Suggested Reading

1. Abdel MP, Trousdale RT, Berry DJ. Pelvic discontinuity associated with total hip arthroplasty: evaluation and management. *J Am Acad Orthop Surg*. 2017;25(5):330-338.
2. Martin JR, Barrett I, Sierra RJ, Lewallen DG, Berry DJ. Construct rigidity: keystone for treating pelvic discontinuity. *J Bone Joint Surg Am*. 2017;99(9):e43.
3. Martin JR, Barrett I, Sierra RJ, Lewallen DG, Berry DJ. Preoperative radiographic evaluation of patients with pelvic discontinuity. *J Arthroplast*. 2016;31(5):1053-1056.
4. Sculco PK, Ledford CK, Hanssen AD, Abdel MP, Lewallen DG. The evolution of the cup-cage technique for major acetabular defects: full and half cup-cage reconstruction. *J Bone Joint Surg Am*. 2017;99(13):1104-1110.
5. Taunton MJ, Fehring TK, Edwards P, Bernasek T, Holt GE, Christie MJ. Pelvic discontinuity treated with custom triflange component: a reliable option. *Clin Orthop Relat Res*. 2012;470(2):428-434.

Chapter 42
Heterotopic Bone

JOSHUA S. BINGHAM
MICHAEL J. TAUNTON

Key Concepts

- Radiographically evident heterotopic ossification (HO) around the hip and knee is an important clinical finding that must be carefully considered before any anticipated surgery.
- Both extrinsic (head injuries, cerebrovascular accidents, burns, ankylosing spondylitis, etc.) and intrinsic factors (injury to the abductor musculature and extensor mechanism, surgical approach, retained bone debris, and hemorrhage, etc.) contribute to the overall risk of HO.
- Patients who have previously formed heterotopic bone in the past are more likely to do so again and potentially to a greater extent after revision surgery.
- Once heterotopic bone is present on radiographs, nonoperative measures are ineffective at impeding progression of the ectopic bone formation.
- HO after joint arthroplasty most often manifests as ectopic bone in the abductor musculature in the hip and along the anterior femur adjacent to the extensor mechanism in the knee (Figures 42.1A-D and 42.2).
- Although isolated heterotopic bone excision is rarely performed, the primary indication is severe restriction in functional range of motion (ROM). Pain is not an indication for isolated excision of HO (Figure 42.3A-C).
- Excision of ectopic bone should not be performed before radiographic maturation of the heterotopic bone. Three-dimensional imaging with CT scan before surgery can define the exact location of HO and help with preoperative planning.
- Surgery through ectopic bone is associated with considerable blood loss. Coagulopathies should be corrected and anticoagulants stopped before surgery.
- External beam irradiation and nonsteroidal anti-inflammatory medications (NSAIDs) have proven extremely effective in reducing and altogether preventing severe HO in high-risk patients after revision surgery. Most surgeons prefer NSAIDs for prevention of HO in moderate-risk patients and external beam radiation in patients at high risk (such as when symptomatic HO is being excised).

Sterile Instruments and Implants

- Routine hip retractors
- Blunt elevators
- Osteotomes
- Bone wax
- Autologous blood recovery system

Positioning

- *Hip:* The patient is placed in a lateral decubitus position, which allows for a more extensile exposure if needed.
- *Knee:* The patient is supine with an ipsilateral bump under the pelvis and tourniquet placed proximally around the thigh.
- Draping should allow for adequate access for any extensile approach.

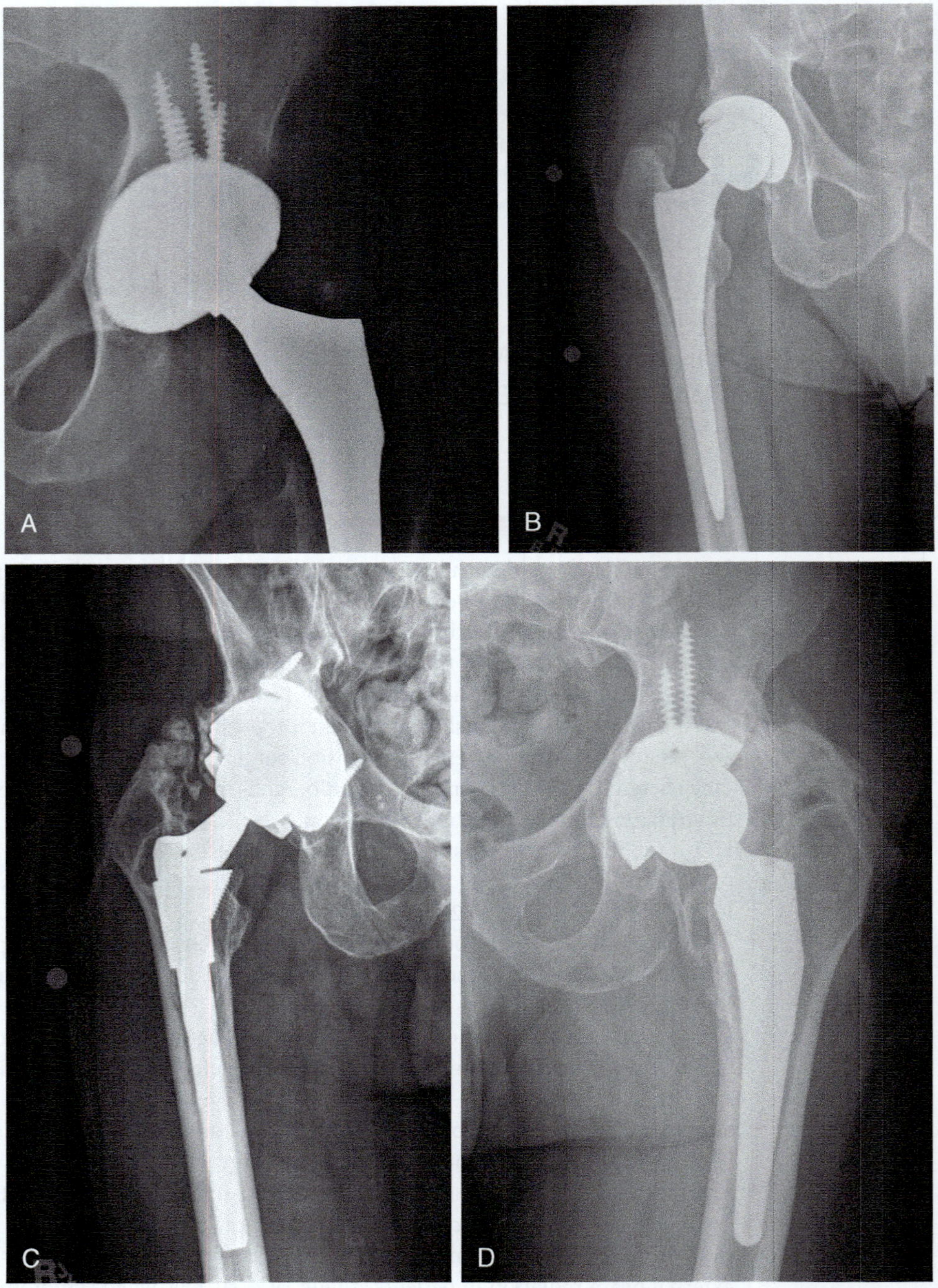

Figure 42.1 | Anteroposterior hip radiographs of heterotopic ossification around the hip. A, Grade I. B, Grade II. C, Grade III. D, Grade IV.

Surgical Approaches

- *Hip:* The preferred approach of the authors in the majority of revision total hip arthroplasty is an extensile posterior approach. However, the operative approach for HO excision should be tailored to the location of the HO. The goal is effective HO excision and preservation of muscle tissue to the degree possible.
- The skin incision is dictated partly by previous incisions but should be based on the planned operative approach.
- In cases with extensive heterotopic bone present, and when wide exposure is needed for complex femoral or acetabular reconstruction, a trochanteric osteotomy can be performed both for exposure purposes and to help protect and maintain the remaining abductor musculature.
- *Knee:* The preferred approach for the authors is an extensile medial parapatellar approach.

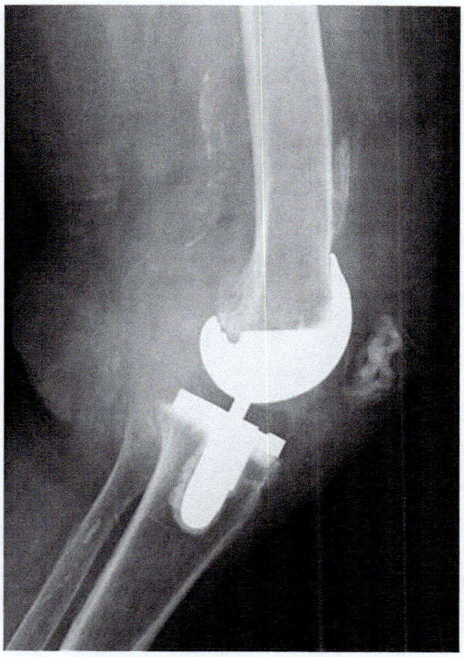

Figure 42.2 | Lateral radiograph of heterotopic ossification along the anterior femur.

- The skin incision is dictated by the previous incisions, but ideally the most lateral usable incision is chosen. If there is any concern for wound issues, there should be a low threshold to involve our plastic surgery colleagues in helping plan the skin incision and to prepare for any subsequent soft tissue procedure that may be required.

Preoperative Planning

- Preoperative orthogonal radiographs (anteroposterior [AP] and lateral) of the involved joint are critical for the appropriate surgical planning.
- Brooker et al classification of HO around the hip based on the AP pelvic radiograph is the most commonly used classification system for Hip HO (Table 42.1 and Figure 42.4):
- A preoperative computed tomography (CT) scan with metal artifact suppression can be helpful in defining the location of the HO and soft tissue structures within or displaced by the mass of ectopic bone. Careful preoperative evaluation may reduce the risk of intraoperative injury of vital structures (Figure 42.5).

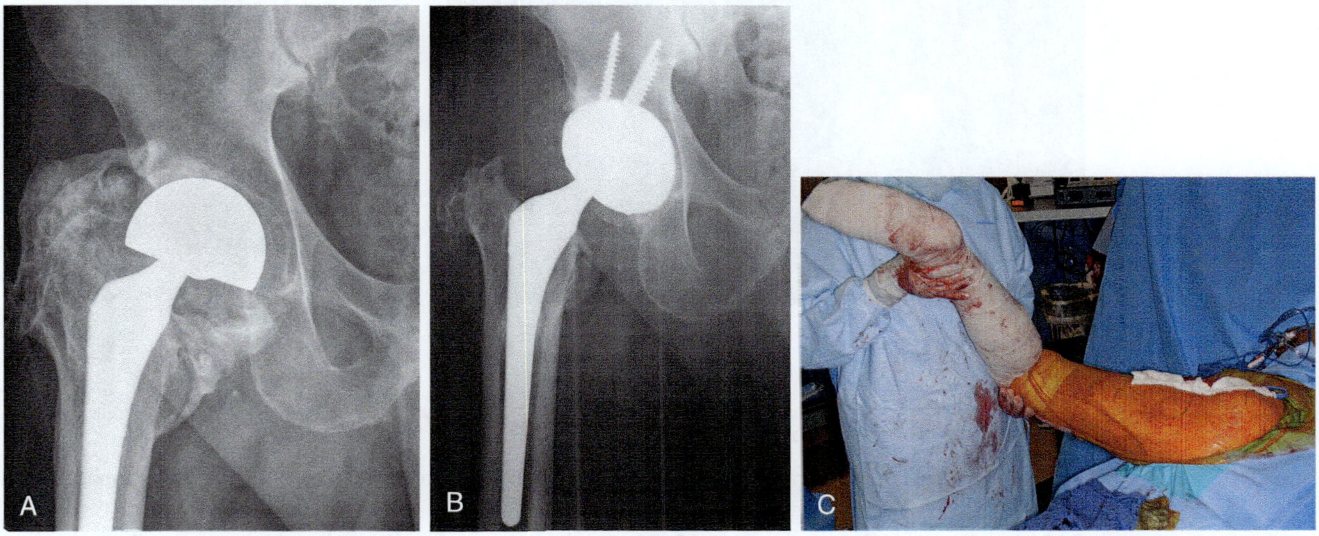

Figure 42.3 | A, Preoperative radiograph of grade IV heterotopic ossification before excision and acetabular revision for severe limited functional range of motion. B, Postoperative radiograph after excision of grade IV heterotopic ossification. C Intraoperative photograph of the improved hip range of motion after excision.

Table 42.1 | Brooker et al Classification of Heterotopic Ossification Around the Hip Based on the Anteroposterior Hip Radiograph

Brooker Classification of Heterotopic Ossification Around the Hip Joint	
Grade	**Description**
I	Islands of bone in the soft tissue
II	Bone spurs arising from the pelvis of proximal femur with at least 1 cm between the bone surfaces
III	Bone spurs arising from the pelvis of proximal femur with less than 1 cm between the bone surfaces
IV	Bridging of pelvis and proximal femur bone spurs; bony ankyloses of the hip

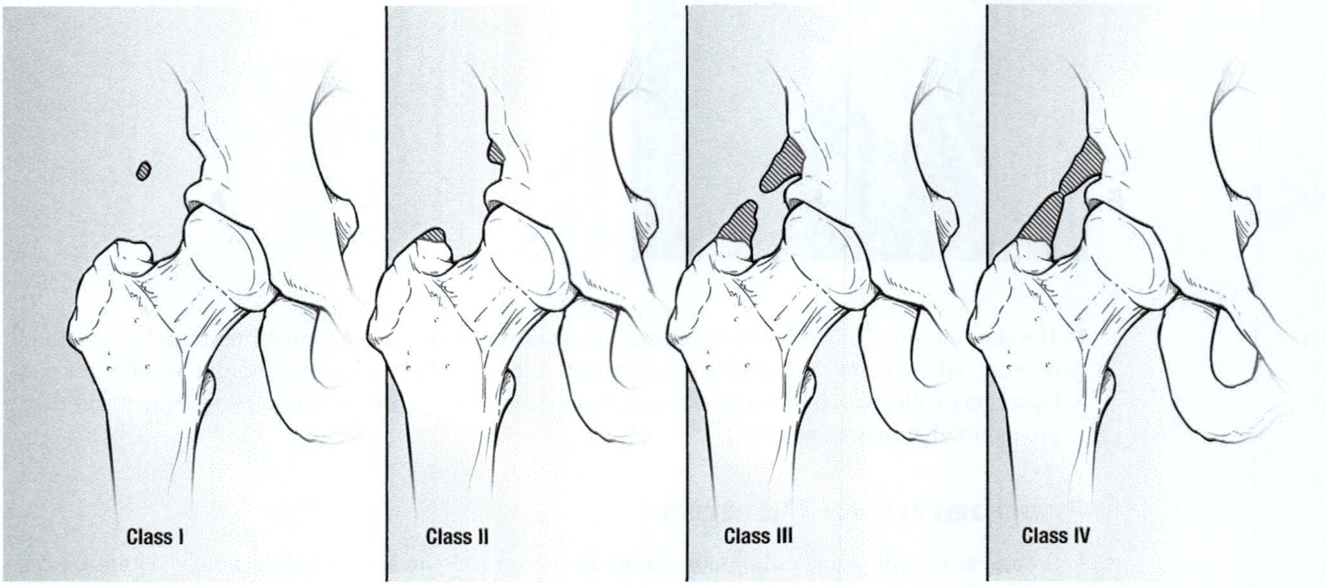

Figure 42.4 | Illustration of the Brooker et al classification of heterotopic ossification around the hip based on the anteroposterior hip radiograph.

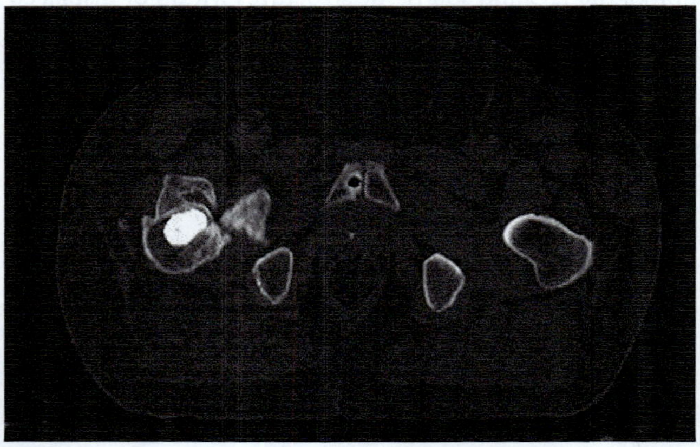

Figure 42.5 | Preoperative CT scan before heterotopic ossification excision to help define HO location and the anatomic relationship of HO to nearby soft tissue structures.

Bone, Implant, and Soft Tissue Techniques

- Isolated surgical excision of HO or revision through HO should not be performed before maturation of the ectopic bone.
- Maturation of HO can take up to 12–24 months to occur. Traditionally a bone scan and serum alkaline phosphatase levels have been used to monitor both the activity and resolution of the pathologic process (Figure 42.6).

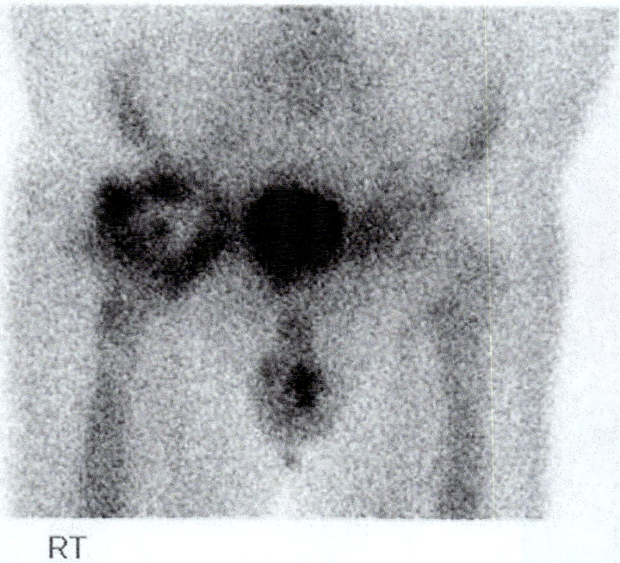

Figure 42.6 | Bone scan of a pelvis demonstrating immature heterotopic ossification. Heterotopic ossification excision should not be performed until after maturation.

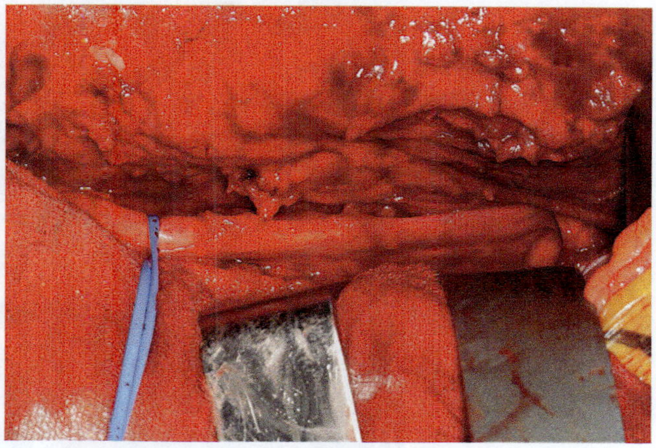

Figure 42.7 | Intraoperative photograph demonstrating careful dissection of the sciatic nerve from the heterotopic ossification before excision.

- In patients with severe HO, careful consideration must be given to the critical soft tissue structures around the ectopic bone. Most commonly the ectopic bone displaces the soft tissue structures from their normal anatomic location, but it can also incarcerate critical structures.
- The surgical approach most commonly used in revision arthroplasty in the setting of HO is the same approach as the index procedure but should be chosen to provide access to the HO.
- After incision, operative dissection though the soft tissue around the ectopic bone should be done slowly and with care as dissection around critical soft tissue structures will increase the risk of traction-related and direct iatrogenic injuries (Figure 42.7).
- Generally there will be a fibrous plan between the ectopic bone and the native soft tissues.
- Sharp dissection of the bone mass should be avoided. Blunt dissection of normal structures away from the ectopic bone at the periphery should be the operative strategy with the use of a blunt elevator. Electrocautery is effective for dividing strong soft tissue attachments to the HO.
- Final separation and removal of the bone mass may require division of the HO mass from underlying host bone with an osteotome or saw. Fresh bone surfaces may be coated with bone wax to reduce bleeding. Some believe this also reduces the risk of HO recurrence (Figure 42.8).
- In addition to removing the ectopic bone, often circumferential excision of the hip capsule around the hip or extensive release of the collateral ligaments in conjunction with resection of any remaining posterior cruciate ligament in the knee is required to maximize improvement in ROM.
- Excision of large amounts of heterotopic bone is accompanied with the risk of destabilizing the hip and potentially creating a permanent limp secondary to inadequate remaining abductor muscle mass. Attention to soft tissue preservation, especially muscle, during the operation is important.
- Preoperatively, the patient should be apprised of the risk of requiring a cane indefinitely after surgery. Unwillingness to use a cane postoperatively is a relative contraindication to surgical excision of HO around the hip.
- There is a propensity for increased blood loss when operating though soft tissue with ectopic bone. Preoperatively any coagulopathies present should be corrected, anticoagulants stopped, and the patient should be typed and cross-matched with blood products available throughout the perioperative period.
- Intraoperatively an autologous blood recovery system can help decrease the need of transfusion.
- In the setting of HO excision around the knee considerable bleeding may also occur around the periosteum. Bone wax can be utilized to help control the bleeding as cautery often is not effective.
- Postoperatively the surgeon should be wary of an increased risk of symptomatic postoperative hematoma.

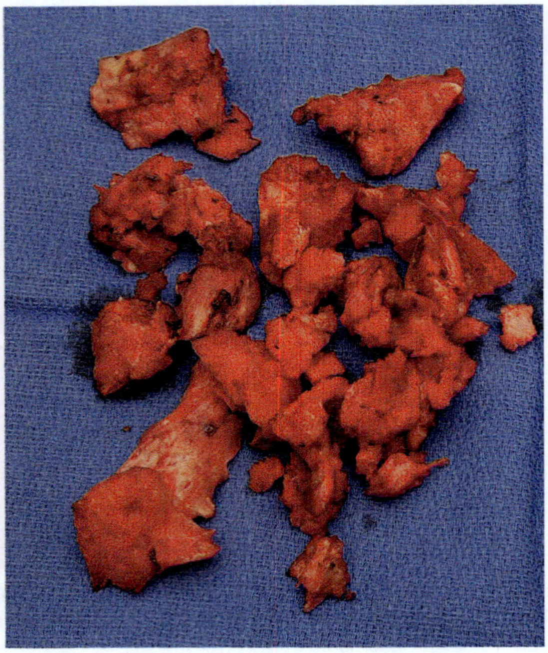

Figure 42.8 | Bluntly dissected heterotopic ossification fragments after excision.

Postoperative Care

- The most common complication after HO excision is recurrence of HO, and often it is more severe than before revision surgery. Without HO prophylaxis, recurrence is almost guaranteed.
- Abductor weakness can be common after HO excision, often necessitating cane use, and is directly related to the amount of abductor mass loss from the heterotopic bone formation and excision.
- Limited ROM around the knee after HO excision is often seen and flexion to 90° should be considered an excellent result. Early physical therapy should be utilized to help maintain ROM after surgery.
- External beam irradiation and NSAIDs have been the most studied and widely utilized interventions for the prevention of HO. Bisphosphonates have previously been used but have been abandoned as these agents only delay the appearance of HO by blocking mineralization of the osteoid matrix.

External Beam Irradiation

- Perioperative single-dose administration of 700 to 800 cGy within 6 hours before surgery or 72 hours postoperatively has been shown to effectively eliminate grade III and IV HO and reduce the rate of grade I and II to 10 to 20% in high-risk patients.
- It is our preference to administer a single dose of 700 to 800 cGy <4 hours preoperatively or <72 hours postoperatively. Preoperative dosing eliminates the concerns for dislocation with transfers in the early postoperative period and is advantageous for both planning and scheduling purposes. However, it does not allow the surgeon to shield newly placed uncemented components from radiation as precisely as does application of shielded postoperative radiation.
- Limited field radiation using an obliquely oriented rectangular portal centered over the joint space and oriented parallel to the acetabular component effectively excludes the ingrowth hip components in most cases, thereby reducing theoretic concern for impaired bone ingrowth of cementless complements (Figure 42.9).
- Relative contraindications for external beam irradiation include patients younger than 40 years and patients with prior radiation for a cancer diagnosis in order to avoid a cumulative effective radiation dose in the toxic range.
- Women of childbearing age should not receive radiation prophylaxis for HO.

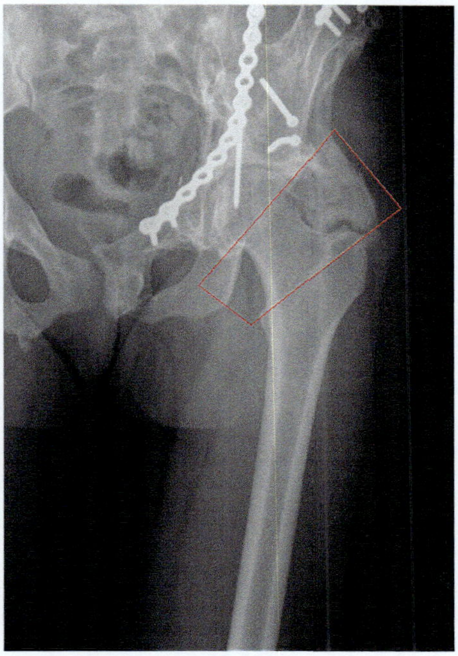

Figure 42.9 | Limited field radiation using an obliquely oriented rectangular portal centered over the joint space excluding the ingrowth hip components.

Nonsteroidal Anti-inflammatory Medications

- Indomethacin 25 mg TID (or once daily 75 mg sustained release) administered for 10 days is the authors' preferred choice for NSAID HO prophylaxis.
- Similar to irradiation, NSAIDs have been shown to effectively eliminate grade III and IV HO and reduce grade I and II to <10% in high-risk patients.
- Prospective controlled trials have failed to show a statistically significant difference between a single dose of postoperative radiation and a daily divided dose of 75 mg indomethacin in preventing HO around the hip.
- Relative contraindications for NSAID HO prophylaxis include end-stage kidney disease, peptic ulcer disease, and a history of prior gastrointestinal bleeding.
- Patients receiving NSAID HO prophylaxis should also receive a gastroprotective agent during their course of treatment.

Chapter 43
Abductor Muscle Repair/ Reconstruction

ADAM HART
RAFAEL J. SIERRA

Key Concepts

- Abductor deficiency following total hip replacement is a major problem that may lead to pain, Trendelenburg gait, and instability. Multiple etiologies should be considered:
  - Prior anterolateral (transgluteal) approach to the hip resulting in
    - Failure of the abductor repair (Figure 43.1A), or
    - Injury to the superior gluteal nerve.
  - Periprosthetic fracture of the greater trochanter occurring intraoperatively or postoperatively (Figure 43.1B).
  - Adverse local soft tissue reaction with destruction of the abductors (Figure 43.1C).
- Abductor deficiency generally presents as 3 distinct clinical scenarios:
  - Moderate abductor deficiency and limp, often with some lateral hip pain, but without total hip arthroplasty instability. This is most commonly seen after hip replacement performed through an anterolateral approach with a failed abductor tendon repair.
  - Severe abductor-related Trendelenburg limp with varying degrees of pain. This may present in the setting of a trochanteric avulsion fracture or when there is complete avulsion of the abductor mechanism from the trochanter.
  - Recurrent dislocations of the hip in association with abductor deficiency. In cases in which there is no apparent etiology for the dislocation, abductor muscle necrosis as seen in cases with severe taper corrosion should be investigated.

Sterile Instruments and Implants

- Perioperative—consider the use of tranexamic acid, local and regional anesthesia
- Heavy Ethibond sutures for tendon reattachment and Fiberwire sutures for tendon reinforcement
- High-speed burr
- Fresh frozen Achilles allograft (when allograft augmentation is planned)

Surgical Approaches

- Anterolateral or posterolateral according to surgeon preference. The authors prefer a posterior approach, splitting the gluteus maximus near its midportion so that a gluteus maximus muscle transfer may be utilized if needed.

Preoperative Planning

- Detailed history and physical examination are essential. Onset and severity of symptoms should be clarified. The operative note from the index surgery should be reviewed to determine the approach, implants, and any pertinent intraoperative findings. The examination should assess the patient's abductor strength, presence of an antalgic gait or Trendelenburg gait, and tenderness over the greater trochanter.

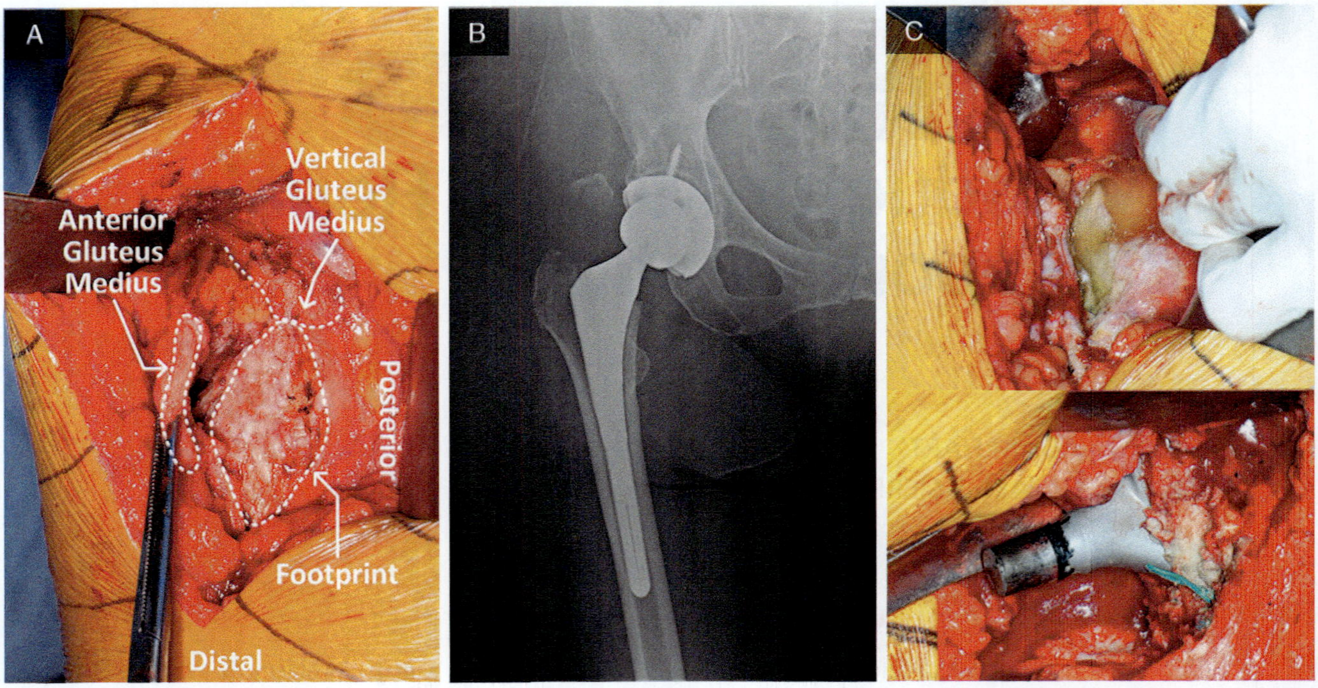

Figure 43.1 | Abductor deficiency etiologies: failure of the anterior head of gluteus medius to heal to the greater trochanter footprint but intact attachment of the vertical head following hip replacement through an anterolateral approach (A), avulsion fracture of the greater trochanter following total hip replacement (B), and large cystic pseudotumor with significant destruction of the abductors secondary to trunionosis (C).

- Radiographs of the hip to assess the current implants and presence of a greater trochanter fracture.
- Magnetic resonance imaging (MRI) evaluation using metal suppression provides valuable information on the tear morphology and status of the gluteal muscles. In particular, fatty infiltration of the abductors should be assessed on the axial T1 sequence (Figure 43.2). Fatty atrophy of the anterior two-thirds of the gluteus minimus is common, whereas significant fatty atrophy of the gluteus medius portends a poor prognosis following repair and may prompt the surgeon to use a muscle transfer.
- An electromyography study is indicated to confirm and quantify a gluteal nerve injury when suspected.

Bone, Implant, and Soft Tissue Techniques

- Abductor repair—When preoperative MRI demonstrates reasonable muscle quality of the gluteus medius, a direct repair with augmentation is the preferred treatment.
    - Exposure is according to the surgeon's preference and may utilize the previous incision. The fascia is opened in-line with the femur distally, and the author's preference is to split the gluteus maximus near its midportion such that a transfer may be performed if needed.

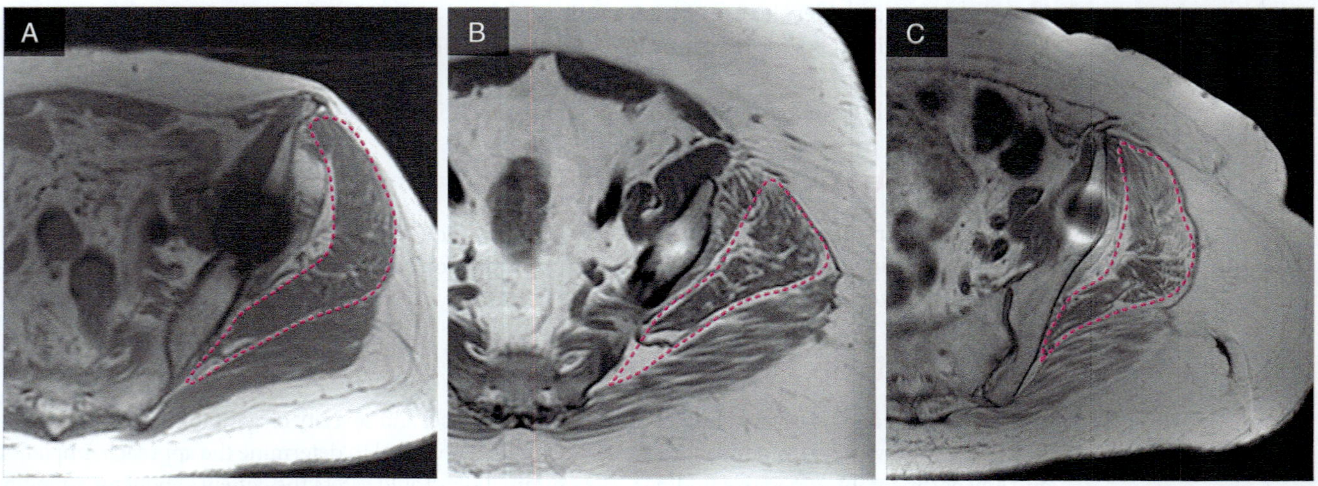

Figure 43.2 | Axial T1 MRI in 3 patients with abductor deficiency demonstrating increasing fatty infiltration from A to C of the gluteus medius (delineated by the dotted lines).

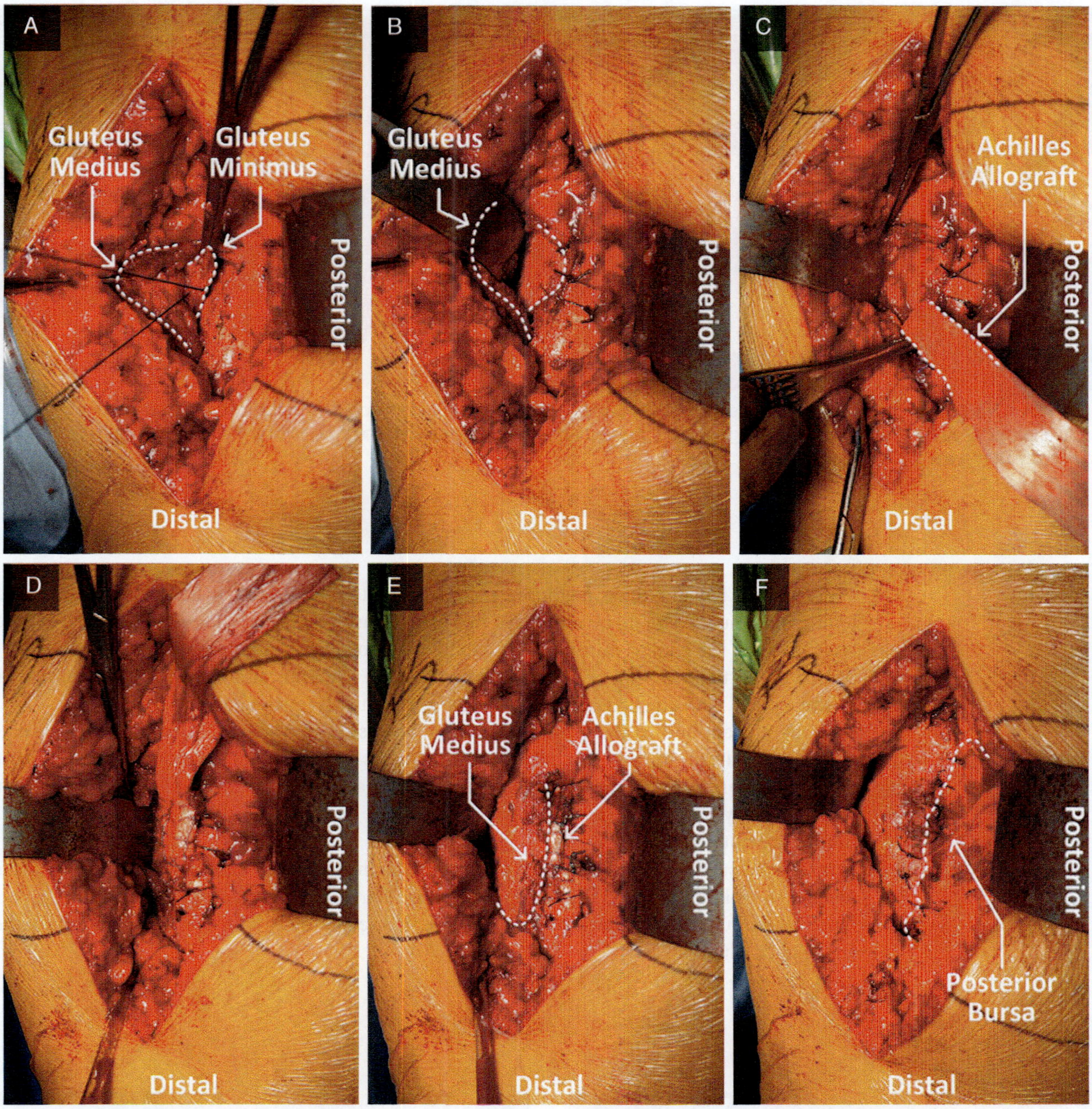

Figure 43.3 | Direct repair of the gluteus minimus and medius with Achilles allograft augmentation. Development of flaps from torn sections of gluteus minimus and medius (A), reattachment of the gluteus minimus with 4 transosseous sutures (B), anchoring of the Achilles tendon to the vastus lateralis (C), reinforcement of the gluteus minimus repair with the Achilles allograft using Krackow sutures (D), reattachment of the gluteus medius (E), and concealing the sutures by covering the repair with bursal tissue (F).

- There is often hypertrophied bursa and scar tissue overlying the greater trochanter—we attempt to divide this tissue to expose the underlying vastus and gluteus medius. This tissue sometimes is useful to close overtop the repair when possible (Figure 43.3F).
- The anterior fibers of gluteus medius are almost invariably detached along the anterior aspect of the trochanter, whereas the posterior (vertical) fibers usually are still attached (Figure 43.1A). Oftentimes, there is fluid around the injured tendon and the attachment site (footprint) of the tendon has a shiny and scarred appearance (Figures 43.4A and 43.5).
- After delineating the portion of the gluteus medius that is torn from the portion that is still well attached, use the cautery to lift the torn tendon and develop a full-thickness flap (Figure 43.3A). The detached muscle and tendon can be further mobilized by gently running a Cobb elevator above and below.

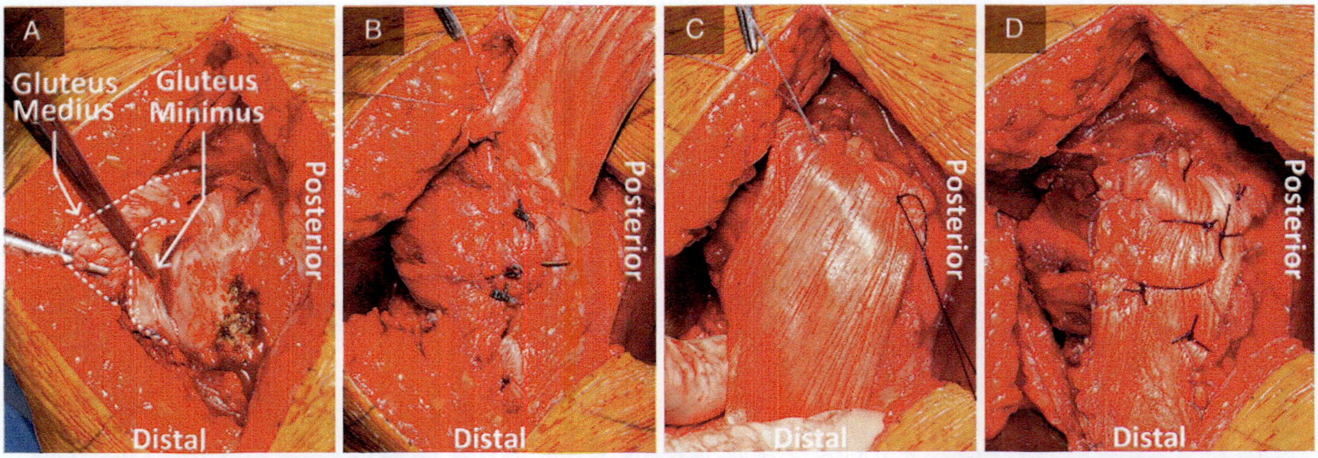

Figure 43.4 | Direct repair of the gluteus minimus and medius with Achilles allograft augmentation. Delineation of the torn tendons with surrounding fluid and scar tissue (A), reattachment of the gluteus minims and Achilles allograft reinforcement (B), folding of the Achilles tendon overtop the repaired gluteus medius (C-D).

- With the torn flap of gluteus medius retracted, the gluteus minimus can be examined. If torn, the tendon and muscle should be mobilized in a similar fashion (Figures 43.3A and 43.4A). Separate attachment of the gluteus minimus is preferable but not always attainable.
- At this point, the footprint of the gluteus medius +/− minimus attachment is now exposed and freshened to a bleeding bed of bone using a 4.5-mm burr (Figure 43.6).
- Allis clamps applied to the tendon flaps should ensure there is sufficient mobility to reach the exposed bone on the trochanter. In rare cases in which the tendons are significantly retracted, a bridging technique using the Achilles allograft (or other allograft or synthetic material) may be used to span the gap. This is rare, and the results of these bridging techniques are not good.
- Transosseous sutures (#5 Ethibond) are placed through the trochanter and passed through the gluteus medius +/− minimus tendon flaps using a Masson-Allen technique (Figures 43.3B and 43.4B).
- Once all the sutures have been passed, they are tied sequentially with the leg in neutral rotation and slight abduction.

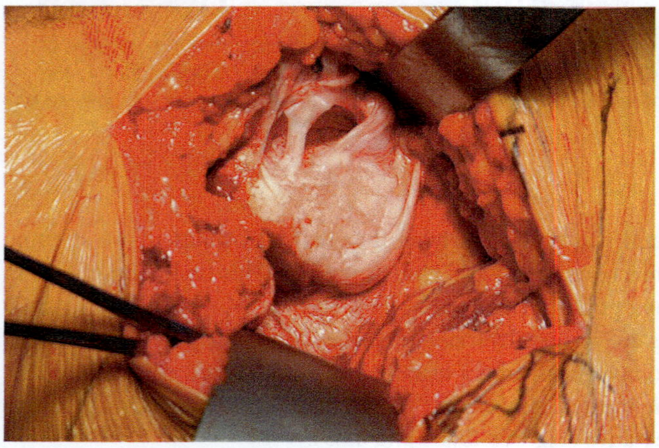

Figure 43.5 | Typical appearance of a chronic abductor deficiency demonstration scarred and atrophied detachment of the anterior portion of gluteus medius with surrounding fluid.

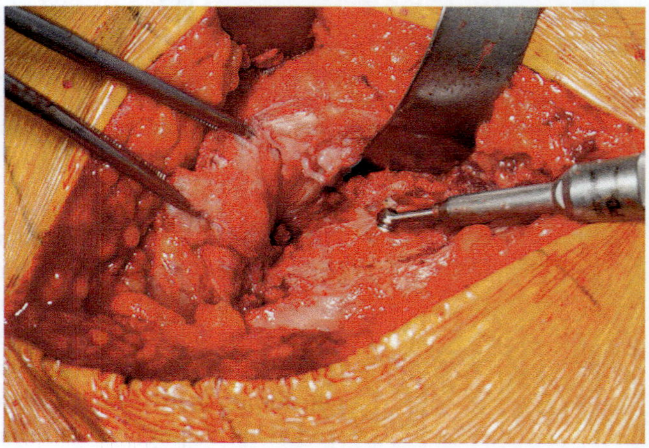

Figure 43.6 | A burr is used to debride the attachment site of the gluteus medius on the greater trochanter.

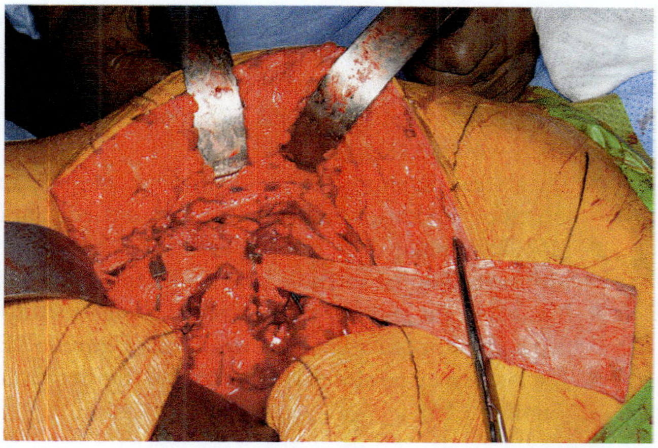

Figure 43.7 | Alternative technique to secure the Achilles allograft using cables and calcaneal bone block.

- Achilles allograft reinforcement—Despite a solid repair of the abductor tendons to the trochanter, augmentation with an Achilles allograft provides additional strength to the repair and is used routinely by the authors.
  - The vastus lateralis fascia and underlying muscle is divided and retracted approximately 4 cm distal to the vastus ridge. The distal end of the Achilles allograft is then placed over the femur and anchored by sutures into the vastus fascia (Figure 43.3C). Alternatively, a calcaneal bone block from the Achilles allograft may be fashioned into a square and countersunk into the femur and secured with 2 cables (Figure 43.7).
  - The Achilles allograft is then draped over the abductor repair and sutured to the tendon using a Krackow suture with FiberWire along the anterior, posterior, and superior boarders (Figures 43.3D and 43.4C).
    - When the gluteus minimus is torn, the allograft may be placed overtop the minimus repair and underneath the gluteus medius repair thereby creating a sandwich between the 2 tendons (Figure 43.3E).
    - After passing the allograft proximally, it may be folded overtop and sutured a second time to the repair for further reinforcement (Figure 43.4C and D).
  - In situations in which the gluteus medius flap is tenuous or cannot reach the trochanter, the allograft (or an alternative synthetic material) may be used to bridge the gap (Figure 43.6).
- Gluteus maximus transfer (Figure 43.8)—In situations in which the gluteal muscles exhibit fatty atrophy on preoperative MRI or have been significantly damaged (for example, a large pseudotumor), a local muscle transfer is recommended. The authors prefer a gluteus maximus transfer; however, tenodesis of the tensor fascia lata and vastus lateralis is an alternative option, especially if the greater trochanter is deficient or fractured.

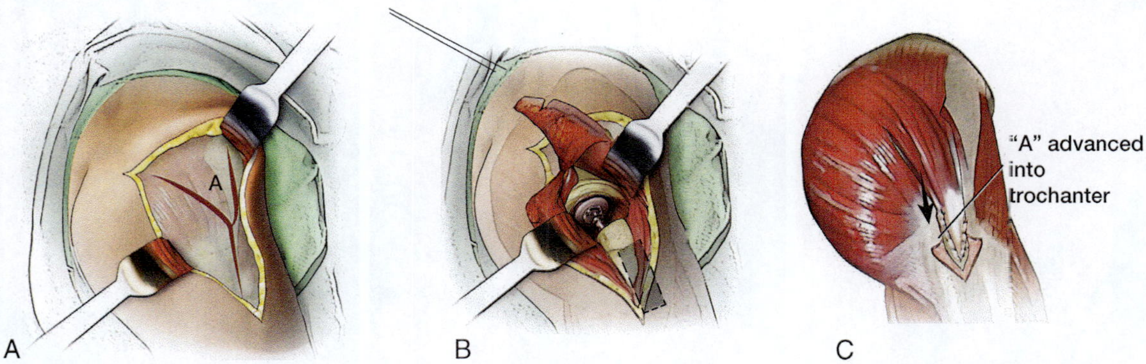

Figure 43.8 | Gluteus maximus transfer: planned division of gluteus maximus (A), attachment of distal flap (B) and proximal flap (C) to the greater trochanter.

- After exposing the hip, the abductors are evaluated and the decision to proceed with a gluteus maximus transfer is confirmed. Any remnant gluteus medius and minimus should be developed into an anterior flap if possible (Figure 43.9A).
- Wide exposure of the gluteus maximus, extending anteriorly to the junction of the tensor fascia lata is required (Figure 43.9B).
- The gluteus maximus was divided near its midportion (during the hip approach) and next at the junction with tensor fascia lata to create a triangular flap (Figure 43.9C).
- Mobilize this flap distally to the trochanter (and ideally to the vastus lateralis) where it is anchored with several nonabsorbable heavy sutures (Figure 43.9D).
- If possible, the anterior portion of the gluteus medius is attached overtop of the gluteus maximus flap and unitized with Krackow sutures (Figure 43.9E and F).
- The fascia may be closed overtop of the transfer distally but will have to remain open proximally (Figure 43.10).

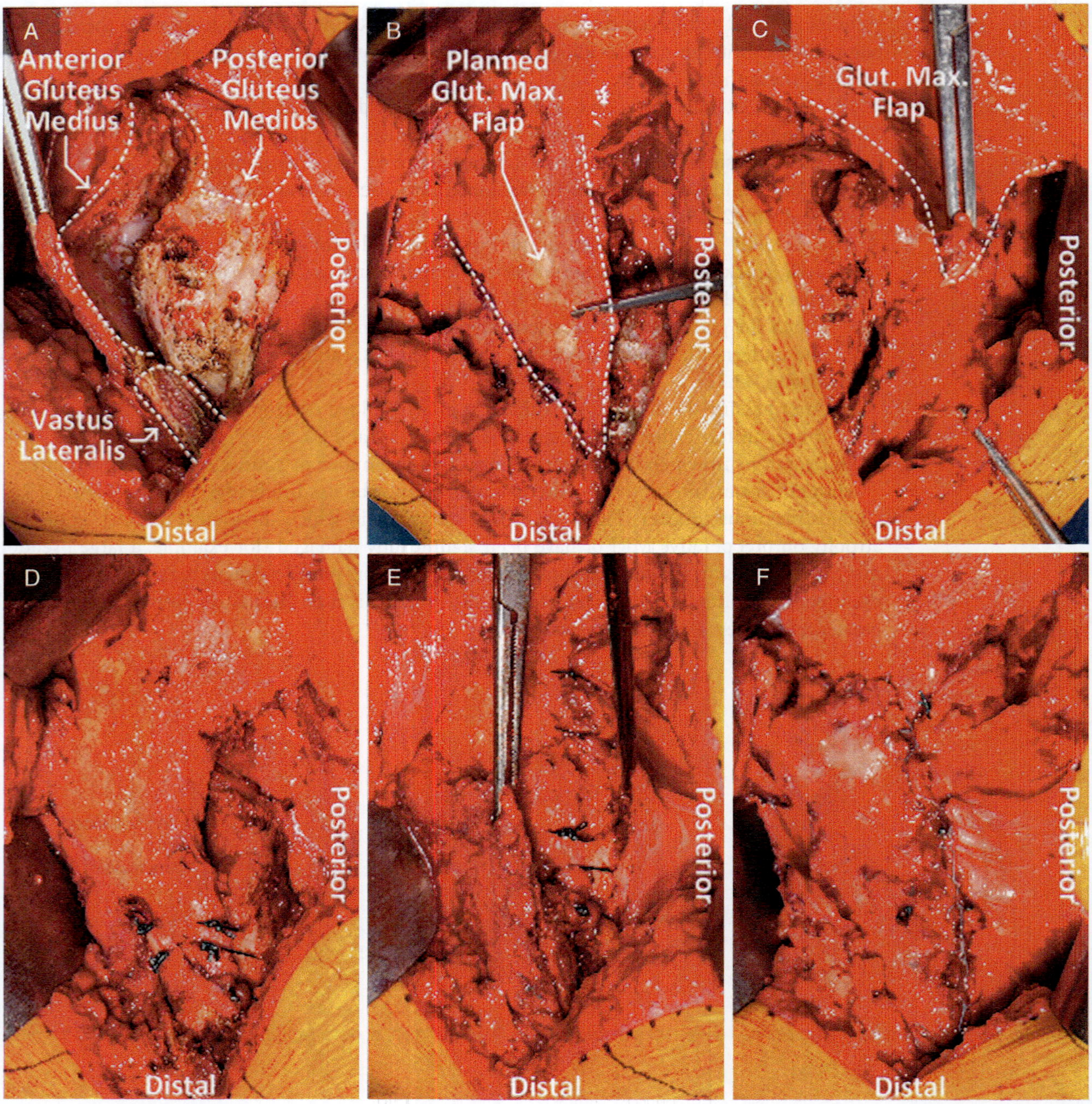

Figure 43.9 | Gluteus maximus transfer. Atrophic and scarred anterior fibers of the gluteus medius created into a flap (A), exposure of the gluteus maximus and planning of a triangular flap (B), creation and mobilization of the flap (C), and attachment to the trochanter (D), closure of the gluteus medius and bursal tissue overtop of the gluteus maximus transfer and unitization with Krackow sutures (E-F).

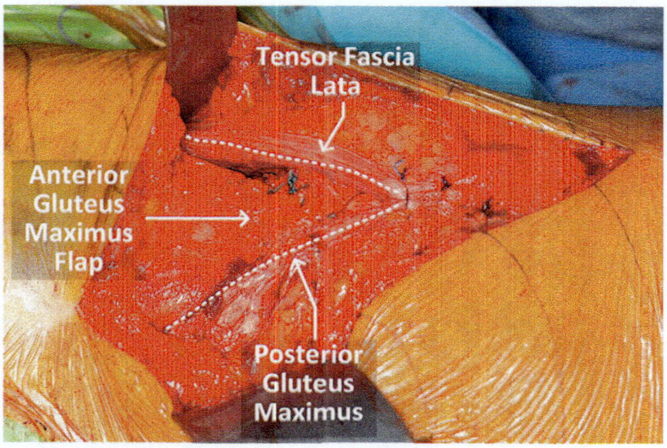

Figure 43.10 | Closure following gluteus maximus transfer.

Postoperative Care

- An abduction pillow is used postoperatively, and the patient is kept in bed until a hip spica cast is placed on the first postoperative day. The hip spica cast maintains the hip in approximately 20° of abduction and 30° of flexion. We apply the hip spica for 6 weeks and then transition to a hip abduction brace for an additional 6 weeks. The patient is toe-touch weight bearing for this period of time.
- Following the spica cast and bracing, physical therapy is initiated for progressive abductor strengthening.

Part III
Primary Knee

Chapter 44
Preoperative Planning/Templating/Limb Alignment for Primary Total Knee Arthroplasty

TIMOTHY B. ALTON
MARK W. PAGNANO

Introduction

- Preoperative planning in total knee arthroplasty helps surgeons visualize the bone cuts and decrease intraoperative errors regarding implant size and alignment (Figure 44.1).
- Preoperative planning can identify the need for nonstandard implants and identify major extra-articular deformities that require osteotomy or an alternative surgical technique.
- Digital templating allows fast, precise, calibrated measurements and digital storage in the electronic medical record for access at the time of surgery.
- Weight bearing radiographs in the anteroposterior and posteroanterior projections are very helpful for accurate planning.
- Full-length radiographs of the hip-knee-ankle are particularly useful when substantial extra-articular deformity is present or suspected and serve as a useful reminder to rule out hip pathology in every patient presenting with knee pain.

History

- Detailed medical history to identify risks for bony abnormalities
  - Prior trauma or infection in hip, femur, tibia, ankle, or foot
  - History of Paget disease, rickets, congenital or developmental conditions
  - Think specifically about extra-articular deformity
- Detailed surgical history focused on lower extremity
  - Prior hip, femur, tibia, ankle, or foot surgery that might impact overall limb alignment or have caused a neurovascular problem.

Physical Examination

- Observe patient standing and walking.
  - Identify and document gait abnormalities, coronal plane deformities, foot drop, pes planovalgus, knee hyperextension, etc.
- Examination of operative knee.
  - Evaluate ipsilateral hip to rule out hip pathology manifesting as knee pain.
  - Evaluate knee range of motion; identify and document preoperative contractures, coronal plane instability, and patellar stability.
  - Carefully examine the skin for open sores and prior incisions, then treat or plan accordingly.

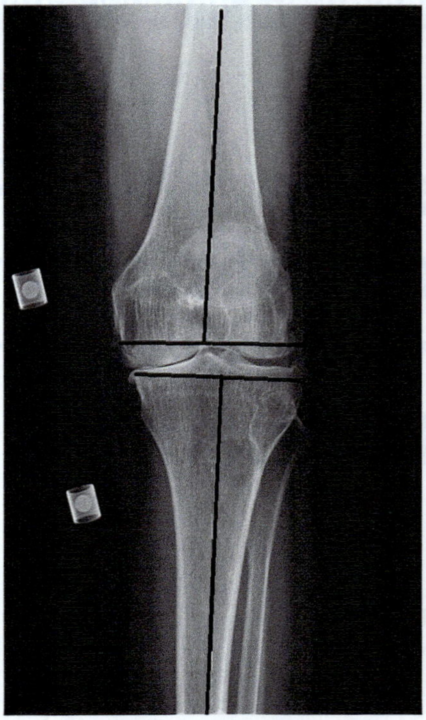

Figure 44.1 | Coronal plane femoral and tibial bone resections drawn on the anteroposterior radiograph.

Radiographs

- Four views
  - Standing AP, PA weight bearing flexed, lateral, and patella sunrise views (Figure 44.2A-D).
  - Consider full-length hip-knee-ankle AP radiographs when evaluating coronal plane deformity (Figure 44.3). Another choice is EOS to image the entire body (Figure 44.4A and B). Full-length radiographs are particularly valuable in patients with substantial extra-articular deformity in whom a decision between intra-articular correction alone or combined osteotomy and total knee are being contemplated.
  - Extra-articular deformities further from the knee joint or smaller in angular deviation are more likely to be correctable with total knee alone ("correction through the joint"). In contrast, those deformities that are closer to the joint or that are larger in angular deviation are more likely to require osteotomy ("correction outside the joint") either staged or combined with the total knee.
  - Various, sometimes confusing, rules have been proposed to determine when osteotomy is required. One very pragmatic method is to template mechanical axis cuts on a hip-knee-ankle radiograph. If the projected femoral cut compromises an epicondyle, then osteotomy is a better choice. On the tibial side, a line is projected from the center of the talus through the center of that part of the tibial shaft that is distal to the deformity. If the proximal extension of that distal tibial shaft line passes outside the tibial plateau, then osteotomy is a better choice. Similarly, if the deformity is very close to the tibial plateau and there is no room for the tibial stem, keel, or pegs, then osteotomy is needed.

Templating

Goals

- To ensure the alignment targets are accurately hit during surgery
  - Visibly draw the projected femoral, tibial, and patellar resection levels preoperatively to act as an intraoperative guide and secondary check. This simple step can occasionally avoid mistakes from human errors such as inadvertently setting a guide for right versus left or confusing 6° and 9°, for instance.
  - Most surgeons continue to use mechanical axis principles and aim to cut both the distal femur and proximal tibia perpendicular to the mechanical axis.
  - Recognition of current tibial slope versus desired correction based on implants to be used (Figure 44.5A and B).

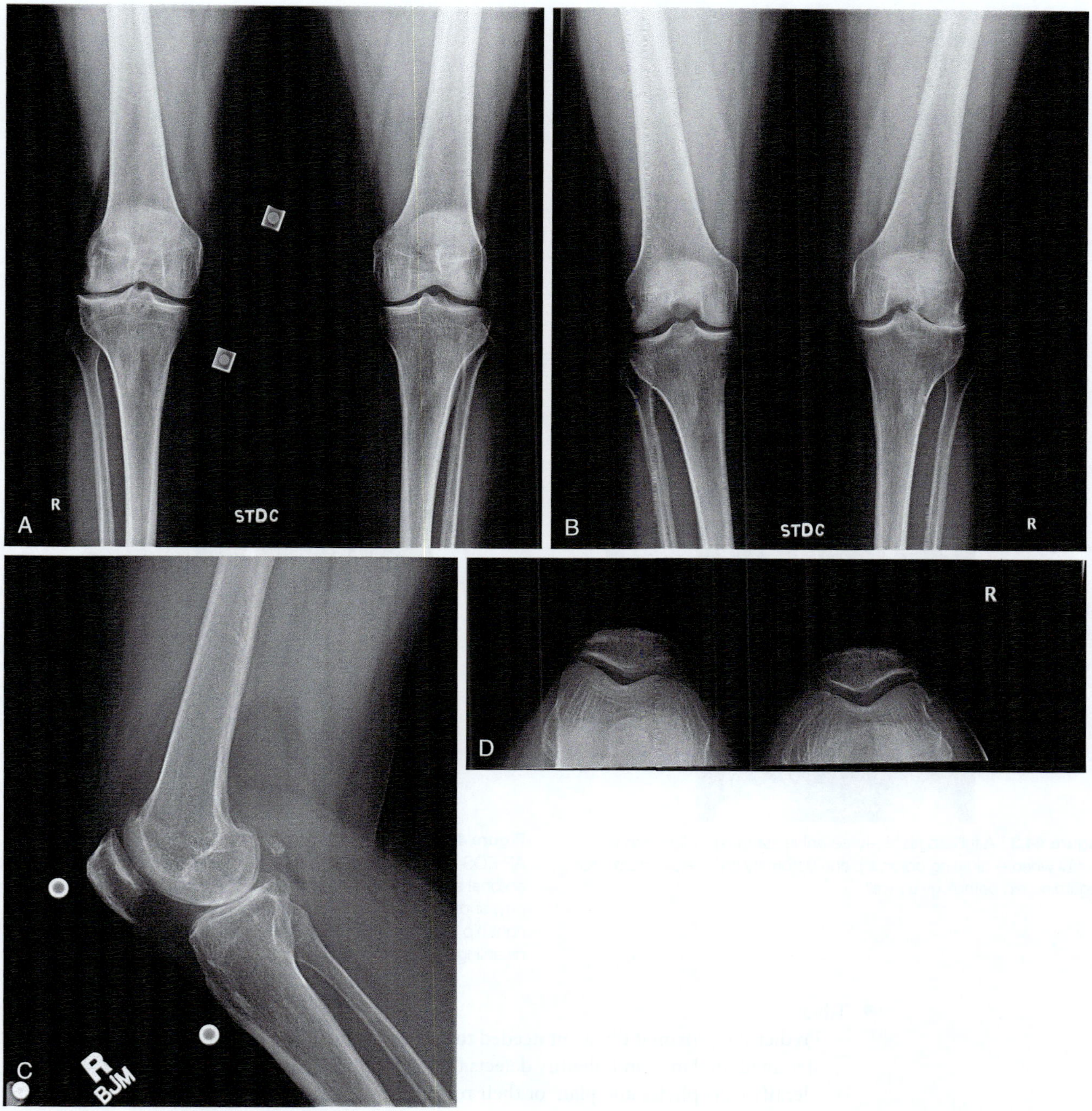

Figure 44.2 | Four views of the knee are ideal for assessment of the patient with knee arthritis and include (A) standing AP, (B) weight bearing PA flexion, (C) lateral, and (D) patellar views. The weight bearing PA flexion view is particularly useful for evaluating patients with suspected lateral compartment arthritis as in this example.

- Identify patients with substantial extra-articular deformity who may require either higher levels of constraint or a combined osteotomy and total knee.
- Correct implant sizing:
  - Decrease risk of oversizing or undersizing femoral or tibial components.
  - Identify excessively thin or thick patellar bone and plan resection accordingly.
  - Streamline implant inventory.
- Assess bone and deformity:
  - Femur:
    - Recognize distal femoral deformity from prior fracture, hypoplastic femoral condyle, retained hardware.
    - Anticipate need for stems (severe flexion contracture, poor distal femur bone quality) and increased constraint (severe coronal plane deformity).
    - Identify posterior osteophytes and plan for their resection.

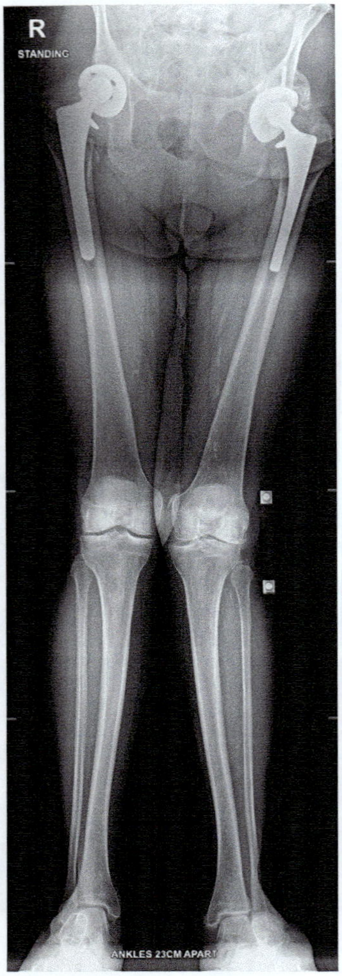

Figure 44.3 | A full-length hip-knee-ankle standing radiograph is useful when evaluating coronal plane deformity and yields information regarding hip pathology as well.

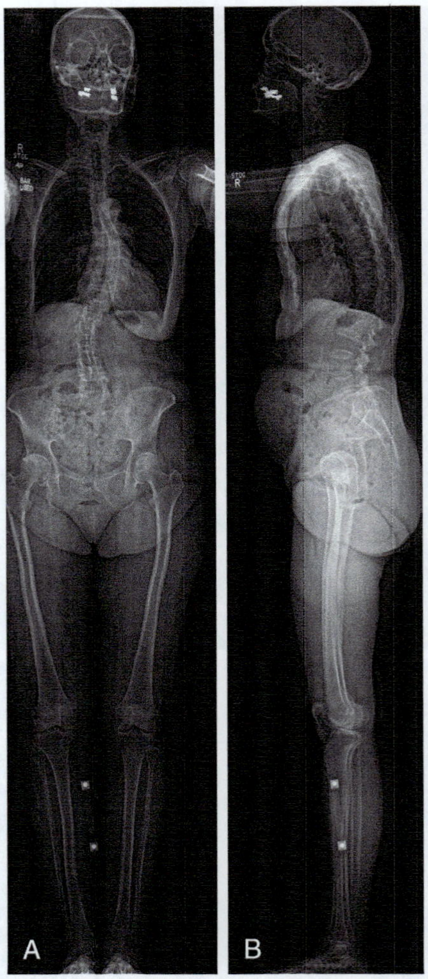

Figure 44.4 | Another contemporary imaging option is EOS. The (A) AP EOS projection and (B) lateral EOS projection can be assessed for coronal and sagittal plane deformity, allows assessment of hip pathology, and can reveal substantial spine deformity. Note the advanced right hip arthritis in this patient presenting with a chief complaint of disabling right knee pain.

- Tibia:
  - Predict the proximal tibial cut needed to correct coronal plane deformity, anticipate need for stemmed implants, and identify defects that may require augments.
  - Identify osteophytes and plan for their resection.

Steps

- Magnification:
  - Determine the magnification of radiograph based on radiographic marker or known dimension of retained implant.
- Lateral radiograph (Figure 44.6):
  - Femoral component:
    - Size based on anteroposterior dimension of the distal femur. Flexion and extension of the component are adjusted until the anterior flange aligns with the anterior femoral cortex, and size is increased until posterior flange replaces resected posterior femoral condyles.
    - Avoid anterior femoral cortical notching.
    - Recreate posterior femoral offset.
    - Identify posterior femoral osteophytes that require resection.
  - Tibial component:
    - Posterior slope adjusted to desired goal based on anatomic axis of the tibia in the sagittal plane, implant manufacturer specifics, and cruciate retaining versus posterior stabilized design.

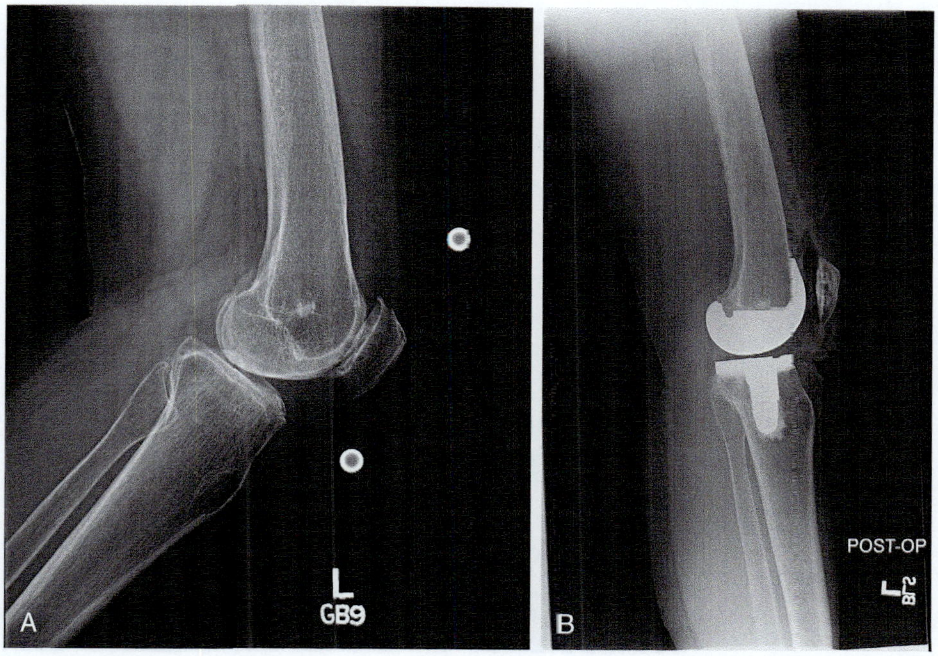

Figure 44.5 | The lateral radiograph should be used to assess appropriate posterior tibial slope by accounting for both patient anatomy and the specific implant. The (A) preoperative lateral radiograph and (B) postoperative radiograph of a patient with a posterior stabilized implant for whom the intended posterior slope was zero.

- Anteroposterior radiograph (Figure 44.7):
  - Tibial component:
    - Size determined based on lateral templating and medial-lateral coverage of the proximal tibia after proposed resection. It is common to adjust to a size larger or smaller at this point.
    - Coronal alignment is typically perpendicular to the mechanical axis (midpoint of tibial plateau to center of the talus).
    - Depth of resection adjusted to optimize the amount of proximal tibial resection.

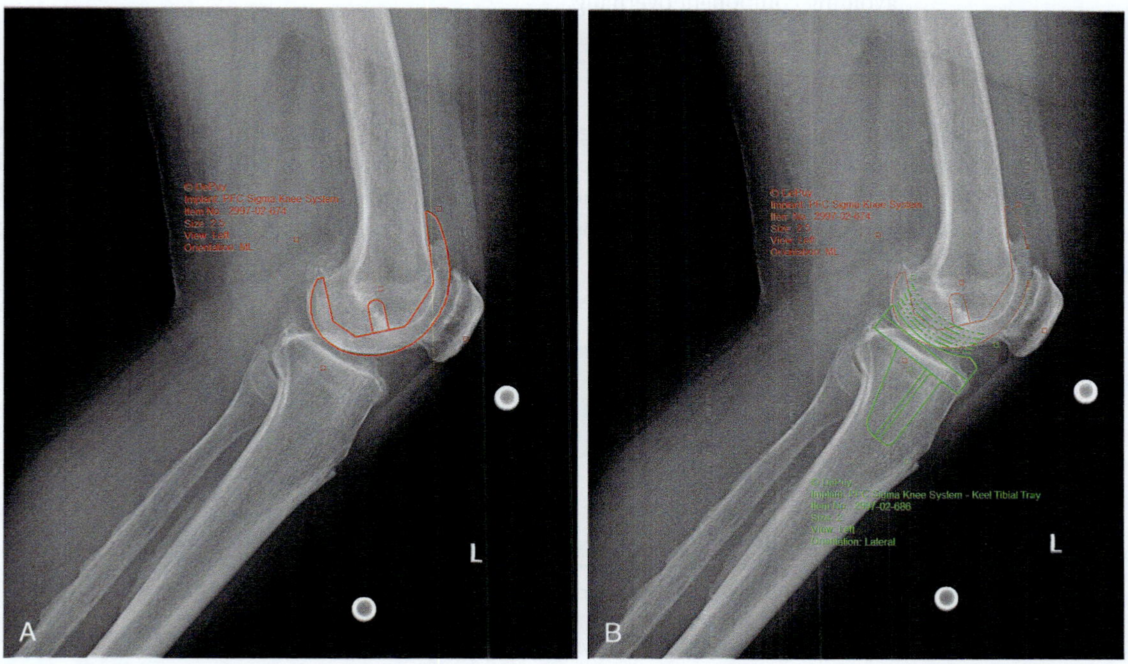

Figure 44.6 | The lateral radiograph is used to assess (A) the femoral component size and identify any posterior osteophytes that should be excised and (B) the posterior tibial slope and any posterior tibial osteophytes.

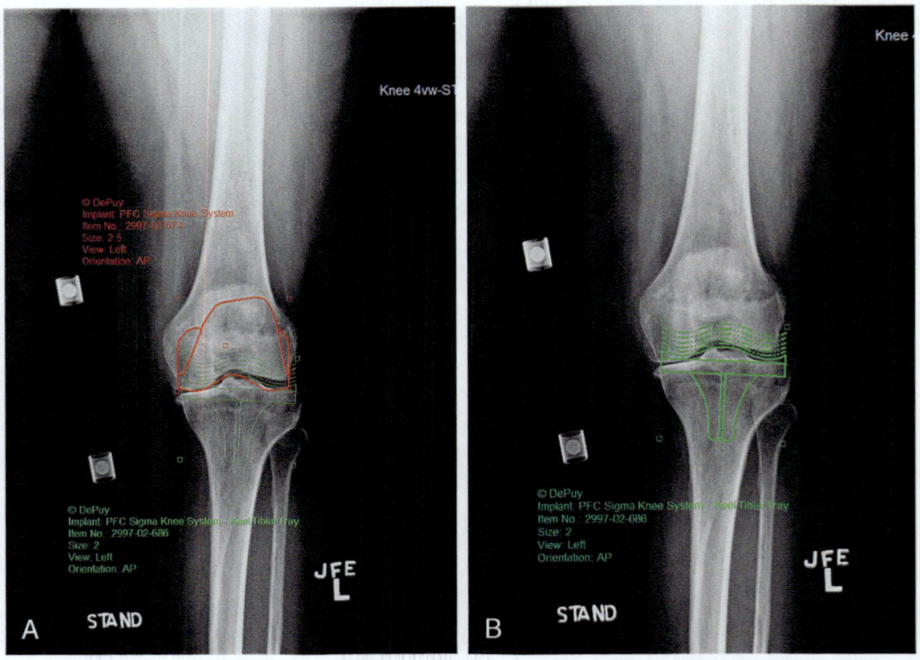

Figure 44.7 | The anteroposterior radiograph is used to assess (A) the size of the tibial component by determining the medial-lateral dimensions of the tibia at the expected depth of the tibial resection and (B) confirm that the previously selected femoral component size will not overhang in the medial-lateral dimension.

- Femoral component:
  - Size determined by lateral templating is then confirmed to ensure it does not grossly overhang in the medial-lateral plane.
  - Coronal alignment adjusted to surgeon preference but typically perpendicular to mechanical axis.
- Patella radiograph
  - The patella resection typically proceeds from the subchondral bone level medially to the subchondral bone junction laterally and results in an asymmetric portion of resected bone (Figure 44.8). The implant size is typically chosen intraoperatively to maximize bone coverage while avoiding component overhang.

Summary

Comprehensive preoperative planning is an important step that helps ensure accurate postoperative limb alignment, appropriate component sizing, and implant choice in the face of substantial extra-articular deformity or other bony abnormalities. The availability of navigation and robotics for TKA in contemporary practice does not supplant the need for careful preoperative evaluation and planning.

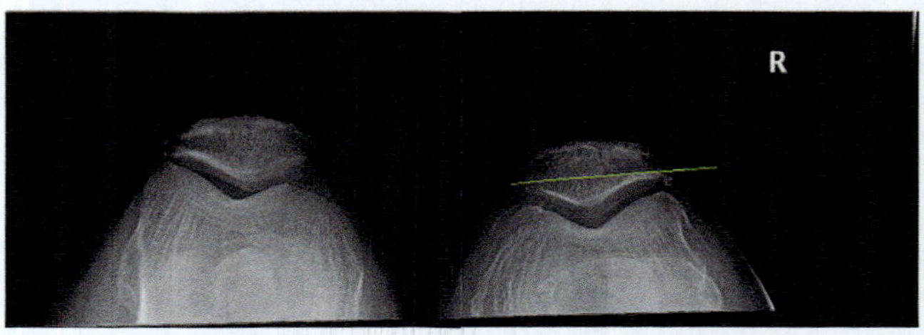

Figure 44.8 | The appropriate patella resection extends from the subchondral bone medially to the subchondral bone junction laterally and results in an asymmetric portion of resected bone.

Section B
Surgical Exposures

Chapter 45
Median Parapatellar Approach

TIMOTHY S. BROWN
MICHAEL J. TAUNTON

Key Concepts

- Supine positioning, with a nonsterile leg holder to help maintain knee flexion and a nonsterile post to prevent passive hip abduction during the operation (Figure 45.1).
- Midline incision, starting approximately 6 cm proximal to the superior pole of the patella and ending just medial to the tibial tubercle.
- Care should be taken to allow adequate closure of the medial capsule—avoid going into vastus medialis obliquus, leave a small cuff of tissue on medial patella, and avoid overrelease medially off the plateau at the distal aspect of the arthrotomy.
- Closure should provide robust support of the capsule at the medial edge of the patella as this area sees the highest stress when flexing the knee postoperatively.

Sterile Instruments and Implants

- Sandbag or other leg positioner to attach to the table under the drapes
- Post to attach to the table proximally to prevent hip abduction
- One bent Hohmann retractor
- One Chandler blunt retractor
- Two curved cobra retractors
- One posterior knee retractor
- Ioban or similar adhesive barrier dressing

Preoperative Planning

- Preoperatively the limb is examined for prior incisions, contractures, and deformity.
- If multiple incisions are present, the lateral-most incision that will allow safe exposure for medial parapatellar approach is selected.
- A good neurovascular examination should be performed and documented before any knee operation.

Bone, Implant, and Soft Tissue Techniques

Introduction

The median parapatellar approach to the knee is the standard and most versatile approach for both primary and revision knee arthroplasty.

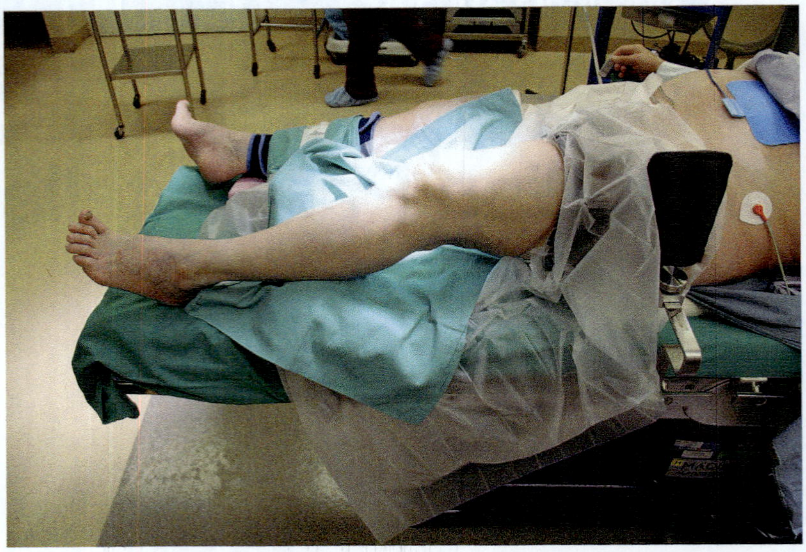

Figure 45.1 | Patient positioning supine for the median parapatellar approach to the knee.

Technique

- Patient positioning (Figure 45.1)
- Draping of the patient involves an extremity drape and 360° coverage of the extremity with barrier dressing (Figure 45.2)
- Skin incision (Figure 45.3)
    - The knee is flexed to 90° and held in place with the positioner.
    - The patella and tibial tubercle are palpated and marked.
    - The incision starts approximately 6 cm proximal to the patella and ends level with and just medial to the tibial tubercle. The incision is directly anterior.
    - The skin is incised with a clean scalpel, which is immediately passed off the field. A deep knife is then used to continue the subcutaneous dissection and identify the quadriceps tendon proximally.
- Deep exposure
    - The correct depth will be level with the vastus medialis obliquus (VMO) fascia medially and the patella more laterally.
    - Full-thickness medial and lateral flaps are raised to provide adequate exposure.
    - A marker is used to draw a horizontal line at the superomedial pole of the patella to guide accurate repair at the time of closure. The arthrotomy can be delineated with the same marker (Figure 45.4).

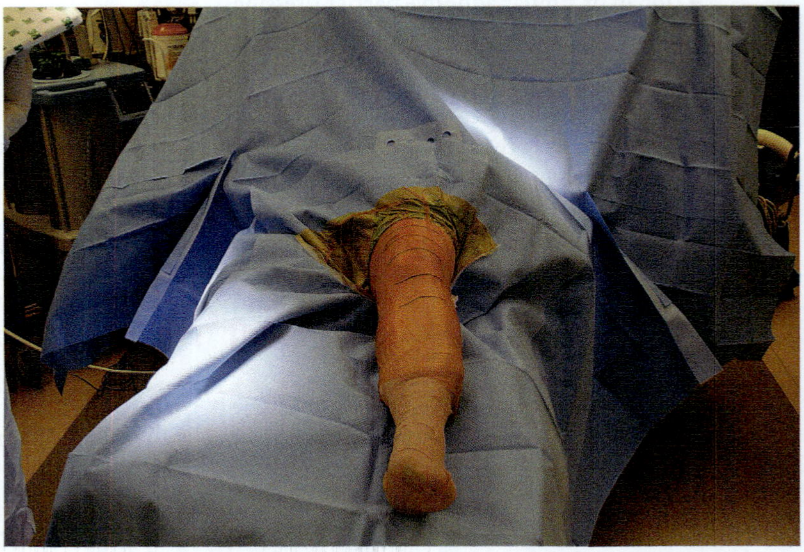

Figure 45.2 | The operative extremity draped and ready for the operation.

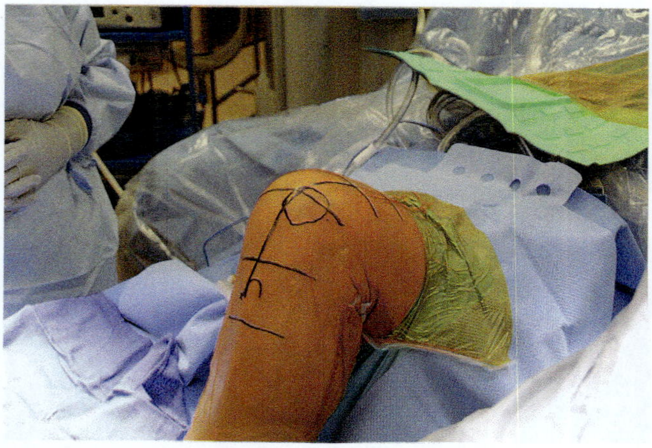

Figure 45.3 | Marking out the skin incision on the patient.

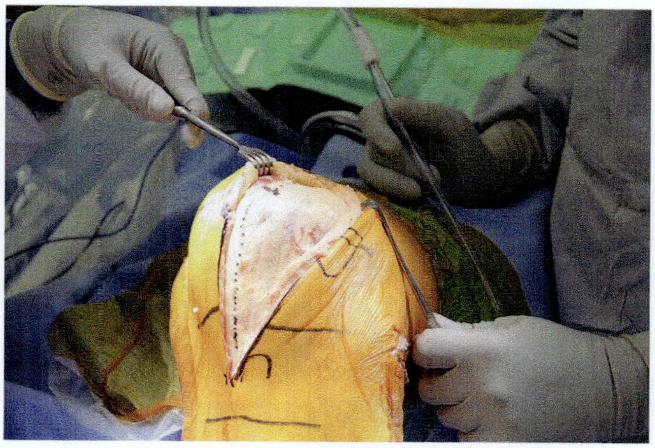

Figure 45.4 | Median parapatellar arthrotomy marked out medially.

- Arthrotomy
  - The arthrotomy is made in flexion, starting proximally and extending distally to the tibial plateau. Care is taken to leave the majority of the quadriceps tendon attached to the patella and to leave a small cuff of tissue for repair on the medial border of the patella.
  - The arthrotomy is extended distally over the tibial metaphysis to perform the medial release. The extent of medial release necessary depends on the deformity and size of the patient (Figure 45.5). A small Cobb elevator is placed under the medial tissues and the release completed to the mid-coronal line.
  - The knee is placed into extension and the infrapatellar bursa released (Figure 45.6).
  - The patella is then subluxated and the fat pad resected with a scalpel (Figure 45.7)
  - With the knee extended, the fat and synovium is removed from the suprapatellar pouch to expose the anterior femur to aid in femoral sizing and to avoid femoral notching.
  - The knee is then flexed to 90° with the patella subluxed, and a bent Hohmann placed under the medial collateral ligament (MCL). A blunt Chandler retractor is placed laterally.
  - Curved cobras are placed medially and/or laterally at the distal femur to provide further exposure if necessary (Figure 45.8).
- Exposure of the tibia
  - The tibia is exposed after resection of the anterior cruciate ligament with the aid of a posterior knee retractor to sublux the tibia anteriorly and put the cruciate ligaments under tension. The knee is hyperflexed and externally rotated, protecting the MCL, limiting tension on the patellar tendon and providing full exposure of the plateau for removal of both menisci and for the tibial resection (Figure 45.9)

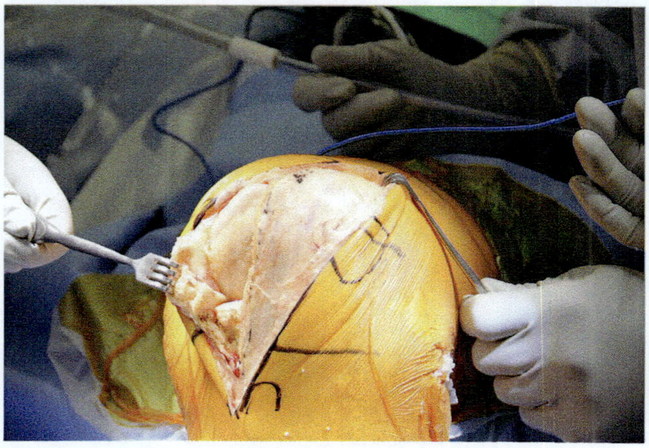

Figure 45.5 | Medial soft tissue release for exposure is performed in flexion.

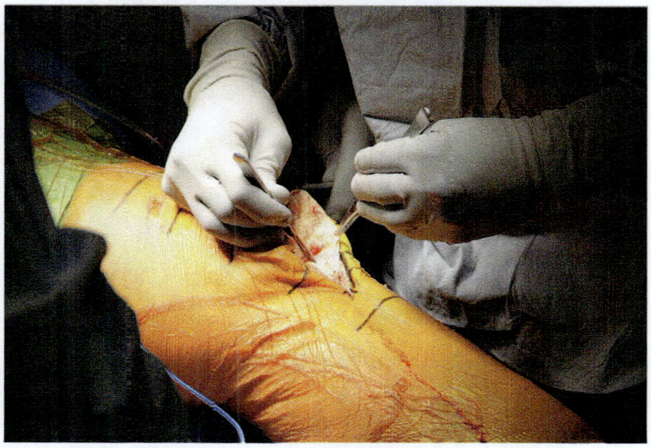

Figure 45.6 | Release of the infrapatellar bursa.

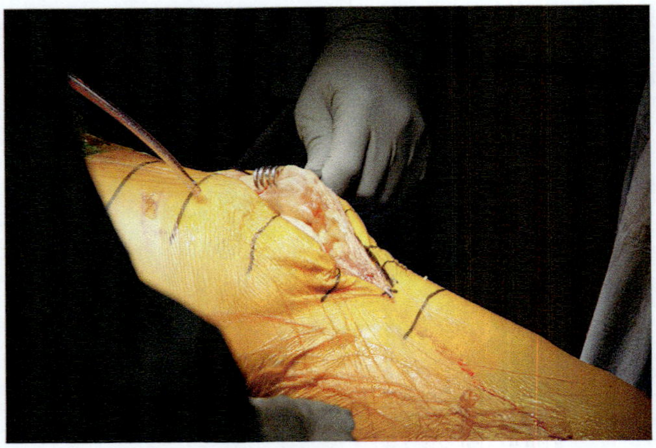

Figure 45.7 I Subluxation of the patella and removal of the fat pad.

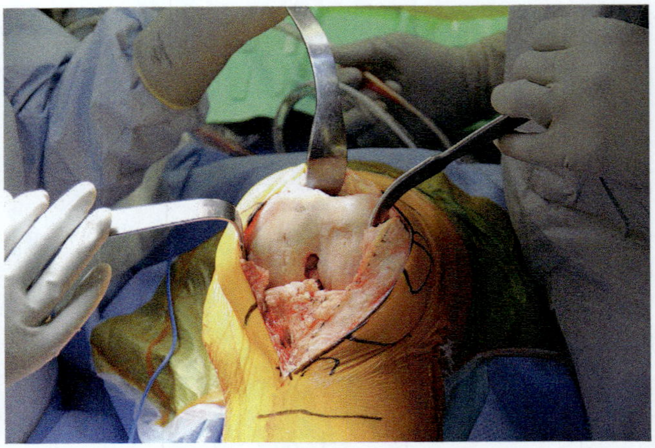

Figure 45.8 I Exposure completed, the distal femur and proximal tibia are ready for resection.

- Bone preparation for arthroplasty
  - The femur, tibia, and patella are prepared in accordance with the surgeon's preferred implant choice using appropriate implant-specific instrumentation.
- Closure
  - Closure begins with repair of the arthrotomy at the area previously marked, near the superomedial pole of the patella and the VMO (Figure 45.10).
  - Closure of the arthrotomy is completed with interrupted size 1 or size 0 Vicryl or a similar strong braided suture (Figure 45.11).
  - The subcutaneous tissues are closed with interrupted 0 and 2-0 suture.
  - The skin is closed with a running 2-0 barbed monofilament.
  - The incision is dressed with 2-octyl cyanoacrylate and a silver-impregnated barrier dressing.

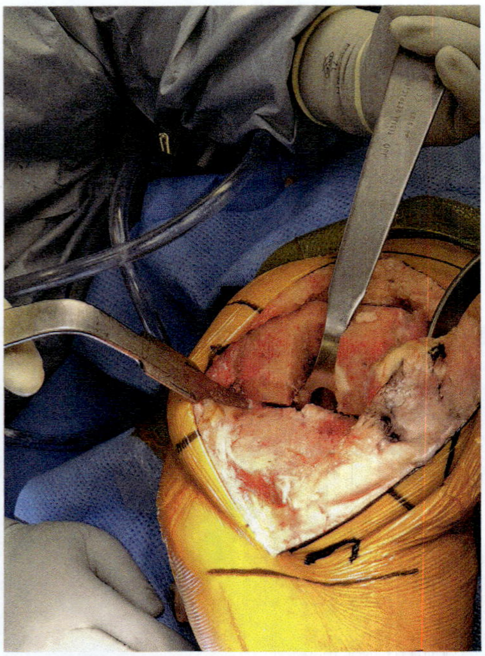

Figure 45.9 I Exposure of the tibial plateau for tibial resection.

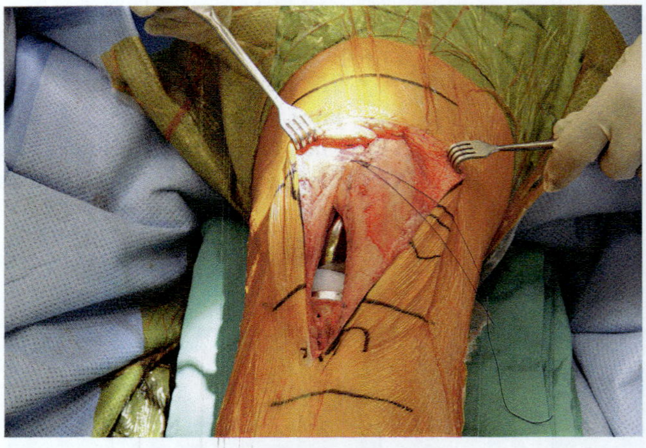

Figure 45.10 I Closure of the medial arthrotomy near the VMO.

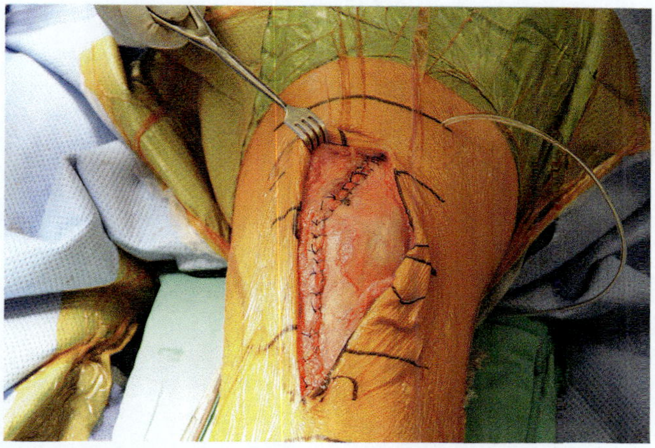

Figure 45.11 | Closure of the arthrotomy with multiple interrupted braided sutures.

Postoperative Care

- Postoperatively the patients are allowed immediate range of motion unless there was a difficulty in closing the incision distally. In these instances, the knee is immobilized in full extension for a period of time before motion is allowed.

Chapter 46
Mid Vastus; Mini Mid Vastus Approaches

HEATH P. MELUGIN
MARK W. PAGNANO

Key Concepts

- Patient is positioned supine without the use of a leg holder or hip rest to give the surgeon maximum intraoperative flexibility to change the position of the knee.
- The skin incision is medial to the midline from 4 cm proximal to the superior pole of the patella ending just medial to the tibial tubercle.
- The intersection of a transverse line marking the superior pole of the patella and a line along the medial patella marks the location where the arthrotomy should intersect the vastus medialis obliquus (VMO) muscle. The arthrotomy is then angled proximally at 50° in line with the fibers of the VMO.
- The arthrotomy closure is started at the clearly defined corner defined by the intersection of the medial arthrotomy and VMO at the level of the superior pole of the patella.
- The sutures closing the VMO muscle itself are specifically not overtightened; instead the VMO muscle belly is simply reapproximated.

Sterile Instruments and Implants

- Two 90° bent Hohmann retractors
- One posterior cruciate ligament (PCL) retractor
- Two Kocher clamps
- One knee retractor
- One ¾-inch curved osteotome
- One mallet
- One lamina spreader
- One large rongeur

Preoperative Planning

- The limb is examined for prior incisions, contractures, patellar immobility, and deformity.
- Neurovascular status of the limb is always documented.
- Four radiographic views of the knee (anteroposterior standing, lateral, posteroanterior flexion standing, and patella view) and a standing, full-length, hip-to-ankle radiograph are obtained and examined.
- Preoperative templating is performed to maximize intraoperative efficiency and determine the proper orientation and level of the bone cuts.

Bone, Implant, and Soft Tissue Techniques

Introduction

- The mid-vastus approach to the knee is a safe and reproducible way to access the knee joint. With this approach there is minimal violation of the extensor mechanism by angling the proximal portion of the arthrotomy along the midsubstance fibers of the VMO when reaching the superior pole of the patella. This minimally invasive approach allows for a smaller skin incision and reliable closure of the arthrotomy.
- Those patients with a very stiff knee, patella baja from any cause, or retained hardware from prior surgery may be better served with a standard medial patellar approach.

Technique

- Positioning and draping
  - The patient is positioned supine on the operating room table (Figure 46.1). No leg holder or hip rests are used to stabilize the knee. This allows the surgeon to have maximum flexibility in changing the position of the knee intraoperatively.
  - A tourniquet is placed on the proximal thigh and the knee prepped and draped in a sterile fashion.
  - Transverse lines are drawn anteriorly on the knee before applying iodine-impregnated drapes to all exposed skin (Figure 46.2).
- Superficial exposure
  - With the knee flexed, a skin incision is made medial to the midline from 4 cm proximal to the superior pole of the patella and extended just medial the tibial tubercle (Figure 46.2).
  - The knee is then placed in extension on the table. A clean scalpel or cautery may be used to develop a medially based skin flap to visualize the VMO, while preserving the overlying fascia. The tissue plane just superficial to the VMO fascia is used to verify correct dissection depth.
  - A lateral skin flap is made to the lateral border of the patella to allow for improved intraoperative patellar mobility.
- Arthrotomy
  - The superior pole of the patella is marked by a transverse line with a marker (Figure 46.3). A longitudinal line from just medial to the tibial tubercle along the medial aspect of the patellar tendon and patella is marked. The location where these 2 lines intersect marks where the arthrotomy should be angled proximally at 50° in line with the fibers of the VMO (Figure 46.4A and B).

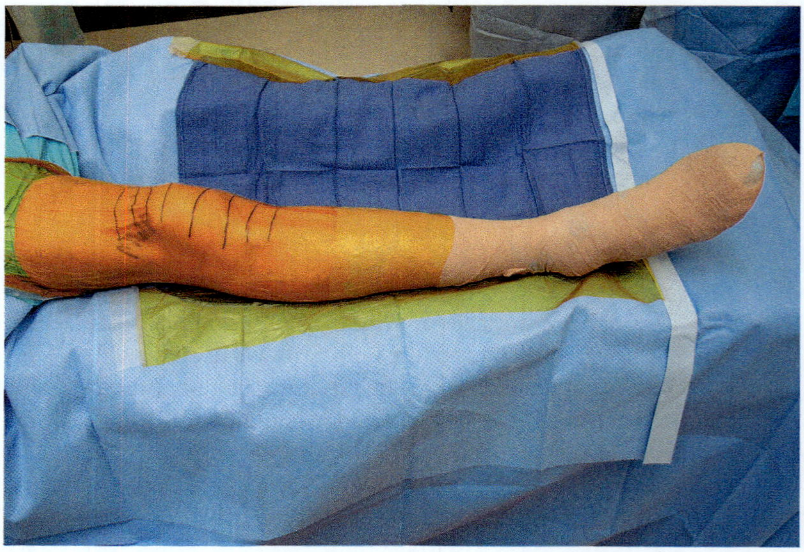

Figure 46.1 | The leg is positioned supine without a leg holder.

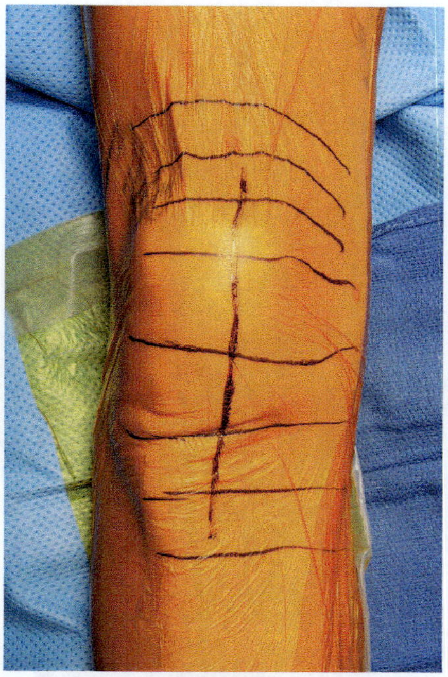

Figure 46.2 | Transverse lines are drawn, and the skin incision is made just medial to midline.

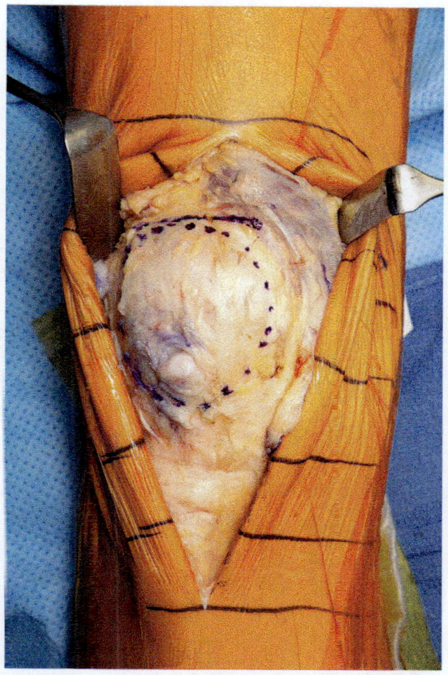

Figure 46.3 | A transverse line is drawn along the superior pole of the patella.

- Using cautery, the arthrotomy is made with the knee in extension creating a distinct corner where the medial arthrotomy and proximal extension into the VMO begins (Figure 46.5).
  - It is extremely important not to begin the angle into the VMO too distal as this will make exposure difficult throughout the case. The proximal extent of the medial arthrotomy should always continue to the level of the superior pole of the patella before being angled into the VMO.
- In the sagittal plane, angle the cautery at 45° toward the medial side when incising tissue along the patella to ensure there is an adequate cuff of tissue to repair.

- Deep exposure
  - The anterior horn of the medial meniscus is released, and the medial soft tissues are released subperiosteally to expose the medial joint line.
  - A Kocher clamp is placed on the medial capsular sleeve just proximal to the medial meniscus to assist with exposure throughout the case.
  - The retropatellar fat pad is removed, and the anterior horn of the lateral meniscus is released.
  - The soft tissue on the lateral proximal tibia is released proximal to the insertion of the patellar tendon.
  - A 90° bent Hohmann retractor is placed in the corner of the arthrotomy at the superior pole of the patella into the lateral gutter to assist with patellar translation (Figure 46.6).
  - The patella is then translated into the lateral gutter, and the knee may be flexed to 90° (Figure 46.7).
    - If there is any difficulty translating the patella, ensure that there are no adhesions between the fascia overlying the VMO and the subcutaneous tissue above it.
  - The femoral canal is drilled, and the intramedullary femoral cutting guide is placed (Figure 46.8).
  - The distal femur is cut first.
  - The rotation of the femur is set by referencing the posterior condyles, although the transepicondylar axis or Whiteside line may also be used.
  - The 4-in-1 finishing guide is then placed, and the bent Hohmann retractors in the medial and lateral gutters are used to expose the anterior femoral cortex.
  - The suprapatellar synovial tissue is excised if synovitic or simply incised with cautery to expose the lateral anterior cortex of the femur to avoid notching.
  - Extending the knee slightly to around 60° decreases tension on the extensor mechanism and assists with exposure while making the anterior femoral cut.
  - Once all femoral cuts are made, a rongeur is used to remove any osteophytes on the femur.

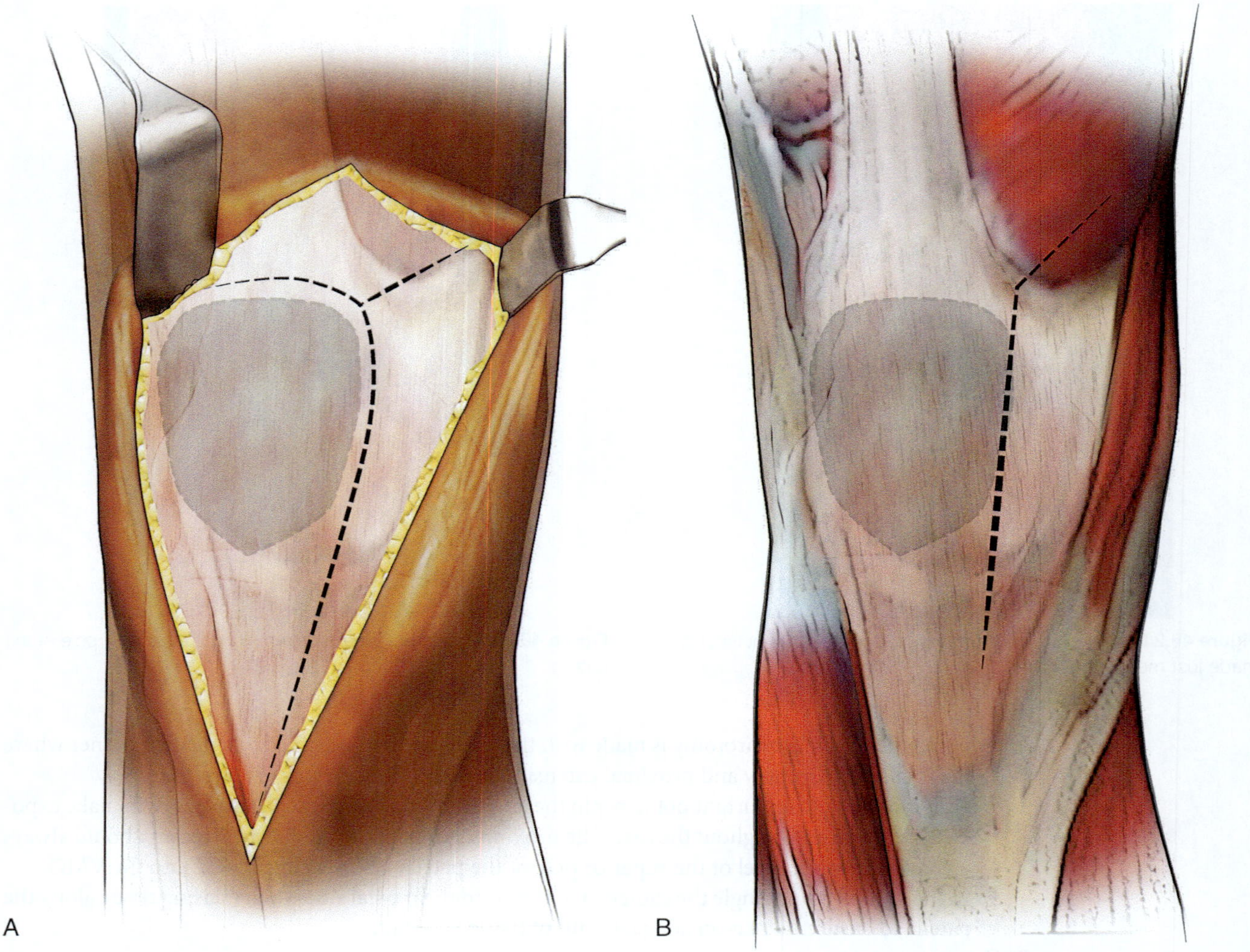

Figure 46.4 | longitudinal line along the medial patella and patellar tendon is drawn until it intersects with the previously drawn transverse line. This marks the location of the angled VMO split. A, Illustration of the relevant anatomy and (B) the anticipated position, angle and direction of the midvastus arthrotomy.

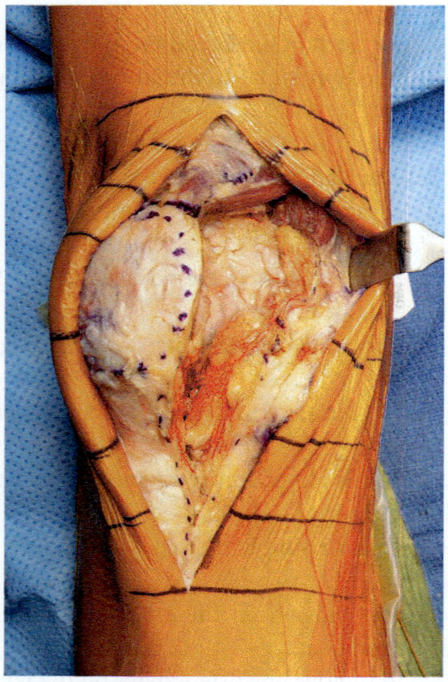

Figure 46.5 | The arthrotomy is completed.

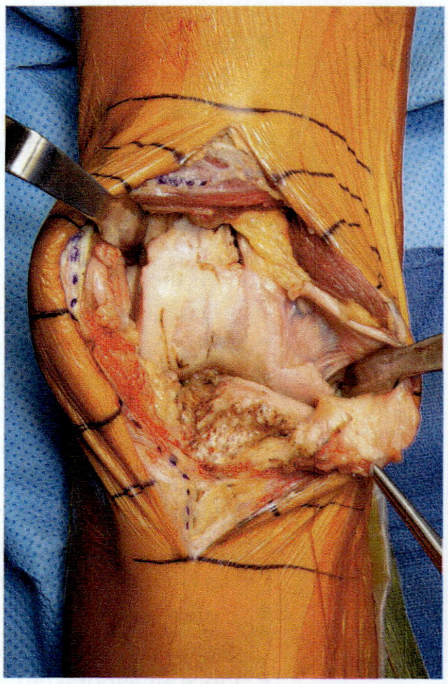

Figure 46.6 | The medial soft tissues are released subperiosteally off the tibia to expose the medial joint line, and the patella is subluxed laterally with the aid of 90° bent Hohmann retractors.

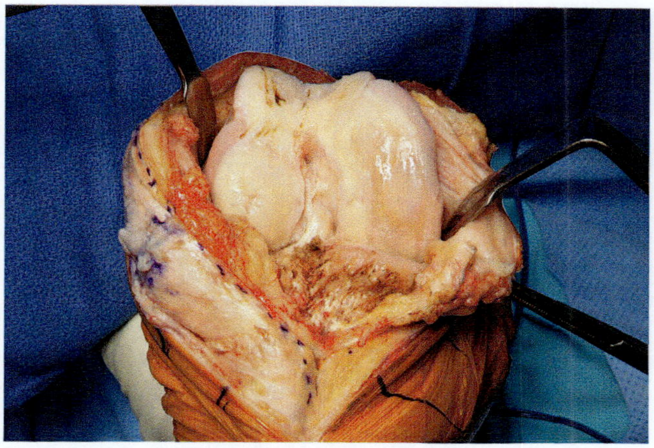

Figure 46.7 | Two 90° bent Hohmann retractors are placed medially and laterally to expose both femoral condyles.

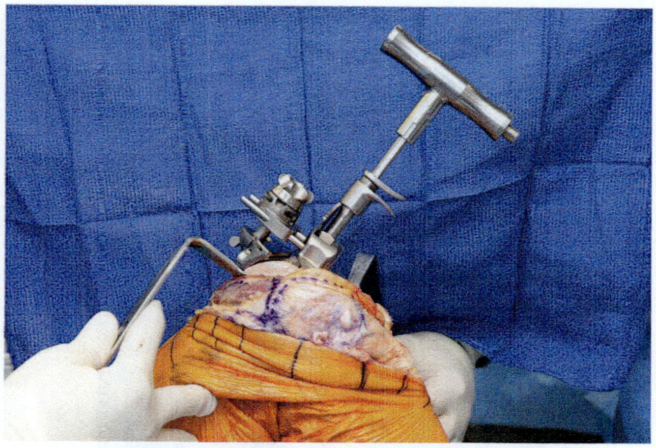

Figure 46.8 | Slight knee extension allows for relaxation of the extensor mechanism and correct positioning of the distal femoral cutting guide.

- Exposure of the tibia
  - The knee is flexed to 90°.
  - A 90° bent Hohmann retractor is placed medially to protect the superficial medial collateral ligament (MCL).
  - Another 90° bent Hohmann retractor is placed under the lateral meniscus and directly adjacent to the lateral tibial bone margin.
  - A PCL retractor is placed posteriorly to sublux the tibia anteriorly and expose its posterior perimeter (Figure 46.9).
  - The anterior cruciate ligament (ACL) tibial footprint is released.
  - The tibial extramedullary guide is placed, and the proximal tibia is cut after verifying correct coronal and sagittal alignment of the cutting block (Figure 46.10).

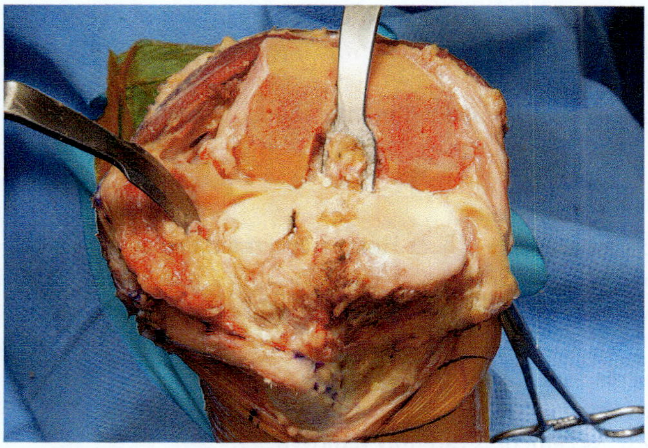

Figure 46.9 | Adequate exposure of the tibia is obtained with 3 retractors.

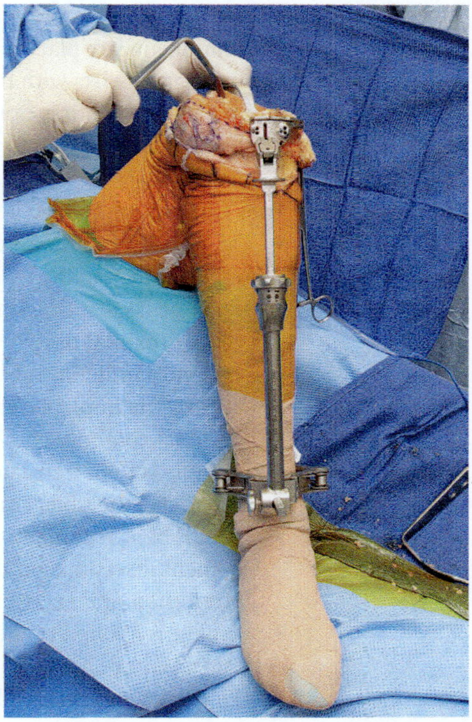

Figure 46.10 | A minimally invasive tibial cutting guide is used.

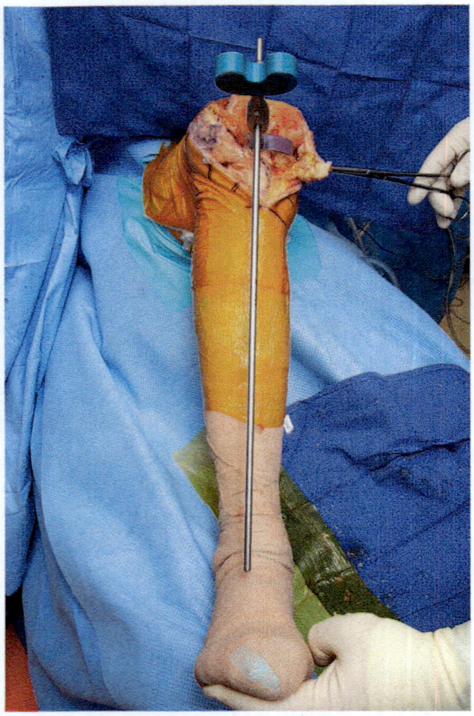

Figure 46.11 | A spacer block or trial components are used to assess the flexion and extension gaps and medial versus lateral soft-tissue balancing based on surgeon preference.

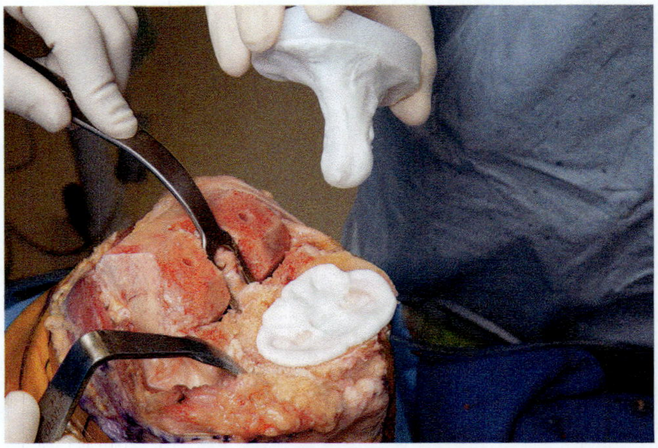

Figure 46.12 | Precoating the entire underside of the tibial implant prevents fluid from entering the implant-cement interface.

- Balancing
  - A laminar spreader is placed laterally, and the medial meniscus, ACL, and PCL (depending on implant design) are excised using cautery. Posterior osteophytes are removed with a slightly curved ¾-inch osteotome and mallet. The same maneuver is performed for the lateral side.
  - Proper balancing is evaluated in flexion and extension using a spacer block and alignment rod (Figure 46.11).
- Patella
  - The patella is cut using a cutting guide after all tibia and femoral cuts are made but before trial components are placed. This allows the entire limb to shorten, which relaxes the extensor mechanism and assists with patellar positioning.
  - Excess synovial tissue proximal to the patella is excised to limit the chance of patellar crepitus or clunk postoperatively.
- Cementing
  - A trial reduction may be performed before cementing.
  - The tibia is cemented first and is exposed using the 2 bent Hohmann retractors placed medially and laterally and the PCL retractor posteriorly to sublux the tibia forward.
  - The bone is cleaned with pulsatile lavage and dried with a lap sponge before placement of cement on the proximal tibia.
  - The entire undersurface of the tibial component is precoated with cement to prevent fluid from entering the implant-cement interface (Figure 46.12).
  - The tibial component is placed, and excess cement is carefully removed.
  - The tibia is then translated posteriorly under the posterior femoral condyles with care not to rock or dislodge the tibial component.
  - The 90° bent Hohmann retractors are placed medially and laterally just proximal to the collateral ligament insertions on the femur. A knee retractor may be placed under the VMO to assist with anterior femoral exposure.
  - Cement is applied to the exposed femur and to the posterior condyles and anterior flange of the femoral component.
  - The patella is cemented last.

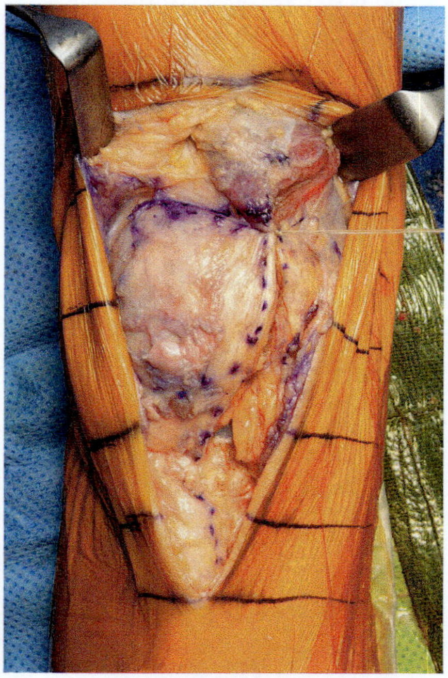

Figure 46.13 | The closure of the arthrotomy begins by reapproximating the corner of tissue created at the intersection of the superior pole of the patella and arthrotomy just medial to the patella.

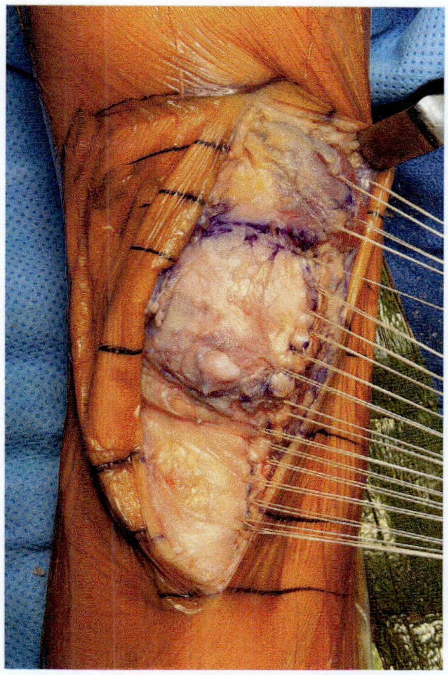

Figure 46.14 | Sutures for the arthrotomy are placed making sure not to overtighten the medial tissues or VMO.

- Closure
  - The wound is soaked with a dilute Betadine solution and thoroughly irrigated with normal saline solution. A periarticular local anesthetic injection typically is done.
  - Proper patellar tracking is ensured and hemostasis is achieved once the cement has cured.
  - The arthrotomy is closed with multiple interrupted 0-Vicryl sutures. Care is taken not to overtighten the sutures placed through muscle while also including the VMO fascia superficially and the joint capsule deeply with each throw of the suture (Figures 46.13 and 46.14).
  - Skin and subcutaneous suture are closed in layers with 0-Vicryl and 2-0 Monocryl followed by a running subcuticular closure. The incision is dressed with 2-octyl cyanoacrylate.
  - A sterile dressing is applied, and the extremity is wrapped with a 6-inch-wide elastic bandage from the foot to midthigh.

Postoperative Care

- Patients meet with physical therapy on the day of surgery and may weight bear as tolerated. Patients typically use a walker for several days before transitioning to a cane. Most are able to discharge from the hospital on postoperative day 1 or 2 as long as they demonstrate an ability to mobilize safely and have adequate pain control. We ask patients to see a physical therapist once a week for 6 weeks to assess range of motion. Strengthening exercises are rarely required.

Chapter 47
Exposure of the Problem Knee: Stiffness, Previous Incisions

KEVIN I. PERRY

Key Concepts

- Previous incisions or soft tissue coverage (Figure 47.1A and B) around a knee increase the risks of wound healing issues and periprosthetic joint infection.
- In patients with compromised soft tissues, early motion must sometimes be delayed to ensure wound healing.
- A sequential approach must be taken to obtain adequate exposure of the stiff knee.
- Stiff knees often require a more extensile approach to protect the integrity of the extensor mechanism. Often a quadriceps snip and occasionally a tibial tubercle osteotomy will be performed to expose the knee.
- Wound complications occur more frequently in patients with previous incisions and tenuous soft tissues around the front of the knee (Figure 47.2).
- If the skin or soft tissues are tenuous after knee replacement, a period of immobilization is wise to promote wound healing.
- Intraoperative use of laser angiography (if available) is useful to determine viability of the skin and soft tissues around the knee and help decide if muscle flap coverage is necessary.

Sterile Instruments and Implants

Instruments

- Standard total knee arthroplasty (TKA) retractors and instruments
- Sagittal saw

Implants

- A full complement of constrained implants (posterior stabilized, varus-valgus constrained, hinged) should be available as the integrity of the collateral ligaments can be compromised during exposure of the stiff knee.

Position

- Supine position on the operating table

Surgical Approaches

- In general, the lateral-most incision that can safely access the knee is used.
- Full-thickness flaps (down to the level of the fascia) are created and typically, a standard, median parapatellar arthrotomy is done.

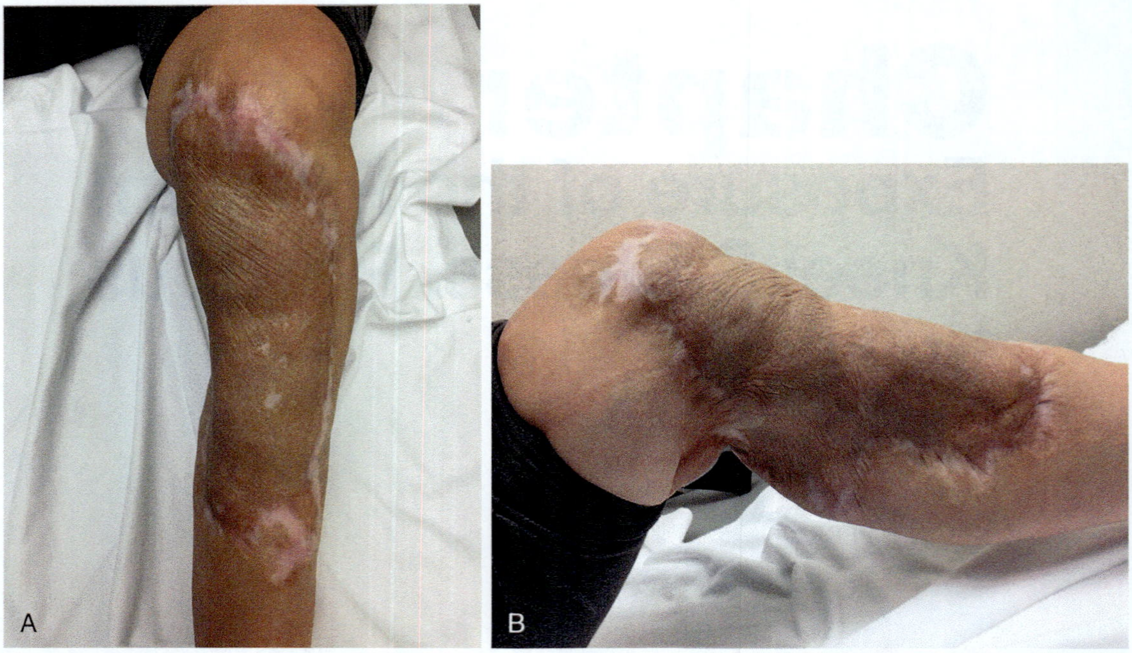

Figure 47.1 | Preoperative AP (A) and lateral (B) photographs demonstrating soft tissue coverage and split-thickness skin grafting around the front and lateral aspects of the knee.

- Extensile exposures may be needed for the stiff knee: these include a quadriceps snip or, in rare cases, a tibial tubercle osteotomy. Those techniques are described in Chapter IV-B-2.

Preoperative Planning

- Anteroposterior (AP), lateral, and sunrise radiographs of the affected knee should be reviewed (Figure 47.3A and B). In addition, ipsilateral views of the hip are obtained to ensure there is no hip arthritis. Significant hip arthritis can lead to difficult knee rehabilitation and most often should be dealt with before TKA.
- Preoperative consultation with a plastic surgeon can be helpful for incision planning and if assistance during exposure or closure of the wound is necessary (Figure 47.4A and B).

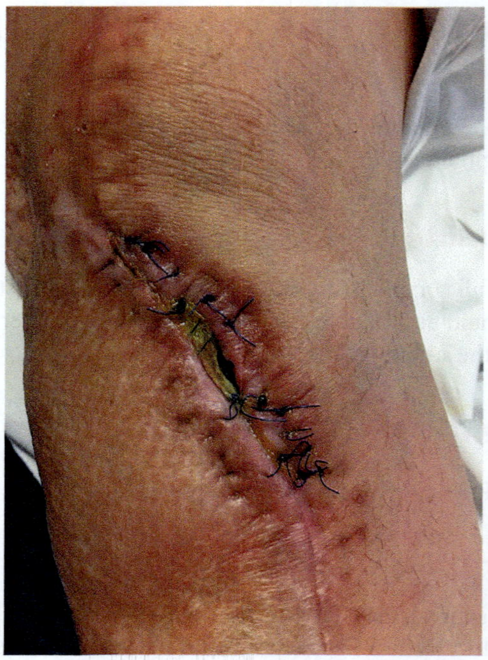

Figure 47.2 | Wound breakdown after TKA with compromised soft tissues.

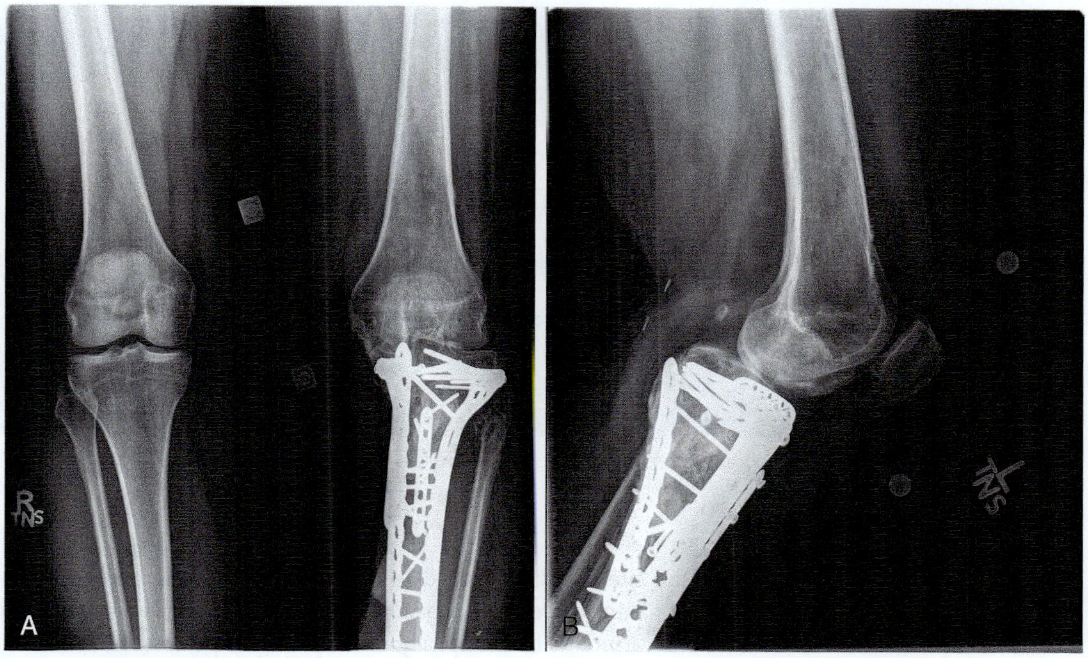

Figure 47.3 | Preoperative AP (A) and lateral (B) radiographs of stiff knee with multiple previous incisions.

- Cessation of smoking and of all nicotine products is imperative to optimize wound healing. We prefer to check a serum cotinine level to ensure patients have been off of all nicotine products for at least 4 weeks preoperatively.
- A full complement of constrained implants (posterior stabilized, varus-valgus constrained, hinged) should be available.

Bone, Implant, and Soft Tissue Techniques

- Photographs of the preoperative range of motion can be helpful to document improvements from preoperative to postoperative motion (Figure 47.5A, B and 47.6A, B).
- A standard release of the superficial and deep medial collateral ligament should be carried out over the proximal tibia.

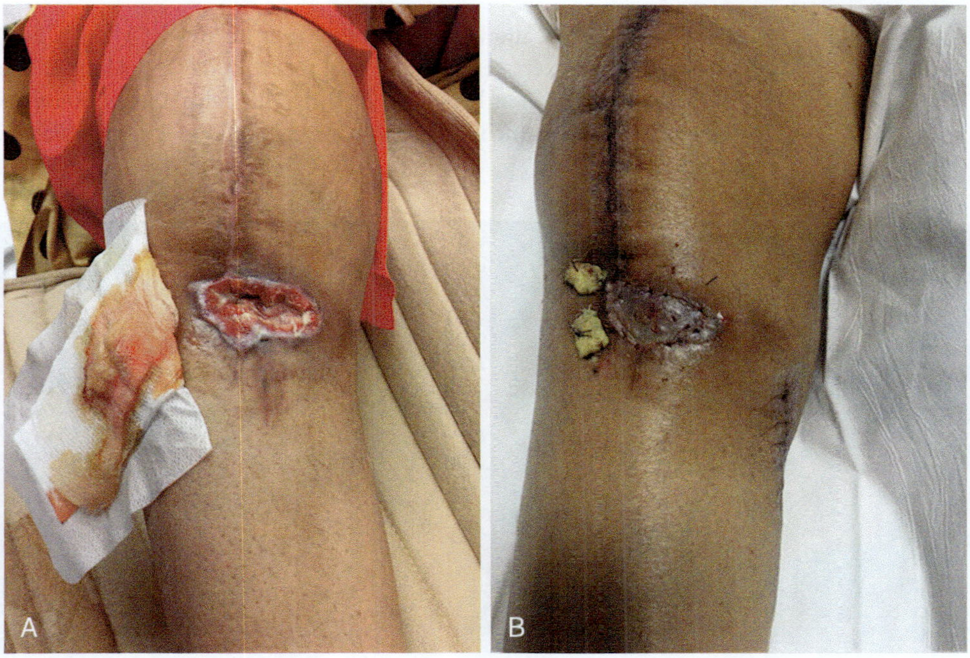

Figure 47.4 | Large soft tissue defect requiring coverage (A) and after soft tissue coverage with plastic surgery (B).

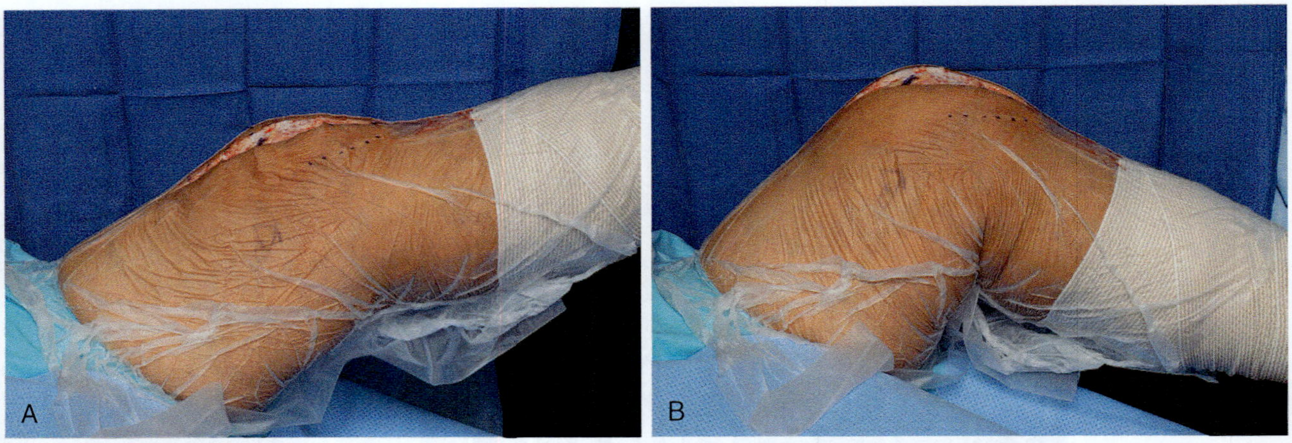

Figure 47.5 | Intraoperative photographs demonstrating preoperative knee range extension (A) and flexion (B).

- The medial and lateral gutters should be developed and the fat pad excised.
- Occasionally, making a provisional patellar resection can help facilitate exposure.
- If the knee still cannot be flexed up, a quadriceps snip is performed (Chapter IV-B-2).
- If the exposure is still inadequate, a tibial tubercle osteotomy is performed (Chapter IV-B-2).
- After committing to a hinged TKA design, peeling the origins of the medial and lateral collateral ligaments off the femur will facilitate exposure, but hinged TKA is used in a judicial fashion in only the extreme cases.
- After adequate exposure, the TKA proceeds in an orderly fashion (Chapter III-C and III-D). Often there is need for increased TKA constraint due to the extensive soft tissue dissection needed for exposure. Constrained implants are described in Chapter IV-C-5.
- Careful closure of the wound is needed, and plastic surgery can assist with primary closure or soft tissue coverage (Figure 47.7A and B).
- Use of laser angiography during closure can determine viability of the soft tissues around the knee and help determine if formal soft tissue coverage is necessary.
- If the soft tissues are tenuous or soft tissue coverage was needed, a posterior-based splint will immobilize the knee and promote wound healing.

Postoperative Care

- Patients are typically allowed weight bearing as tolerated.
- Range-of-motion exercises begin on postoperative day #1 as long as the soft tissues allow it. Formal physical therapy is often beneficial in these difficult patients. Return visits to the clinic early and often can help determine if a formal manipulation under anesthesia is warranted.

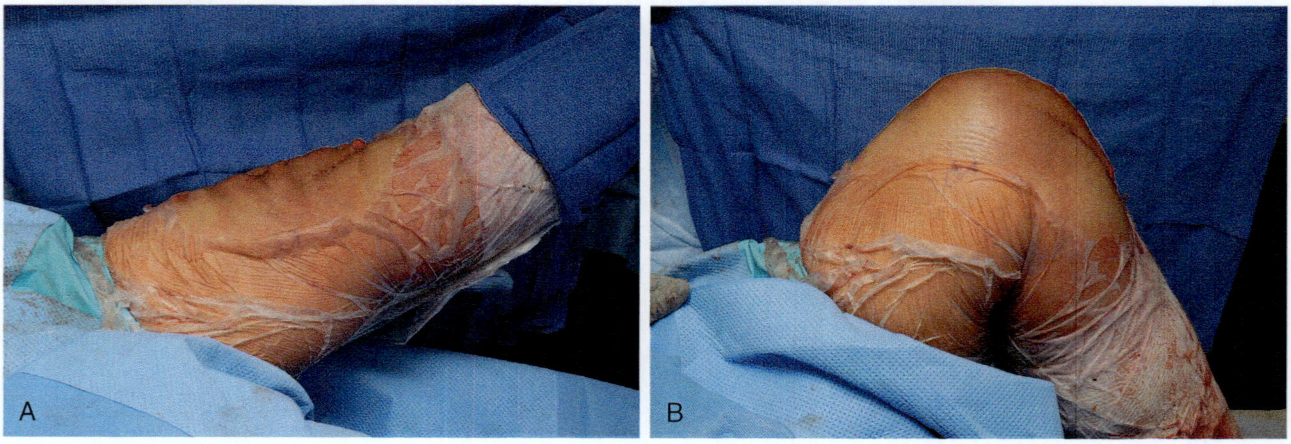

Figure 47.6 | Intraoperative photographs demonstrating post-TKA extension (A) and flexion (B).

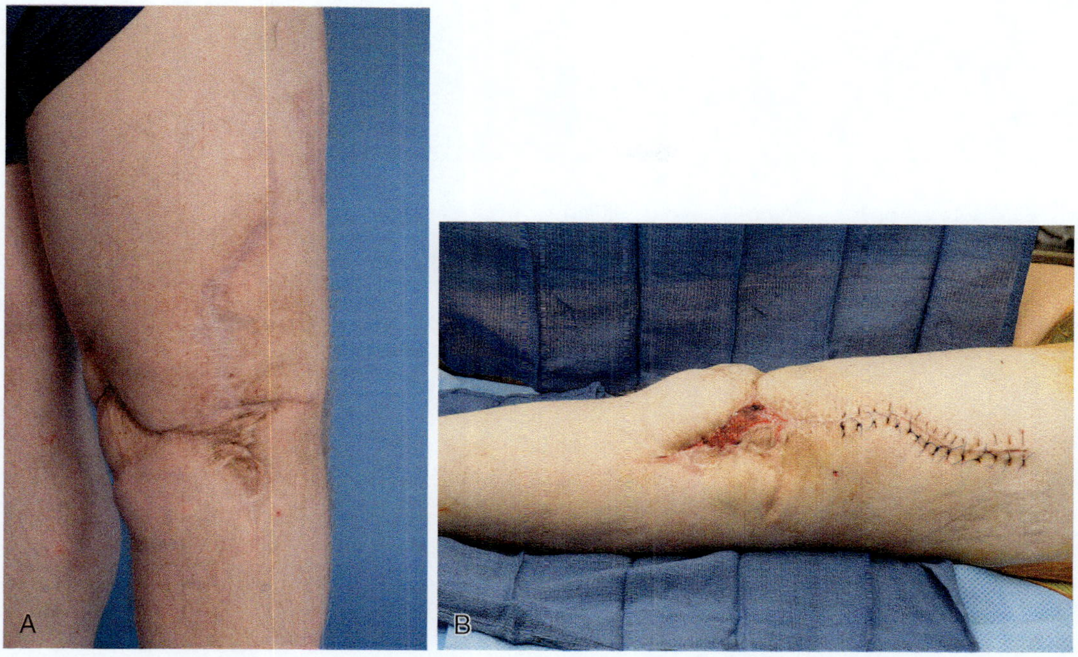

Figure 47.7 | Preoperative photograph of knee with multiple prior incisions (A) requiring complex primary closure (B).

- When the skin closure is tenuous, keeping the leg out straight for a few days or more promotes healing of the soft tissues.
- If a rotational flap, free flap, or split-thickness skin graft (STSG) was done, the leg is typically immobilized for 10 to 14 days of the flap and the STSG is closely monitored.

Chapter 48
Unicompartmental Knee Arthroplasty

RAFAEL J. SIERRA
MARK W. PAGNANO

Key Concepts

- Medial unicompartmental arthroplasty (UKA) is a good option for those patients with isolated advanced medial compartment degenerative arthritis (best if bone on bone) with acceptable patellofemoral cartilage damage.
- Compared with total knee arthroplasty (TKA), a UKA is typically a smaller operation, has a quicker recovery, and can deliver a little better function because both cruciate ligaments are preserved.
- In an experienced surgeon's hands, the long-term survivorship of UKA with either mobile or fixed bearing designs rivals that of TKA.
  - Fixed versus mobile bearing design choice depends on surgeon preference and relative experience with the technique.
  - Medial mobile bearing design is contraindicated in patients with an incompetent anterior cruciate ligament (ACL), previous upper tibial osteotomy, and when difficulty is anticipated in balancing the medial side appropriately.
  - For the mobile bearing UKA, we recommend obtaining a stress view in valgus or a PA flexion view to determine integrity of the lateral compartment and to determine that the varus deformity is correctable. A fixed deformity indicates a structurally shortened medial collateral ligament (MCL) and likely an incompetent ACL and should be contraindication to a mobile bearing UKA.
  - Some surgeons including one of the authors (MWP) will use a weightbearing PA flexion view of the knee as a surrogate for the valgus stress x-ray in determining the integrity of the lateral compartment.

Indications

- A UKA is indicated in all age groups when isolated advanced bone-on-bone arthritis is present in the medial compartment.
- The ideal candidate is a patient with a varus deformity that is passively correctable with good range of motion and minimal patellofemoral arthritis (>100° of flexion < 15° flexion contracture, <15° varus deformity, not severe patellofemoral arthritis especially if involving the lateral facet).
- The best results of UKA have been reported in patients with anteromedial osteoarthritis and an intact ACL.

Sterile Instruments and Implants

- Routine knee retractors
- Surgeon's choice of unicompartmental knee arthroplasty system (with instrumentation)

Positioning

- Patient can be positioned supine on the operating room table.
- For mobile bearing UKA, the leg is placed in a leg holder and draped free hanging at approximately 100° of flexion and with slight hip flexion about 20°.

Surgical Approaches

- UKA can be inserted through different approaches to the knee. A medial parapatellar approach most of the time is not necessary and less invasive approaches can be used. This includes a subvastus or a midvastus approach based on surgeon's expertise and preference.

Preoperative Planning

- Depending on the surgical technique used, AP and lateral radiographs are sufficient to plan for implant placement. The lateral x-ray for a mobile bearing UKA will help determine the size of the femoral component to be used, and the lateral tibial radiograph could give some insight as to the size of the tibial component as well. The final decision of the tibial component will be made intraoperatively.

Bone Implant and Soft Tissue Techniques

Mobile Bearing Unicompartmental Arthroplasty

Femur First Technique

- Verify that that ACL is intact. Verify that the lateral compartment cartilage does not have any central defects. Always consent for TKA.
- Mark the entry of an intramedullary femoral guide approximately 1 cm anteromedial and superior to the intercondylar notch. Use the rod pusher to position the rod intramedullary (Figure 48.1). The IM rod is placed as a guide for flexion of the femoral component. The femoral component should be flexed approximately 10° from sagittal plane of the femur.
- Preparation of the femur. Remove the femoral osteophytes. Mark the center of the femoral guide with a marking pen in the center of the femoral condyle (Figure 48.2). Alternatively you can use the technique described by Shakespeare et al by measuring the distance from the lateral aspect of the

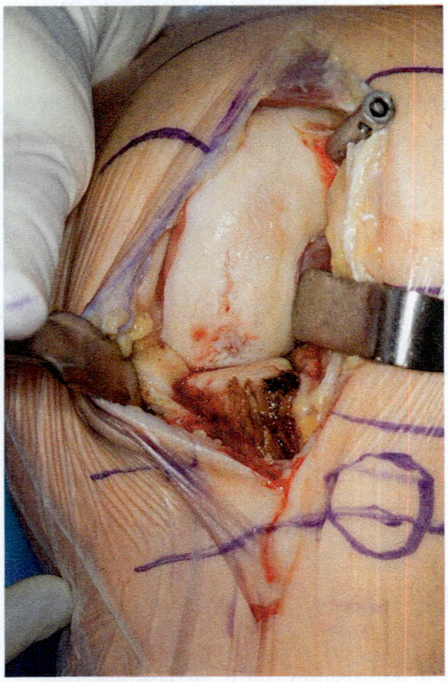

Figure 48.1 | The intramedullary guide has been placed in the appropriate position above the notch. It can be used to retract the patella.

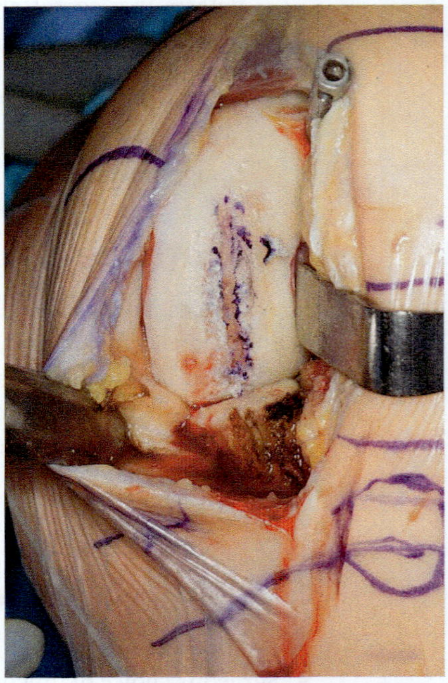

Figure 48.2 | The center of the medial femoral condyle has been marked.

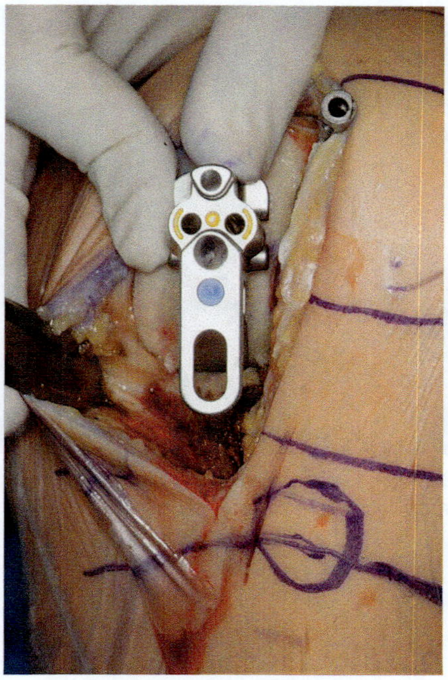

Figure 48.3 | The curved femoral guide then is decoupled from the femoral guide and used to position and drill the femoral component in place.

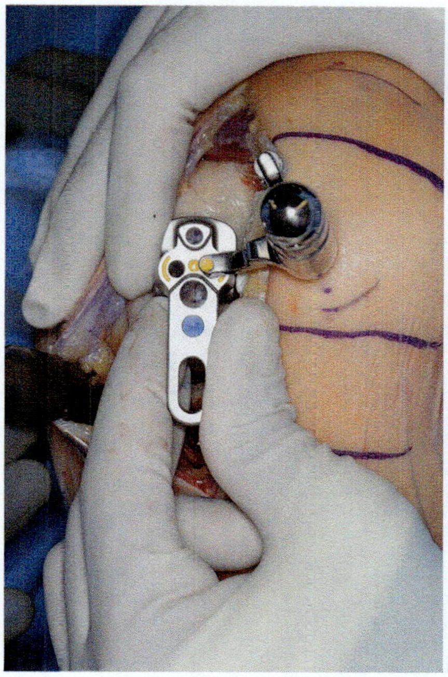

Figure 48.4 | The femoral guide is then coupled to the intramedullary guide using the linking guide.

medial condyle as 13, 14, or 15 mm for a small, medium, or large components respectively. This will ensure that the meniscal bearing is seated 2 mm lateral from the lateral aspect of the wall of the tibial tray. The curved femoral guide then is decoupled from the femoral guide and used to position and drill the femoral component in place (Figure 48.3). The femoral guide is linked to the intramedullary guide. This will allow appropriate positioning in the flexion and extension plane (Figure 48.4). Be sure the guide is seated on bone and make the drill holes that coincide with the marked center of the condyle. Drill the anterior smaller hole, make sure that the guide is in the center of the condyle, and then drill the 6 mm drill hole thereafter (Figures 48.5 and 48.6). Place the guide of the posterior femoral resection (Figures 48.7 and 48.8). Complete your posterior resection. Protect the ACL and MCL.

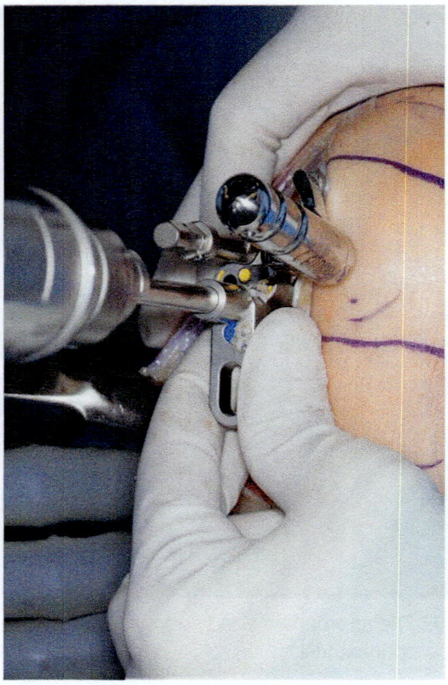

Figure 48.5 | The 6 mm drill is used to prepare the larger hole for the femoral guide.

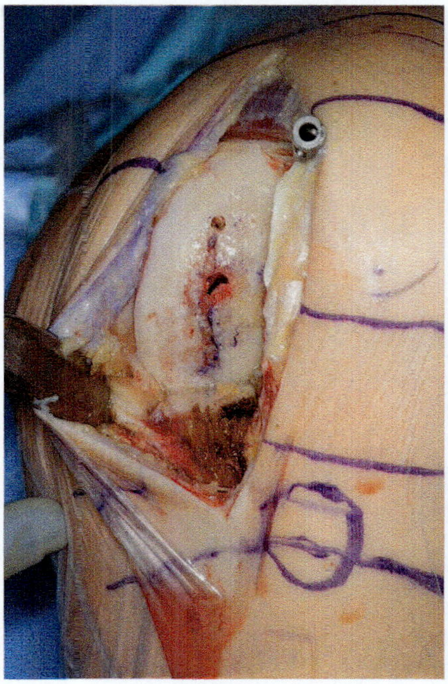

Figure 48.6 | The femoral guide holes match the center of the medial femoral condyle.

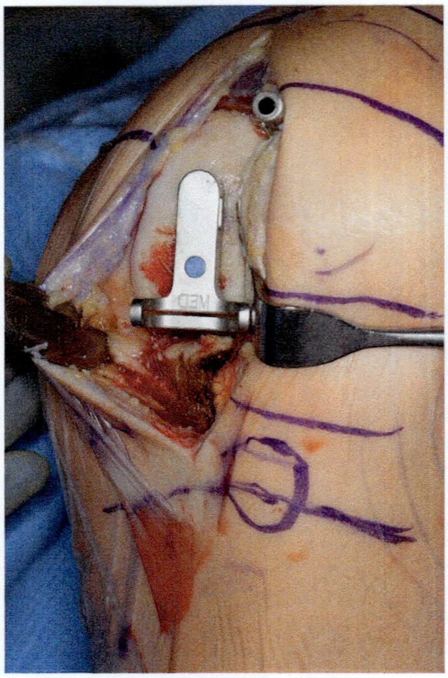

Figure 48.7 | The distal femoral resection guide is placed and the posterior femoral resection is verified.

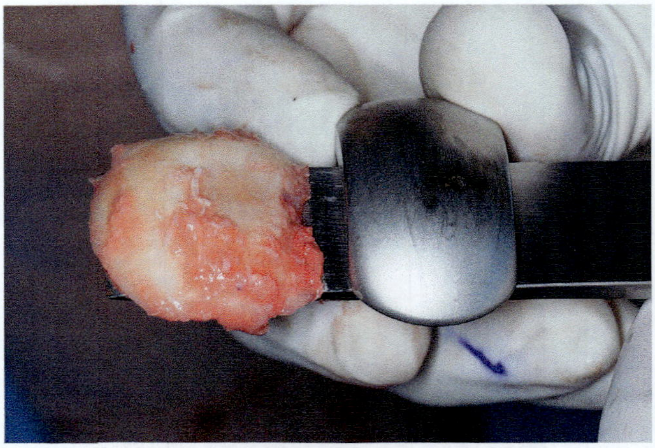

Figure 48.8 | The posterior femoral resection should match the posterior femoral condylar implant if the sizing is correct and the resection has been performed without allowing the saw to deflect off the bone.

- Mill the distal femur. Begin milling the distal femur with a zero spigot. Remove the subsequent osteophytes and remaining bone and then place your femoral component as a trial (Figure 48.9). Subsequent millings are performed after tibial resection. Apply the spherical gauge around the femoral trial (Figure 48.10). Place the extramedullary tibial guide parallel to the long axis of the tibia. The extramedullary guide will cut the tibia with 7° of posterior slope if against the anterior aspect of the tibia. Use the G-clamp to clamp the tibial guide with the zero resection bloc and pin the tibial guide in place with one nonheaded pin (Figures 48.11 and 48.12). In order to avoid overresection of the tibia, change the zero guide for the +2 as your initial resection. Remove the G-clamp and check for resection level with the C-guide. Start with your vertical resection, stay medial to the ACL, and aim the blade toward the head of the femur but also use your trial femoral component as your guide

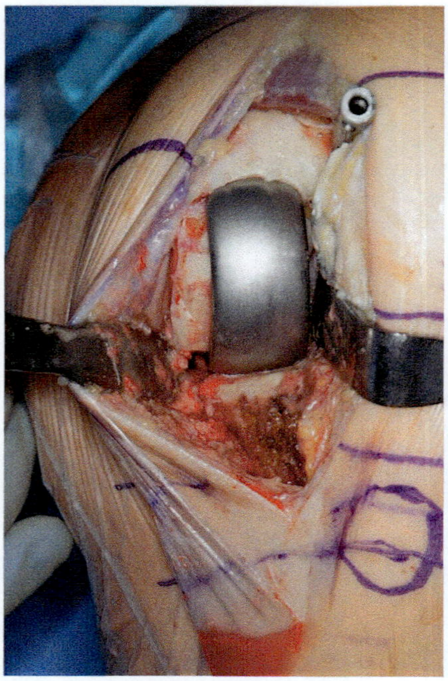

Figure 48.9 | The femoral component is then placed after the initial milling with the 0 spigot.

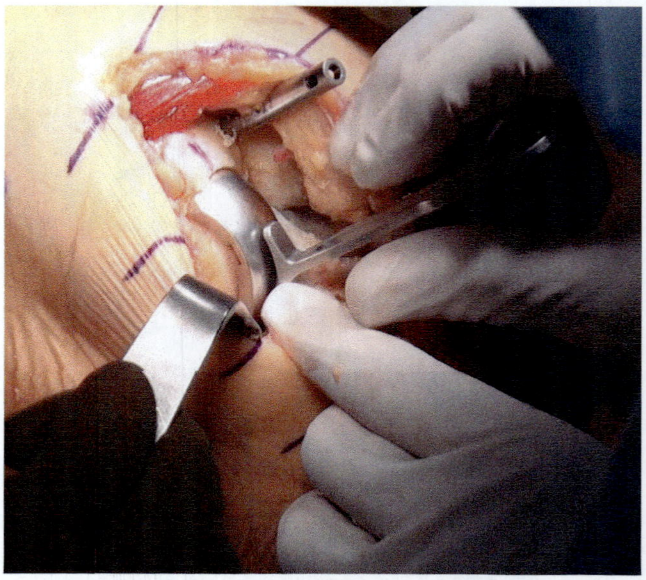

Figure 48.10 | The appropriate sized spoon is then placed around the femoral component trial.

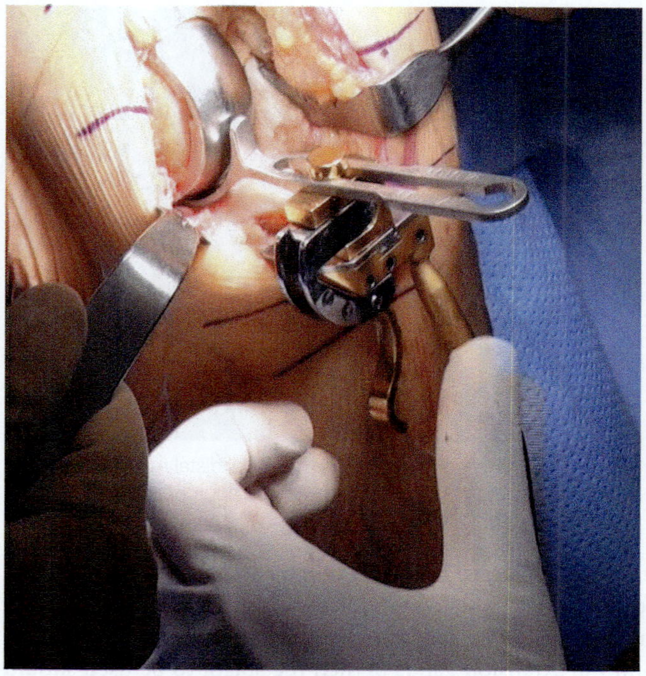

Figure 48.11 | The G-clamp is then used to couple the spoon to the tibial guide to aid in determining the depth of tibial resection.

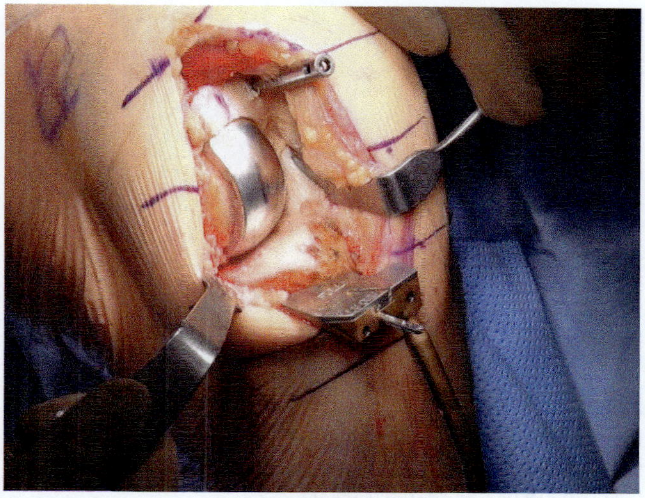

Figure 48.12 | The tibial guide is then pinned at the appropriate depth.

of internal and external rotation of the tibial cut. Subsequently make your horizontal cut, assuring protection to the MCL and the tibial spine (Figure 48.13). Remove the tibial bone. Verify that enough bone has been removed. If necessary recut with the 0 cutting guide. Place a tibial trial and assess the flexion extension gaps. The 3 mm feeler gauge should be easily inserted and removed without much extra force into the flexion space at 100° of flexion (Figure 48.14). Remove the 3 mm feeler gauge and bring the knee into extension and determine the extension gap. Establish the extension gap with the knee in approximately 20° of extension rather than full extension because of posterior capsular tightening. The gap is usually smaller and a thinner, metal feeler gauge should be used (Figure 48.15). If the 1 mm gauge is unable to be inserted in extension, then the gap is considered to be zero but could also be tighter than zero.

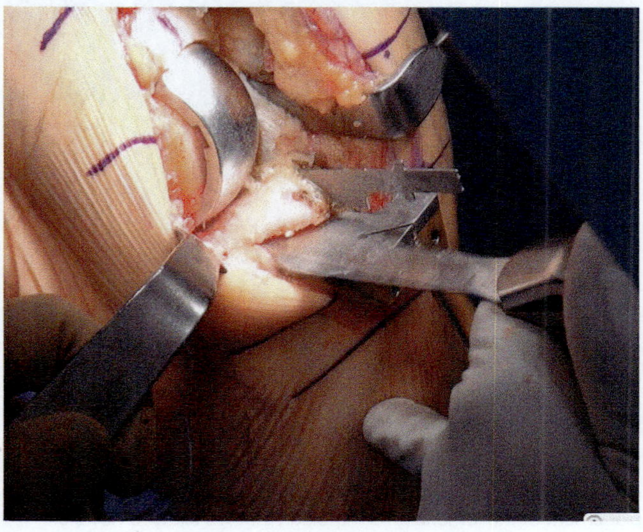

Figure 48.13 | First the vertical and then the horizontal cuts for the tibial bone resection are made.

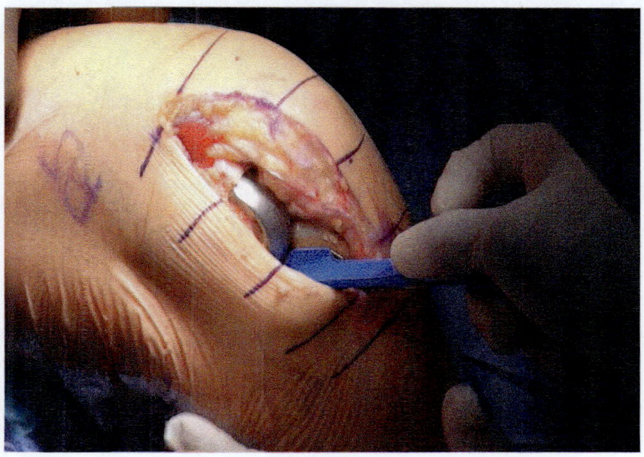

Figure 48.14 | The flexion space should fit a 3 mm feeler gauge with relative looseness.

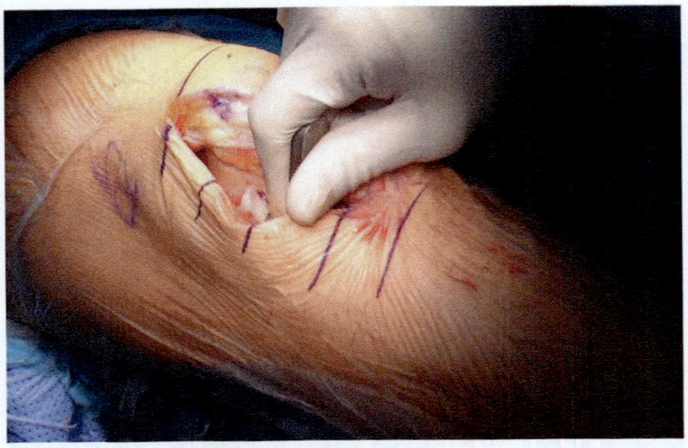

Figure 48.15 | The extension space is then trialled with a 1 mm metal gauge. The most common scenario is that the extension space will not allow insertion of the metal gauge

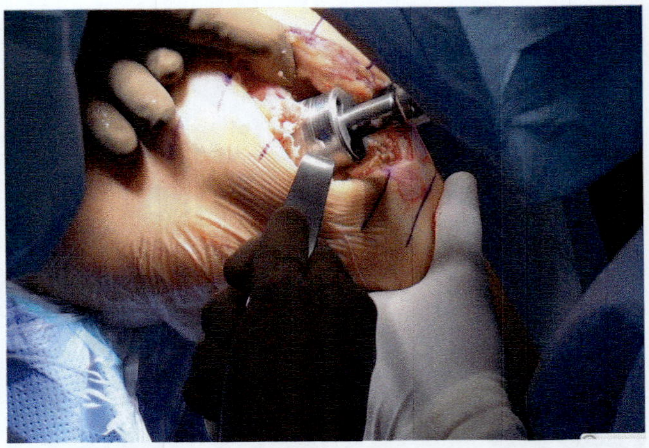

Figure 48.16 | After calculating the additional distal resection required, the femoral bone is milled with the appropriate sized mill.

- The spigots used for milling the distal femur are increased in 1 mm intervals and are numbered based on this. The formula for calculating the amount of bone to be removed from the distal femur is as follows: The thickness of bone to be removed equals the flexion gap in mm minus the extension gap in mm. So if the flexion gap is 3 mm and the extension gap is 0, then the spigot to be used should be the 3 spigot. Verify that the flexion and extension gaps are even before proceeding (Figures 48.16 and 48.17).
- Retrial the flexion and extension gaps until even. If the flexion space is still more than the extension space, then mill more distal femur using a new spigot. The spigot should reference off the initial spigot used. In other words, if the space after retrialling is still 2 mm tighter in extension than in flexion, and the first spigot used was a 3 mm spigot (as discussed above), then the next spigot should be a 5 mm spigot.
- Never leave the feeler gauge inside the flexion space when bringing the knee into extension until the gaps have been balanced.
- Completing femoral preparation: Use the femoral trimming guide to remove anterior and posterior osteophytes by using the drill and lightly tapping posteriorly with a mallet to remove the posterior osteophytes (Figure 48.18).
- Sizing the tibial component trial insertion: The tibial template is placed so that the posterior and medial margins are lined up with the posterior and medial edges of the tibial plateau using the tibial hook to ensure there is adequate placement. Pushing the tibial component posteriorly against the

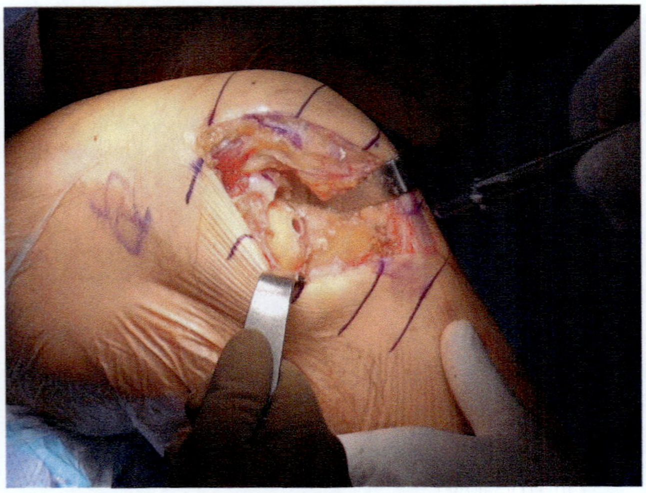

Figure 48.17 | The distal femur has been milled an additional 3 mm.

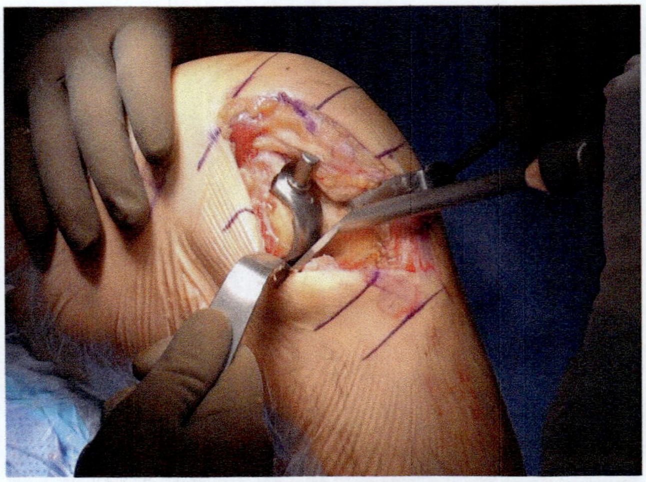

Figure 48.18 | After repeat trialling, and verification of equal flexion and extension spaces, the medial meniscus is removed followed by placement of the femoral finishing block that will allow removal of bone from the anterior and posterior aspects of the femoral condyle to prevent femoral/polyethylene impingement.

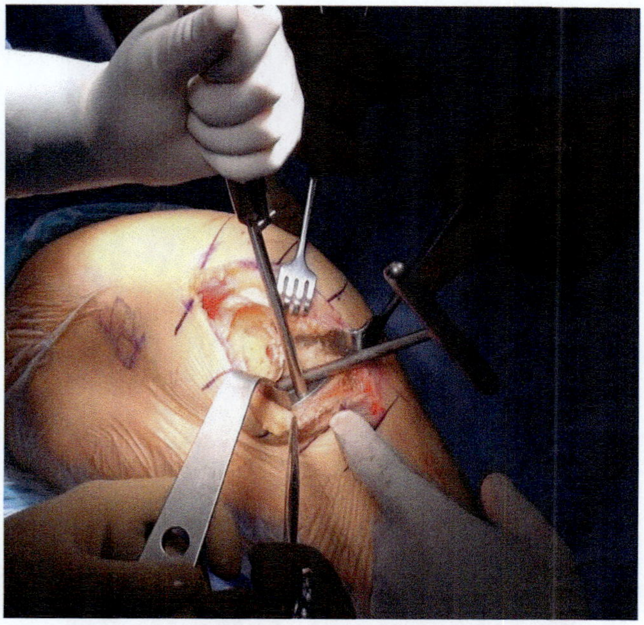

Figure 48.19 | The tibial component is sized using the T-handle to verify that the posterior aspect of the tibial trial is at the level of the posterior tibial cortex.

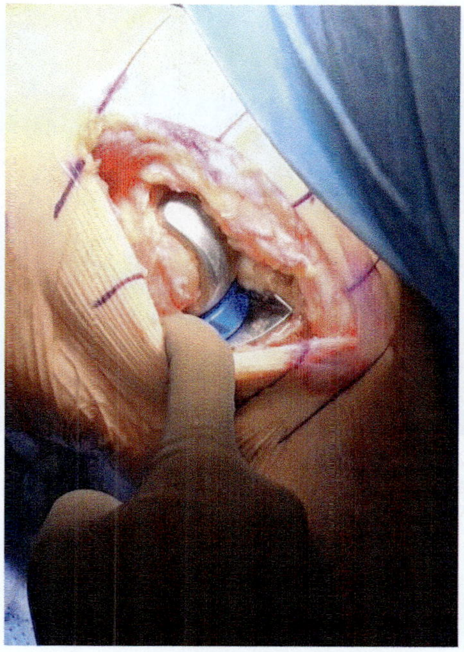

Figure 48.20 | The trial implants and mobile bearing polyethylene trial are in place.

hook that holding onto the posterior aspect of the tibial bone will prevent under-coverage of the posterior plateau that in turn could lead to subsidence (Figure 48.19). Up to 2 mm of overhang medially has been reported to be acceptable; however, the author prefers no overhang if possible.

- Insert the femoral and tibial trials and check range of motion. The trial polyethylene should be placed by hand. It should require some thumb pressure to insert, but if extreme force is needed, then the gap is too tight and further balancing is required (Figure 48.20).
- The tibial and femoral components can then be cemented into place. The author uses 1 batch of heated cement to fix both the tibial and femoral components at the same time. After the implants have been placed, placing the feeler gauge and placing a slight varus load will ensure that the implants are down on bone (Figures 48.21 and 48.22).

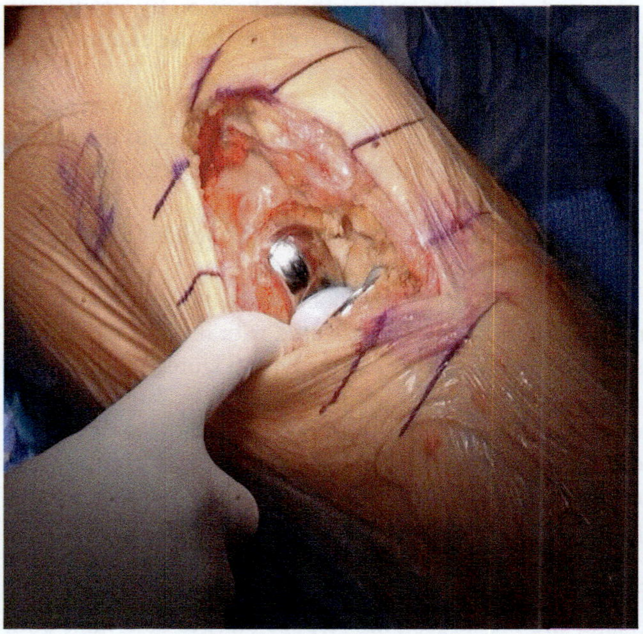

Figure 48.21 | The cemented implants and polyethylene are shown in extension.

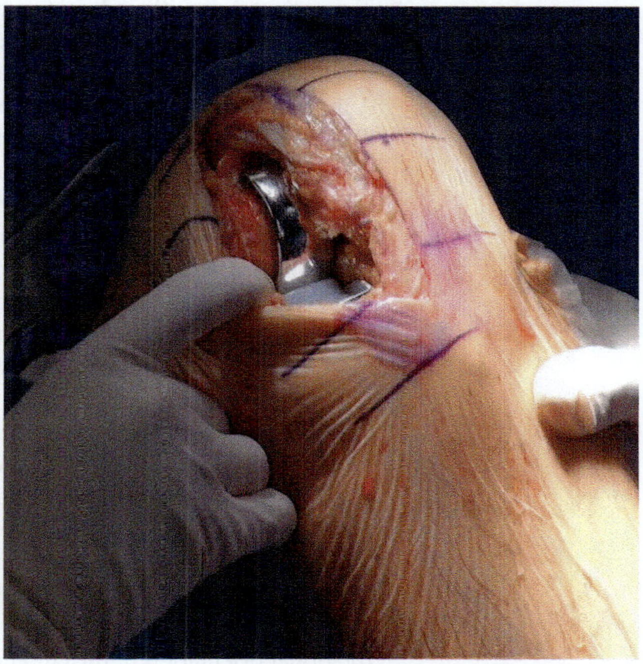

Figure 48.22 | The cemented implants and polyethylene are shown in flexion.

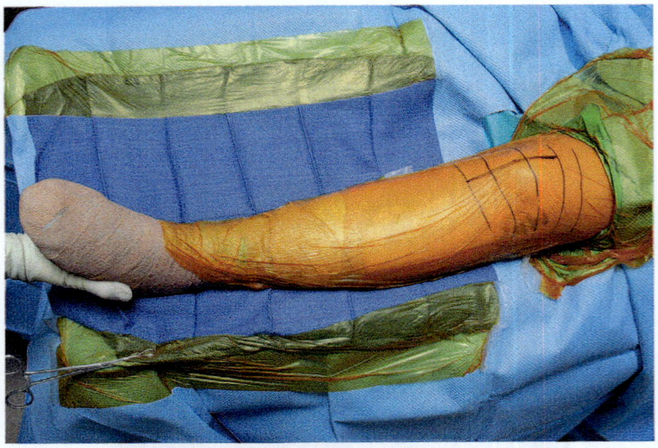

Figure 48.23 | Patient is positioned supine on the operating table with the feet at the end of the bed to facilitate use of intraoperative fluoroscopy.

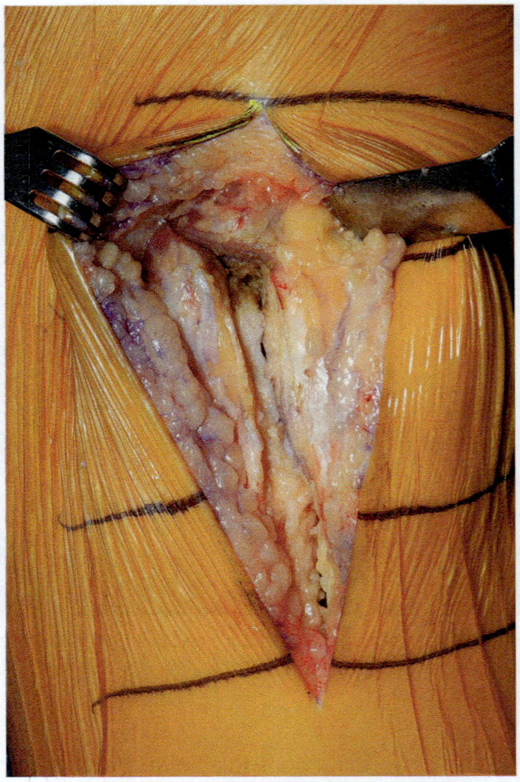

Figure 48.24 | A mini-midvastus approach with a 2.5 cm split in the vastus medialis is done.

- Remove excess cement from the edges of the implant, and irrigate the wound thoroughly. Close the arthrotomy and perform routine closure specific to the chosen approach; apply sterile dressing.
- Postoperative care: The patient is allowed to weightbear as tolerated.

Fixed Bearing Unicompartmental Arthroplasty Technique

- The patient is positioned supine on a standard operating table with no knee or leg positioning devices. The patient is brought as far distal on the table as possible to facilitate the use of intraoperative fluoroscopy that must include a view of the ipsilateral hip (Figure 48.23).
- A mini-midvastus arthrotomy is performed (Figure 48.24).
- The deep portion of the MCL is released and a Coker-clamp is placed just proximal to the medial meniscus to facilitate exposure throughout the procedure (Figure 48.25). A small portion of the retropatellar fat pad can be excised for visualization.
- Identify and debride the anvil osteophyte on the anterior tibia, if present, as this will limit full extension and be a source of painful impingement postoperatively (Figure 48.26).
- The extramedullary alignment guide is introduced into the medial joint space. Before pinning, the position of the guide and the overall limb alignment are quickly assessed with intraoperative fluoroscopy (Figure 48.27). Sequential views of the ankle (Figure 48.28), the knee (Figure 48.29), and the hip (Figure 48.30) are obtained.
- This extramedullary system has the dramatic advantage that it simultaneously allows the surgeon to set the limb alignment before any bone cuts are made; links the femoral and tibial cuts to ensure that they are parallel in extension; and ensures a perfect extension gap resection with a measured resection of the distal femur to match the implant and a minimal thickness cut of the tibia (Figure 48.31).
- The guide is removed and the proximal tibial pins are left in place. The 3° posterior slope tibial guide is placed and the knee is flexed to 90° (Figure 48.32).
- The vertical tibial cut is carried out freehand, and the surgeon has responsibility to determine both rotational orientation of the cut and the midline position of the cut. Most surgeons are best served

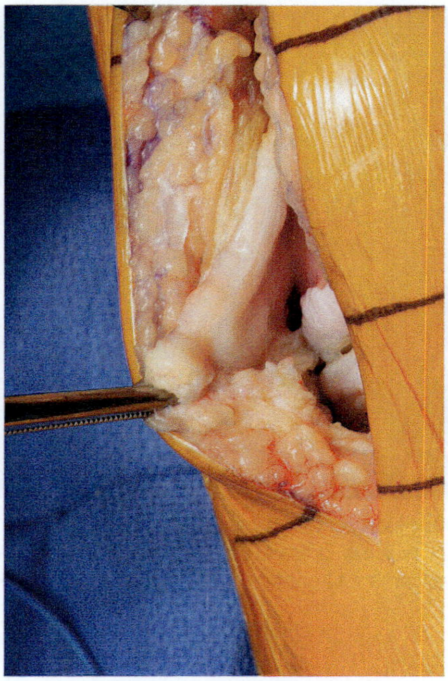

Figure 48.25 | A coker-clamp is placed just proximal to the medial meniscus and serves as a useful retractor throughout the case.

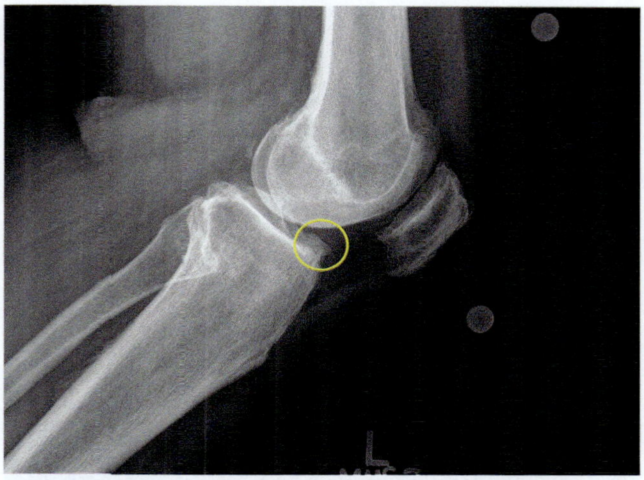

Figure 48.26 | The anterior tibial or anvil osteophyte is important to identify and remove to allow full, pain-free knee extension postoperatively.

to flex the knee to exactly 90° of flexion and to also flex the ankle to 90° in an effort to reproducibly assess knee position (Figure 48.33).

- The midline position of the cut is typically adjacent to the medial femoral condyle and often abuts the ACL insertion. The rotational position of the cut is akin to positioning a tibial component for TKA in that the saw might be described as aligned with the junction of the medial and middle thirds of the tibial tubercle (Figure 48.34).

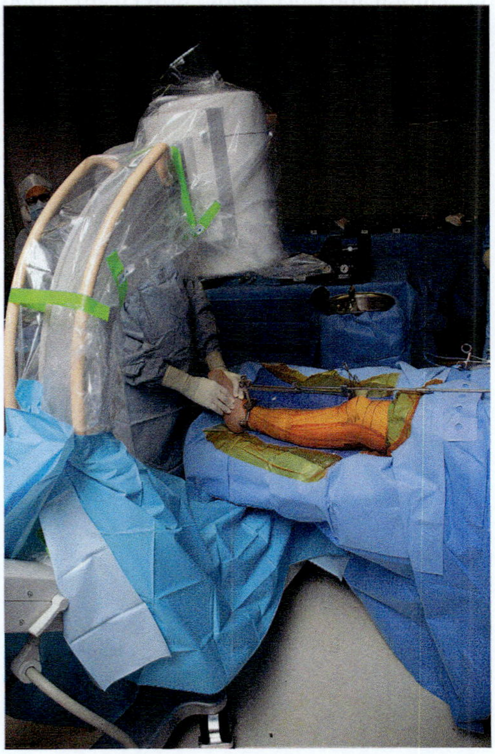

Figure 48.27 | The extramedullary alignment guide is introduced into the medial joint space and C-arm fluoroscopy is used to assess overall limb alignment and quickly correct it before pinning the guide.

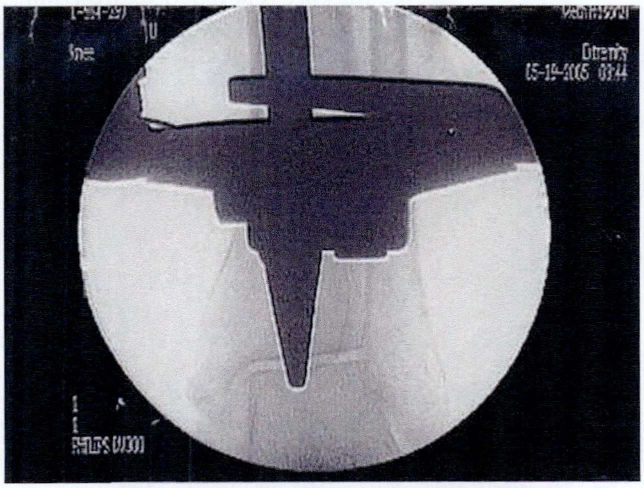

Figure 48.28 | Fluoroscopy confirms that the guide is positioned over the center of the talus.

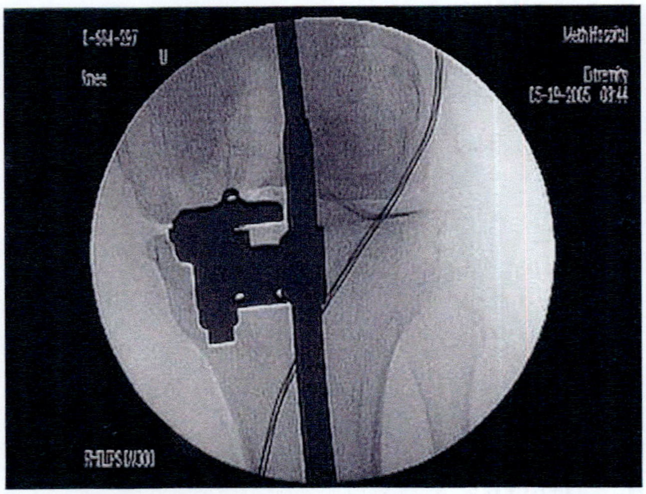

Figure 48.29 | Fluoroscopy confirms the guide is positioned over the center of the knee.

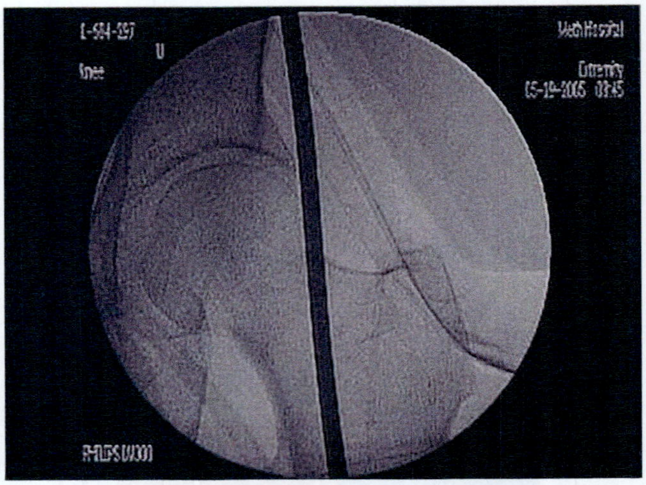

Figure 48.30 | Fluoroscopy confirms the guide rod passes just lateral to the femoral, which is indicative of slight mechanical axis varus, which is the alignment target for medial unicompartmental knee arthroplasty.

- In the typical patient with isolated advanced medial compartment degenerative arthritis, the surgeon will note that there is still full-thickness articular cartilage on the posterior portion of the tibial resection (Figure 48.35).
- It is important to fully fill the tibial space from posterior to anterior while also avoiding medial overhang. The flat tibial sizing plate is left in place and the knee is flexed to 90° (Figure 48.36).
- The appropriate size femur will extend to the subchondral bone anteriorly but never encroach on the articular cartilage (Figure 48.37). It is better to have a small amount of bone exposed anteriorly than to have any overlap with the cartilage.
- Femoral rotation is determined methodically because the flat surface of the femoral sizing guide is resting on the flat surface of the tibial sizing plate. As long as the patella is reduced in the trochlea and the knee is flexed to 90° the co-linear nature of the femoral and tibial guides now ensures appropriate rotation in flexion.

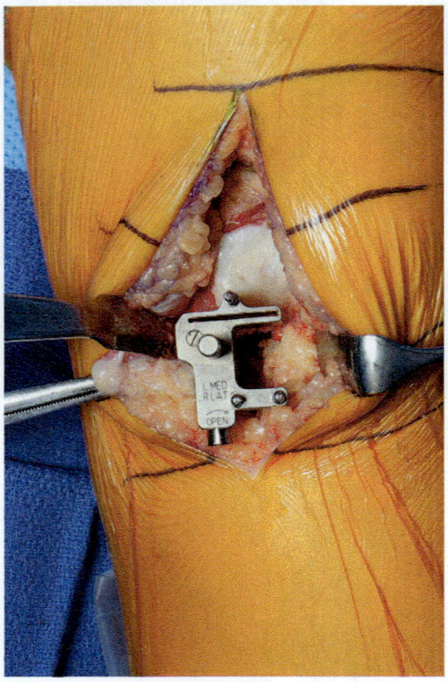

Figure 48.31 | The cutting guide is pinned and the distal femoral cut completed.

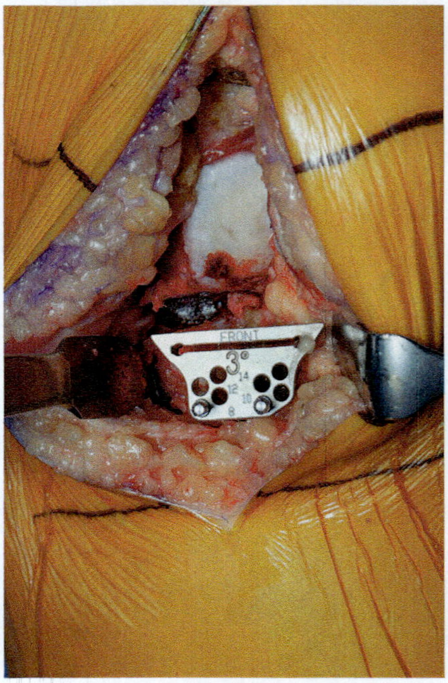

Figure 48.32 | The proximal tibial guide is placed on the tibial pins. The 3° posterior slope guide is routinely selected as is the minimal thickness depth setting.

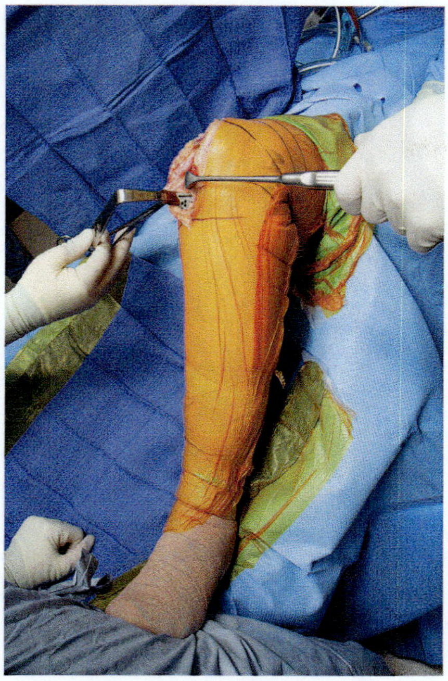

Figure 48.33 I For reproducibility the tibial cut is best made with the knee at 90° of flexion and the ankle at 90°.

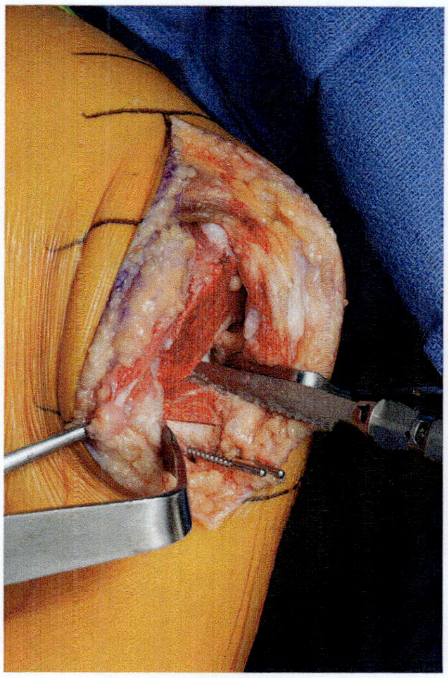

Figure 48.34 I The vertical portion of the tibial cut impacts sizing and also sets the rotation of the tibial component. This cut abuts the medial femoral condyle and often grazes the tibial attachment of the anterior cruciate ligament. Rotationally the vertical cut is often aligned with the junction of the medial and middle thirds of the tibial tubercle.

- The medial meniscus is excised with electrocautery. The midline osteophytes and posterior osteophytes are removed with a curved osteotome (Figure 48.38).
- The intercondylar notch is inspected and any osteophytes are removed with a curved osteotome. Using the same osteotome, a vertical impression is made in the proximal tibia to accommodate the fin of the tibial trial (Figure 48.39).
- The femoral trial and the tibial insert are placed and the knee brought to 90° of flexion (Figure 48.40).

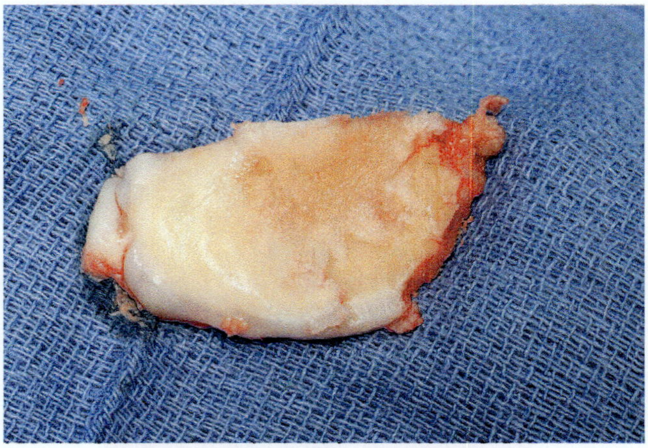

Figure 48.35 I The resected tibia typically has full-thickness articular cartilage posteriorly.

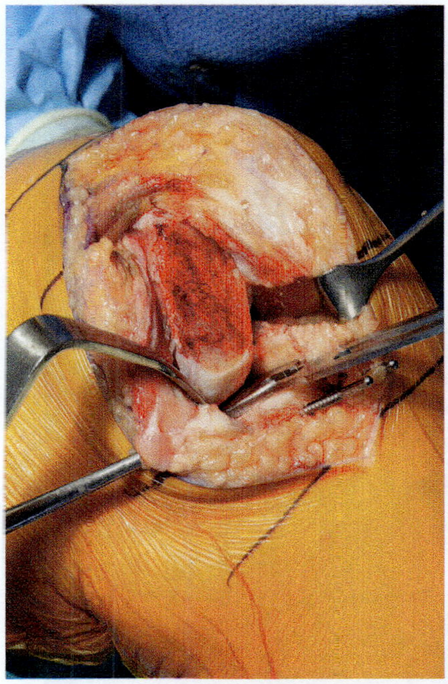

Figure 48.36 I The tibia is sized to prioritize filling the space from posterior to anterior maximally without medial tibial overhang. Occasionally the vertical cut is re-done to fit the next larger tibial implant

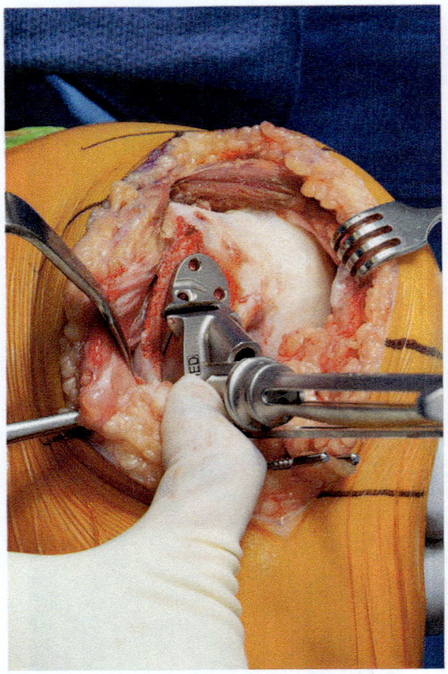

Figure 48.37 | The femoral component should extend to the subchondral bone anteriorly but never encroach on the cartilage. Femoral sizing and rotation is facilitated by leaving the flat tibial sizing plate in place and flexing the knee to 90°. Femoral rotation is methodically set by allowing the flat portion of the tibial sizing plate and the flat posterior surface of the femoral guide to mate at 90° of flexion. This works well provided that the patella is reduced in the trochlea and not subluxed laterally.

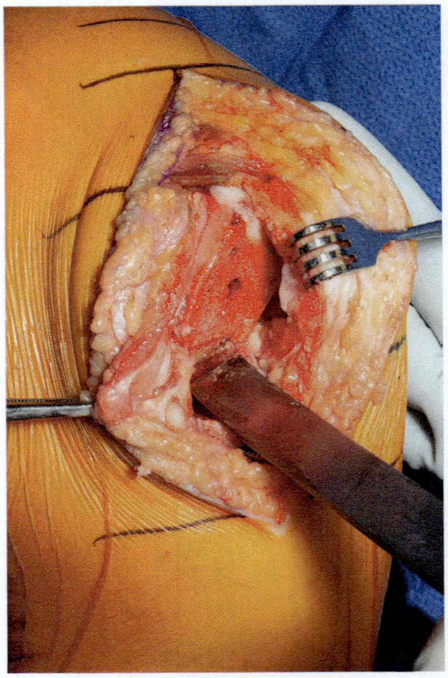

Figure 48.38 | Osteophytes are removed posteriorly and along the intercondylar notch medially and laterally with a curved osteotome.

- The flexion and extension gaps are then assessed with a 2 and 3 mm spacer block (Figure 48.41). The ideal gaps are 2 mm and symmetric, but it is likely acceptable for the flexion gap to be 3 mm. If the flexion gap is <2 or >3 mm, then the tibia can be recut and this is facilitated by leaving the tibial pins in place until this trial has been done. For a tight flexion gap (<2 mm) the tibia is recut with more posterior slope (5° guide instead of the standard 3°), and this solves the issue quickly and accurately.

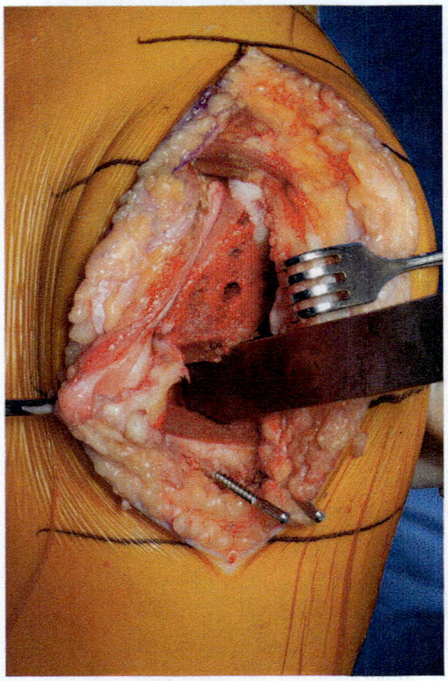

Figure 48.39 | A vertical slot is made for the tibial fin.

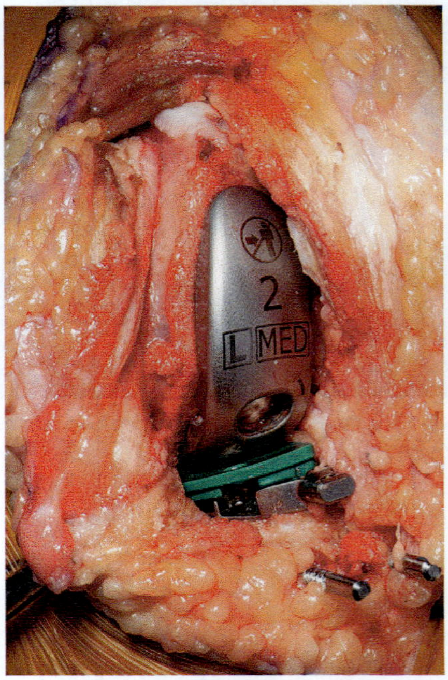

Figure 48.40 | The femoral and tibial trials are assembled and the knee is assessed at 90° of flexion.

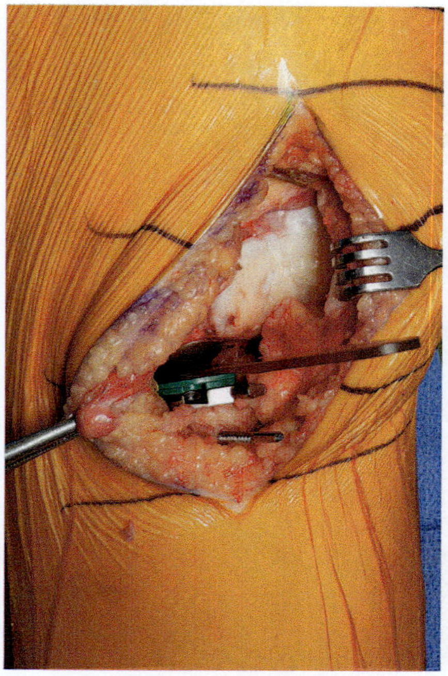

Figure 48.41 | A spacer block with 2 and 3 mm increments is used to assess flexion and extension gap balance. Ideal balance is 2 mm and symmetric gaps.

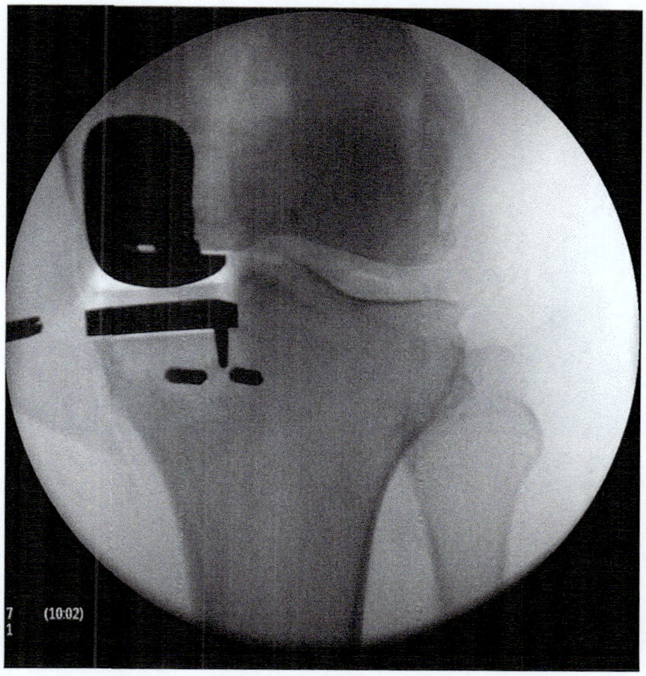

Figure 48.42 | C-arm fluoroscopy confirms final trial component position with attention to ensure no overhang of the tibia medially, co-linearity of the femoral and tibial components in extension, and appropriate tibial varus-valgus (ideal is often 1° of varus not neutral).

- Once perfect balance is obtained, the final trial component position is assessed under c-arm fluoroscopy to ensure no overhang of the tibial component; co-linearity of the femur and tibia in extension; appropriate tibial varus-valgus orientation (ideal is often 1° of tibial varus not neutral) (Figure 48.42).
- Trial components are removed, the knee is irrigated with pulsatile lavage, and a periarticular local anesthetic injection comprising ropivacaine, ketorolac, and dilute epinephrine is performed (Figure 48.43).

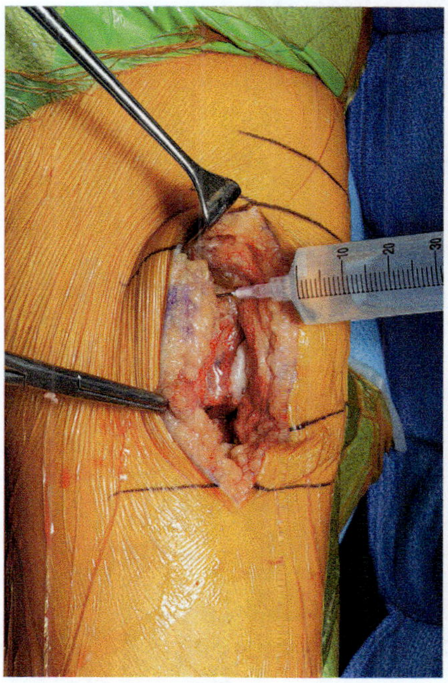

Figure 48.43 | A periarticular local anesthetic injection is performed prior to cementing.

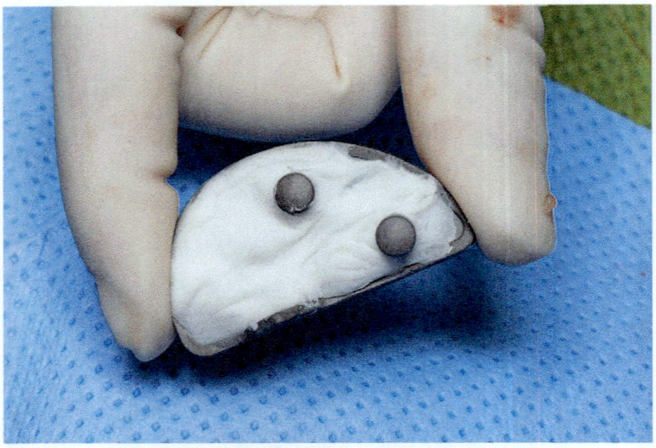

Figure 48.44 I The tibial implant is precoated with cement to prevent fluid infiltration at the implant-cement interface.

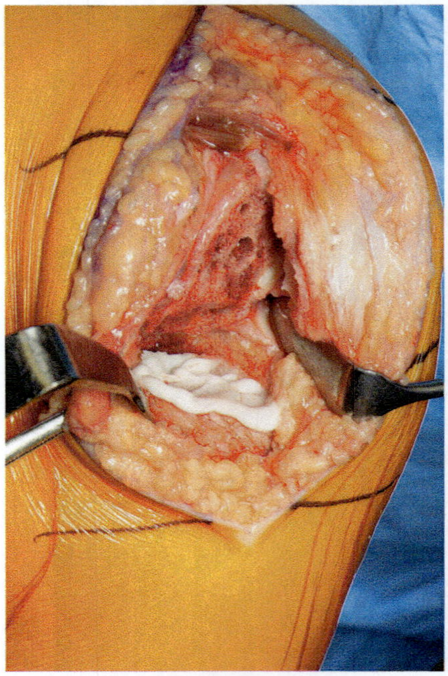

Figure 48.45 I A small amount of additional cement is hand pressed into the proximal tibia.

- The components are cemented using 1 batch of simplex bone cement mixed with 1.2 g of powdered gentamicin. The tibial cementing is done methodically by precoating the entire underside of the tibial component with cement on the back table (Figure 48.44) and then pressurizing a small amount of cement into the proximal tibia by hand using care not to leave excessive cement posteriorly (Figure 48.45).
- The tibia is inserted by hand, the posterior portion is seated first, and then the impactor is used to gently impact the tibia fully starting slightly posterior to ensure full seating (Figure 48.46). Excess cement is carefully removed with a curved cement remover.
- The femoral component is initially inserted at about 95° of flexion and then brought out to about 80° of flexion for final impaction (Figure 48.47). The real tibial insert is then placed with the knee at 90°

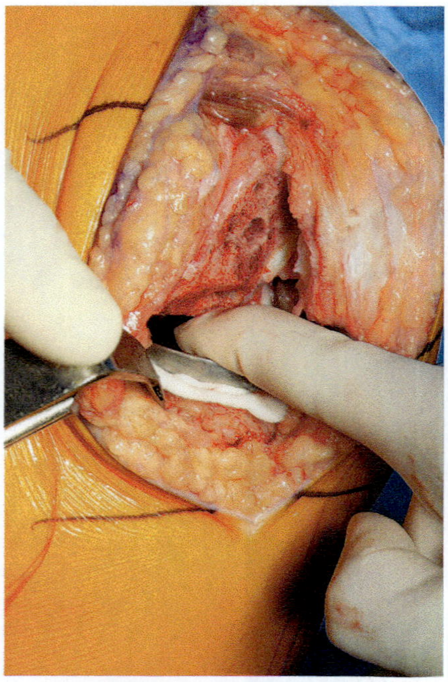

Figure 48.46 I The tibia is impacted starting posteriorly to ensure full seating.

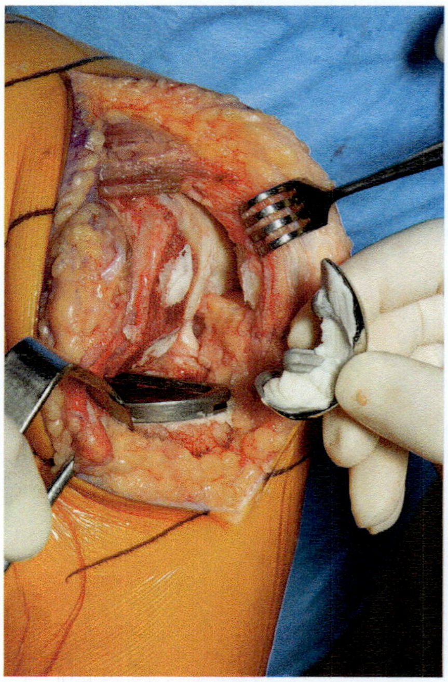

Figure 48.47 I The femoral component is precoated with cement, the femoral lug holes filled with cement, and then the component impacted into place.

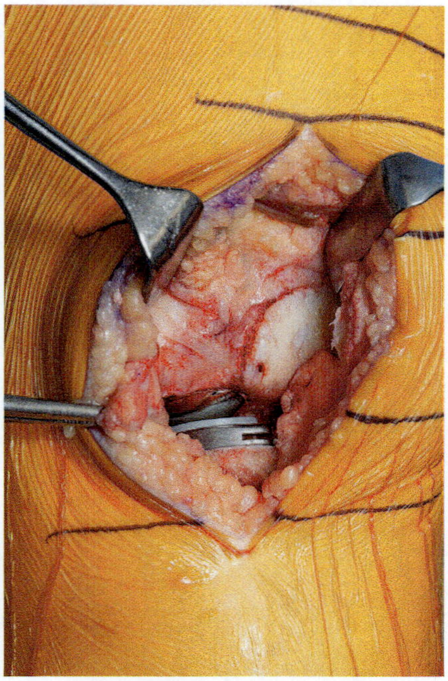

Figure 48.48 | The knee is brought to extension but not hyperextension to avoid posterior tibial lift-off while the cement cures.

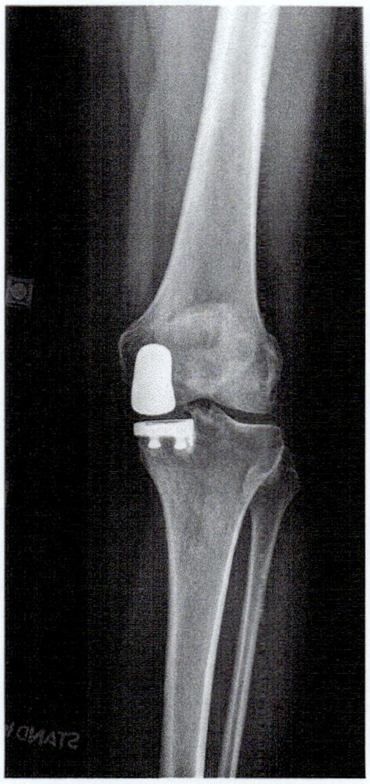

Figure 48.49 | Postoperative anteroposterior view of a typical fixed bearing medial unicompartmental knee arthroplasty.

of flexion and letting the weight of the femur force the posterior dove-tail into place before impacting anteriorly for final seating.

- The knee is gently brought to extension deliberately avoiding hyperextension while the cement is curing (Figure 48.48).
- The wound is then closed in multiple layers using absorbable sutures and a running subcuticular skin closure. A sterile dressing and compressive wrap is applied and then the tourniquet is deflated. Postoperative radiographs are obtained routinely (Figure 48.49).

Final Thoughts for Fixed Bearing UKA

- Avoid overcorrection of the mechanical axis. The overall limb alignment should remain in slight mechanical varus to avoid overloading the lateral compartment.
- Carefully review the preoperative lateral radiograph for the presence of an anterior tibial anvil osteophyte, which must be removed to ensure full extension.
- In order to facilitate exposure, try various combinations of knee flexion, external rotation of the tibia, and valgus stress. Often small changes in one of those parameters can markedly improve visualization.
- Most patients will recover uneventfully with little supervised physical therapy. More often it is necessary to prevent UKA patients from overdoing activities in the early postoperative period.
- Consider the routine use of intraoperative fluoroscopy to confirm accuracy of the bone cuts, colinearity of the femoral and tibial components in extension, and overall limb alignment before cementing takes place.

Chapter 49
Patellofemoral Arthroplasty

R. KYLE MARTIN
DIANE L. DAHM

Key Concepts

- Patellofemoral arthroplasty (PFA) is indicated for a specific subset of patients with degenerative arthritis whose pattern of symptoms localizes to the anterior knee and occurs primarily during activities that load the knee in flexion. This may include climbing up and down stairs, rising from a seated position, squatting, kneeling, and/or navigating uneven surfaces.
- Outcomes of PFA can be optimized with proper surgical indications, appropriate implant selection, and meticulous surgical technique.
- PFA can be considered a definitive procedure for older patients with isolated patellofemoral arthritis. This may offer advantages over total knee arthroplasty (TKA) such as decreased blood loss, shorter hospital stay, and improved range of motion. PFA can also be utilized as an "interim" procedure for relatively young patients with advanced symptomatic patellofemoral arthritis and early tibiofemoral arthritis who wish to postpone TKA (Figure 49.1).

Surgical Indications

- Isolated, advanced, primary patellofemoral degenerative arthritis
- Patellofemoral arthritis with trochlear dysplasia
  - These patients have a relatively low reported rate of progression of tibiofemoral arthritis and are well suited for PFA.
  - Patellofemoral malalignment is common in this population and may be addressed by way of implant selection and positioning or with concomitant bony or soft tissue realignment procedures.
- Posttraumatic patellofemoral arthritis
- Radiographic evidence of patellofemoral joint space narrowing
  - Patients with "normal" low-flexion-angle axial radiographs exhibit inferior results versus those with visible patellofemoral joint space narrowing.
- Failure of a comprehensive nonoperative management program

Contraindications

- Moderate or advanced tibiofemoral chondromalacia
- Inflammatory arthritis
  - PFA can be considered if there is no clinical or radiographic evidence of synovitis or inflammatory arthropathy in the operative knee.
- Post septic arthritis
- Morbid obesity
- Significant coronal plane malalignment (>5°-10° varus/valgus)
- Significant patella baja (<0.8 Caton-Deschamps Index)
- Significant flexion contracture (>5°-10°)

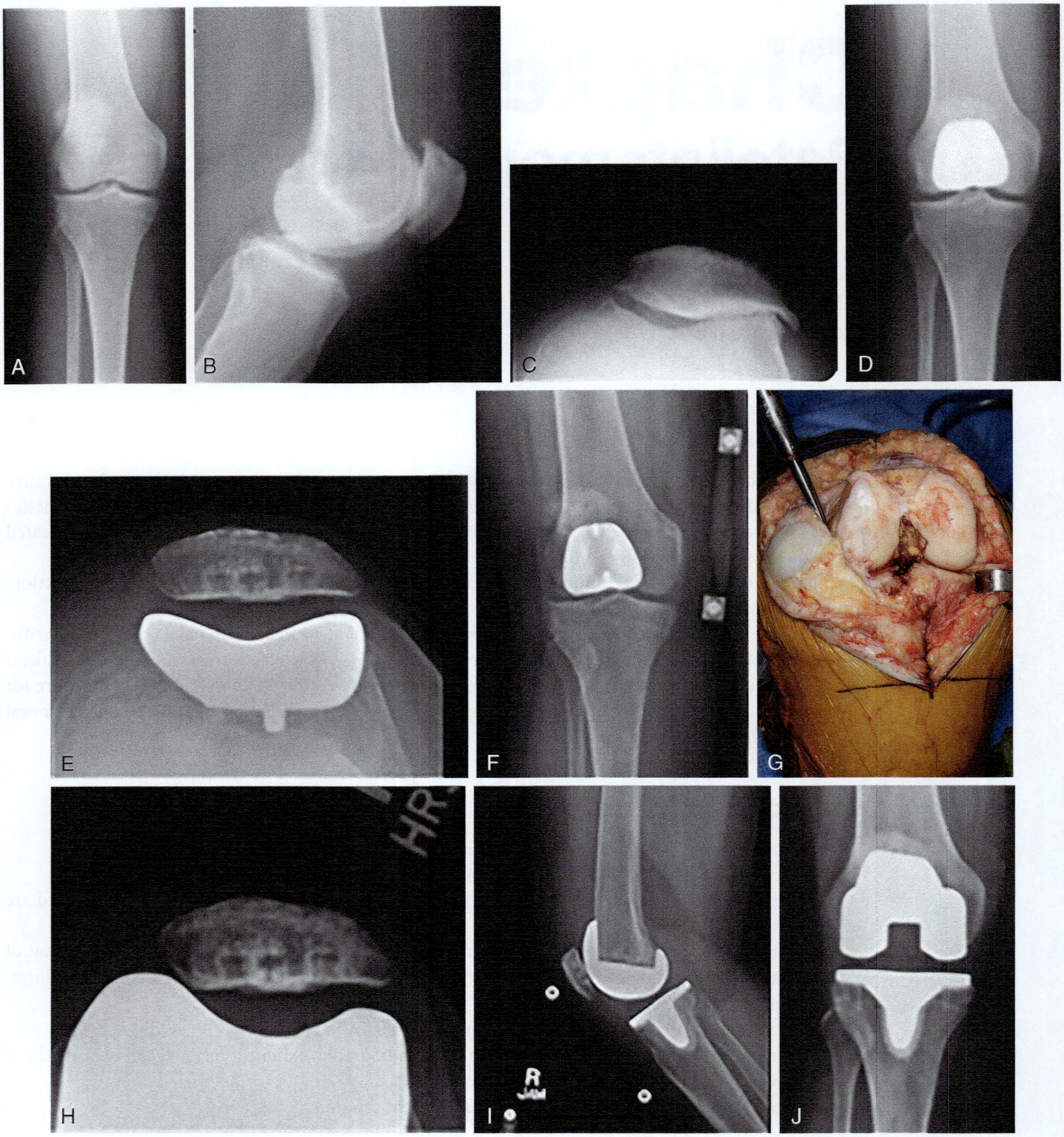

Figure 49.1 | Preoperative AP, lateral, and Merchant radiographs (A-C) and postoperative AP and Merchant (D and E) radiographs of a 50-year-old woman with advanced patellofemoral arthritis who underwent PFA. Progression of tibiofemoral arthritis occurred 12 years post PFA (F) and subsequent conversion to TKA was performed (G-J).

Imaging

- Radiographs: Standing anteroposterior (AP), posteroanterior (PA) flexion, lateral, Merchant, and long-leg standing hip-to-ankle radiographs (Figure 49.2).
- Magnetic resonance imaging (MRI) may be necessary to rule out significant (grade 3-4) tibiofemoral chondromalacia (Figure 49.3).
- Computed tomography (CT) may assist with preoperative planning, specifically regarding the need for concomitant tibial tubercle osteotomy (TTO) in the setting of significant lateral patellar subluxation/dislocation (Figure 49.4).

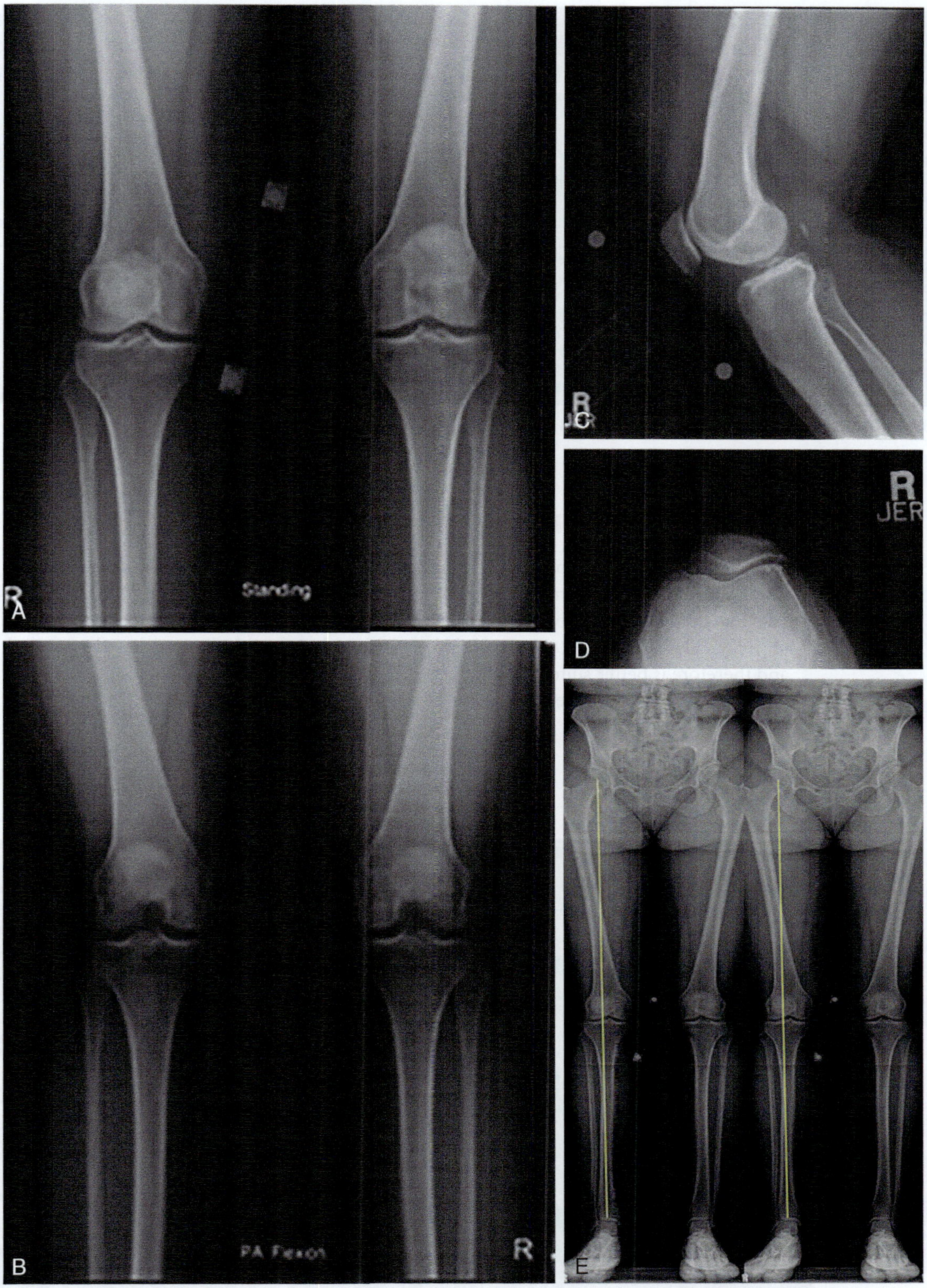

Figure 49.2 | AP (A), PA flexion (B), lateral (C), Merchant (D), and hip-to-ankle standing radiographs (E) of a 58-year-old woman demonstrating isolated patellofemoral arthritis with neutral mechanical axis.

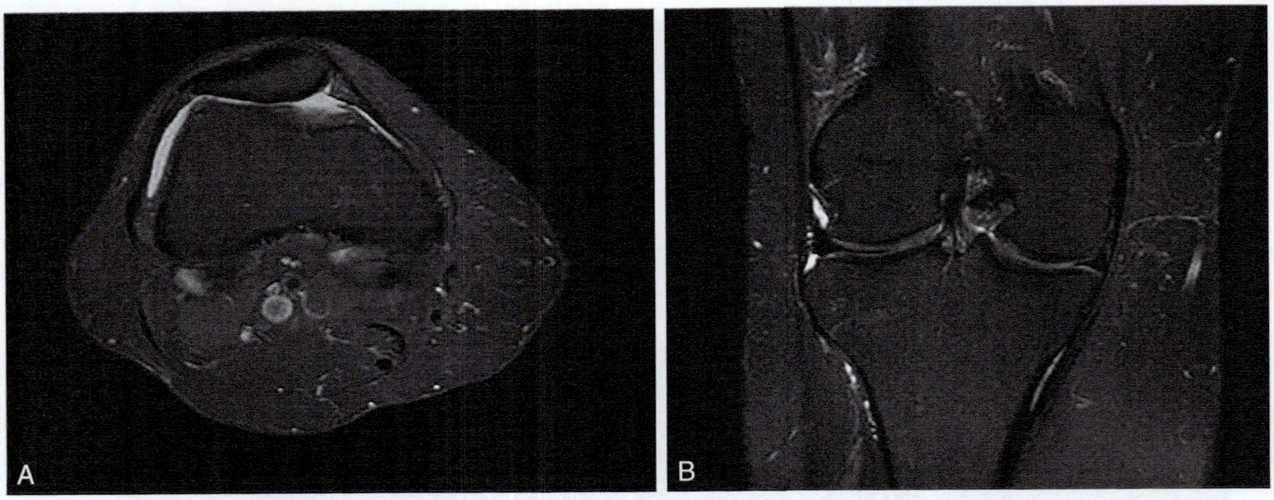

Figure 49.3 | Axial (A) and coronal (B) MRI confirms isolated patellofemoral disease.

Surgical Technique

- Choice of implant: Most patients with isolated patellofemoral degenerative arthritis have trochlear dysplasia and exhibit internal rotation of the distal femur. The authors prefer an implant that utilizes an onlay design owing to belief that it provides a more reproducible outcome for these patients than an inlay design (Figure 49.5). The inlay prosthetic design typically matches the patient's anatomy and therefore is better suited for patients with posttraumatic arthritis or those with low-grade or no trochlear dysplasia (Figure 49.6).

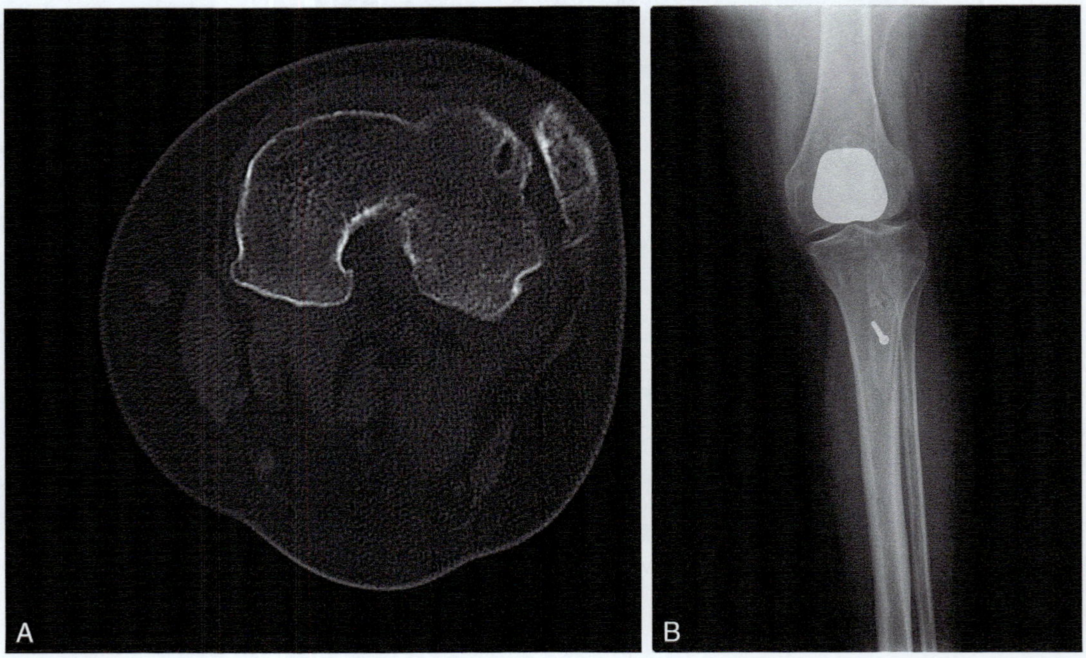

Figure 49.4 | CT confirms high- grade trochlear dysplasia (A), and the patient required tibial tubercle osteotomy and medial patellofemoral ligament reconstruction in addition to PFA (B).

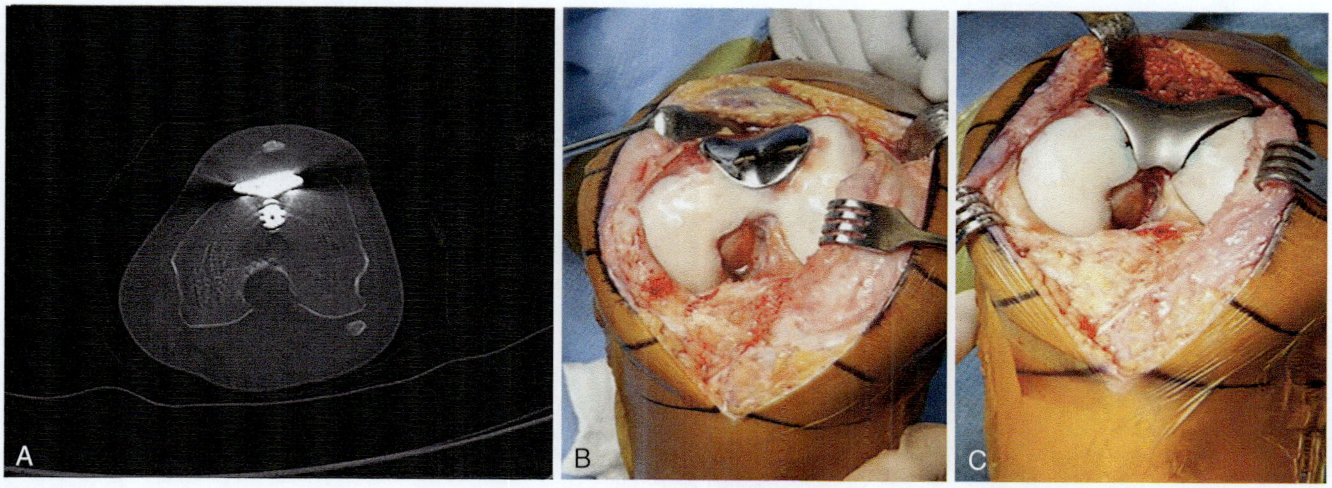

Figure 49.5 | Axial CT (A) and intraoperative photograph (B) of an inlay component that required conversion to an onlay PFA (C) due to persistent "J sign".

Preoperative Planning

- Trochlear component: Consider anteroposterior and medial-lateral sizing. In the setting of patella alta, ensure that the proximal extent of the prosthesis is adequate for proper tracking. If there is no apparent engagement of the patella in the trochlea on lateral radiograph, consider tibial tubercle distalization, either staged or in conjunction with PFA. If the patella is tracking or subluxating laterally, in general, a trochlear component with a wider proximal geometry will be less likely to require a combined realignment procedure.
- Patellar component: For extensive patellar wear resulting a very thin patella, consider leaving the patella unresurfaced or performing a staged bone grafting procedure (Figure 49.7).

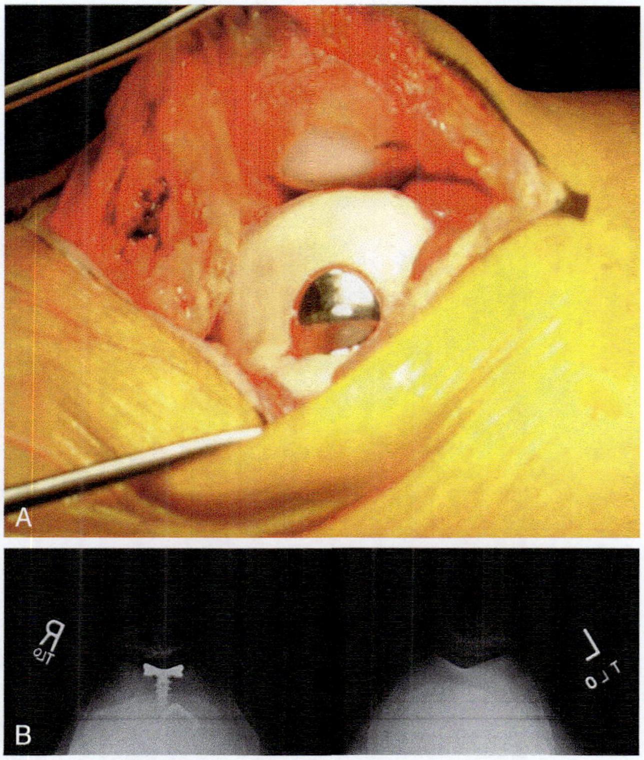

Figure 49.6 | Surgical (A) and Merchant radiographic (B) images of an inlay prosthesis in a patient with no evidence of patellofemoral malalignment. (From Cannon A, Stolley M, Wolf B, Amendola A. Patellofemoral resurfacing arthroplasty: literature review and a description of a novel technique. *Iowa Orthop J.* 2008;28:42-48.)

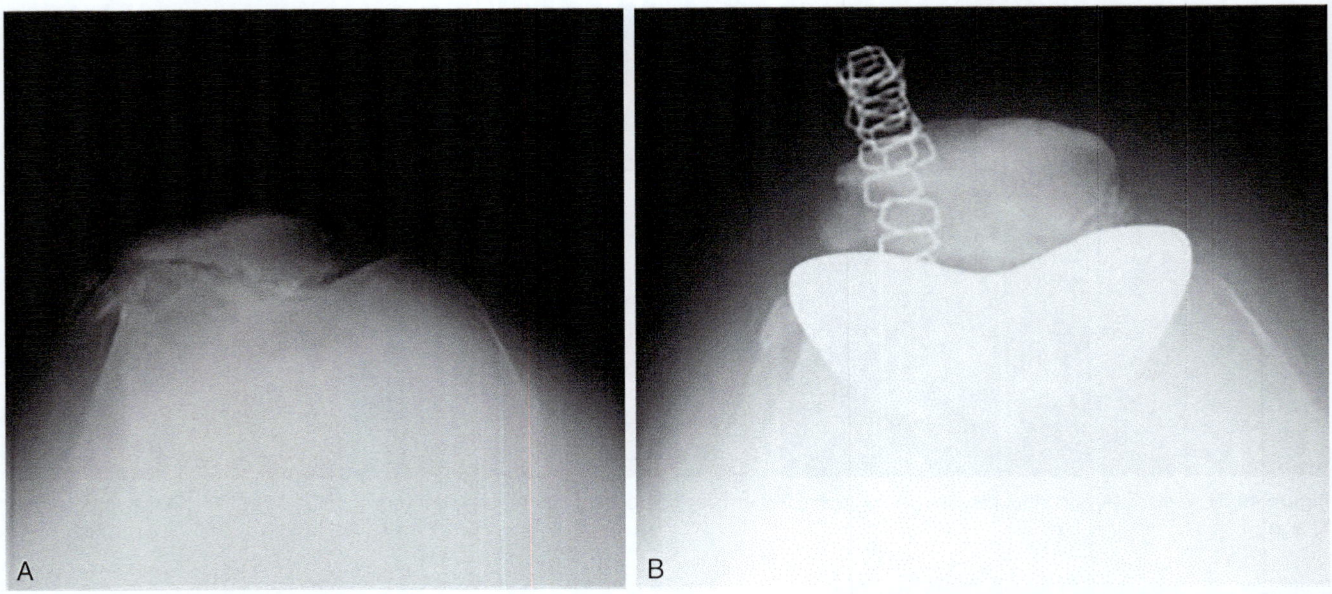

Figure 49.7 | Preoperative (A) and postoperative (B) Merchant radiographs of a very thin patella that required bone grafting at the time of PFA, with planned staged resurfacing.

Positioning

- Supine positioning with use of padding under the ipsilateral hip to achieve neutral limb rotation (patella facing straight up).

Surgical Approach

- Standard medial parapatellar (shown), midvastus or subvastus approach, with preservation of the medial meniscus and intermeniscal ligament. A portion of the fat pad may be excised as needed to achieve improved exposure (Figure 49.8).
- Excise peripheral osteophytes.
- Expose the distal anterior femur immediately adjacent to the proximal extent of the trochlea.

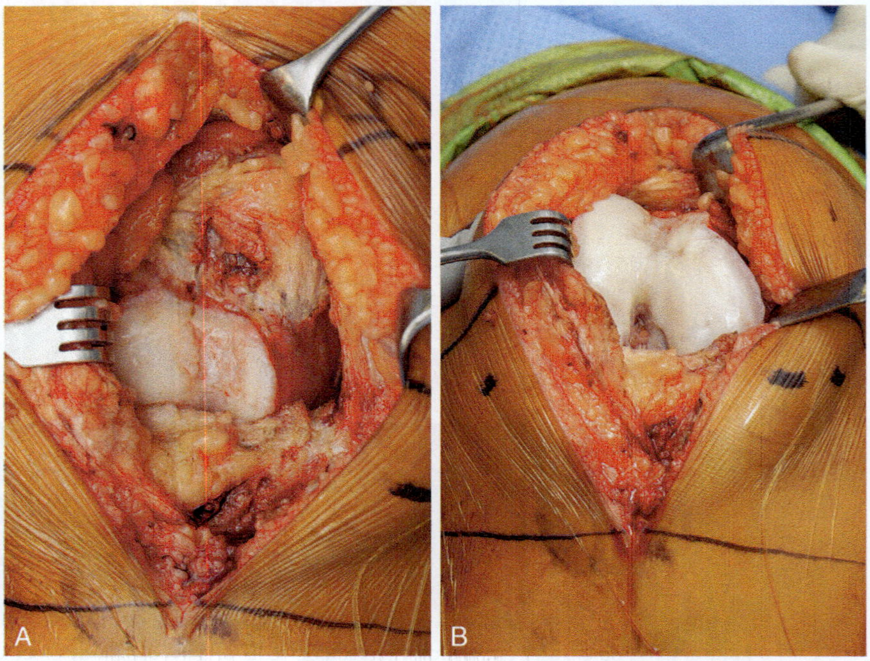

Figure 49.8 | Intraoperative exposure (A and B) via medial parapatellar arthrotomy, preserving the menisci and intermeniscal ligament.

Preparation of the Femur

- Ensure appropriate trochlear component alignment in the sagittal, axial, and coronal planes
  - Sagittal plane positioning: Anterior femoral cut is performed parallel to the distal anterior femoral cortex (Figure 49.9).
    - Avoid notching of the anterior distal femur (prosthesis too extended).
    - Distal extent of the implant should not extend beyond the intercondylar notch to prevent impingement on the anterior cruciate ligament in extension.
    - Avoid excessive component flexion to prevent notch impingement and "catching" of the patella on the proximal flange of the prosthesis. Risk is greatest in patients with patella alta (Figure 49.10).
- Axial plane positioning: Component rotation should match the transepicondylar axis with slight external rotation considered desirable for most onlay designs. Rotation can also be set using a guide to allow for a perpendicular orientation to the long axis of the tibia (Figure 49.11). Specifically, internal rotation of the trochlear component should be avoided.
- Coronal plane (varus-valgus) positioning (Figure 49.12)
  - Symmetric prostheses: Should be placed perpendicular to the long axis of the femur.
  - Asymmetric prostheses: These designs have a built-in lateral tracking angle and thus should be placed perpendicular to the mechanical axis in most cases. The implant should be flush or slightly recessed to the articular cartilage distally, medially, and laterally when possible.
  - Slight lateral translation of the trochlear component can be performed in cases of significant lateral patellar tracking. Lateral overhang of the prosthesis should be avoided, however (Figure 49.13).

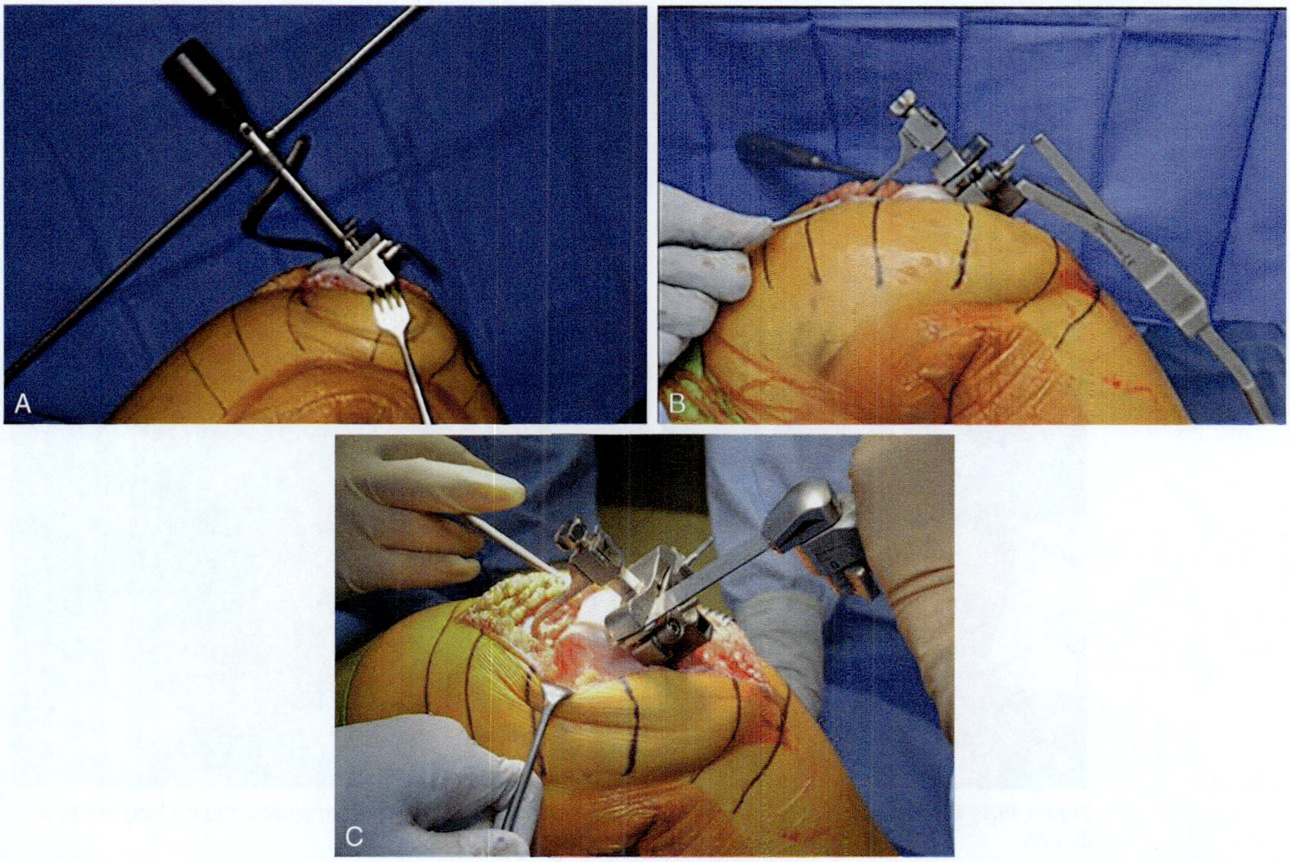

Figure 49.9 I The anterior femoral cut is performed parallel to the distal anterior femoral cortex using an alignment rod (A). Alternatively, sagittal alignment may be determined through direct contact with the distal anterior femoral cortex (B). Intraoperative photograph of anterior femoral cut (C).

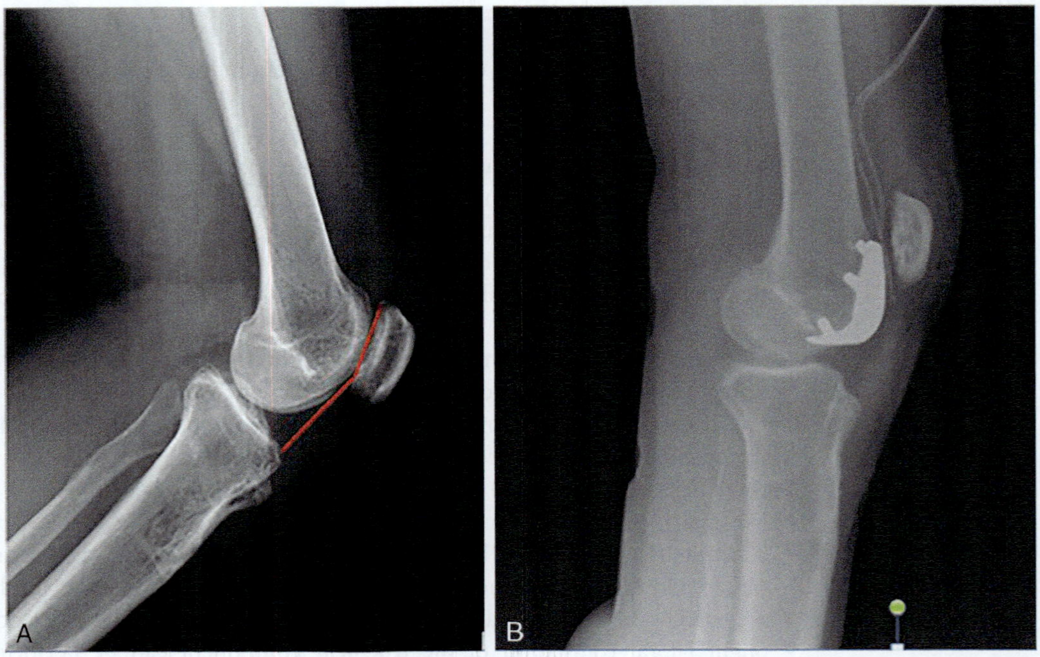

Figure 49.10 | Preoperative lateral radiographs demonstrating patella alta (A) and a somewhat flexed trochlear component at risk for having the patella "catch" on the superior flange during motion (B).

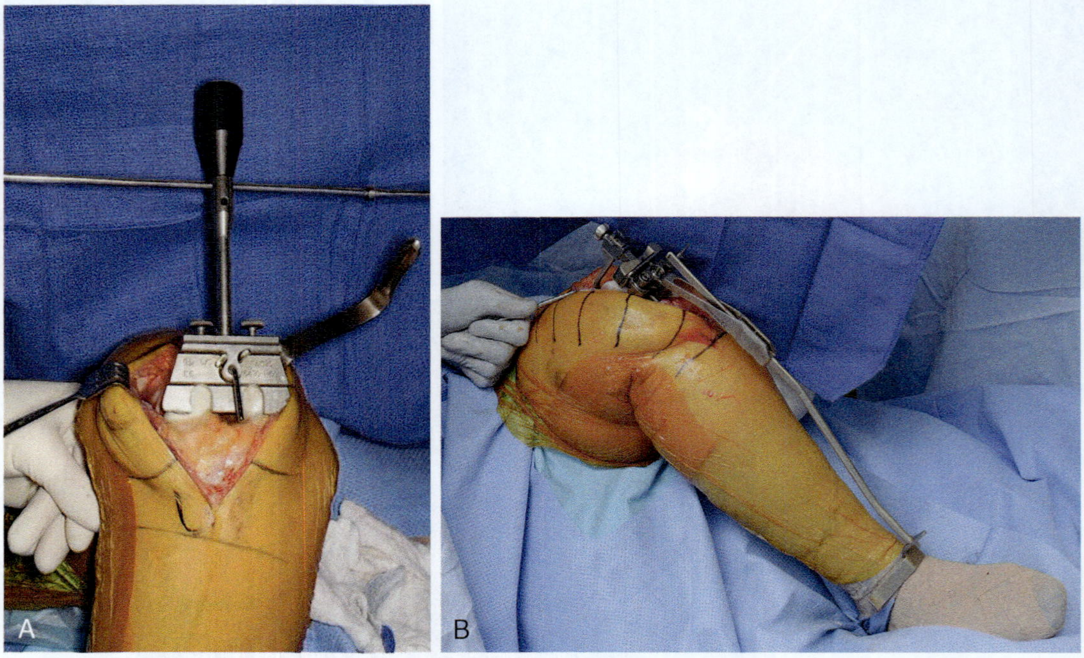

Figure 49.11 | Axial plane alignment parallel to the transepicondylar axis (A) and perpendicular to the long axis of the tibia (B).

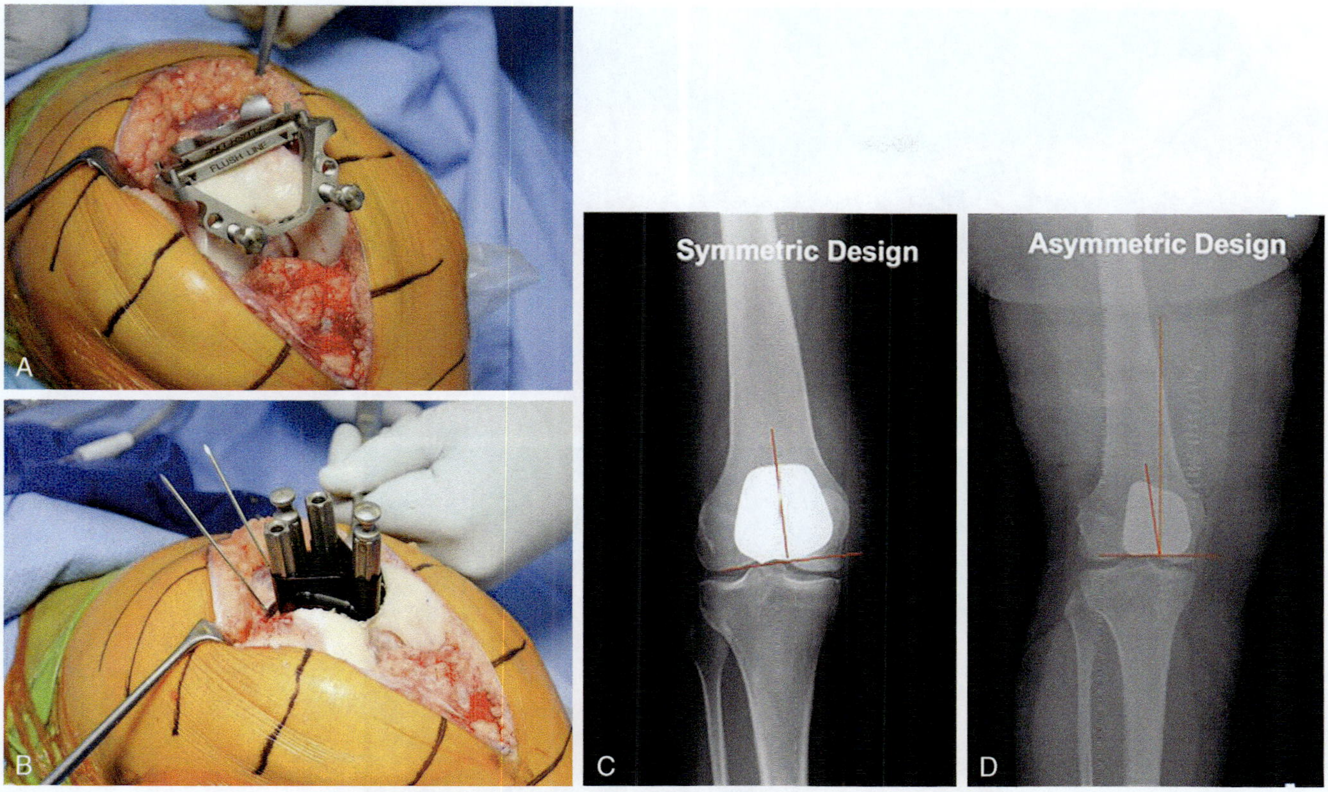

Figure 49.12 | Medial and lateral trochlear edges are flush with articular cartilage (A and B). Symmetric prostheses placed perpendicular to the long axis of the femur (C). Asymmetric prosthesis placed perpendicular to the mechanical axis (D).

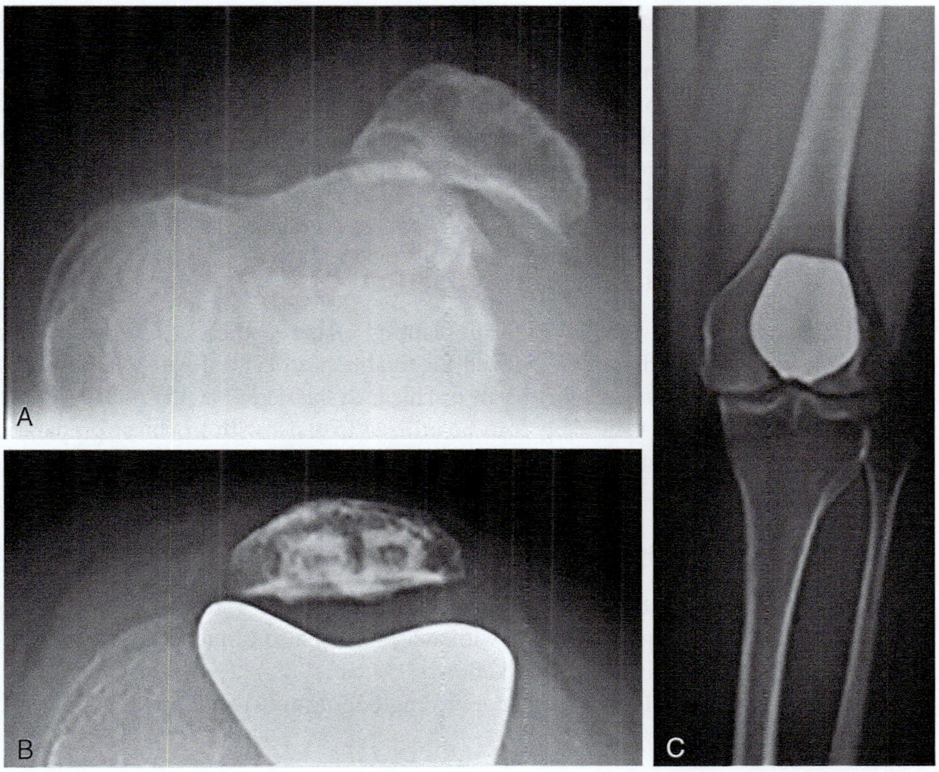

Figure 49.13 | Preoperative (A) and postoperative (B and C) radiographs of a patient with severe lateral patellar tracking and symptomatic lateral overhang of laterally placed PFA component.

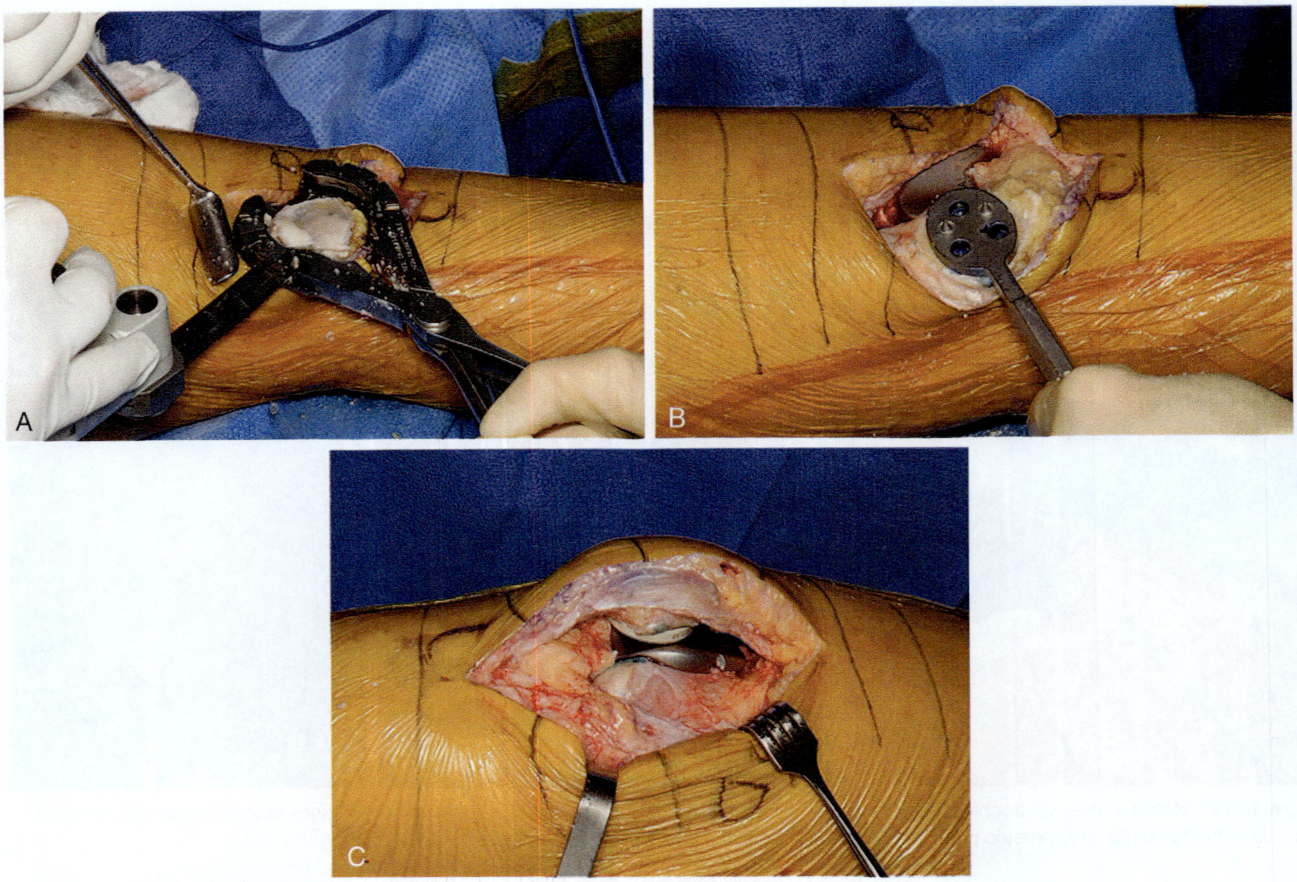

Figure 49.14 | Preparation of the patella with a cemented, pegged, all poly-ethylene component (A-C).

Patellar Preparation

- An attempt should be made to recreate the original patellar thickness; however, "over stuffing" is acceptable and desired in cases of very thin patellae with significant wear (Figure 49.14A-C).
- The patellar component can be medialized slightly to improve patellar tracking.
- Lateral retinacular release is performed when necessary, taking care to avoid branches of the superior lateral geniculate vessels.

Alternative Techniques

- General techniques for implanting inlay prostheses include reproducing the native trochlear anatomy and are best utilized for treatment of central patellofemoral degenerative arthritis in patients with low-grade or absent trochlear dysplasia or patellar malalignment.
- Robotic technology can be utilized to assist with trochlear preparation; however, comparative outcome data are lacking versus standard techniques.

Postoperative Care

- Protected weight bearing until able to perform a straight leg raise with satisfactory quadriceps control
- Early range of motion with assistance of a continuous passive motion machine as needed
- Aggressive edema and effusion control
- Emphasis on hip and core strengthening and avoidance of pelvic tilt

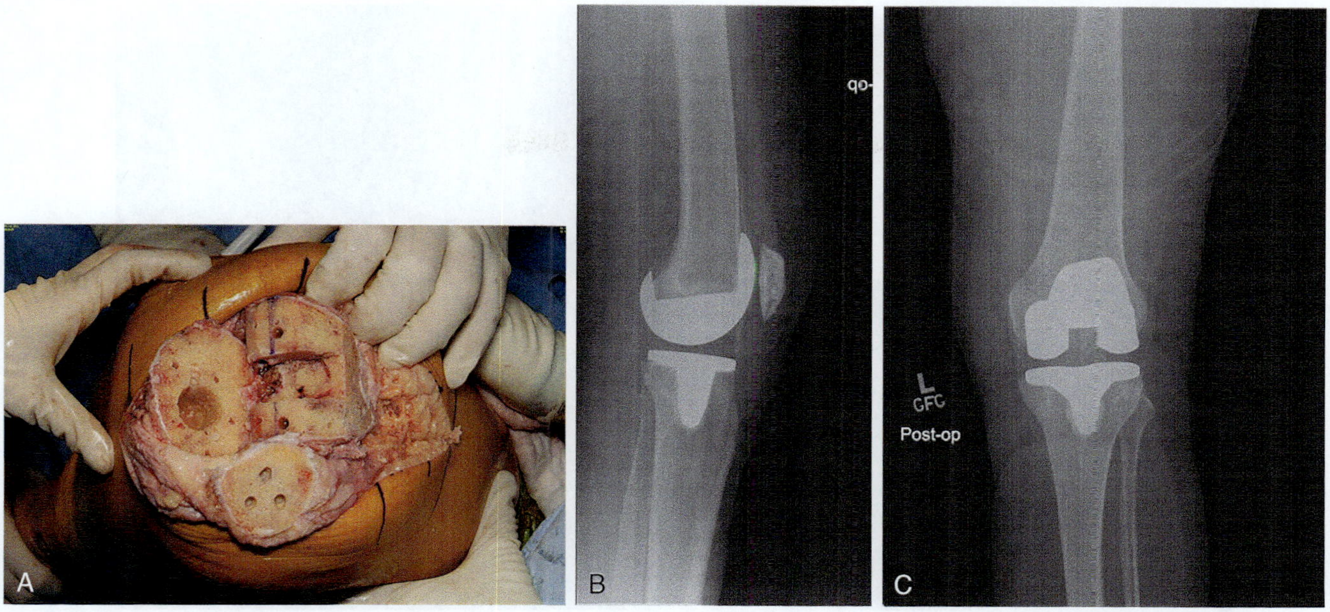

Figure 49.15 | Intraoperative photograph of a patient undergoing conversion from PFA to TKA (A). Postoperative lateral (B) and AP (C) radiographs demonstrating satisfactory conversion with primary TKA implants.

Results

- Outcomes are dependent on proper patient selection and surgical technique.
- Compared with TKA, patients undergoing PFA experience less blood loss, shorter hospitalization, and improved range of motion (not statistically significant).
- Patients with trochlear dysplasia exhibit less progression of degenerative arthritis than those without trochlear dysplasia and therefore represent ideal candidates for PFA.

Complications

- Progression of tibia femoral degenerative arthritis.
  - Most common in patients with obesity, varus malalignment, and no evidence of trochlear dysplasia.
  - Revision to TKA yields results that are relatively comparable with primary TKA (Figure 49.15).
  - Occasionally, femoral stems may be required, particularly in the event of bone loss encountered on removal of the trochlear component (Figure 49.16).
- Patellar component maltracking: Most commonly due to implant malpositioning or failure to correct significant patellar malalignment (Figure 49.17).

Patella Fracture

- Associated risk factors include low body mass index, increased bone resection, decreased patellar thickness, and larger trochlear size (Figure 49.18).

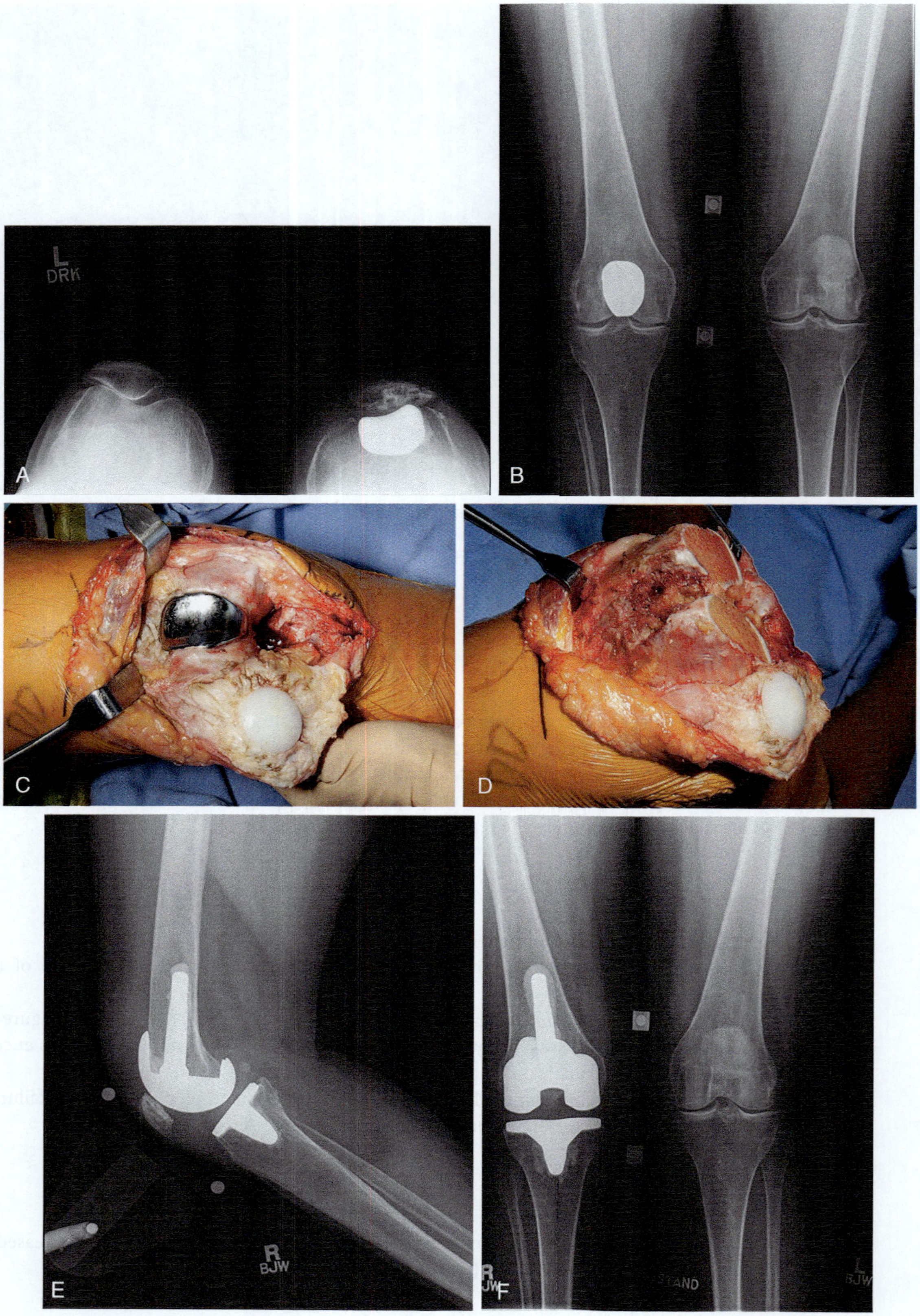

Figure 49.16 | Preoperative Merchant (A) and AP (B) radiographs of failed PFA due to maltracking. Intraoperative photographs of the conversion (C and D). Postoperative lateral (E) and AP (F) radiographs after conversion of PFA to TKA requiring stemmed components.

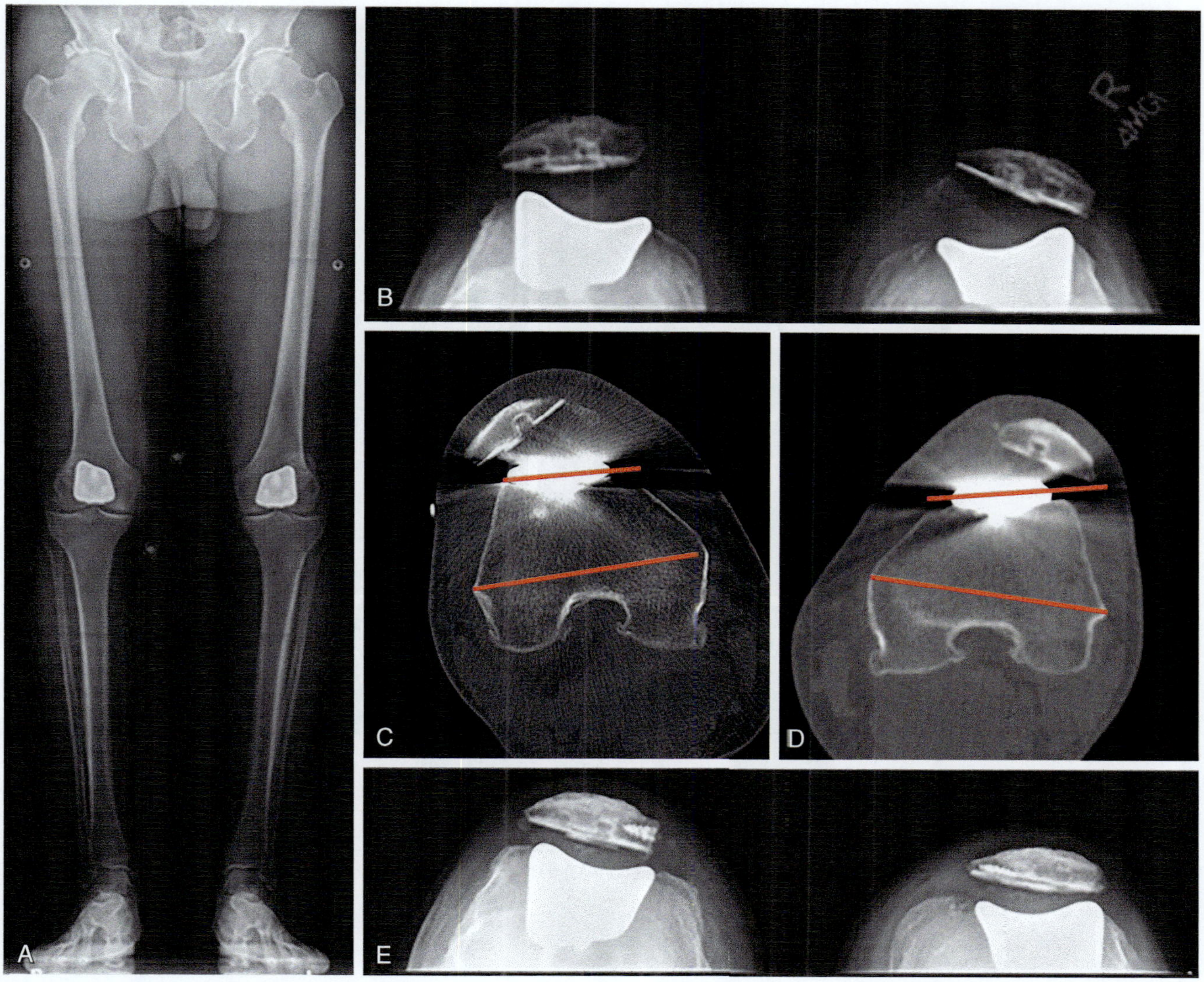

Figure 49.17 | Full-length standing AP (A) and Merchant (B) radiographs of a patient with patella instability following bilateral PFA. Axial CT (C and D) shows evidence of medial patellofemoral ligament insufficiency. The trochlear components are positioned in internal rotation relative to the transepicondylar axis, further contributing to instability. Merchant view (E) showing correction of patella alignment and tracking following medial patellofemoral ligament reconstruction and TTO.

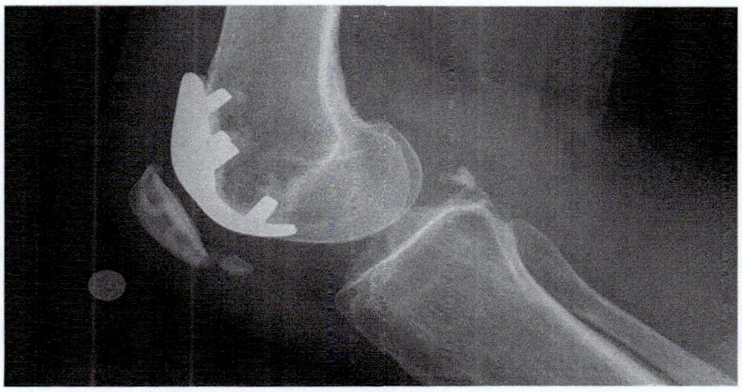

Figure 49.18 | Lateral radiograph showing post-PFA marginal inferior pole patella fracture.

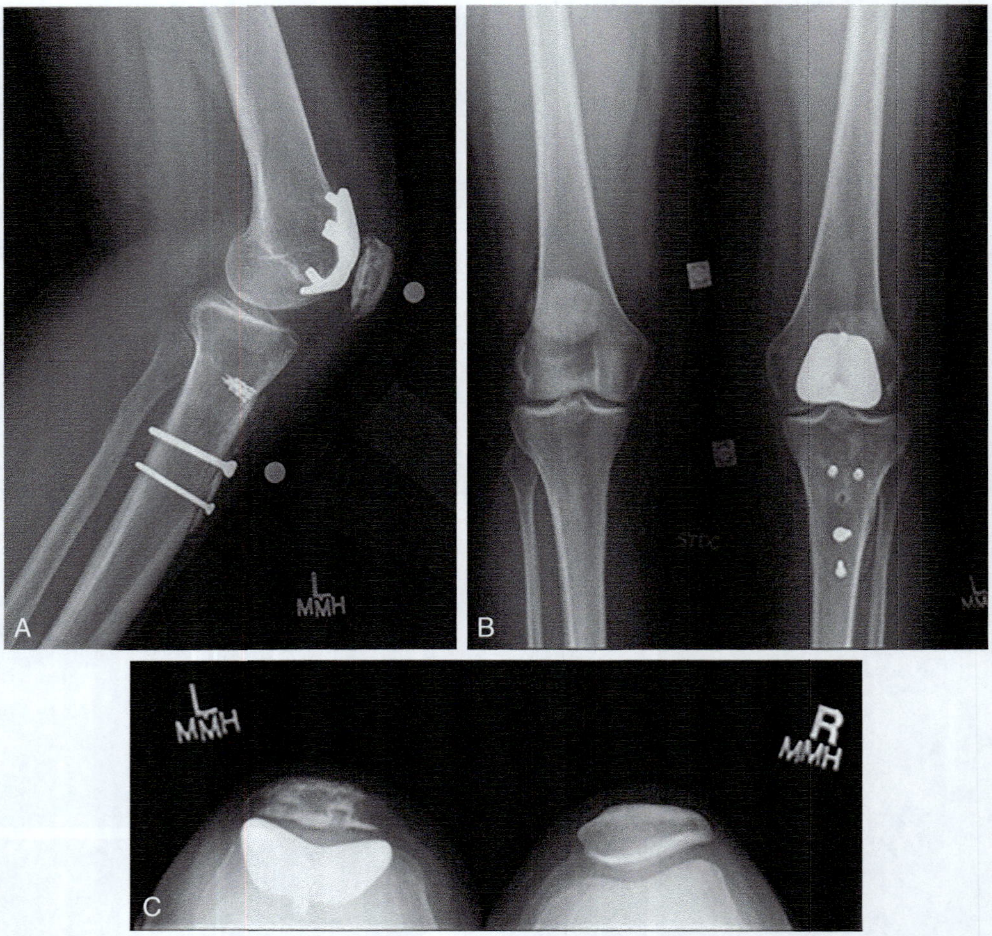

Figure 49.19 | Lateral (A), AP (B), and Merchant (C) radiographs of tibial tubercle distalization osteotomy performed for significant patella alta.

Pearls

- Proper patient selection is key.
- Irrigate tibiofemoral cartilage every 10 minutes to avoid cartilage cell death.
- Choose an onlay-type prosthesis for patients with trochlear dysplasia and/or significant patellofemoral malalignment.
- Consider tibia tubercle distalization for significant patella alta (Figure 49.19).
- In the case of patellofemoral arthritis with isolated chondral lesions on the medial or lateral femoral condyles, consider combined osteochondral autograft transfer system procedure (Figure 49.20).

Pitfalls

- Avoid PFA in patients with significant patella baja.
- Avoid PFA in obese patients with varus alignment and no trochlear dysplasia.
- Consider nonoperative management in patients who do not exhibit radiographic evidence of advanced patellofemoral arthritis but show evidence of patellofemoral joint space narrowing.

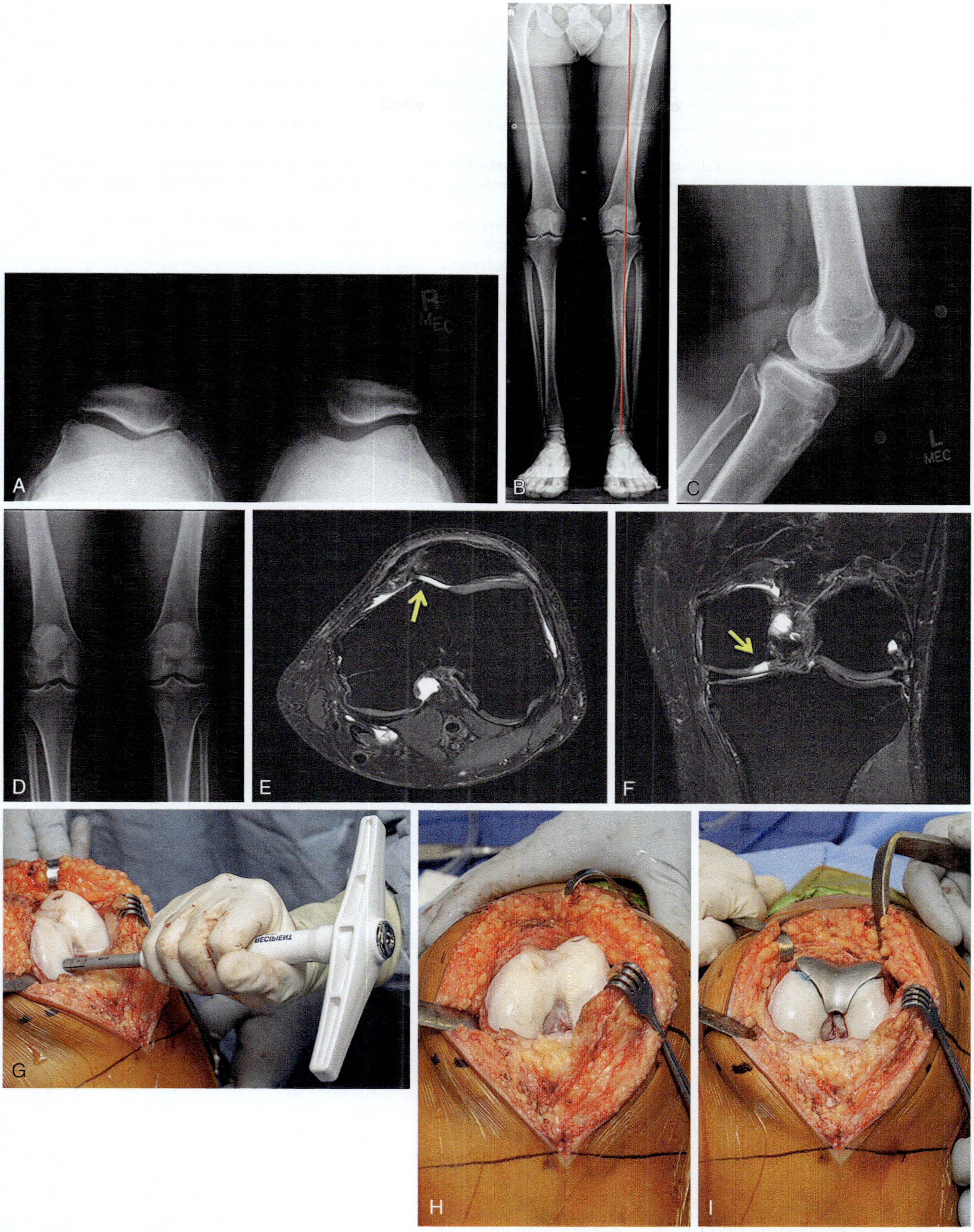

Figure 49.20 | Merchant (A), hip-to-ankle (B), lateral (C), and AP (D) plain radiographs showing patellofemoral arthritis with normal alignment and absence of tibiofemoral degeneration. MRI demonstrating patellofemoral (E) and focal medial femoral condyle cartilage lesion (F). Intraoperative photographs of osteochondral autograft transplantation performed at the same time as PFA (G-I).

Suggested Reading

1. Cannon A, Stolley M, Wolf B, Amendola A. Patellofemoral resurfacing arthroplasty: literature review and a description of a novel technique. *Iowa Orthop J.* 2008;28:42-48.
2. Davies AP, Vince AS, Shepstone L, Donell ST, Glasgow MM. The radiologic prevalence of patellofemoral osteoarthritis. *Clin Orthop Relat Res.* 2002;(402):206-212; PMID:12218486.
3. Dejour D, Le Coultre B. Osteotomies in patello-femoral instabilities. *Sports Med Arthrosc Rev* 2007;15(1):39-46; PMID:17301701.
4. Dahm DL, Kalisvaart MM, Stuart MJ, Slettedahl SW. Patellofemoral arthroplasty: outcomes and factors associated with early progression of tibiofemoral arthritis. *Knee Surg Sports Traumatol Arthrosc.* 2014;22(10):2554-2559. doi:10.1007/s00167-014-3202-3.
5. Dahm DL, Al-Rayashi W, Dajani K, Shah JP, Levy BA, Stuart MJ. Patellofemoral arthroplasty versus total knee arthroplasty in patients with isolated patellofemoral osteoarthritis. *Am J Orthop (Belle Mead NJ).* 2010;39(10):487-491; PMID:21290009.
6. King AH, Engasser WM, Sousa PL, Arendt EA, Dahm DL. Patellar fracture following patellofemoral arthroplasty. *J Arthroplasty.* 2015;30(7):1203-1206. doi:10.1016/j.arth.2015.02.007. Epub February 18, 2015.
7. Thienpont E, Lonner JH. Coronal alignment of patellofemoral arthroplasty. *Knee.* 2014;21(suppl 1):S52-S57.

Chapter 50
Total Knee Arthroplasty: Posterior Cruciate Retaining and Substituting Implants

ASHTON H. GOLDMAN
ROBERT T. TROUSDALE

Key Concepts

- Both posterior stabilized (PS) and cruciate retaining (CR) knees can be successful when appropriately balanced.
- With removal of the posterior cruciate ligament (PCL), the increased flexion gap must be managed by a combination of slightly increasing the distal femoral resection and decreasing posterior slope of the tibial resection.
- Midflexion instability can occur if the joint line is markedly elevated. This can be seen with excessive distal femoral resection. Some argue this is more common with a PS design.
- Flexion instability is different from midflexion instability and is a result of a flexion/extension mismatch. This can be a result of undersizing the femoral component, excessive tibial slope, or incompetence of the PCL. Some argue this is more common with a CR design.
- Anteroposterior sizing tends toward undersizing with modern systems and must be avoided.
- Patella resurfacing may decrease reoperation but can invite unintended risks (avascular necrosis, fracture, over/understuffing).

Sterile Instruments and Implants

- Knee retractors
- Implants: femoral PS or femoral CR component per surgeon preference
- PS femur—small oscillating saw blade or reciprocating saw blade for box cut
- Modular or monoblock tibial component that appropriately mates with the femoral component
- Patella component if needed
- Dilute betadine
- Local joint anesthetic cocktail

Surgical Approaches

- Median parapatellar approach—The standard extensile approach to the knee that can easily be augmented with a quadriceps snip or tibial tubercle osteotomy if required.
- Midvastus approach—Splits the vastus medialis in line with its fibers starting at the top of the patella thereby sparing the quadriceps tendon. Because it is less extensile in the revision setting, it is more commonly used with medial unicompartmental knee arthroplasty.
- Subvastus approach—minimally invasive quadriceps tendon sparing approach. Elevates the vastus medialis from the intramuscular septum and is less extensile than other approaches.

Preoperative Planning

- A standing long limb alignment view
  a. Shows the degree of deformity and other deformities/arthroses (i.e., hip, ankle)
  b. Establishes entry point for the entry drill into the canal. This is especially important on the valgus/deformed knee
  c. Can be used to determine the appropriate distal femur valgus resection angle if desired
- A standing posteroanterior flexion (Rosenberg) view sometimes demonstrates significant arthrosis not seen on an anteroposterior (AP) view
- The AP view is appropriate for tibial sizing for templating.
- The lateral view aids with sizing the femur for templating.
- Optimization in terms of smoking cessation, diabetes management, and nutrition may aid in postoperative wound complications
- Previous scars—Blood supply is from medial to lateral. Using the most lateral scar that allows access to the knee is ideal. If a medial incision is used, a lateral flap with potentially compromised blood flow risks wound healing problems. Transverse incisions can be ignored.

Bone, Implant, and Soft Tissue Techniques

- After the knee is exposed, an entry drill goes into the femur to identify the intramedullary cavity (Figure 50.1). Keep one hand on either condyle and ensure visualization of the distal anterior femoral cortex in order not to perforate. The entry spot can be determined by several means:
  - AP plane: Approximately 1 cm above the PCL insertion, which is approximately at the most anterior portion of the medial femoral condyle wear pattern.
  - ML plane: Just medial to the femoral AP axis (Whiteside line), or in a deformity case it can be found in line with the femoral canal on the standing long limb alignment view.
  - If a step drill (wider than the intramedullary alignment rod) is used, it is ok to enter in the deepest part of the trochlea; however, one must ensure the hole is large enough not to change the distal femoral valgus angle.
- The intramedullary rod enters the canal. Be careful to not hit the anterior cortex with the intramedullary rod as this can cause the cutting jig to go into flexion. Allowing the rod to ride along the posterior cortex helps protect the guide from going into flexion.

The Distal Femoral Cut Sets the Joint Line in Extension

- The goal is to reestablish the joint line by resecting the same amount of bone as the implant is thick: typically 8 to 9 mm.
- Elevation of the joint line changes the axis of rotation of the medial collateral ligament (MCL) and lateral collateral ligament (LCL) and can cause these ligaments to become unbalanced in midflexion, thereby causing instability.

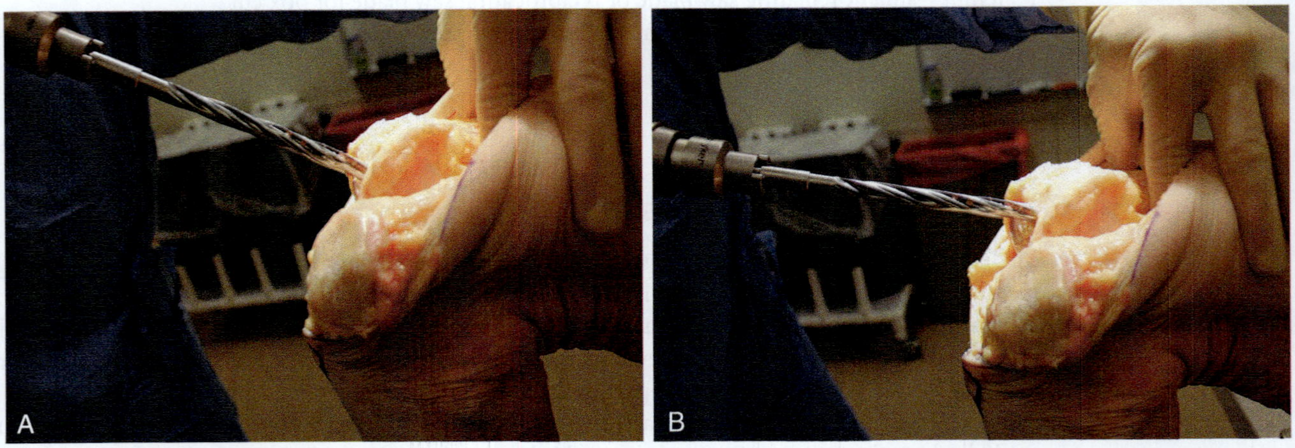

Figure 50.1 | Placement of the entry drill. A, With your hand extended posterior femoral perforation and risk to neurovascular structures can occur. B, Correct alignment of the entry drill colinear with the femoral canal.

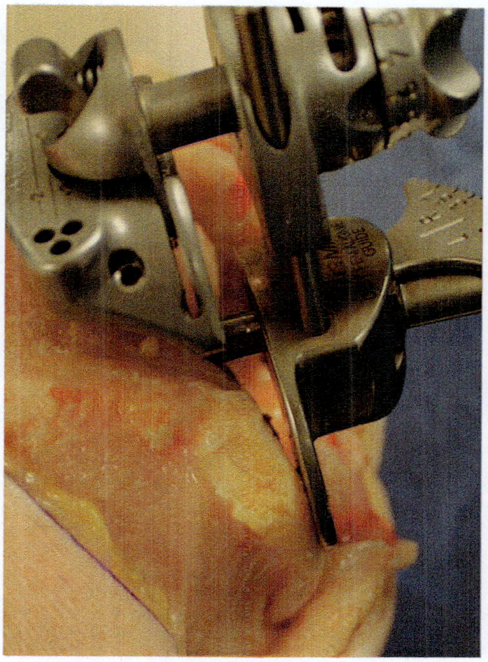

Figure 50.2 | Excessive medial osteophytes can displace the distal femoral resection distally thereby underresecting the distal femur. Removal of excessive medial osteophytes allows the distal femoral resection guide to sit flush on the distal femur.

- For significant preoperative flexion contracture, 1 to 2 mm additional can be taken off the distal femur to allow easier balancing.
- Be careful not to flex the distal femoral cutting jig or have it resting on prominent osteophytes (Figures 50.2 and 50.3).
- Figure 50.4: Ensure removal of enough bone from the trochlea to have a flat distal femoral cut.

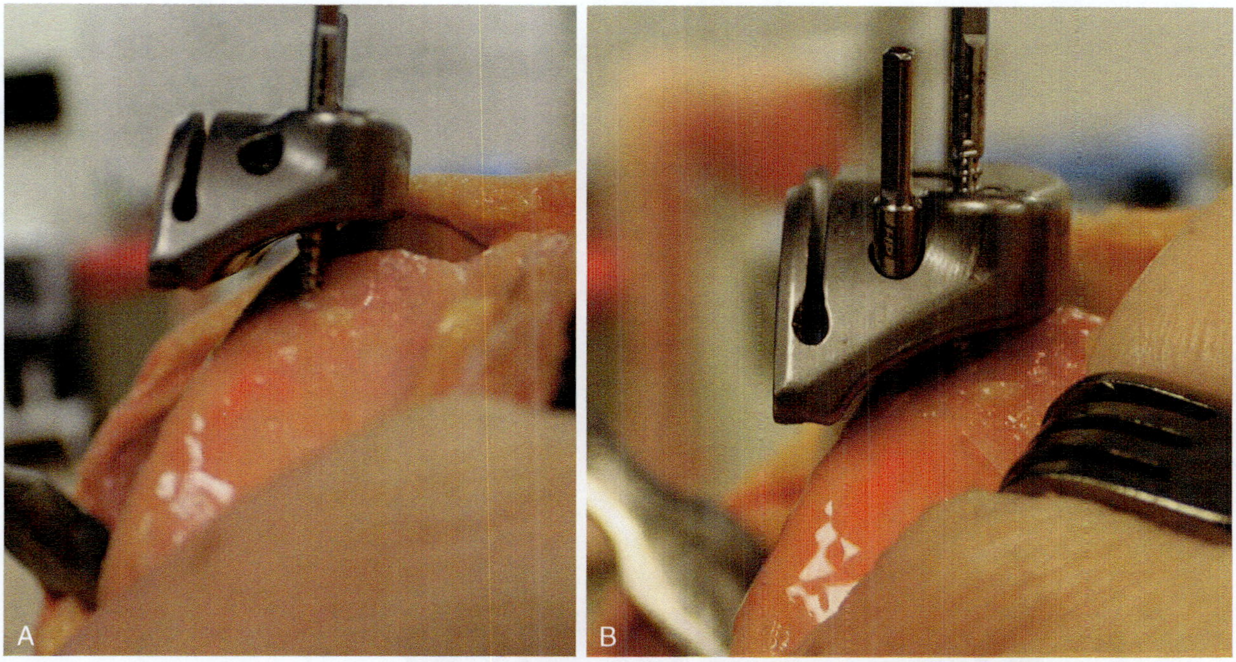

Figure 50.3 | Distal femoral resection typically is done perpendicular to the femoral axis. A, Correct placement of distal femoral resection guide resting on the anterior femur. B, Flexion of the distal femoral resection guide: note how it hugs the end of the distal femur.

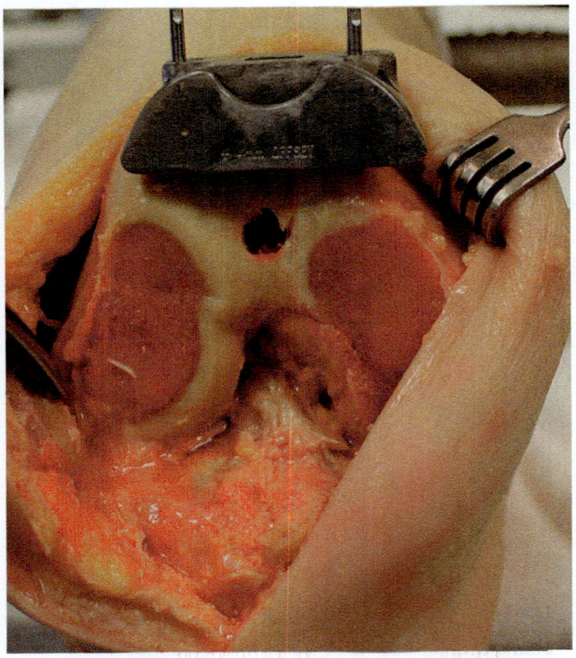

Figure 50.4 | Inadequate level of distal femoral resection. Failure to remove trochlear cartilage is a sign of inadequate distal femoral resection. This leads to distalization of the component and overstuffing of the patellofemoral joint. Adequate resection of the trochlea will remove the trochlear cartilage and reveal a completely flat surface.

Femoral Anterior, Posterior, Chamfer Cuts

- Most current systems utilize a 4-in-1 femoral cutting jig.

Rotation/AP Sizing

- Whiteside line, the epicondylar axis and posterior femoral condyles are all useful for setting rotation. Correct rotation is perpendicular to the Whiteside line, parallel to the epicondylar axis, and 3° to 5° of external rotation from the posterior condylar axis (Figure 50.5).
- Internal rotation risks patellar maltracking. This may be more dramatic with older symmetric femoral component designs. Excessive external rotation will tighten the lateral joint space in flexion (Figure 50.6).

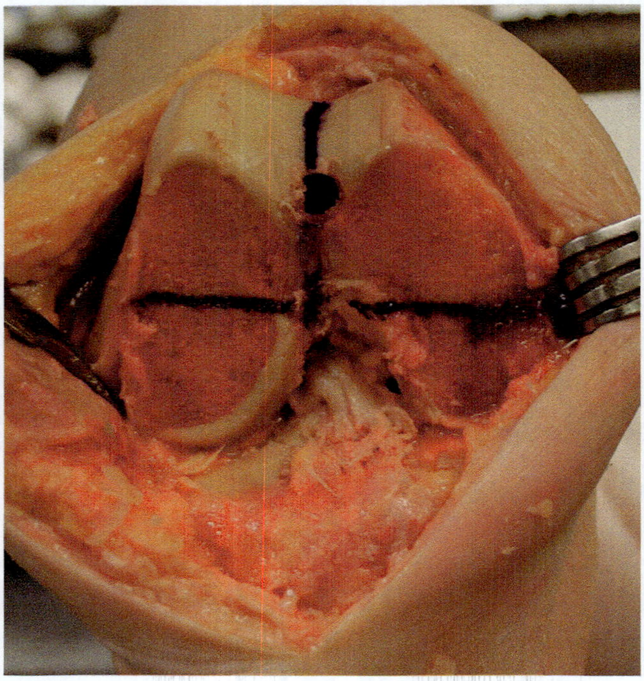

Figure 50.5 | Demonstrates alignment markings for femoral rotation. The vertical line through the deepest portion of the trochlea extending to the center of the femoral head is Whiteside line. The line from the LCL origin to the deepest part of the MCL origin is the transepicondylar axis (perpendicular to Whiteside' line). The posterior condylar axis often is internally rotated 3° to 5° relative to these lines.

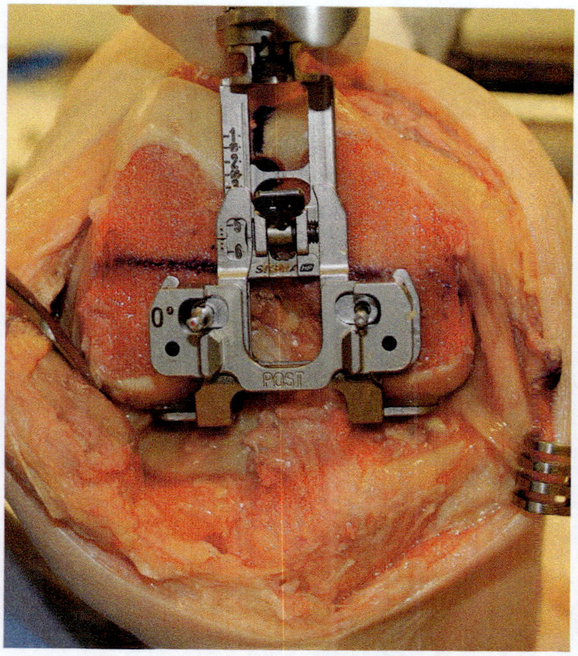

Figure 50.6 | When placing the AP sizing guide, abundant lateral cartilage can excessively externally rotate the femoral component (as compared with the epicondylar axis and Whiteside line) thereby overresecting the posterior medial condyle and elevating the medial joint line in flexion. This can cause instability.

- Anterior referencing (Figure 50.7) uses the anterior cortex of the femur as the base for sizing, meaning the implants will grow in the flexion space with increasing size. This minimizes the risk for femoral notching but may increase the risk for flexion instability in the CR designs if undersized owing to inadequate restoration of the posterior condylar offset. If between sizes, use the larger size and plan to downsize if flexion space is too tight.
- Anterior referencing systems allow one to set the rotation with the identified landmarks. Increasing the external rotation from 3° to 5° allows opening of the medial side, which can be useful in the extremely tight varus knee.
- Posterior referencing (Figure 50.8) sets the size and rotation off the posterior femoral condyles. Be careful to identify thick cartilage caps remaining on the posterior condyles as this can give excessive internal or external rotation if severe. If not sized appropriately, there is a significant risk of notching the anterior femoral cortex. Posterior referencing may minimize flexion instability in a CR design.
- To prevent notching, measure the femoral size on the upslope of the lateral distal femur ridge.

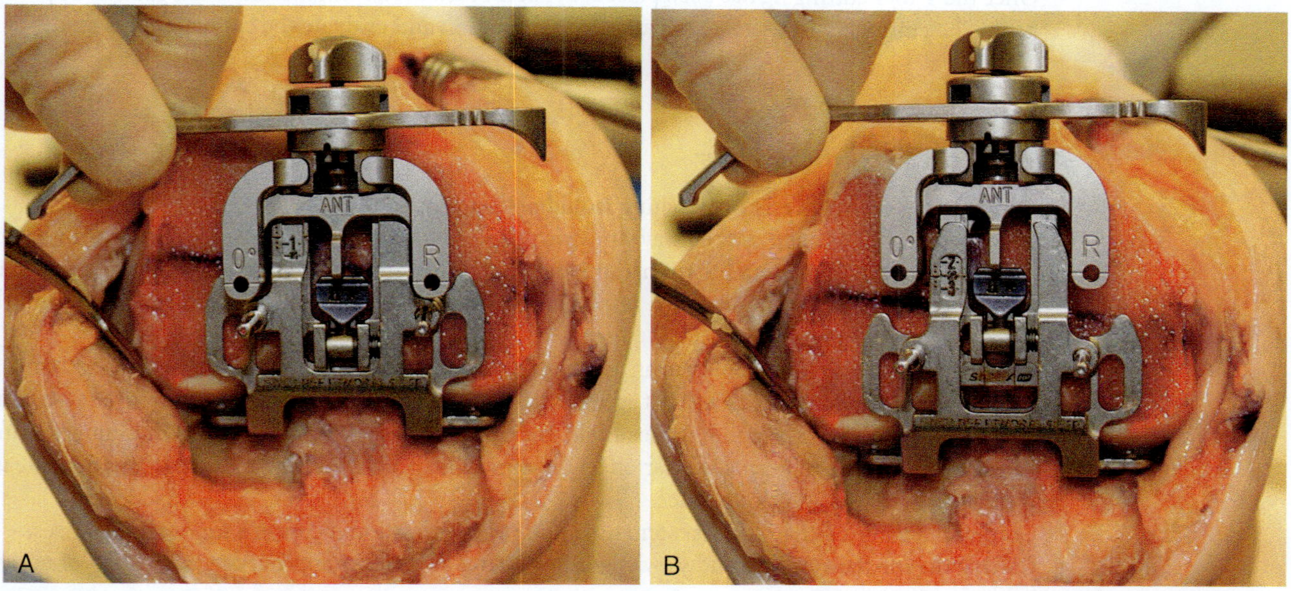

Figure 50.7 | Anterior referencing for sizing (A). As sizes increase (B) the distance from the anterior femoral stylus to the pin holes on the sizing guide remain constant. The variable resection is on the posterior femoral condyles. Undersizing will have excessive posterior condylar resection thereby increasing the flexion gap and potentiating a flexion-extension mismatch. However, the risk of notching with this technique is decreased.

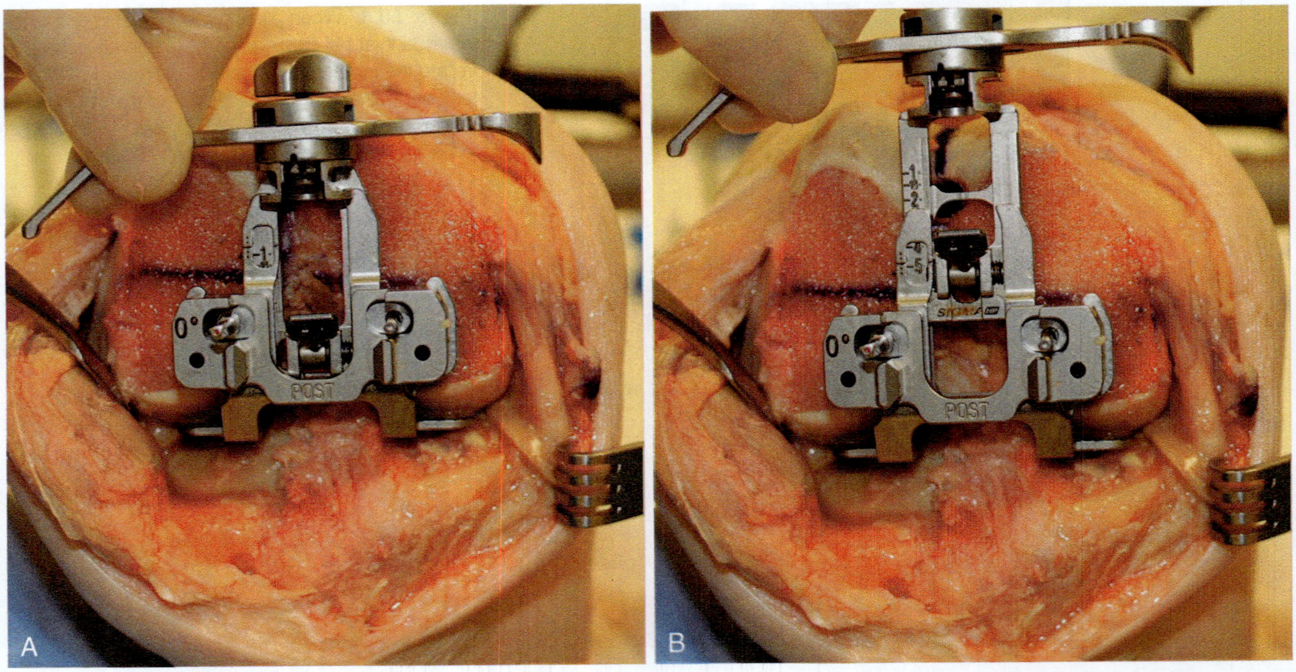

Figure 50.8 | Posterior referencing for sizing (A). As sizes increase (B), the amount of posterior condylar resection stays constant as can be noted by the constant location of the pinholes in relation to the posterior femoral condyles. With this technique, one must always check that the anterior femoral resection does not notch the femur, and if suspected, upsize the femoral component making the necessary accommodations on the resection guide to maintain a stable posterior condylar offset.

- In the valgus knee, the hypoplastic lateral femoral condyle will tend to force the measuring jig into internal rotation if it is utilized. This is exaggerated when significant cartilage remains on the posterior medial femoral condyle. One should ignore the posterior lateral condyle for rotation and sizing in the valgus knee.
- It is important to note that, with abundant posterolateral condylar cartilage, the sizer may cause excessive external rotation of the flexion axis and also give the most accurate representation of size in the varus knee.
- Conversely, if both posterior condyles are worn, the femur has a tendency to be undersized as most systems do not take into account the worn cartilage. When in doubt, always choose the larger femoral size.
- Once the 4-to-1 cutting jig has been placed, a spacer block used to fill the extension gap can be placed below the cutting jig to estimate the appropriate rotation and evaluate the cut before it is made.

Making the Cuts

Avoid Notching the Femur

- Using an angel wing to ensure notching would not occur is useful.
- It is important to understand the ways in which the femoral implant system you choose grows with each size. Femoral components from some manufacturers grow both anteriorly and posteriorly in the AP plane (anterior or posterior referencing), whereas some systems grow purely posteriorly (anterior referencing system).
  - If there is concern for notching in an anterior referencing system, anteriorize the cutting jig 2 mm. It may be prudent to upsize as well if it appears there will be an overzealous posterior condylar resection.
  - If posterior referencing and, for example, the sizes increase 4 mm per size (2 mm anterior and 2 mm posterior), to keep condylar offset the same, anteriorize the jig 2 mm thereby only increasing 2 mm on the anterior surface.
- Cutting the anterior chamfer first sometimes aids at visualization if concern for notching arises.
- Cutting the medial side first and slowly working lateral also allows appropriate assessment of notching before it occurs.
- A successful anterior femoral resection demonstrates a "grand piano" shape if rotation is correct. This cut sets the rotation of the component (Figure 50.9).

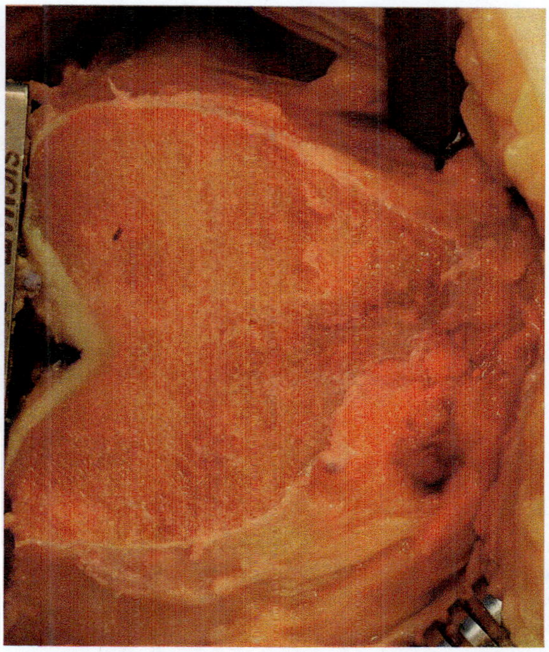

Figure 50.9 | Adequate resection of the anterior femur reveals the "grand-piano sign" whereby the anterior femur appears as a grand piano.

Posterior Condyles

- A resection that appears to be more than 8 mm above eburnated bone is excessive, and the component is likely undersized or, much less commonly, excessively rotated in one direction.
- Ensure retractors are placed at the level of the MCL medially and LCL laterally to prevent iatrogenic transection.
- As soon as the condyles "jump," the cut is complete.
- Anterior chamfer cuts sometimes put the skin at risk. Be sure to use retractors to protect the skin.
- Posterior chamfers risk the collateral ligaments as well as the tibial plateau if the saw dives too deep.

Box Cut (Posterior Stabilized Only) (Figure 50.10)

- Avoid undercutting the medial and lateral femoral condyles while performing the box cut as it can significantly weaken the condyles and risk fracture.
- Placing an osteotome on top of the tibia protects the saw from plunging into the tibia.
- An oscillating saw or a long, thin, rigid reciprocating saw can be used.

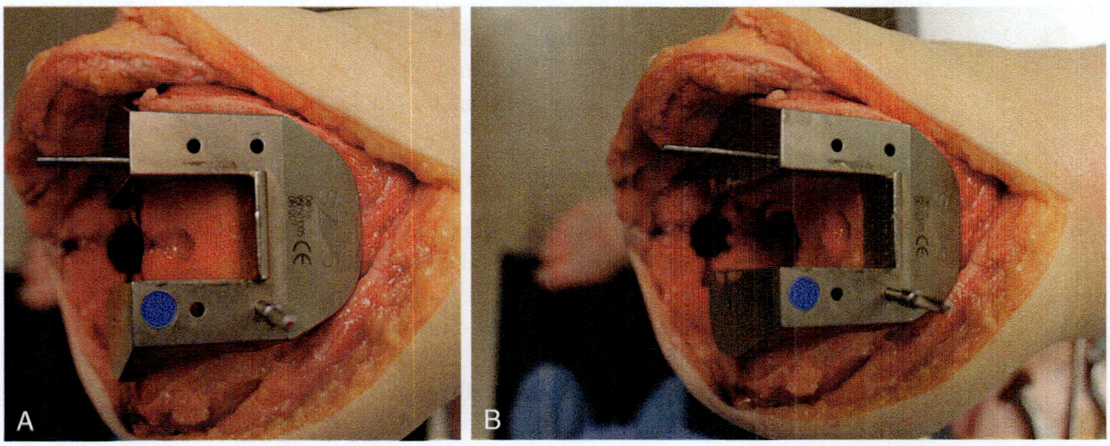

Figure 50.10 | Before (A) and after (B) femoral box cut. Care must be taken to not undercut the femoral condyles or cut into the tibia when performing this cut.

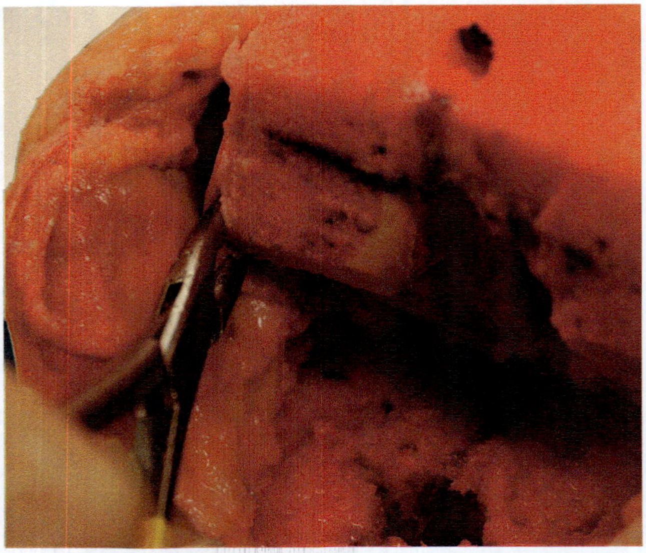

Figure 50.11 | Always look for an osteophyte under the insertion of the popliteus. Failure to remove this bone can cause impingement or postoperative snapping.

- An inadequate box cut may prevent implant seating.
- When finishing the femur, be sure to remove osteophytes from along the popliteus insertion as it can cause postoperative snapping (Figure 50.11).

The Tibial Cut Affects Both the Flexion and Extension Gaps

- Resection depth is important for bone preservation.
  - If significant deformity is not present, 2 mm off the involved side can be used; conversely, 8 mm off the unaffected lateral side is appropriate as well.
  - If there is a significant varus deformity present, chasing this resection may lead to an overzealous lateral resection necessitating a very thick polyethylene insert.
  - Likewise, 8 mm off the lateral side can be utilized accounting for the maintained cartilage in all varus knees.
  - For a valgus knee or one without any deformity, a more conservative 6 to 8 mm is utilized as these knees are more easily correctable.

Tibial Slope (Figure 50.12)

CR designs maintain the PCL for rollback and require posterior slope cut into the tibia, usually between 3° and 7°.

- A pin or angel wing can be placed along the medial tibial plateau to estimate and set the slope for a CR knee.
- Overzealous slope can cause laxity in flexion and subsequent flexion instability.
- PS designs use cam engagement for rollback and typically require a slope between 0° and 3°.
- Less posterior slope in part makes up for the increased flexion gap after removal of the PCL.

Tibial Alignment (Figures 50.13-50.15)

- Extramedullary tibial alignment: A line connecting the second metatarsal, extensor hallucis longus tendon, center of the talus, distal anterior tibial crest, medial one-third of the tibial tubercle, and PCL insertion can be used to assist with alignment. Any or all of these landmarks can be used.
- Intramedullary tibial alignment can be utilized in tibias that are not bowed.
- The cutting jig should be placed appropriately. Ensure that the central marking of the tibial resection is placed in the correct rotation between the tibial tubercle and the PCL insertion. If the jig is placed too far medial, a valgus cut will be made.
- With the jig in place an alignment rod can be placed proximally and a radiograph can be useful to ensure it aligns with the center of the femoral head.

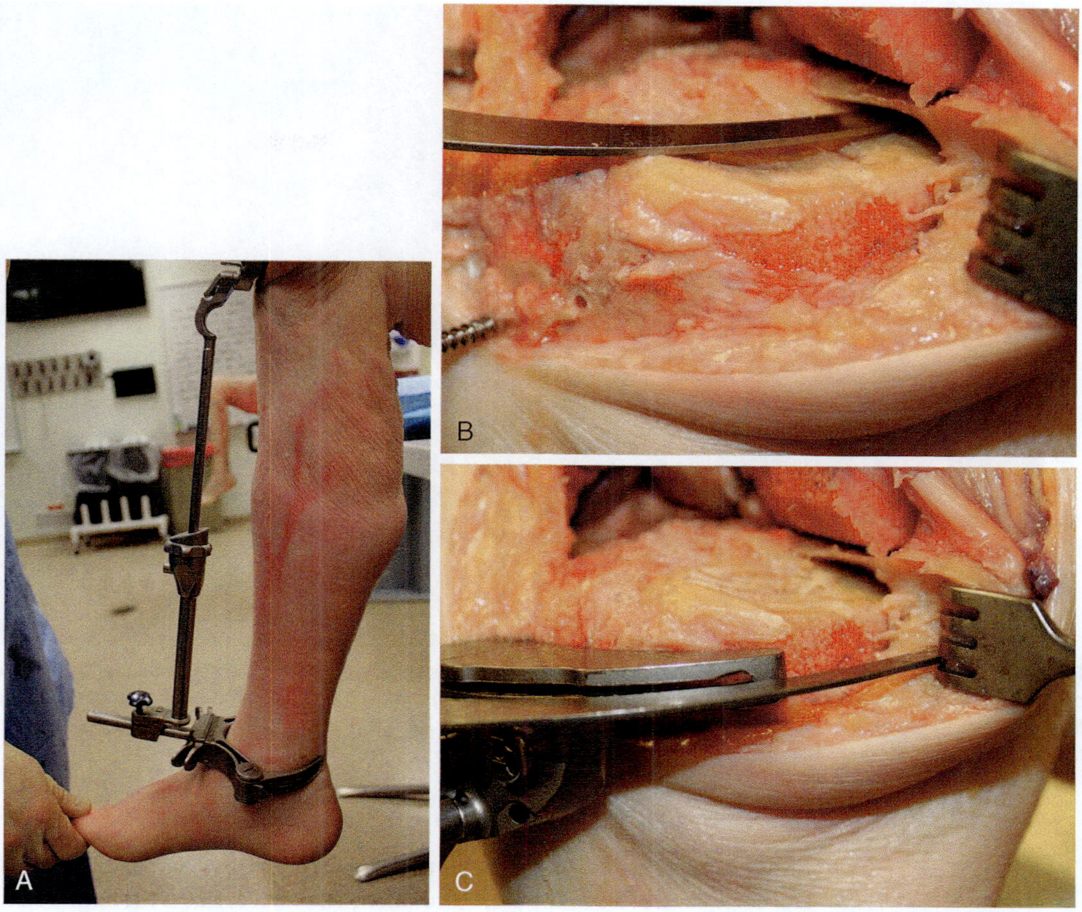

Figure 50.12 | Determining tibial slope. A, Comparison between the tibial alignment rod and the tibia from a sagittal view. If they are parallel, the slope will be 0°. If the distance between the ankle and the alignment rod is increased at the ankle, posterior slope is anticipated. B, Assessment of native slope from intact cartilage anteriorly and posteriorly allows for proper assessment of native slope, which is the goal in a CR knee. C, Removing more bone anteriorly than posteriorly thereby confirming removal of slope, which is required in a PS design.

Performing the Tibial Cut

- Protection of the patellar tendon laterally and MCL medially is essential. If a CR design is planned, an osteotome driven into the bone in front of the PCL protects it from transection.
- Leaving the pins for the tibial resection guide in place until verifying full extension is achieved avoids having to place multiple pin holes and creating stress risers in the tibia if it needs to be recut.

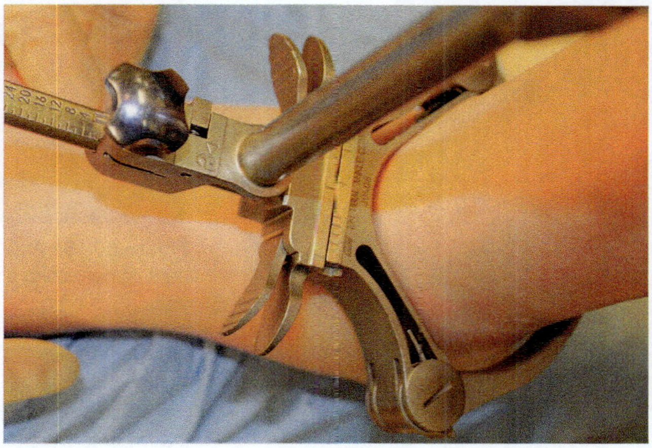

Figure 50.13 | Appropriate placement of the tibial alignment rod distally. Slight medialization of the extramedullary tibial alignment rod will help align the jig with the center of the talus. This medialization helps find the true center as it accounts for the fibula.

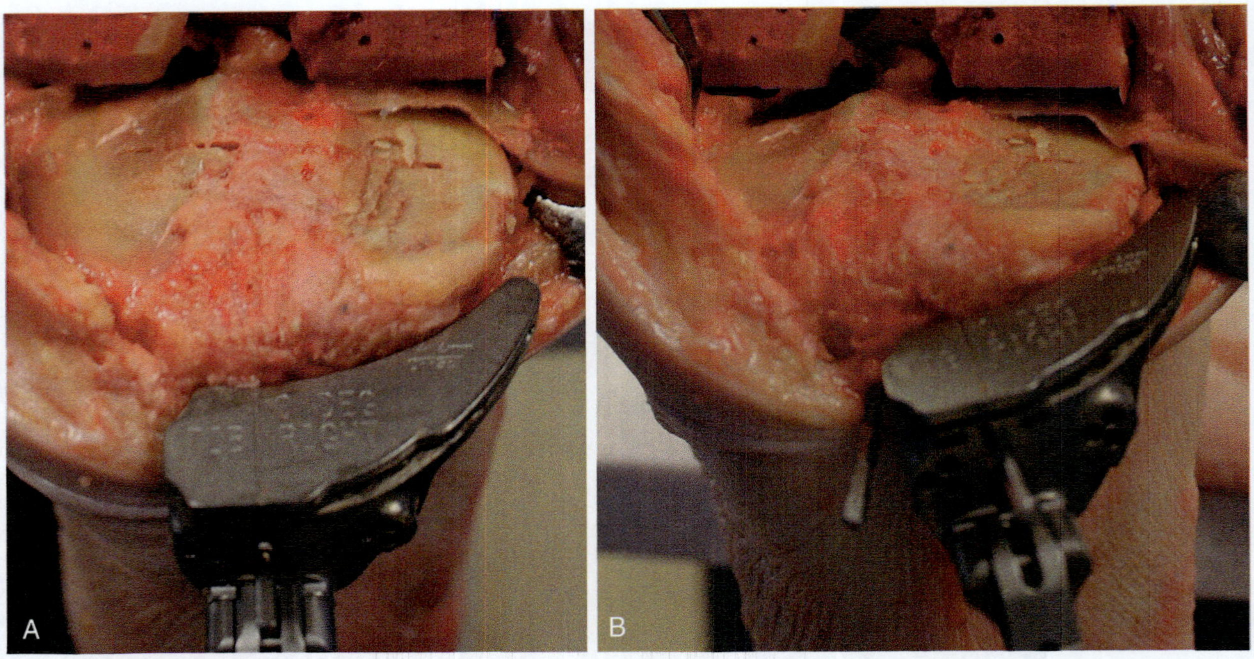

Figure 50.14 | Proximal placement of the tibial extramedullary alignment jig. A, Correct placement with planned rotation. The central axis of the cut should be over the medial aspect of the tibial tubercle and pointing toward the PCL. Removal of anterior osteophytes allows the jig to sit flush. B, Medial placement of the jig will preferentially cut more valgus. As one places the guide medially the planned slope turns into overresection of the lateral tibial plateau.

Tibial Sizing/Rotation (Figure 50.16)

- Ensure complete view of the lateral tibial cortex for sizing. Set the tibia size based on the posterolateral cortex and place in the correct rotation. The correct size is the largest size that does not overhang medially. Given the larger medial tibial plateau, uncoverage in the posteromedial corner of the tibia is expected if correct rotation is achieved. Anatomic designs attempt to minimize that medial uncoverage and may help prevent internal rotation of the tibial component.

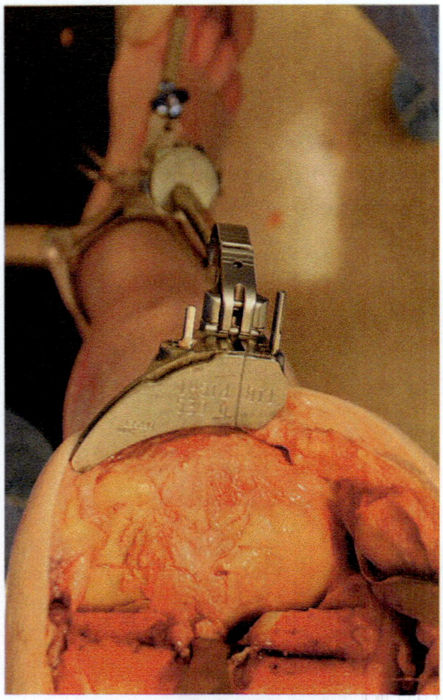

Figure 50.15 | Axial view of an appropriate tibial resection for a mechanically aligned knee. A line connecting the PCL insertion to the medial third of the tibial tubercle, overlying the distal aspect of the anterior tibial spine, extensor hallucis longus, and the second metatarsal.

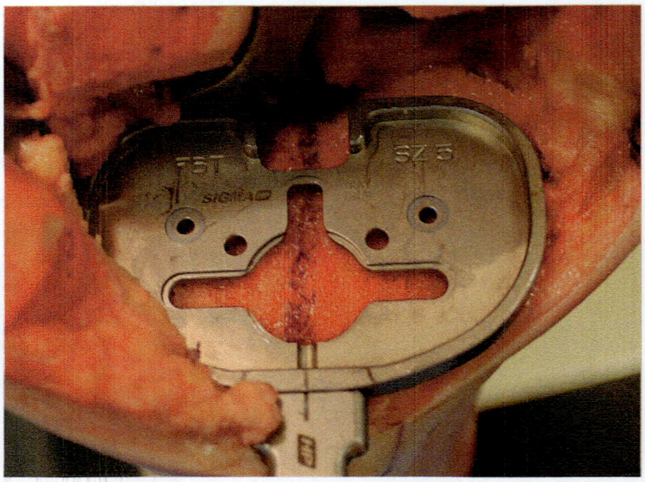

Figure 50.16 | Appropriate sizing and rotation of the tibial component. When sizing the tibia, ensure correct rotation to promote optimal tracking of both the femoral-tibial articulations and the patellofemoral joint. Place the trial in the posterolateral corner of the tibia and set in appropriate rotation. The correct rotation can be a line connecting the PCL insertion to the medial one-third of the tibial tubercle. This line is parallel to the lateral tibial wear pattern. The correct size has minimal if any posterolateral overhang. If using a symmetric design, uncovered bone can be expected on the posteromedial tibial plateau.

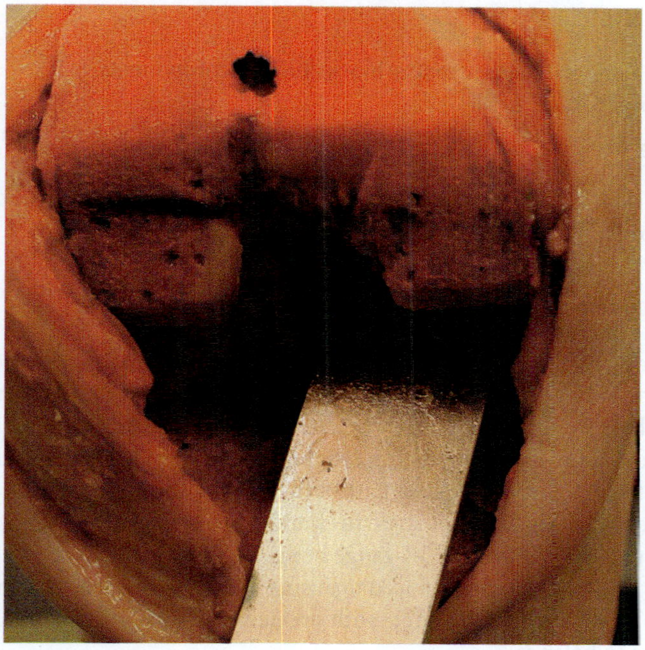

Figure 50.17 | Removing posterior osteophytes and releasing posterior capsule. A tight posterior capsule needs to be released, and osteophytes need to be removed so the MCL and LCL can be appropriately tensioned in extension. Narrow osteotomes should be avoided. Broad instruments as shown are safer to protect against inadvertent neurovascular injury.

- Internal rotation of the tibia increases the risk of patellar maltracking.
- Correct rotation of tibial component can be determined with a line from the PCL to the medial one-third of the tibial tubercle. Conversely, a line parallel to the plane of the lateral tibial wear strip can be used.

Clearing the Joint

- Complete removal of the meniscus on both the medial and lateral sides is important to prevent postoperative entrapment.
- Clearing any bony prominences around the popliteus insertion helps prevent postoperative impingement.
- Removal of posterior osteophytes is critical to allow accurate evaluation of the extension gap. A broad curved osteotome is safer to use than more narrow instruments in the posterior aspect of the knee as the likelihood of puncturing a vital structure is less. Posterior capsule release also allows a more accurate representation of how the medial and lateral structures are influencing the extension gap (Figure 50.17).
- Removal of the PCL opens the flexion gap by a few millimeters. Figure 50.18 demonstrate this concept.

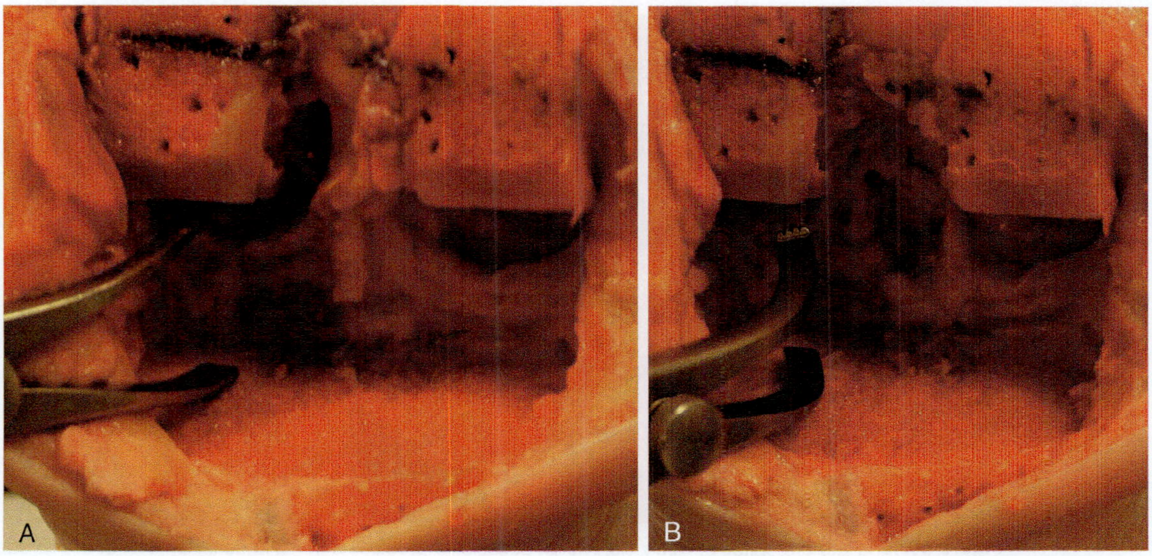

Figure 50.18 | Before (A) and after (B) PCL resection. Notice the increase in flexion gap created with removal of the PCL. This is compensated for either by a slight increase in resection of the distal femur or decreasing posterior slope of the tibia as compared with a CR knee.

Balancing

- Balancing can be done with either spacer blocks or trial components.
- Osteophyte removal is done first.
- In a tight varus knee, a reduction osteotomy (of the medial tibial plateau) can be useful to help balance the knee.
- A medial release 1 cm distal to the tibial cut surface including the insertion of the semimembranosus to the insertion of the PCL aids in balancing.

Performing Releases

- Anterior structures are preferentially tight in flexion; posterior structures are tighter in extension.
- If releasing a portion of the MCL, place an elevator perpendicular to the fibers and gently roll your hand to lift the fibers from the tibia. Likewise, they may be elevated with electrocautery.
- One contemporary approach to balancing a tight MCL is a multiple puncture technique using an 18-gauge needle to perforate the tightest part of the ligament from inside out.
- For a valgus knee, palpating the tight structures and gradually releasing them throughout the arc of motion with either a #15 blade or an 18-gauge needle is appropriate.
- For the CR knee, the PCL must be balanced to ensure appropriate roll back. If it is too tight in flexion, partial elevation off its femoral insertion with an elevator, knife, or cautery can help relax enough fibers for the knee to balance.

Patella

- Patella resurfacing reduces the risk of reoperation but may not improve outcome.
- Patella resurfacing risks fracture, over/understuffing, and avascular necrosis.
- Removal of osteophytes and denervation may be all that is needed in some cases in which the patella is minimally worn or if reconstruction is challenging (overly thick or excessively thin patella).
- Removal of fat/synovium over quadriceps tendon is essential in the PS knee design to prevent patellar clunk or crepitus (Figure 50.19).
- A free hand cut from the osseochondral junction on the medial side to the lateral osseochondral junction avoiding violation of the insertion of the quadriceps and patellar tendon is ideal.
- To achieve a symmetric patella, more bone is removed medially than laterally as the dome of the patella is on the medial side. A preoperative assessment of the sunrise view gives some idea of how the cut should look.
- Measure the patella in 4 quadrants to ensure an even cut and refine as needed.

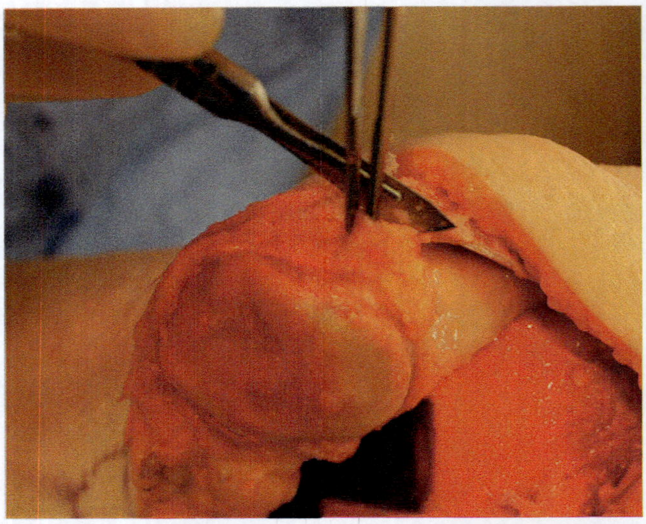

Figure 50.19 I Patella crepitus or rarely clunk is an occasional problem with PS knees. Removal of the fibrous tissue that lies just proximal to the patella on the undersurface of the quadriceps tendon may lessen the risk of postoperative patellar clunk.

Implantation

- Cement bonds best to other cement. Placing cement on the undersurface of the entire tibial component as well as directly on the tibia minimizes the risk of aseptic loosening or debonding due to blood or fat globules in the cement mantle at the cement-implant interface.
- Sclerotic areas can be punctured with a pin to help with cement interdigitation. Furthermore, sclerotic bone from the keel can be removed that may prevent appropriate implant seating (Figure 50.20).
- Placing cement on the posterior and anterior femoral component may avoid postoperative cement voids.
- Holding the leg and components very still during setting of cement is important.
- A dilute Betadine solution may be useful following implantation to prevent postoperative infection.
- A local anesthetic injected around the joint in the surrounding tissues aids with postoperative pain control.

Postoperative Care

- The patient is weight bearing as tolerated following the procedure and is provided multimodal analgesia with acetaminophen, tramadol, and an opioid pain medication for breakthrough pain.
- Individualized deep venous thrombosis prophylaxis in the form of aspirin 81 mg bid, aspirin 325 mg bid, prophylactic lovenox (40 mg daily), or Coumadin are all options while weighing an individual patient's risk of clotting against their propensity for bleeding.
- In cases in which wound healing is a concern, keeping the knee straight for several days helps avoid these issues. A bulky soft dressing for 1 to 2 days postoperatively is recommended.

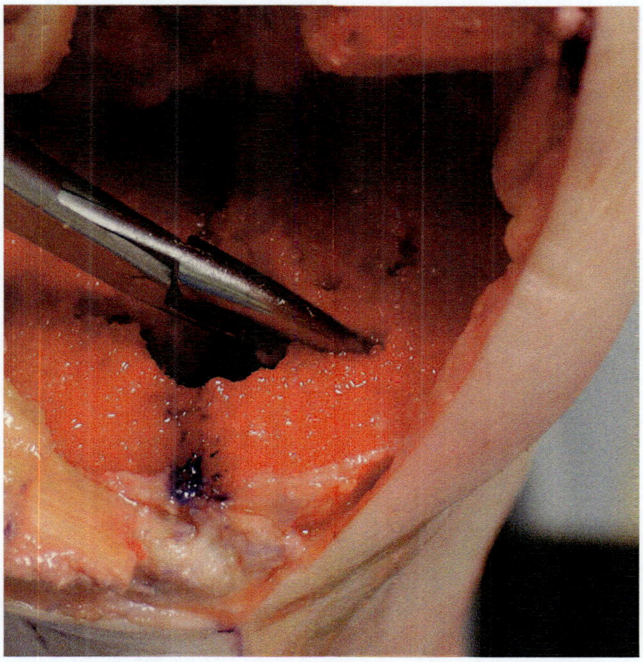

Figure 50.20 | Removal of sclerotic bone from the keel. If there is sclerotic bone in the keel area, slightly enlarging this will allow the component to sit flush against the tibia. If this is not performed, it can lift the tibia and place the final component into more valgus. Lastly, this ensures there will not be a defect in the cement mantle, which may be thin as a result of sclerotic bone.

Chapter 51
Flexion Gap Balancing Techniques in Primary Total Knee Arthroplasty

NICHOLAS A. BEDARD
MICHAEL J. TAUNTON

Key Concepts

- The goal of this technique is a stable knee replacement in both flexion and extension with neutral mechanical alignment of the knee.
- The gap balancing technique relies on the re-creation of neutral mechanical alignment and ligament balancing in extension creating a balanced extension gap before femoral posterior condylar resection.
- It is important to resect the proximal tibia perpendicular to the mechanical axis of the tibia as this cut will determine the femoral component rotation.
- With equal tension on the medial and lateral ligamentous structures of the knee in flexion the femur is sized and rotated to create a balanced flexion gap. The flexion gap must equal the size of the previously established extension gap.

Sterile Instruments and Implants

- Sandbag to position leg under the drapes.
- Post to attach to table proximally to prevent hip abduction.
- Two bent Hohmann retractors.
- One posterior knee retractor.
- Lamina spreader or implant-specific tensioner.
- Total knee arthroplasty (TKA) implant.

Preoperative Planning

- Clinical examination of the patient evaluating for fixed or correctable deformities of the knee, range of motion, and prior incisions.
- Review of the anteroposterior, lateral, and patellar view radiographs to evaluate the arthritis pattern, bone quality, and bone deformities.
- Evaluate weight-bearing long-leg radiographs to plan the distal femoral and proximal tibia cut. The proximal tibia cut is drawn on the long-leg radiographs at 90° to the mechanical axis of the tibia. The angle between the anatomic and mechanical axes of the femur is also measured to determine the magnitude of valgus for the distal femoral cut to ensure the cut is perpendicular to the mechanical axis of the femur (Figure 51.1).
- The planned bony resections and amounts of bone planned to be removed should be noted to help ensure re-creation of a neutral mechanical alignment and a perpendicular tibial resection.

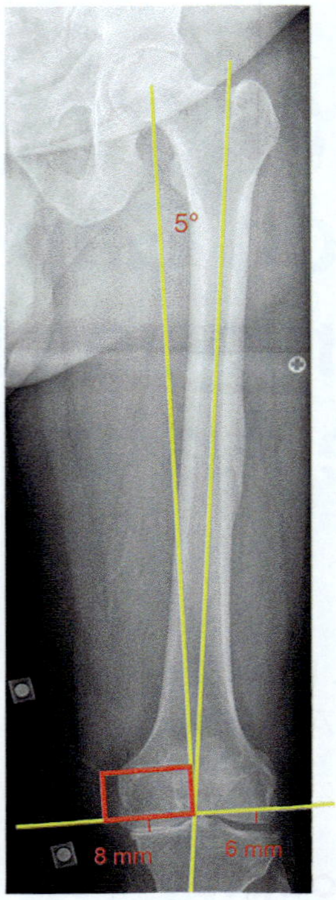

Figure 51.1 | Standing long-leg radiograph demonstrating the anatomic and mechanical axes of the femur. The magnitude of difference between these axes, in this case 5°, is used for the angle of the distal femoral resection to ensure the cut is perpendicular to the mechanical axis of the femur.

Bone, Implant, and Soft Tissue Techniques

Introduction

- One of the primary goals of TKA are symmetric and balanced extension and flexion gaps. The magnitude of bone resection, ligament balancing, tibial slope, and femoral component rotation all contribute to the size and balance of the flexion gap. The 2 primary techniques for determining femoral component rotation and balanced flexion and extension gaps are the gap balancing technique and the measured resection technique. This chapter will focus on a gap balancing technique, of which there are many. Our preferred gap balancing technique relies on first establishing neutral mechanical alignment in extension, then establishing a balanced ligamentous extension gap. The "thickness" of the flexion gap is then altered to match the thickness of the extension gap. This helps prevent altering the joint line in extension and may improve overall knee kinematics. The posterior condylar resection and thus the femoral component rotation is set based on ligament tension, not the posterior condylar axis, as is standard in many measured resection techniques.

Gap Balancing Technique

- Positioning
  - Patient is positioned supine on the operative table.
  - Examination of the knee under anesthesia is performed.
  - A sandbag and lateral hip rest are positioned on the table to assist with keeping the knee in flexion and the leg from abducting during procedure.
- Exposure
  - Surgical exposure of the knee is obtained utilizing the medial parapetallar approach as described in previous chapters.

- Distal femoral cut
  - The distal femoral cut is made utilizing an intramedullary guide.
  - The amount of valgus in the distal femoral cut is modified depending on the preoperative planning and distal femoral alignment.
  - The amount of distal femoral resection should equal the thickness of the femoral implant and is typically around 10 mm off the more distal side of the knee (usually medial).
- Proximal tibia cut
  - The proximal tibia is then exposed with knee flexion, external rotation to take the tension of the patellar tendon and subluxation of the tibia.
  - Proximal tibia resection is made using an extramedullary cutting guide to create a cut at a 90° angle to the mechanical axis of the tibia in the coronal plan. The amount of sagittal slope incorporated into the resection is determined by the implant utilized. The depth of proximal tibia resection is generally 8 to 10 mm off the unaffected side and is approximately 2 mm off the affected side (Figure 51.2). Our preference is to aim for a neutral slope relative to the lateral plateau of the tibia.
  - Residual bony defects of the tibia should rarely be corrected with additional tibia resection. Rather, such defects can be filled with cement, screws in cement technique, bone grafting, or metal augments depending on the size and location of the defect.
- Extension gap balancing
  - Soft tissue structures can be tented over femoral or tibial osteophytes resulting in excessive tension of these structures. Therefore, femoral and tibial osteophytes should be removed before any soft tissue releases.
  - The knee is then brought into extension, and the extension gap is assessed utilizing either spacer blocks or a tensioning device.
    - If utilizing spacer blocks the symmetry of the extension gap should be assessed with valgus- and varus-directed forces.
    - If utilizing a tensioning device, such as laminar spreaders, then symmetry of the extension gap is assessed with the device itself and no further stress needs to be applied to the knee.
  - Alignment rods placed through the extension block handle assess the alignment of the extremity. Our goal is a mechanical axis that passes from the center of the hip through the center of the knee to the center of the ankle (Figure 51.3). This check must be completed before any ligamentous release.

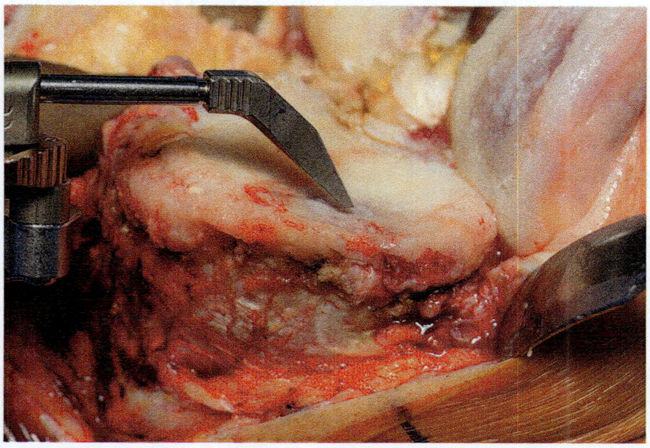

Figure 51.2 | Intraoperative photo measuring the planned proximal tibial resection, in this case planning for a minimal resection of the affected medial tibial plateau.

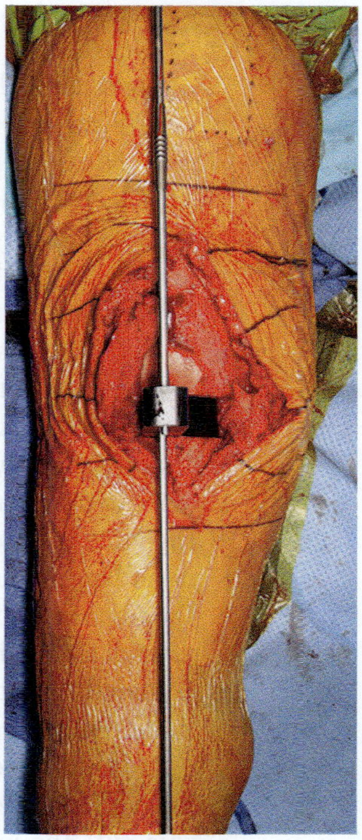

Figure 51.3 | Intraoperative photo with spacer block in extension with alignment rod through the spacer block demonstrating a mechanical axis passing from the center of the hip through the center of the knee to the center of the ankle.

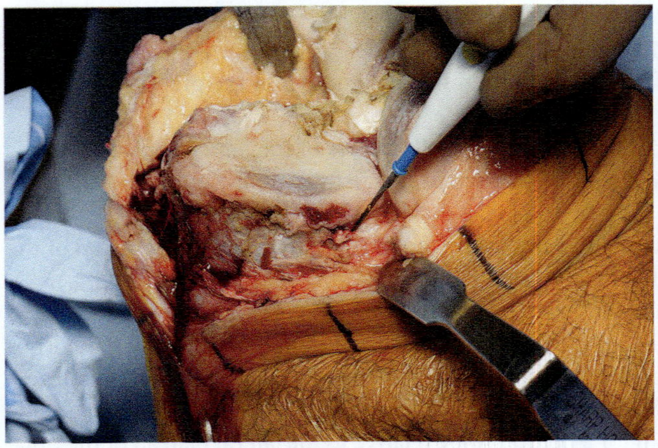

Figure 51.4 | Intraoperative photo of electrocautery being used to release the posterior oblique ligament and semimembranosus insertion to help balance the extension gap when the medial side remains tight in extension.

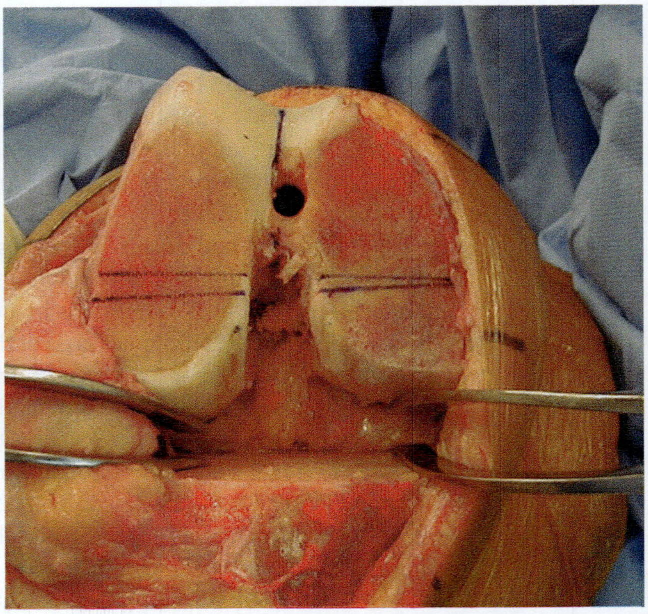

Figure 51.5 | Intraoperative photo demonstrating lamina spreader being utilized to equally tension the medial and lateral sides of the flexion gap.

- If the extension gap is tighter than the thinnest TKA construct both medially and laterally, a decision needs to be made to resect either more distal femur or proximal tibia. If there was a substantial preoperative flexion contracture, it is likely that more distal femoral resection is required.
- Ligamentous releases are performed as necessary to obtain a knee that fully extends and has a rectangular space between the proximal tibia and distal femur and appropriate lower extremity alignment.
  - If the knee is tight medially or laterally in extension and the angles of the bony resection are confirmed to be correct, then posterior-based structures of the knee should be targeted for release.
  - Tight medially
    - Further exposure of the posteromedial tibia with electrocautery can be performed with release of the posterior oblique ligament and semimembranosus insertion if necessary to balance the extension gap (Figure 51.4).
  - Tight laterally
    - With the lateral side of the knee tensioned, the tight structures on the posterior lateral aspect of the knee are palpated and tight structures are partially released using a #15 blade to pie crust the tight structure from the inside out. Rarely should the popliteus tendon be released at this stage as it primarily affects the flexion gap.
- Once the knee is balanced in extension with appropriate alignment, the goal is to balance the flexion gap by duplicating the dimensions of the extension gap.

- Anterior and posterior femoral cuts
  - The knee is brought to 90° of flexion, and the collateral ligaments are equally tensioned using either lamina spreaders or implant-specific tensioners (Figure 51.5).
  - The femoral component size is measured with reference from the anterior aspect of the lateral femoral shaft. The appropriate size femoral component is chosen to maintain the desired posterior condylar offset to allow for a flexion gap that is symmetric to the extension gap and to avoid femoral notching (Figure 51.6).
    - In general, we prefer to set the flexion gap to be 1 to 2 mm tighter than the extension gap.
  - Anterior and posterior cutting block is positioned. This should be parallel to the proximal tibia cut. The proximal tibia cut is what determines your femoral component rotation in the gap balancing technique. However, the transepicondylar axis and anteroposterior axis of the femur can be used as a secondary check of femoral component rotation before completing your femoral cuts.

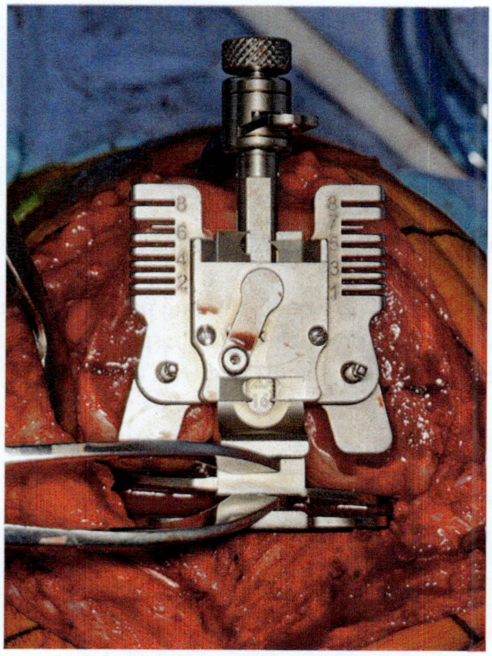

Figure 51.6 I Intraoperative photo of sizing the femoral component with reference to the anterior aspect of lateral femoral shaft and using an implant-specific tensioner to ensure desired posterior condylar resection.

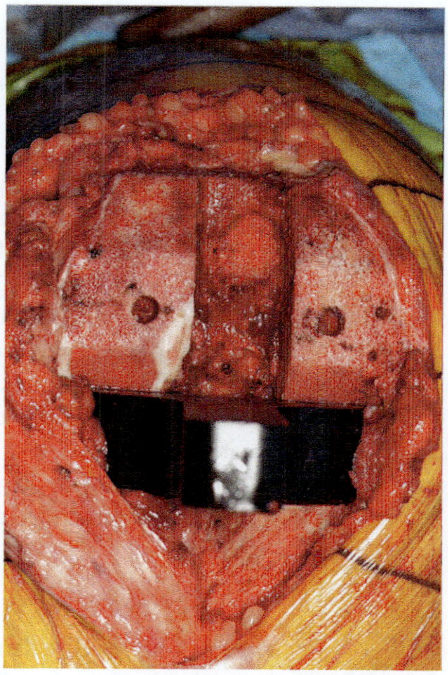

Figure 51.7 I Intraoperative photo of a spacer block inserted into the flexion gap to ensure appropriate sizing and balancing.

- If the AP cutting block does not have saw captures, the spacer block can be reinserted to double check the symmetry of the flexion gap before bony resection.
- Anterior and posterior femoral cuts are made.
- The flexion gap should be balanced and symmetric to the extension gap. This can be again assessed with lamina spreaders or a spacer block (Figure 51.7).
- Any asymmetry of the flexion gap should be addressed with ligament releases. This should be a rare occurrence. The surgeon could choose to note the imbalance at this point and choose to do further balancing of ligaments at the time of trialing.
  - In flexion, anterior-based structures can be released.
  - If tight medially, superficial medical collateral ligament can be released further distally with periosteal elevator or electrocautery (Figure 51.8).
  - If tight laterally, additional pie crusting can be performed to the tight structures as described earlier.

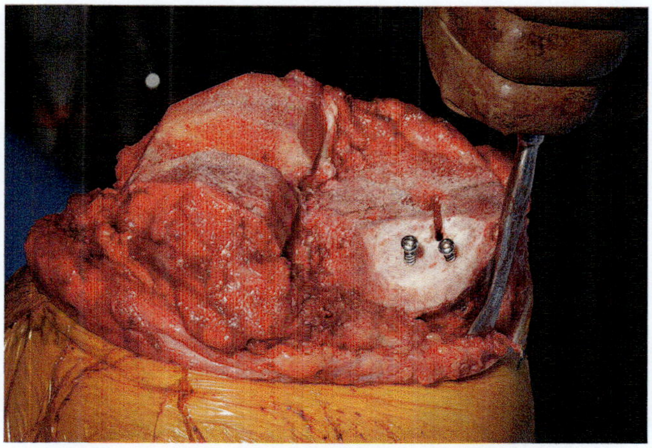

Figure 51.8 I Intraoperative photo of a periosteal elevator being utilized to further release the superficial medial collateral ligament to help balance the flexion gap.

- Final bone cuts
  - Chamfer and box cuts (if using a posterior stabilized knee) are made per implant design.
  - If the patella is to be resurfaced, this can be done before or after balanced flexion and extension gaps are obtained.
- Trial components
  - Trial components are placed and the knee is taken through a range of motion to ensure that full flexion and extension are achieved.
  - The knee is inspected for varus/valgus instability in flexion and extension as well as anteroposterior stability in flexion.
  - The goal should be normal laxity of <2 mm of opening between femur and polyethylene insert in both the lateral and medial compartments with varus and valgus forces, respectively.
  - Any residual tightness in either flexion or extension can be addressed with additional soft tissue releases as previously described.
- Final components
  - Final components are cemented into place.
  - Closure is performed as described in previous chapters.

Postoperative Care

- Patients with a well-balanced and stable knee are made weight bearing as tolerated, and begin working on knee range of motion immediately.
- Mobilization is started the same day of surgery.
- Prophylaxis against venous thromboembolism should be given per the surgeons' protocol.

Chapter 52
Kinematic or Anatomic Alignment Techniques in Primary Total Knee Arthroplasty

ASHTON H. GOLDMAN
MARK W. PAGNANO

Key Concepts

- Kinematic (anatomic) alignment is a true measured resection technique whereby the general goal is to restore the limb to its prearthritic alignment and maintain the native joint line position and inclination throughout the arc of motion. Some believe this minimizes the need for soft tissue releases and creates a more natural feeling knee.
  - The senior author's fundamental premise is that, within some reasonable boundaries, priority should be given to placing the femoral component such that it mimics the 3-dimensional position of the native femur. Within boundaries of ±2 or 3° of varus the tibia is then positioned to accommodate that femoral position and achieve ligamentous balance in both flexion and extension.
  - Anatomic alignment is individualized for each patient, and although it can be performed simply and pragmatically, it is not a cookbook approach. Definitively it is not just leaving varus knees in varus or cutting every tibia in slight varus; instead, it is a deliberate attempt to incrementally adjust the femoral and tibial cuts to mimic the individual patient's anatomy without straying great distances from established norms of alignment.
- In our practice, kinematic/anatomic principles are applied only to varus and neutral knees. It is the senior author's opinion that many valgus knees have inherent bony deformities that make mechanical alignment a better choice for the valgus knee.
- Studies show that neutral mechanical alignment ±3° is a safe boundary in terms of long-term durability. Deliberately aiming for a target beyond ±3° is not recommended, so the technique should have clear boundaries.
  - It is the senior author's contention that, although modern cemented implants seem to tolerate some mild deviations from mechanical alignment, at some point there is a mechanical limit because we are using biomaterials, including metal, plastic, and bone cement. For that reason, we have established 2 to 3° of deviation as the reasonable boundary within which we will adjust component position.
- In the typical varus knee, standard mechanical alignment techniques routinely overresect the lateral tibial plateau in both flexion and extension relative to normal anatomy (Figure 52.1). As a consequence, additional external rotation of the femoral component (typically 3°) is routinely needed to balance the knee in flexion and the distal femur is cut in less valgus to balance in

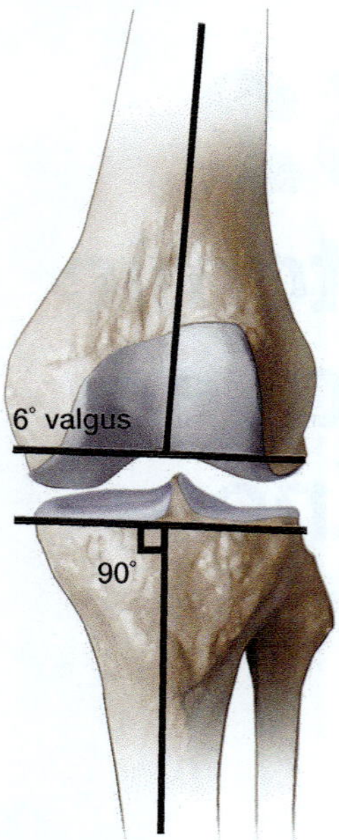

Figure 52.1 | An illustration demonstrates the relative overresection of the proximal lateral tibia and the alteration of the distal femoral joint line that is routinely forced when following mechanical axis alignment principles as compared with the native anatomy of the knee.

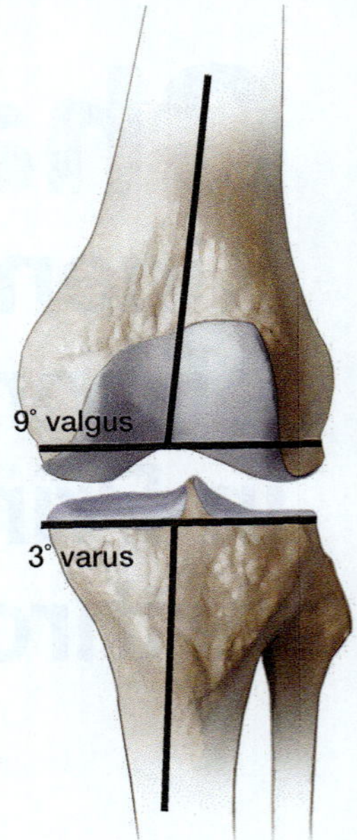

Figure 52.2 | An illustration demonstrates the typical native anatomy of the knee with the proximal tibial joint surface in slight varus and the distal femur in valgus. The values represented in the figure are mean values; surgeons should be aware of the range of individual variability. Note that contemporary kinematic or anatomic alignment techniques typically account for that individual variability rather than preselecting an average, mean, or generic target.

extension. The combination of relative overresection and additional external rotation elevates the medial joint line in both flexion and extension (thereby risking midflexion instability) and decreases posterior femoral offset (limiting ultimate range of motion). Anatomic alignment principles seek to limit those systematic deviations from native anatomy and produce a better balanced total knee arthroplasty without the routine need for medial ligamentous releases (Figure 52.2)

- With this technique, because the tibia is not relatively overresected laterally in flexion, the appropriate femoral rotation is most often 0° relative to the posterior condylar axis. Zero degrees femoral rotation will mimic the native femur.

- Before attempting anatomic alignment, a surgeon must be confident in his/her ability to make precise bone cuts in slight varus/valgus or should use surgical navigation or robotics to achieve that precision.

Sterile Instruments and Implants

- Routine knee retractors
- Wide and narrow rongeurs for osteophyte removal
- Total knee system with following qualities:
  - Favorable trochlear design
  - Ability to make fine varus/valgus adjustment
  - Posterior referencing for both femoral sizing and rotation

Surgical Approaches

- Medial parapatellar, midvastus, and subvastus approach are all appropriate for this technique.

Preoperative Planning

- The senior author has both a simple, pragmatic planning process and a more complicated, mechanistic approach.
- A full-length standing radiograph of the lower limbs is preferred in all cases; is optional for the simple, pragmatic planning process; and is required for the more complicated, mechanistic planning approach.

Simple, Pragmatic Planning

- For knees with preoperative varus deformity or neutral alignment:
  - On the anteroposterior (AP) radiograph the distal femoral valgus angle is measured by defining the angle between the distal femoral subchondral bone and the center of the femoral canal. Typically, this will measure about 5 or 6° but is variable. The distal femoral resection angle is set to match this measured angle, but if the angle exceeds 8°, we pragmatically dial that back to 7 or 8° (Figure 52.3)
  - On the AP radiograph the proximal tibial varus inclination is measured by defining the proximal tibial subchondral bone laterally and medially and the long axis of the tibia. If there is some medial bone loss, then an estimate of the original joint inclination can typically still be made by referencing unworn regions or looking at the contralateral knee (Figure 52.4)
    - The limit for varus position is 2 or 3° of varus, but the goal is to mimic what was present before arthritis.
    - Therefore, if the tibia measures 0° varus cut it at zero (Figure 52.5)
    - If it measures 2° varus, cut it at 2° varus (Figure 52.6)
    - But if it measures 5° of varus, then dial that back to 2 or 3° varus.
  - Femoral rotation is set parallel to the posterior condylar axis, as this mimics the anatomic orientation of the native femur in flexion. This means the guide is typically set at 0° external rotation as opposed to the traditional 3° external.

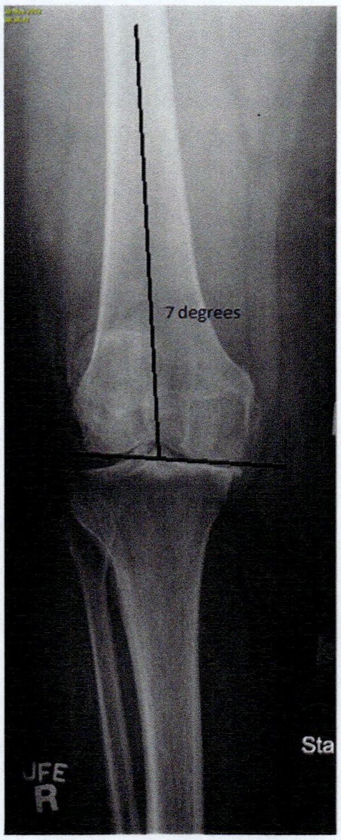

Figure 52.3 | On the AP radiograph the distal femoral valgus angle is measured. Typically, this will measure about 6 or 7° but is variable. The distal femoral valgus resection angle is set to match this measured angle, but if the angle exceeds 8° we pragmatically dial that back to 7 or 8°.

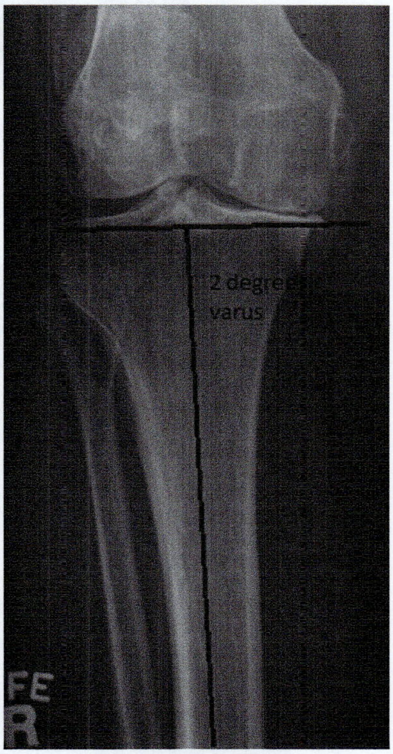

Figure 52.4 | On the AP radiograph the proximal tibial varus inclination is measured by defining the proximal tibial subchondral bone laterally and medially and the long axis of the tibia. If there is some medial bone loss, an estimate of the original joint inclination can typically be made by referencing unworn regions or looking at the contralateral knee. The proximal tibia is then cut to match the measured varus inclination up to a maximum of 3° varus; so in this example the angle measures 2° and the tibia would be cut at 2° varus.

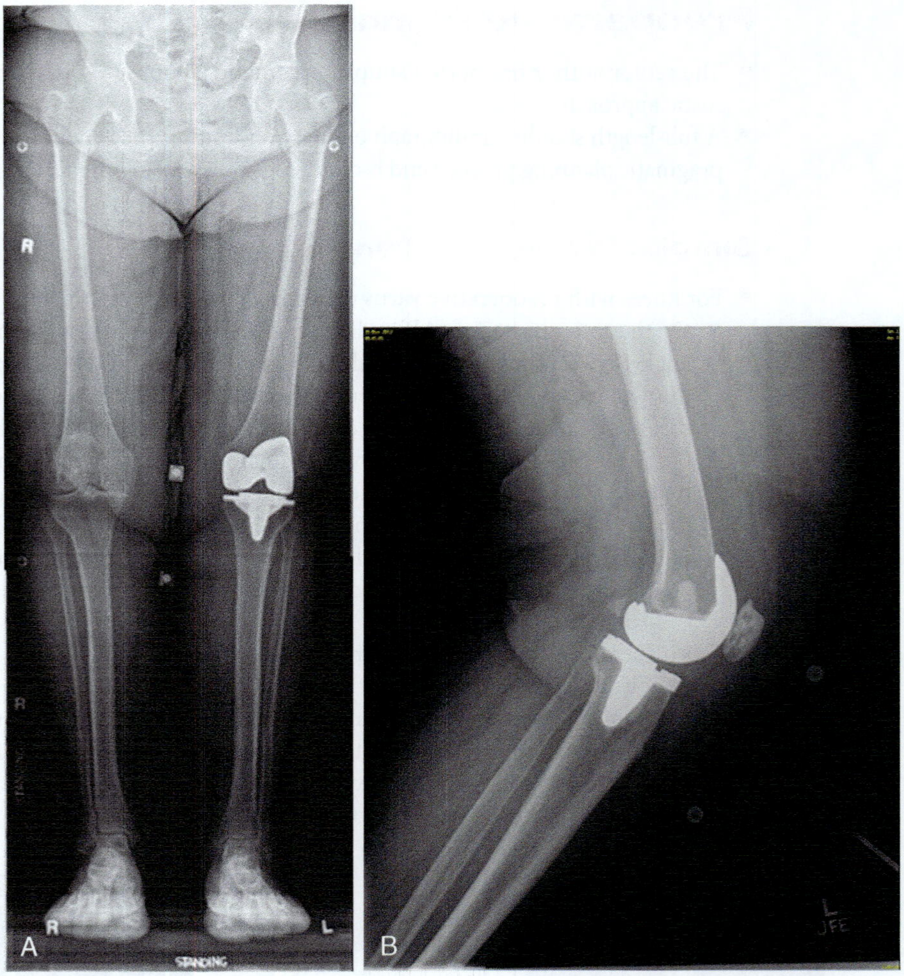

Figure 52.5 | Postoperative radiographs including (A) AP and (B) lateral views of the knee, which demonstrate a case in which the anatomic measurement of the distal femur was 6° valgus and the proximal tibia was 0° varus.

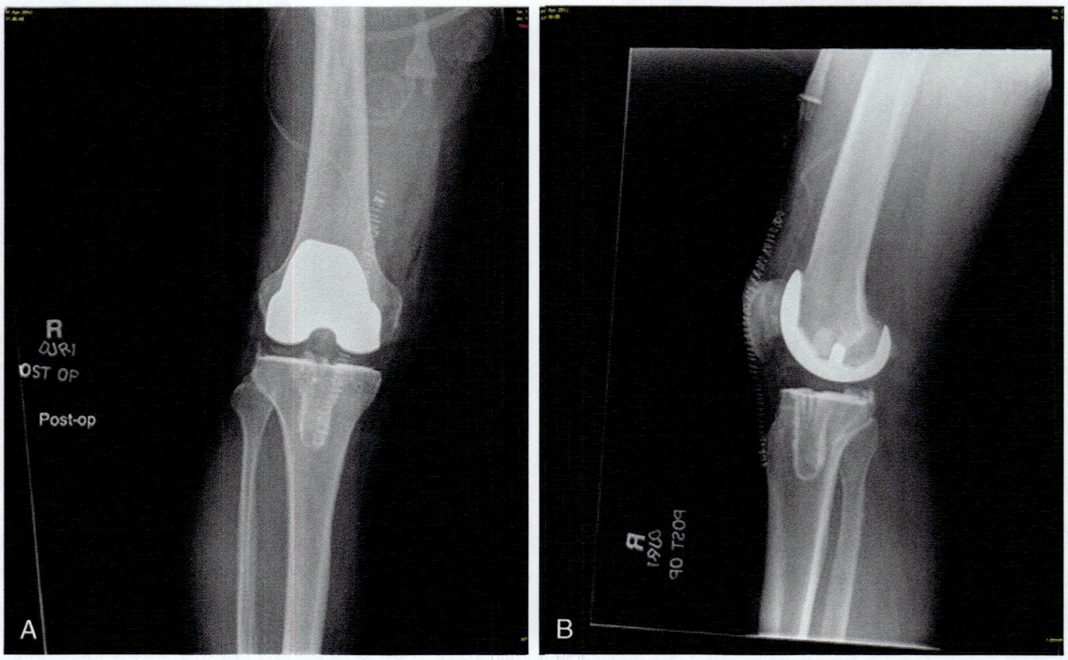

Figure 52.6 | Postoperative radiographs including (A) AP and (B) lateral views of the knee, which demonstrate a case in which the anatomic measurement of the distal femur was 7° valgus and the proximal tibia was 2° varus.

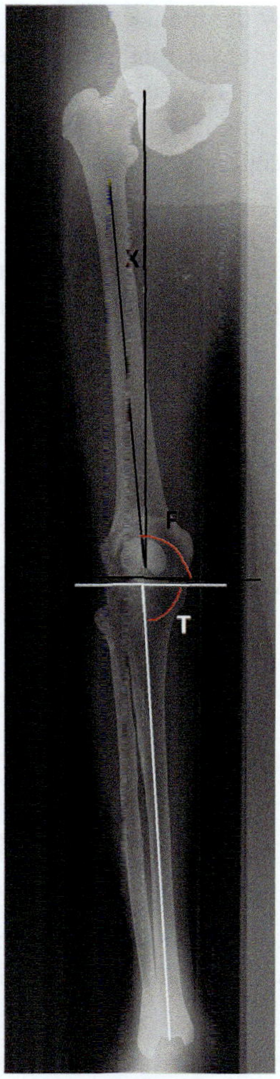

Figure 52.7 | More complex preoperative planning can be undertaken by using hip-knee-ankle radiographs to calculate several values and thus ensure that the chosen targets for anatomic alignment fall within widely accepted parameters of ±3° relative to the mechanical axis. X is the angle that represents the femoral mechanical axis. F is the angle that represents the distal femoral anatomic valgus. T is the angle that represents the proximal tibial anatomic varus inclination. A surgeon who wishes to remain within some traditional "safe harbors" might use these measurement to ensure: (1) the chosen distal femoral cut is within ±3° of femoral mechanical axis; (2) the proximal tibial varus cut is within ±3° of tibial mechanical axis; and (3) the combination of the 2 cuts results in a knee within ±3° of the measured mechanical axis on the individual patient's hip-knee-ankle radiograph.

More Complex, Mechanistic Planning Process

- Hip-Knee-Ankle (HKA) Alignment = Tibial Joint Line Angle (T) + Femoral Valgus Angle (F) – Femoral Anatomic Axis Angle (X) (Figure 52.7)
- Preoperative planning is helpful in anatomic or kinematic alignment for understanding boundaries within ±3° from neutral alignment (HKA = 177 – 183).

Fundamentally, this more complex process ensures that the target for overall limb alignment is within ±3° of the mechanical axis and that both the femur and tibia are individually within ±3° of mechanical alignment as well.

- F boundary = <98° (in other words no distal femur is ever cut in >8° valgus)

Calculate F by the medial subtended angle between femoral shaft and distal femoral subchondral bone.

- X = Angle between the mechanical and anatomic femoral axis. In mechanical alignment this would be the distal femoral resection angle.
- In kinematic alignment the X is not used for distal femoral resection but only to estimate HKA. The distal femoral resection angle in kinematic alignment = F−90.
- T boundary = 87 to 90° (in other words no tibia is ever cut in >3° varus).

Calculate T by the medial subtended angle between the center of the ankle and a line crossing the subchondral bone of the medial and lateral tibial plateau.

- T + F − X = HKA is used to estimate preoperative limb alignment (HKA < 180 = varus, HKA > 180 = valgus).
- Ensure all preoperative measurements are within boundaries; if not, make adjustments accordingly for both F and T.
  - If the F is greater than or equal to 99, change this to be within boundaries (i.e., 98°). The new planned distal femoral resection angle is 98−90 = 8°.
  - Likewise, if T is outside 87 to 90, make adjustments to ensure a cut is made in this range.
- Examples:

Radiographic Parameter	Degrees	In Bounds	Surgical Plan
F (variable)	97	Yes	97 = 7° distal femoral resection
X (fixed)	6	N/A	6°
T (variable)	89	Yes- 1° varus	89 = 1° varus cut
HKA (F + T − FAA)	180	Yes	180°
F (variable)	99	No	Change to 98 = 8° distal femoral resection
X (fixed)	7	N/A	7
T (variable)	86	No	Change to 87 = 3° varus cut
HKA (F + T − X)	178	Yes	178°

Bone, Implant, and Soft Tissue Techniques

- After initial exposure and removal of osteophytes, conduct a stress examination to examine the competency of the ligaments as well as the degree of cartilage loss. If the ligaments are markedly abnormal, a standard mechanical axis total knee arthroplasty is performed.

Distal Femoral Resection

- Set the distal femoral resection jig at the planned resection angle (FV-90). The cut should be made at a thickness that accounts for the cartilage loss and matches the thickness of the implant (most often 8 or 9 mm in contemporary knee designs).
- Calipers can be used to measure the resection. The intact cartilage and bone resected from the lateral condyle should be equal to the thickness of the implant (minus the thickness of the sawblade). The medial resection is often thinner than the implant because of cartilage loss.

AP Sizing/Femoral Finishing

- AP sizing should be set to 0° external rotation relative to the posterior femoral condyles. The goal is to have symmetric posterior condylar resections equal to the implant thickness. Additional external rotation raises the medial joint line in flexion and can cause instability.
- Note that older symmetric femoral designs had less favorable trochleas thereby necessitating additional external rotation of the femoral component to improve patellar tracking. With modern side-specific femoral components, additional external rotation is not required assuming appropriate tibial rotation, appropriate lateral translation of the components, and medialization of the patella dome.
- Posterior referencing for size and rotation ensures consistent posterior femoral resection.
- Set the AP sizer against the posterior condyles, adjust the external rotation to zero, and fix it in place.
- Measure the AP size to avoid notching anteriorly. Place the appropriate 4-in-1 cutting jig.
- If notching is predicted, increase the size of the proposed implant. Ensure an understanding of the system used. The change between sizes will either grow anteriorly, posteriorly, or in both directions. Therefore, the placement of the cutting jig may need to be moved in the AP plane to ensure a stable flexion gap.
- After completing femoral resections, ensure the posterior condyles match the thickness of the implant accounting for cartilage loss and the kerf of the saw blade.

Tibial Preparation

- Align the tibial resection guide in the standard fashion for a 0° mechanical axis resection. The height of the resection is set to a 9- to 10-mm resection off the high/unworn cartilage side to account for the thickness of the implant.
- For either cruciate-retaining (CR) or posterior-stabilized (PS) components, use the slope that is standard for the implant configuration. For a CR component, matching the native slope with an angel wing is preferred (usually 5-7°). Likewise, a 0° posterior slope is preferred for a PS to make up for the flexion space increased with PCL sacrificing.
- Accounting for the length of the tibia, make fine adjustments in the varus/valgus at the ankle to match the preoperative plan. If the tibia was measured within boundaries, a symmetric cut on the tibia (accounting for cartilage loss) would be expected.
- While adjusting varus/valgus at the ankle, longer tibias will require more angular correction, whereas shorter tibia will need less.
- Some systems can provide values on degree change with respect to varus/valgus angular marks at the ankle to simplify the process.
- Conversely, one can set the guide at a varus/valgus angle by visually matching the native joint line while compensating for bone loss and cartilage loss. Use the ankle guide to ensure it is within appropriate boundaries.
- Resect the tibia in standard fashion protecting the local structures.

Trialing/Balancing

- Ensure all osteophytes are removed. Be sure the posterior osteophytes are removed to avoid inappropriate tensioning of the medial and lateral ligaments in extension.
- If within the boundary of 0 to 3° tibial varus, some additional balancing can be done with fine adjustments of the tibial resection thereby minimizing soft tissue release and allowing these structures to remain in their native orientation and tension:

  If both flexion & extension spaces are symmetrically tight, resect 2 mm more tibia.
  If only the flexion space is tight, add 2 degrees more slope to the tibial resection.
  If flexion space is too loose, decrease slope and use a thicker polyethylene insert.
  If medial side tight, add 1 degree of tibial varus (do not exceed 3 degrees total).
  If cuts are correct and still unbalanced, perform soft tissue releases as needed.

Postoperative Care

- A standard postoperative course with early mobilization, range-of-motion exercises, pain control, and deep vein thrombosis chemoprophylaxis is appropriate.

Section D
Primary TKA in Specific Conditions

Chapter 53
Varus Knee Deformity

KAPIL MEHROTRA
DANIEL J. BERRY

Key Concepts

- Balancing the varus knee begins with making bone cuts that restore neutral (or near-neutral) mechanical alignment to the knee, followed by soft tissue management to obtain even (or near-even) soft tissue tension on the medial and lateral sides of the knee.
- In the great majority of cases, soft tissue management consists of sequential releases of tight soft tissue structures on the medial side of the knee in an iterative manner.
- Overrelease of medial soft tissues is a constant concern and should be avoided to minimize risk of instability.
- Constrained implants providing extra varus/valgus stability are reserved for severe cases.

Sterile Instruments and Implants

Sterile Instruments

- Routine knee arthroplasty retractors
- Periosteal elevator
- 18-gauge needle
- Electrocautery
- Small oscillating saw

Implants

- Routine knee arthroplasty instrumentation.
- In cases with notable bone loss: metal augments to make up for bone deficiencies and implants to protect fixation.
- In cases of severe deformity: constrained implants with stems to protect fixation.

Position

- Supine on operating table
- Tourniquet on the thigh well above area of knee incision

Surgical Approaches

- Use the surgeon's routine preferred knee exposure in most cases: usually this will be medial parapatellar.
- In more severe deformities, use medial parapatellar approach even if surgeon usually uses a different exposure for patients with minimal deformity.

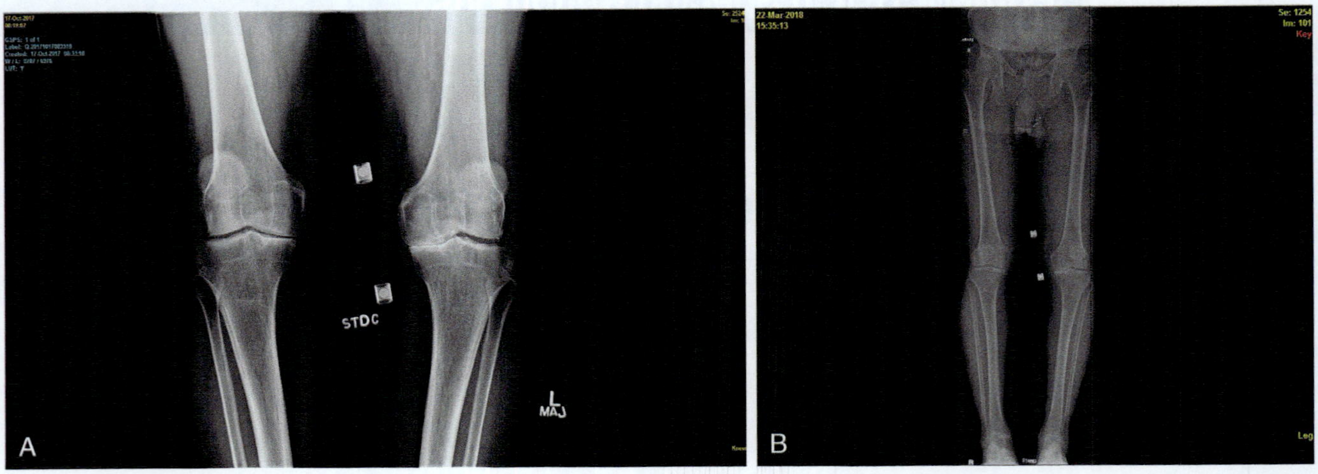

Figure 53.1 | A, Standing weight-bearing knee films. B, Longstanding hip to ankle radiograph to evaluate limb alignment and to use for preoperative planning.

Preoperative Planning

- In addition to performing routine preoperative total knee arthroplasty (TKA) orthopedic and medical evaluation, carefully evaluate the degree to which the varus deformity is correctable with valgus stress and the degree to which lateral structures are stretched out with varus stress. This will provide an idea of the amount of soft tissue balancing that will be required.
- Obtain long-standing hip to ankle radiographs to plan the bone cuts required to restore neutral or near-neutral mechanical limb alignment (Figure 53.1A and B).
- Measure the tibiofemoral angle (angle created between the anatomic axis of the tibia and femur) to determine the severity of the varus deformity.
- Evaluate for medial femoral condyle or medial tibial plateau bone deficiencies.
- Identify posterior osteophytes on the lateral radiograph.
- Template femoral and tibial component size.
- Consider the need for augments, stems, or constrained implants.

Bone, Implant, and Soft Tissue Techniques

Bone Preparation

- After routine exposure via medial parapatellar exposure, make bone cuts on femur and tibia per the surgeon's routine method, either measured resection or flexion gap balancing methods (see Chapters 2, 50, and 51).
- Make sure during routine exposure the dissection around the medial proximal tibia is in the subperiosteal plane. This protects the medial collateral ligament (MCL), which can be adherent to medial osteophytes and also provides a good soft tissue sleeve for later repair.
- If bone deficiency is present, it is usually of the medial tibia in the varus knee. Make bone cuts to avoid excessive tibial resection. If the medial tibia is notably deficient, plan to fill the deficiency rather than resecting much extra bone. Usually the bone loss will be filled with a medial metal tibial block augment (Figure 53.2A-D). Very mild deficiencies may be filled with cement. Realize some mild bone deficiencies will be removed after resection of medial tibial osteophytes (Figure 53.3A and B).
- Remove medial and posterior femoral osteophytes and medial tibial osteophytes (Figure 53.4). This helps relax the medial soft tissues that are tented by these structures.
- Assess medial and lateral soft tissue tension and flexion and extension gaps with trial implants, blocks, or soft tissue tensioning devices per the surgeon's preference.

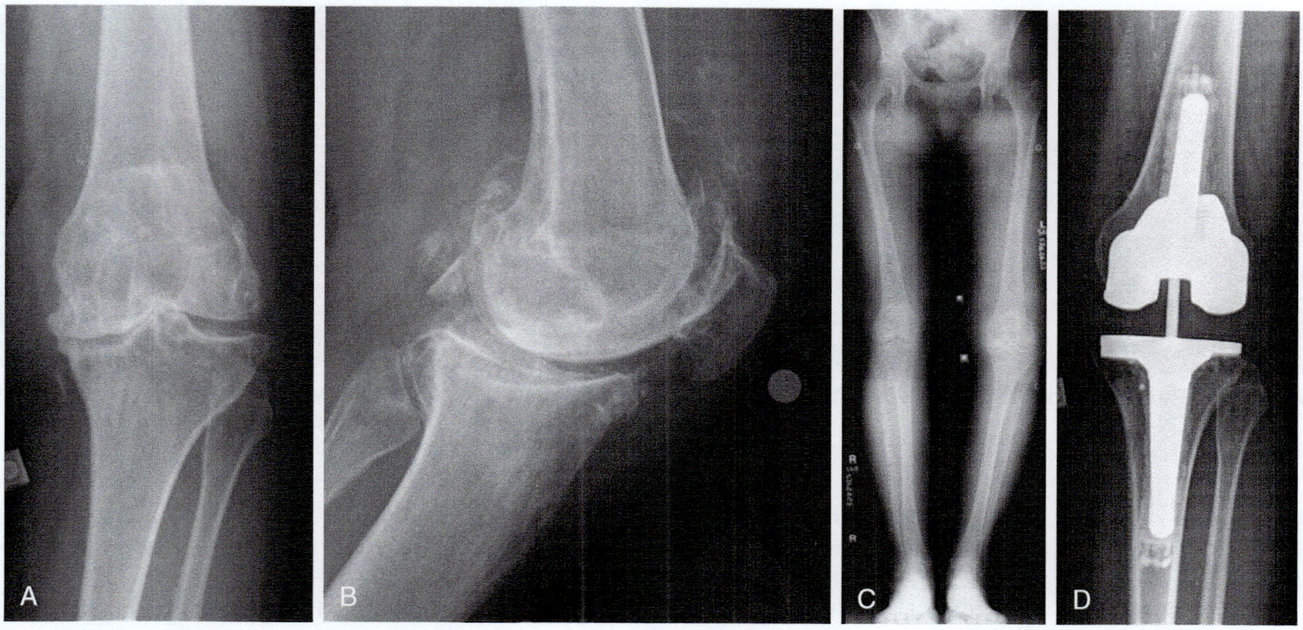

Figure 53.2 | A-C, AP and lateral knee and longstanding hip to ankle radiographs of patient with varus left knee deformity and medial-tibial bone erosion. D, Radiograph after TKA using medial tibial metal block augment to make up for medial tibial bone loss.

- In cases of mild deformity, no further soft tissue releases other than routine exposure and osteophyte removal may be needed. However, in most cases of substantial varus deformity further releases usually are needed and may be performed in an iterative manner.
- Begin by releasing the deep MCL at its attachment near the tibial plateau. This may already have been done with routine exposure and osteophyte removal. Carefully protect the superficial MCL during this process by retracting it away from the tibia with a periosteal elevator that has been placed deep to the superficial MCL and passed in the subperiosteal plane on the medial proximal tibia. Assess soft tissue balance.

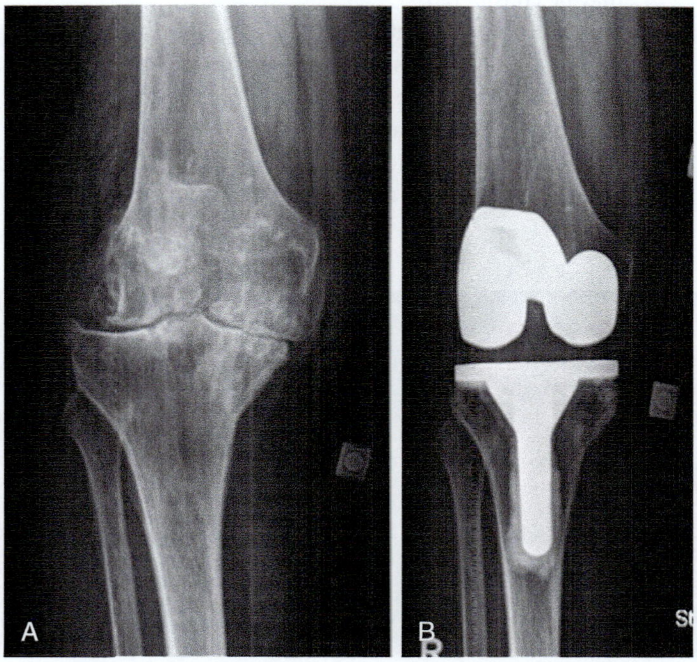

Figure 53.3 | A, Radiograph of patient with varus knee deformity and moderate medial tibial bone loss. B, Radiograph after TKA. The bone deficiency was removed with standard tibial bone resection.

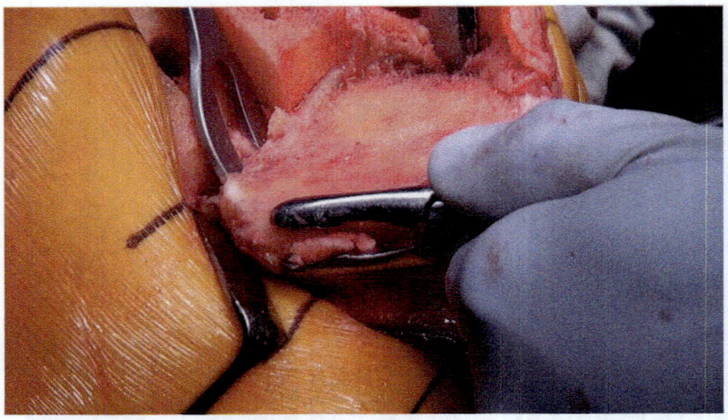

Figure 53.4 | Removing medial tibial osteophytes with a rongeur.

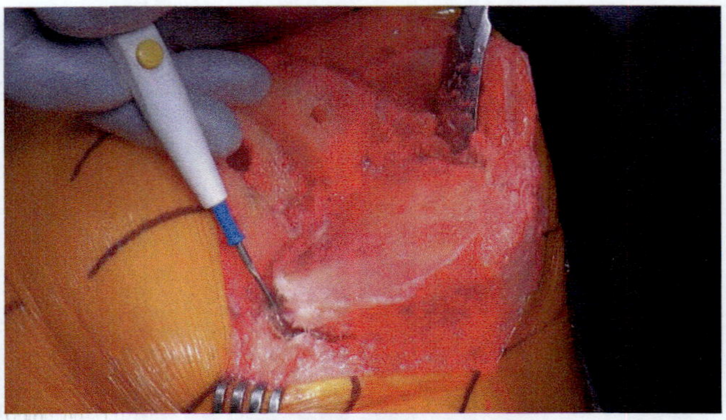

Figure 53.5 | Using electrocautery to release the posterior-medial soft tissue attachments near the tibial plateau. This is mainly the semimembranosus tendon insertion.

- Next, if needed, carry dissection around the proximal posteromedial tibia in the subperiosteal plane with electrocautery to take down the semimembranosus insertion (Figure 53.5). Reassess soft tissue balance.
- Next, if needed, judiciously elevate the medial soft tissue sleeve that includes the upper attachments of the superficial MCL with a periosteal elevator, working from proximal to distal (Figure 53.6). More severe deformities require more release and modest deformities less release. Be very careful with this step: too much release will completely release the superficial MCL, which may cause medial-sided knee instability. In general, the tissues of big men with dense periosteum tolerate more medial subperiosteal stripping than do those of women with less dense periosteum. More posterior stripping helps provide more release when the knee is selectively tight medially in extension, and more anterior release helps provide more release when the knee is selectively tight medially in flexion. Reassess soft tissue balance.
- Next, if the knee is still tight medially, careful "pie crusting" release of the MCL itself using an 18-gauge needle (which acts like a tiny knife blade) may be performed (Figure 53.7). Release the MCL under tension with the 18-gauge needle at different levels from anterior to posterior. Avoid overrelease. About 5 to 15 perforations at different levels of the MCL (proximal to tibial) are usually sufficient. Reassess soft tissue balance.
- If the above-mentioned measures still do not lead to balanced soft tissues, the following methods may be considered:
  - Downsizing and laterally translating the tibial component and resecting extra medial tibia (Figure 53.8A and B). This decompresses the medial soft tissue structures. With a trial in place, trim the medial tibial bone that is not needed to support the downsized component using a rongeur or small oscillating saw.
  - Sliding medial epicondylar osteotomy. A thin wafer (approximately 0.5 cm thick) that incorporates the adductor attachments and MCL origin is made with a small oscillating saw (Figure 53.9).

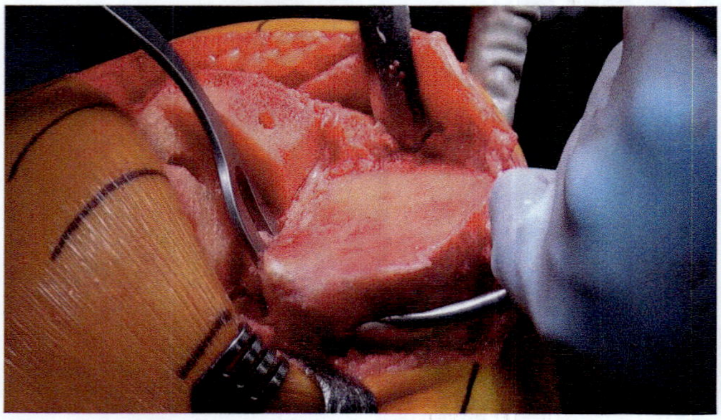

Figure 53.6 | Judicious elevation of the medial soft tissue sleeve including fibers of the superficial medial collateral ligament insertion with a periosteal elevator.

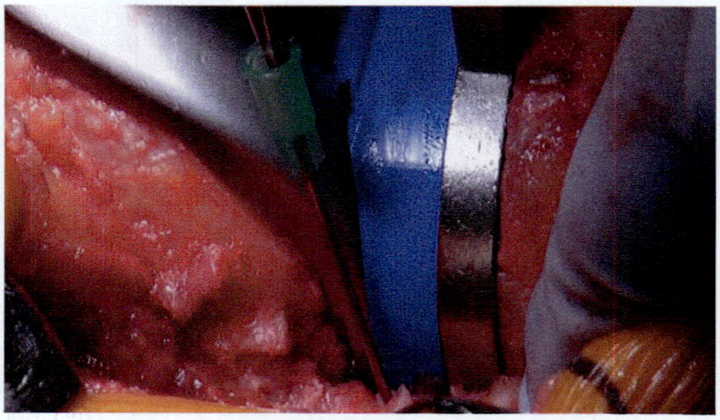

Figure 53.7 | Release of the medial collateral ligament using an 18-gauge needle to pie crust the ligament at different levels.

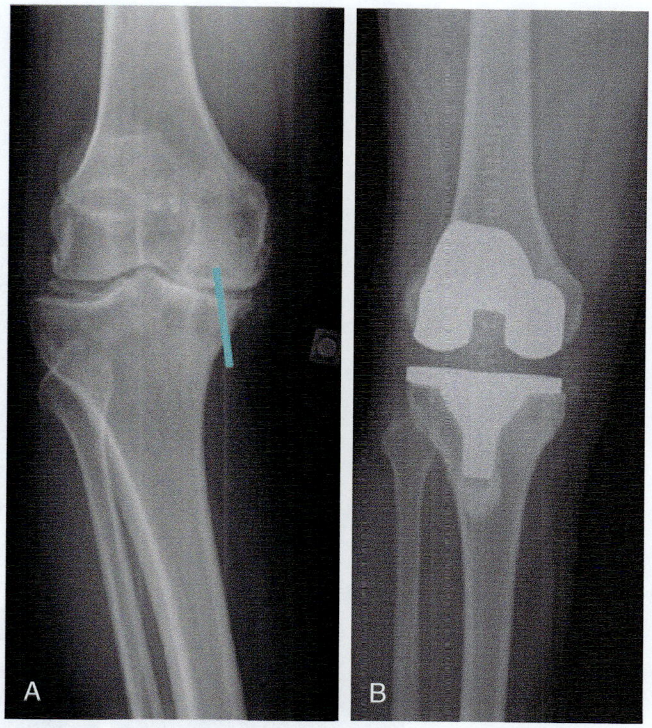

Figure 53.8 | A, Radiograph of patient with varus knee deformity. The line shows where bone can be resected to reduce medial collateral ligament tension. B, Radiograph after TKA with osteophyte resection, resection of a small amount of medial tibial plateau, and modest lateral translation of the tibial component.

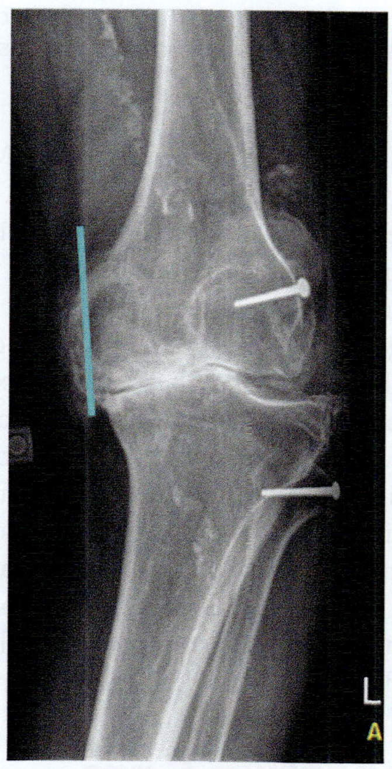

Figure 53.9 | Radiograph of patient with varus knee deformity showing where a sliding medial epicondylar osteotomy could be performed.

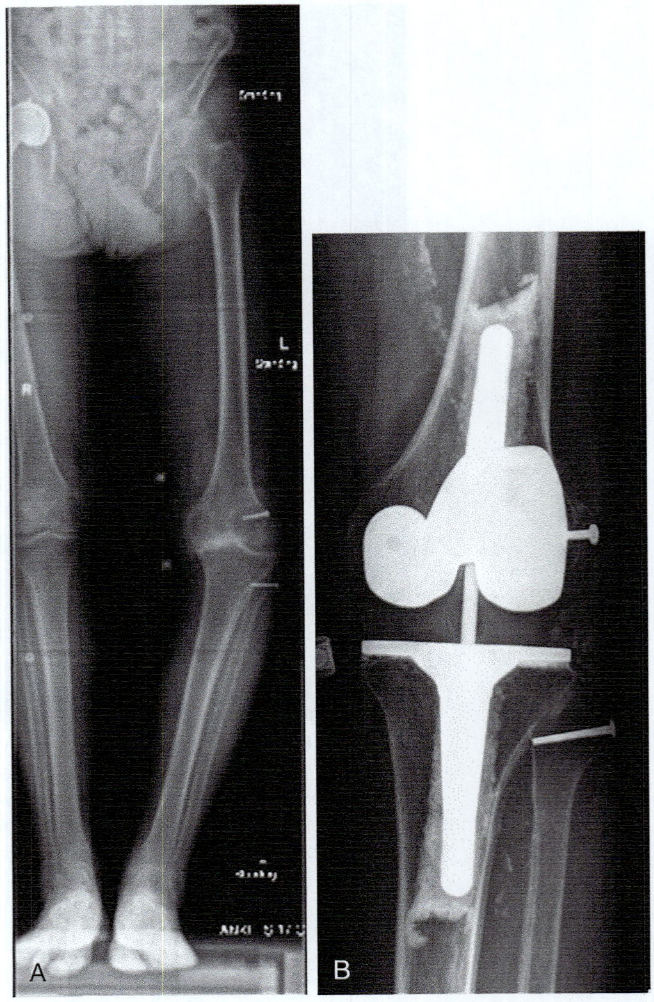

Figure 53.10 | A, Hip to ankle standing radiograph of an 89-year-old patient with notable varus knee deformity and previous lateral collateral ligament injury. B, Knee radiograph after TKA with constrained condylar implant. Note short stems were used to offload increased interface stresses.

This allows the MCL to slide distally. Make sure proximal soft tissue attachments are retained to provide dynamic tension on the MCL. A small amount of the distal osteotomy fragment may be trimmed away if it is too close to the joint. After retensioning the knee, the epicondylar osteotomy fragment is reapproximated to its new position in its bed with heavy sutures. Make sure the osteotomy fragment is stable and does not subluxate posteriorly after suture fixation.

- If the surgeon has performed whichever of the above-mentioned iterative release he or she prefers, and if the lateral side is still excessively lax, the lateral soft tissues may be very stretched or damaged and further medial releases may risk global knee instability. In such cases, which are usually the most severe deformities, the surgeon may choose to use extra constraint with a constrained condylar, or rarely, a hinged implant (Figure 53.10A and B).
- A constrained condylar implant may also be considered after notable medial release in the older, lower-demand patient to protect the released soft tissues with an "internal splint."
- Closure is routine and in layers. Careful attention to good reapproximation of the medial soft tissue sleeve to its bed distally is important in these cases to prevent wound drainage in this area. Placing the most distal sutures in place before tying them helps grasp the medial soft tissue sleeve effectively.

Postoperative Care

- In most cases, postoperative care follows routine TKA protocol with weight bearing as tolerated and early active knee range of motion.

Chapter 54
Valgus Knee Deformity

KAPIL MEHROTRA
MARK W. PAGNANO

Key Concepts

- Mild to moderate valgus knee deformities often can be corrected with soft tissue balancing by selectively releasing tight structures on the lateral side.
- A very pragmatic approach to lateral releases is the inside-out multiple-puncture or "pie-crust" release. This is further simplified if the surgeon tensions the lateral side in extension, palpates the lateral structures to identify the tightest, and sequentially punctures the tightest remaining structure with a #15 blade until adequately released.
- Severe valgus deformities result in stretching of the medial collateral ligament (MCL) and may require a constrained knee prosthesis.
- A tiny subgroup of patients with large, fixed deformity may require a lateral epicondyle wafer osteotomy.
- In contemporary practice, about 95% of valgus knees are amenable to the multiple-puncture technique; 5% of patients, particularly the elderly, are better served with deliberate undercorrection and use of a constrained knee; and a rare subset of younger patients with large, fixed deformity may require epicondylar osteotomy.

Sterile Instruments and Implants

Instruments

- Routine knee retractors (e.g., bent Hohmann retractors, Z retractors, Chandler retractors, Pickle fork)
- Large and small oscillating saw
- Osteotome (3/4 inches curved, broad straight)
- Lamina spreaders
- Spacer blocks and alignment rods
- Patella caliper
- Cobb elevator

Implants

- Cemented femoral, tibial, and patellar components (with instrumentation)
- Constrained condylar implant design should be available for fixed deformities

Position

- Supine
- Thigh tourniquet

Surgical Approaches

- Anterior midline incision starting 3 to 5 cm above the proximal pole of the patella to the distal end of the tibial tubercle.
- Median parapatellar arthrotomy or a midvastus arthrotomy if correctable deformity.
- Lateral parapatellar arthrotomy is not used in our practice but is described by others for use in the valgus knee.

Preoperative Planning

Physical Examination

- Inspect the skin for any previous incisions. If less than 5 cm from the planned incision, it should typically be incorporated into the total knee incision.
- Evaluate overall limb alignment in both the coronal and sagittal planes:
    - Assess if the valgus deformity is correctable.
    - Look for any recurvatum or flexion contracture.
    - Determine the integrity of the posterior cruciate ligament and the MCL.
    - Patients at highest risk for a postoperative peroneal nerve injury are those with substantial combined valgus deformity and flexion contracture.

Radiographs

- Measure the tibiofemoral angle (angle created between the anatomic axis of the tibia and femur) to determine the severity of the valgus deformity (Figure 54.1).
- In the valgus knee a weight-bearing posteroanterior flexed-knee radiograph will often reveal more substantial arthritis than the standard anteroposterior radiograph (Figure 54.2A and B).
- Look for medial joint space widening, which may indicate MCL laxity.

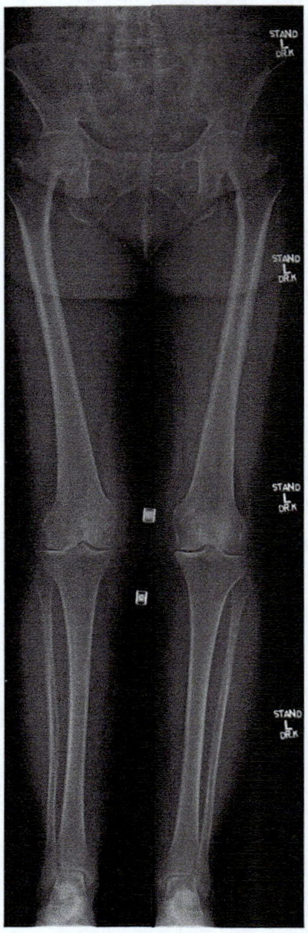

Figure 54.1 I A full-length standing radiograph that includes the hip-knee-ankle is useful in assessing the overall limb alignment and the presence or absence of extra-articular deformity.

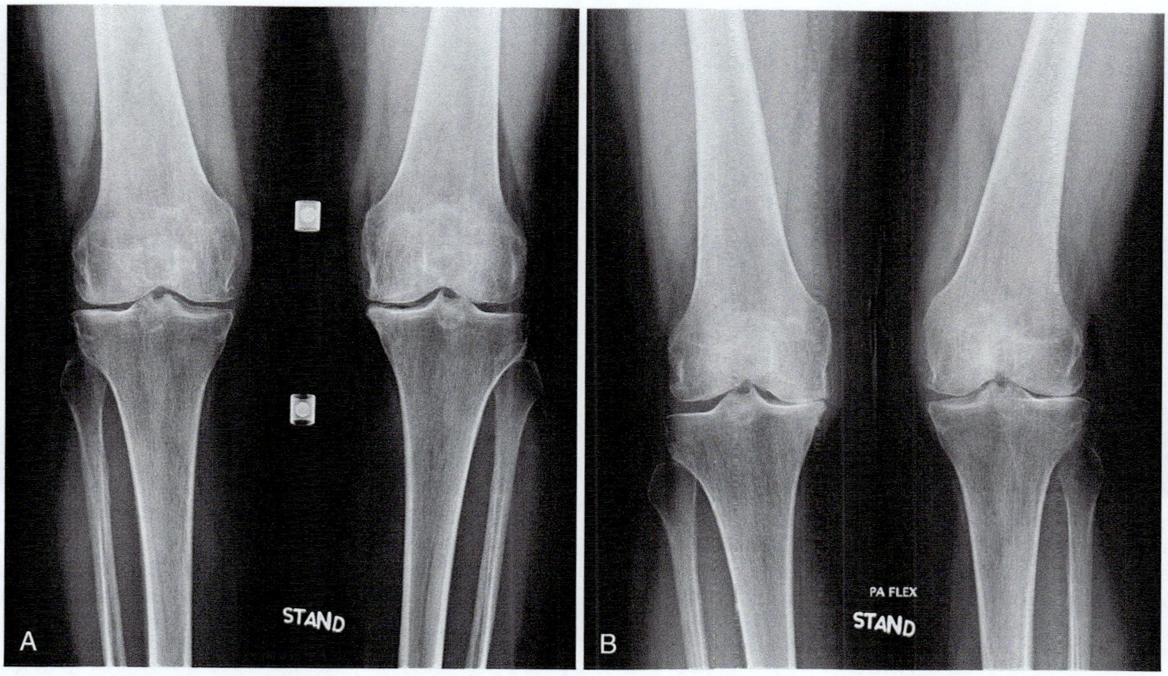

Figure 54.2 | A, A typical standing anteroposterior radiograph often underestimates the extent of lateral compartment degenerative arthritis. B, A weight-bearing posteroanterior view of the same knee reveals advanced lateral compartment degenerative arthritis with grade 4 bone-on-bone changes laterally.

- Evaluate for lateral femoral condyle or lateral tibial plateau bone deficiencies.
- Many patients with valgus deformity will also have substantial concomitant patellofemoral degenerative arthritis visible on a merchant or skyline radiograph.
- Identify posterior osteophytes on the lateral radiograph.
- Template femoral and tibial component size.
- Consider the need for augments, stems, or constrained implants.

Bone, Implant, and Soft Tissue Techniques

Exposure

- Median parapatellar approach (see Section III B, Chapter 1 for details of the surgical exposure).
- Limited subperiosteal elevation of the medial soft tissue should be performed. Extensive medial release will contribute to the medial-sided laxity and will add to the complexity of soft tissue balancing.

Bone Cuts

- The amount of initial distal femoral resection matches the thickness of the implant. In the presence of a substantial flexion contracture, resecting more distal femur subsequently may be required to obtain full extension.
- Whiteside line or the transepicondylar axis of the femur should be used to set femoral component rotation. Setting femoral rotation relative to the posterior condyles can be misleading in the valgus knee because the worn posterior condyle on the lateral side forces the femoral sizing and rotation guide into internal rotation. This will result in internal rotation of the femoral component and exacerbate patellar maltracking. If the posterior condyles are used to set rotation, then choosing 5° of external rotation is more often correct (as opposed to the typical 3° in the varus knee).
- The depth of tibial resection typically is less than that of a varus knee. In many circumstances it is still possible to identify an area of intact cartilage/normal lateral tibial plateau and to measure from that point. In other circumstances the surgeon can reference from the medial side. In most cases the appropriate depth will lead to a skim-cut across at least a portion of the worn lateral tibial side.

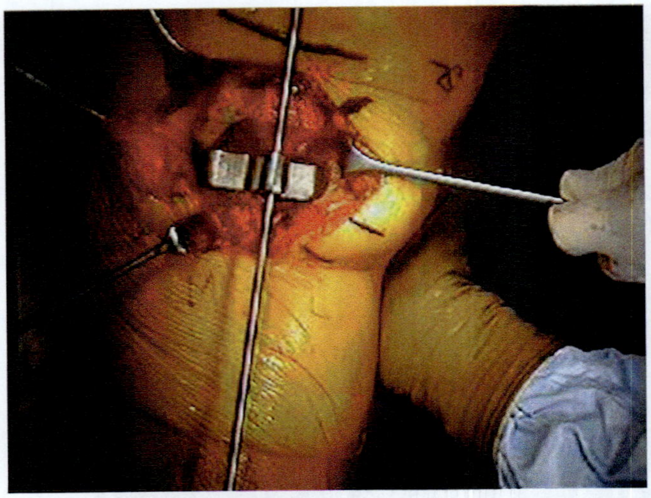

Figure 54.3 | A spacer block and alignment rod are useful in assessing the relative balance of the medial side versus the lateral side in both extension and flexion. The alignment rod is useful in estimating the overall limb alignment after correction has been obtained.

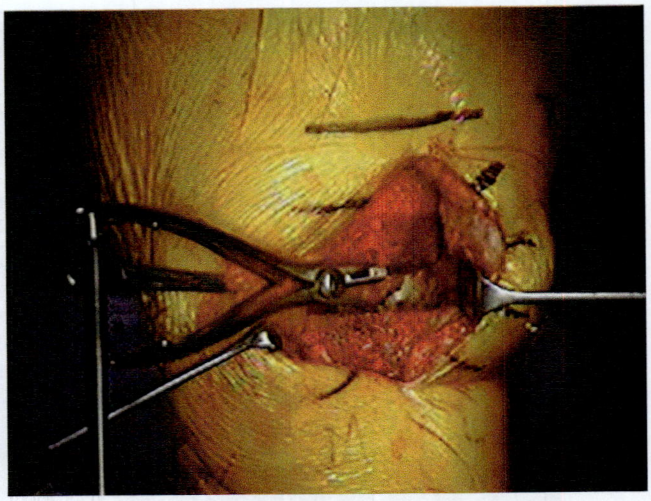

Figure 54.4 | A lamina spreader placed in the extension space is useful to tension the lateral-sided structures in the valgus knee. As the lateral structures are progressively released the lamina spreader can be further tensioned until the requisite balance has been obtained.

- Typically it is better to error in resecting too little proximal tibia than to take too much in the valgus knee.
- Assess the alignment of the bone cuts and the flexion/extension gap balance with the use of spacer blocks and extramedullary guide rods.

Soft Tissue Balancing

- With the spacer block in place, the medial and lateral joint stability is assessed in full extension with varus and valgus stress (Figure 54.3).
- Valgus knees often demonstrate a tight lateral side relative to the medial side.
- Steps of the "Inside-Out" technique as described by Ranawat et al.
  - Remove peripheral osteophytes.
  - Extend the knee and distract the joint with a laminar spreader (Figure 54.4).
  - Palpate the tight lateral structures.
  - Use a #15 blade to puncture (pie crust) the lateral-sided structures, starting with the tightest structure first and progressing with multiple punctures (Figure 54.5).
  - Avoid release of the popliteus at this stage (Figure 54.6).

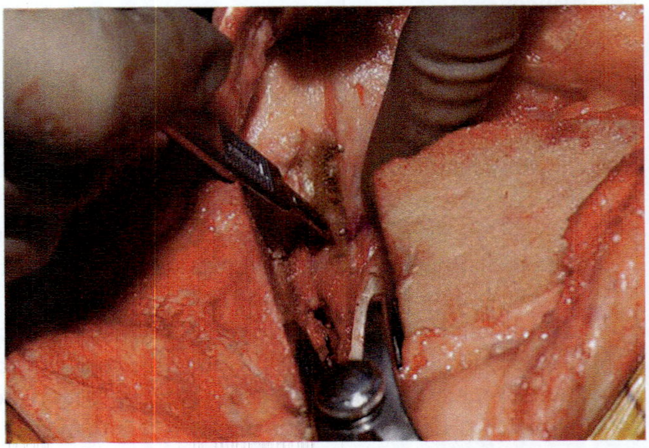

Figure 54.5 | The multiple puncture technique, or pie-crust release, is the most frequently employed method to release the tight lateral structures in the valgus knee. The surgeon can palpate the lateral structures from inside the knee joint and readily determine which band of tissue is under the greatest tension.

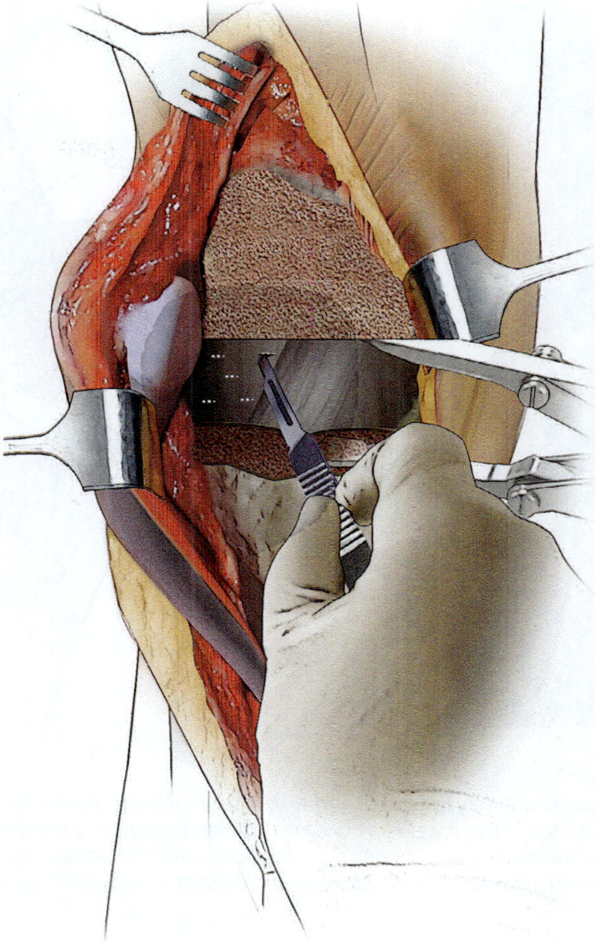

Figure 54.6 | Starting with the tightest structure, a #15 blade is used to puncture the lateral-sided tissue multiple times until an adequate release has been obtained. The lamina spreader can be further tensioned to stretch the lateral side and the adequacy of balance assessed with the spacer block and confirmed with trial components.

- A second laminar spreader can then be placed in the lateral joint space and tensioned to stretch out the lateral side. Reassess the medial and lateral joint stability with the spacer block in extension. If it is still tight laterally, then repeat the earlier steps until symmetric extension gaps are achieved.
- If there continues to be asymmetry with the lateral side tight, then the popliteus tendon may be fully released.
- If there is still asymmetry, then the final release (typically reserved for patients with large fixed valgus deformity and flexion contracture) is a lateral epicondylar osteotomy. A thin wafer of bone that includes the lateral epicondyle and the femoral attachments of the LCL and popliteus is created with use of a broad, flat osteotome. In most circumstances the posterior-lateral capsular attachments to the bony wafer can be left intact so that the fragment does not migrate (Figure 54.7A and B).
- Once the knee is balanced in extension, then trial components are inserted and the knee is assessed in flexion to ensure that it has not been overreleased. With the knee in a "figure-of-4" position (flexed 90°, varus stress applied by allowing the hip to fully externally rotate) the cam of a posterior-stabilized knee should not sublux or dislocate. If it does the knee is overreleased, at risk of postoperative dislocation, and the surgeon is best served to choose a varus-valgus constrained implant instead (Figure 54.8).

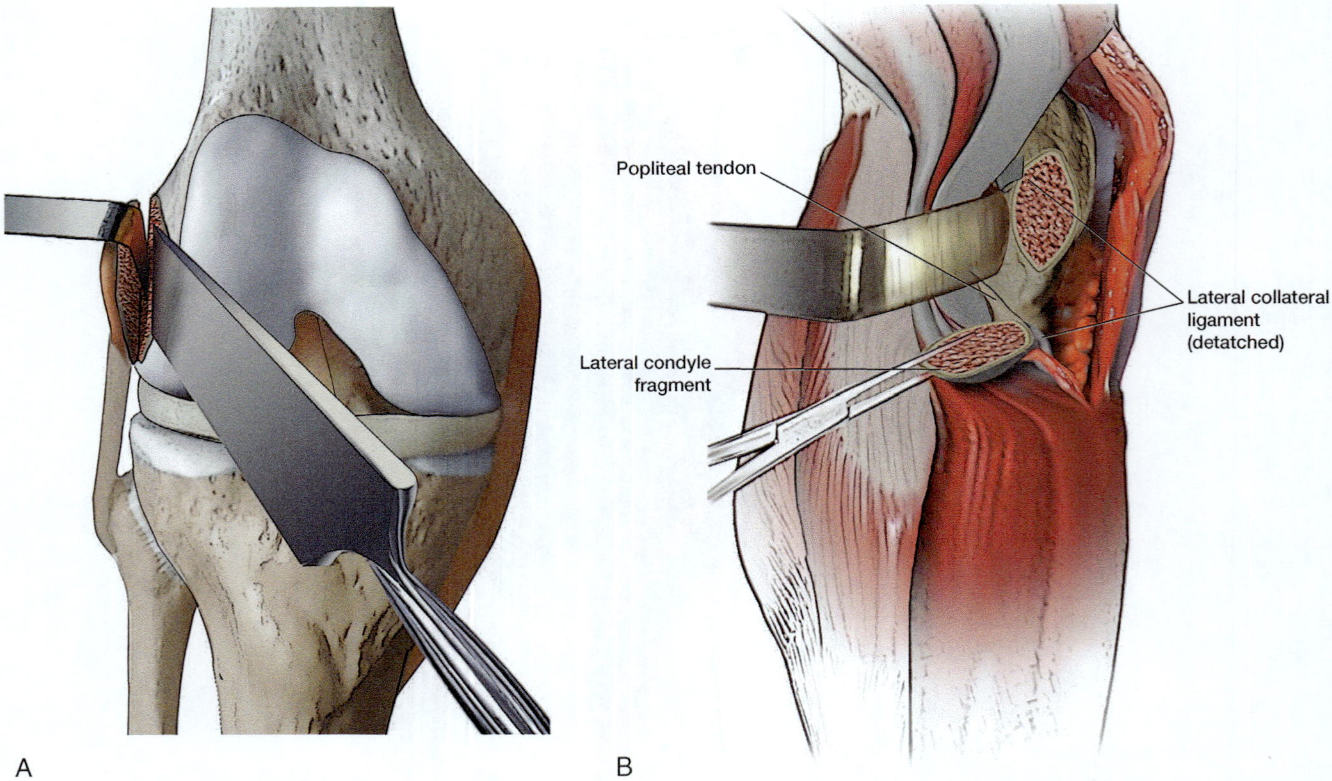

Figure 54.7 | In younger patients with very large fixed valgus deformity a lateral epicondylar osteotomy may be needed to fully balance the knee. A, A broad, thin osteotome is used to free a wafer of bone from the lateral femoral epicondyle to which is attached the lateral collateral ligament and the popliteus tendon. B, The osteotomized fragment is allowed to retract proximally and posteriorly as needed to balance the knee. The fragment can be tacked down in this new position with sutures to prevent subsequent migration postoperatively.

Implant Selection

- If the MCL is deficient, or if the lateral side is inadvertently overreleased, then a varus-valgus constrained implant may be necessary (Figure 54.9).
- A varus-valgus constrained implant can also be a good choice in elderly patients with combined fixed valgus and flexion deformities as these patients are at particular risk of peroneal nerve palsy if a full release is done (Figure 54.10). In this subgroup the valgus deformity is deliberately left slightly undercorrected and the varus-valgus constrained knee design helps make up for that asymmetry (Figure 54.11).

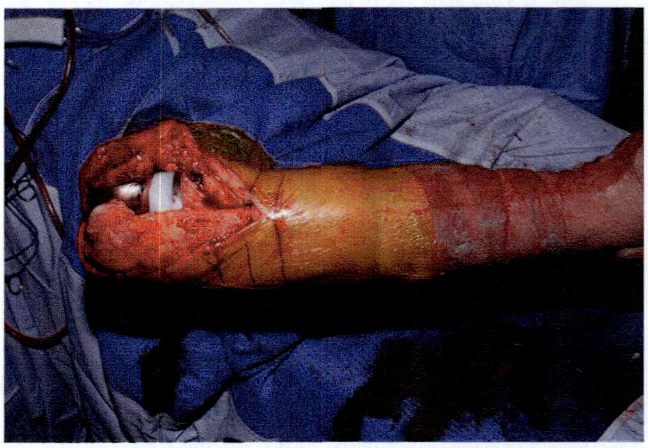

Figure 54.8 | After obtaining correction in extension, it is useful to confirm that the lateral side has not been overreleased in flexion, which might predispose to subsequent subluxation or dislocation postoperatively. Trial components are assembled, and the knee is deliberately brought into the so-called figure-of-4 position by flexing the knee to 90°, lifting the limb by the foot, and allowing the hip to maximally externally rotate thus imparting a substantial valgus stress on the knee. If the knee appears to sublux or the tibial post of a posterior-stabilized implant drops out of the femoral box, then the surgeon should consider a switch to a constrained knee design with a taller and more conforming tibial post and femoral box.

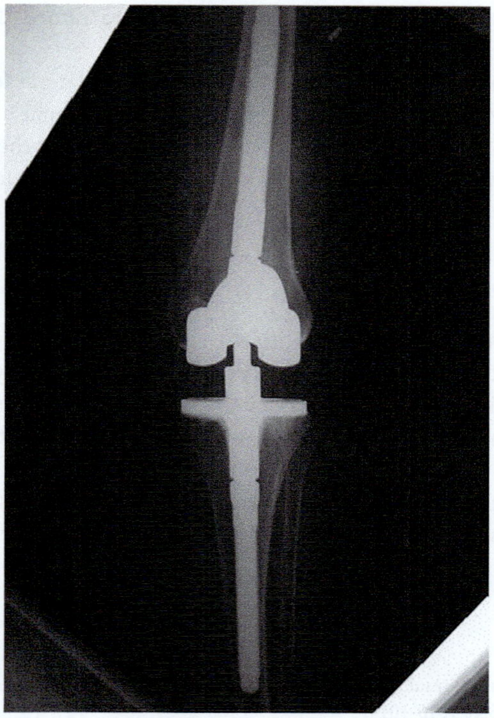

Figure 54.9 | A varus-valgus constrained implant is used when there is some remaining flexion gap asymmetry and is also used in some elderly, lower-demand patients when large deformities are deliberately left only partially corrected in an effort to minimize risk to the peroneal nerve.

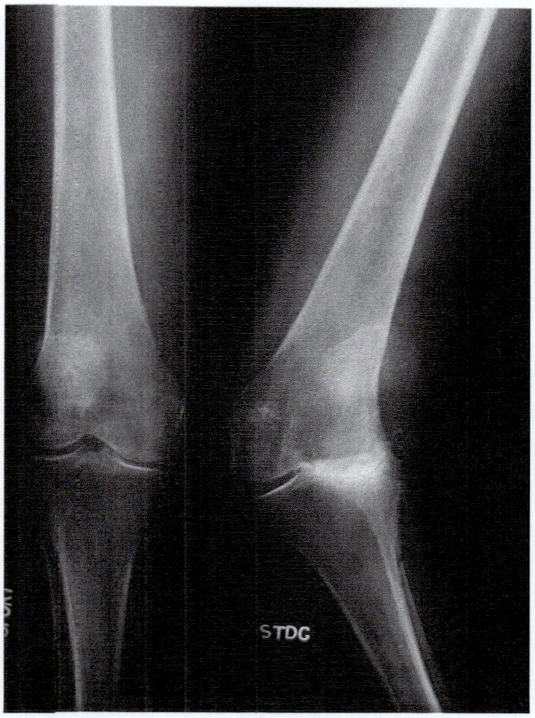

Figure 54.10 | Anteroposterior standing radiograph of an elderly patient with a large fixed valgus deformity for whom deliberate under-correction of the deformity and use of a varus-valgus constrained implant was chosen.

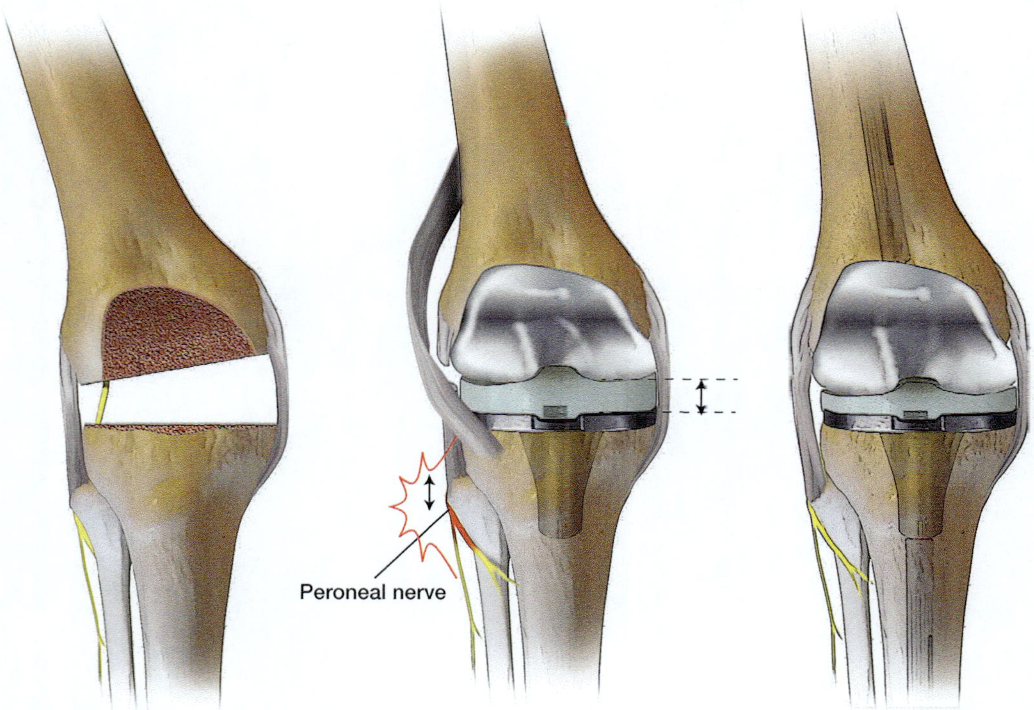

Figure 54.11 | Illustration of the situation in which complete correction of a fixed valgus deformity via lateral soft-tissue release would lengthen the limb and place the peroneal nerve at risk of stretch injury. Instead the lateral soft tissues are partially corrected and the varus-valgus constrained implant is relied upon for ultimate stability.

- Even when the MCL is intact in patients with severe valgus deformities, it may be extremely difficult to achieve adequate soft tissue balancing.
- On very rare occasions, augments may be considered in patients with a hypoplastic lateral femoral condyle or deficient lateral tibial plateau. We will routinely consider resecting an additional 2 mm of proximal tibia if it eliminates the need for a tibial augment. Alternatively, we also consider the use of metaphyseal sleeves or cones in selected cases with tibial bone loss to bypass the proximal defect and avoid cutting away additional proximal tibia.

Postoperative Care

- We typically avoid peripheral nerve blocks that would interfere with the early postoperative assessment of peroneal nerve function in the patient with substantial preoperative valgus deformity.
- The operative extremity is monitored for any signs of peroneal nerve palsy. This is especially important in the patient with a combined flexion and valgus deformity that was corrected at the time of surgery.
- If there are any concerns about postoperative neurologic deficit, the knee is flexed to 30°, the hip maintained in extension, and the surgical dressings are loosened to minimize tension on the sciatic and peroneal nerves.

Suggested Reading

1. Clarke HD, Fuchs R, Scuderi GR, Scott WN, Insall JN. Clinical results in valgus total knee arthroplasty with the "pie crust" technique of lateral soft tissue releases. *J Arthroplasty*. 2005;20:1010-1014.
2. Clarke HD, Schwartz JB, Math KR, Scuderi GR. Anatomic risk of peroneal nerve injury with the pie crust technique for valgus release in total knee arthroplasty. *J Arthroplasty*. 2004;19:40-44.
3. Kanayima T, Whiteside LA, Nakamura T, Mihalko WM, Steiger J, Naito M. Ranawat Award paper: effect of selective lateral ligament release on stability in knee arthroplasty. *Clin Orthop and Relat Research*. 2002;304:24-31.
4. Krackow KA, Mihalko WM. Flexion-extension gap changes after lateral structure release for valgus deformity correction in total knee arthroplasty: a cadaveric study. *J Arthroplasty*. 1999;14:994-1004.

Chapter 55
Flexion Contracture

STEPHEN M. PETIS
MATTHEW P. ABDEL

Key Concepts

- Flexion contractures are not uncommon before total knee arthroplasty (TKA), occurring in patients with varus and valgus gonarthrosis.
- A flexion contracture of greater than 5° to 10° requires complete surgical correction, as residual contractures after TKA can lead to reduced function and walking ability.
- The etiology can be multifactorial; however, it is more common with more severe knee deformities, posttraumatic and inflammatory arthritis, prior surgery (i.e., knee arthroscopy, high tibial osteotomy), and neuromuscular disorders.
- The sagittal plane deformity is typically corrected first through bone resection and removal of osteophytes and releasing shortened soft tissue.
- It is important to perform maneuvers that preferentially open the extension gap and do not affect the flexion gap, as this can lead to a flexion-extension gap mismatch.

Sterile Instruments and Implants

Instruments

- Routine knee retractors
- Laminar spreaders
- Blunt soft tissue elevators (i.e., Cobb elevators)

Implants

- Cruciate-retaining or posterior-stabilized TKA system
- Varus-valgus constrained devices and hinged knee options for severe (30° or greater) contractures
- Femoral and tibial stems
- Consider metaphyseal cones if increasing constraint is utilized

Positioning

- Supine

Surgical Approaches

- A midline incision with a medial parapatellar arthrotomy is performed in almost every instance.
- Rarely, a lateral arthrotomy may be considered for severe valgus gonarthrosis.

Preoperative Planning

- A full complement of knee radiographs is recommended, including a long-leg hip-knee-ankle radiograph (Figure 55.1), standing anteroposterior (AP) radiograph (Figure 55.2), standing posteroanterior (PA) flexion radiograph (Figure 55.3), lateral radiograph (Figure 55.4), and patellar views (Figure 55.5).

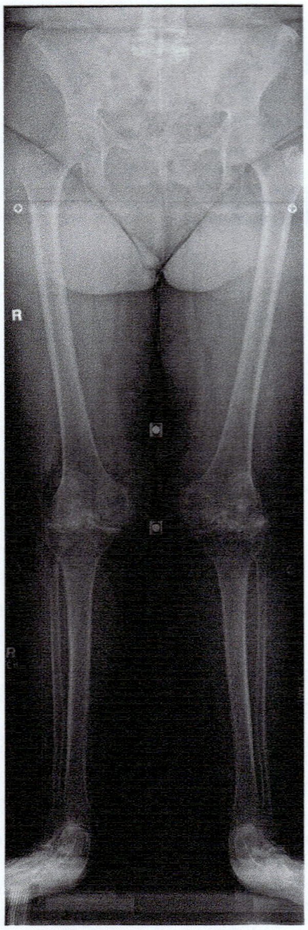

Figure 55.1 | Standing long-leg hip-knee-ankle radiograph of a 71-year-old woman with bilateral valgus gonarthrosis and 20° flexion contractures.

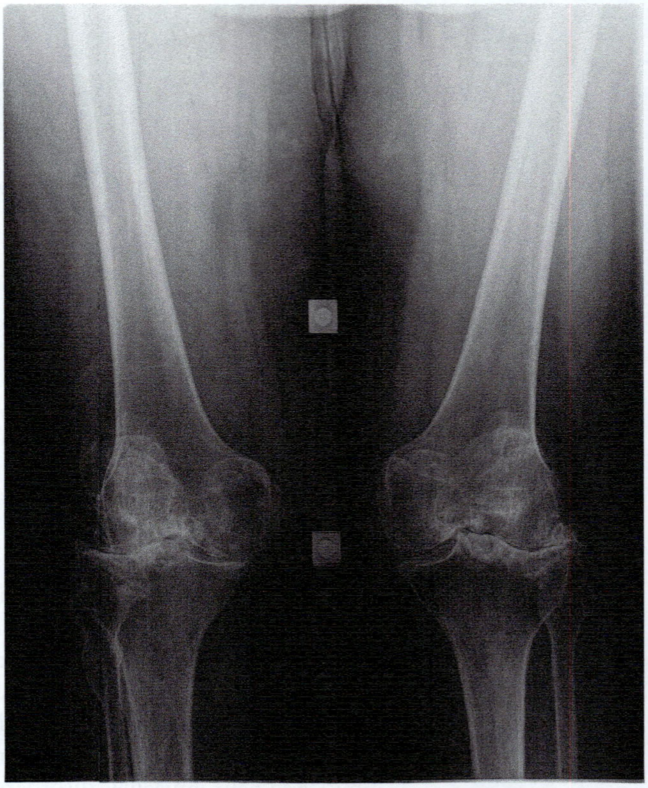

Figure 55.2 | Standing AP knee radiographs of the aforementioned patient.

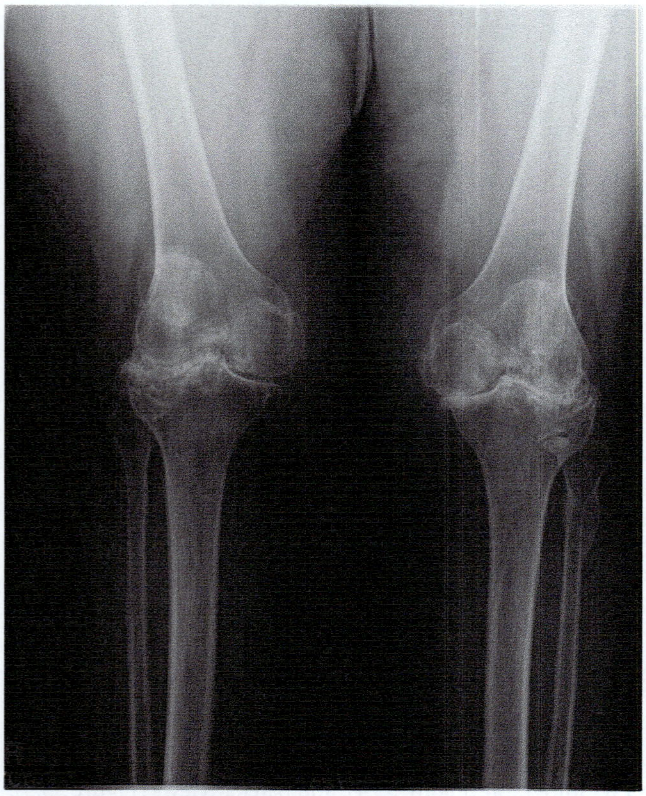

Figure 55.3 | Standing PA flexion knee radiographs of the aforementioned patient.

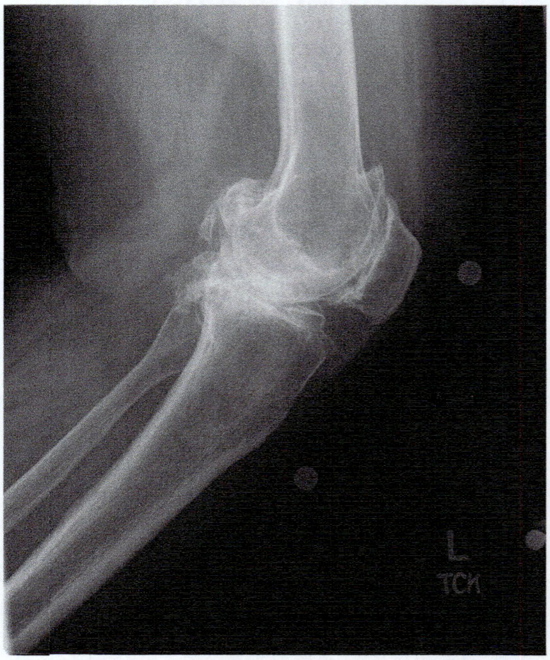

Figure 55.4 | Lateral knee radiograph of the aforementioned patient.

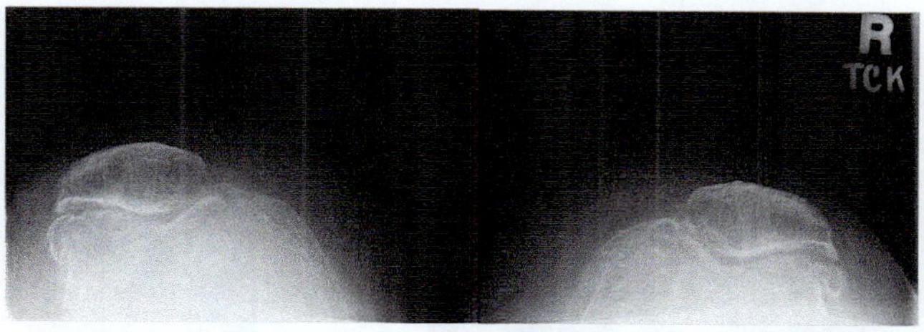

Figure 55.5 | Bilateral patellar views of the aforementioned patient.

The radiographs are used to anticipate areas of the knee that will require releases to improve the flexion contracture (i.e., posterior osteophytes [Figure 55.6]/loose bodies [Figure 55.7]) or bone deformities that will have to be addressed (i.e., tibial slope, intra-articular posttraumatic deformities) (Figure 55.8).

- A physical examination should document the degree of passive correction of the flexion deformity to anticipate the degree of surgical correction/releases required.
- It is important to document a complete neurovascular examination, as correction of a severe flexion contracture (particularly in combination with a large fixed valgus deformity) may result in a traction neuropraxia.

Bone/Implant/Soft Tissue Techniques

- While the patient is under anesthesia, assess and document the degree of the flexion contracture and consider documenting with an intraoperative picture (Figure 55.9).
- Perform a midline incision with a medial parapatellar arthrotomy and excise any scar tissue in the suprapatellar pouch, medial and lateral gutters, and intrapatellar area that may be present in patients with previous surgery.
- For flexion contractures >15°, additional bone is routinely resected from the distal femur (Figure 55.10) to preferentially open the extension space early in the procedure (i.e., an additional 2 to 4 mm of bone) (Figure 55.11).

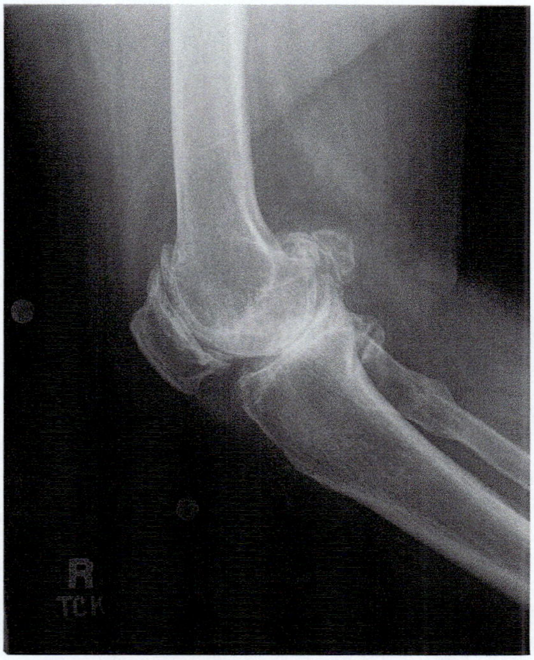

Figure 55.6 | Lateral radiograph of a patient revealing significant posterior osteophytes and a large loose body, both contributing to the lack of extension. As such, both must be removed at the time of TKA to minimize distention on the posterior capsule, thus promoting full extension.

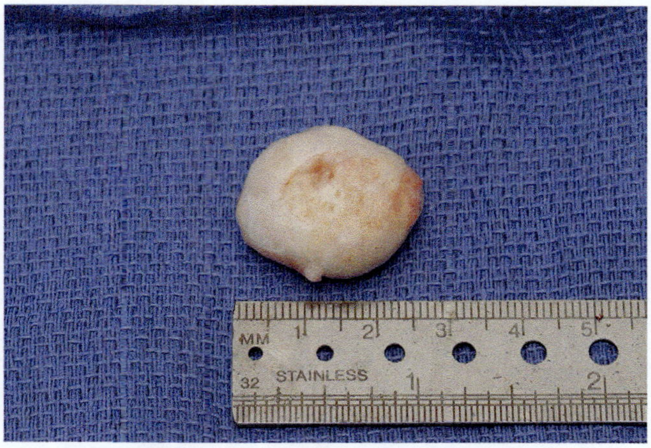

Figure 55.7 | Intraoperative picture of a large posterior loose body distending the posterior capsule.

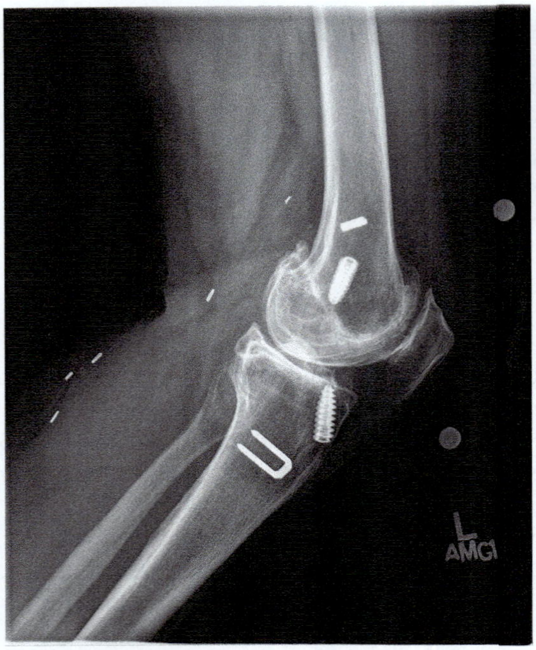

Figure 55.8 | In this posttraumatic knee with a 15° flexion contracture, the excessive posterior tibial slope will have to be corrected at the time of the TKA in an effort to equalize the flexion and extension gaps.

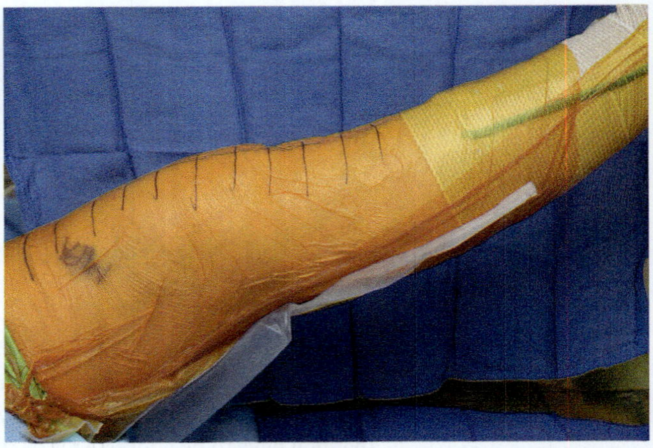

Figure 55.9 | An intraoperative photograph of a 61-year-old man with a 10° flexion contracture noted before incision in the operating room while the patient is under anesthesia.

- It is critical not to cut excess posterior slope with the tibial cut, as this can inadvertently cause tightness in extension and laxity in the flexion space.
- After the femoral cuts are completed, posterior femoral osteophytes should be removed with a marked osteotome (Figure 55.12) as they can cause posterior capsular contractures (Figure 55.13).
- After the femoral and tibial cuts are completed, flexion-extension blocks can help identify areas of tightness that require releasing for optimal coronal and sagittal plane balancing (Figure 55.14A and B).

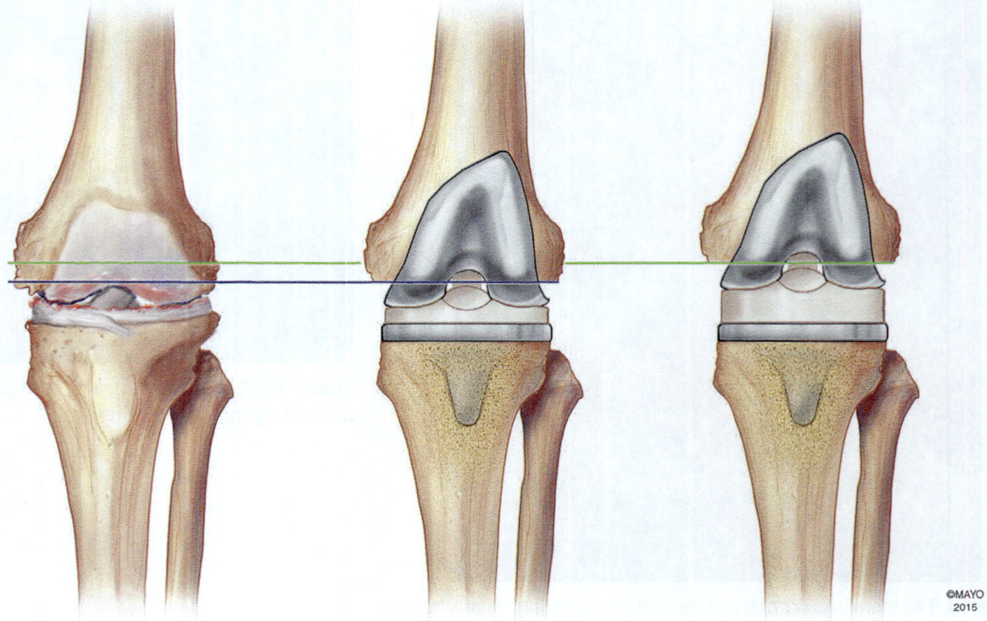

Figure 55.10 | An illustration showing the need for additional distal femoral resection in increments of 2 mm for flexion contractures >20° in patients without significant posterior osteophytes or loose bodies. (Used with permission of Mayo Foundation for Medical Education and Research. All rights reserved.)

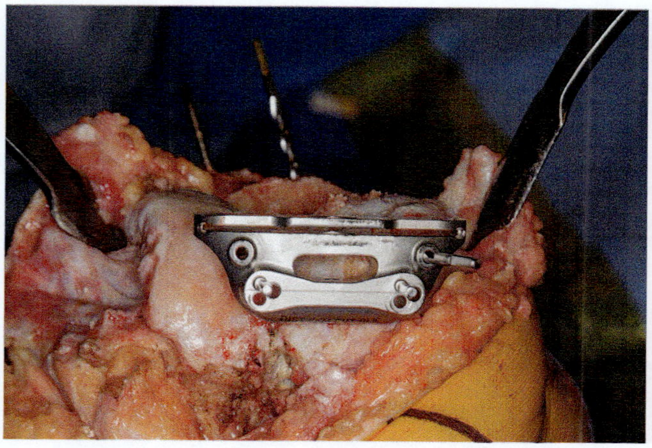

Figure 55.11 | In this particular case, the distal femoral cutting jig was proximalized by 4 mm given a 25° preoperative flexion contracture.

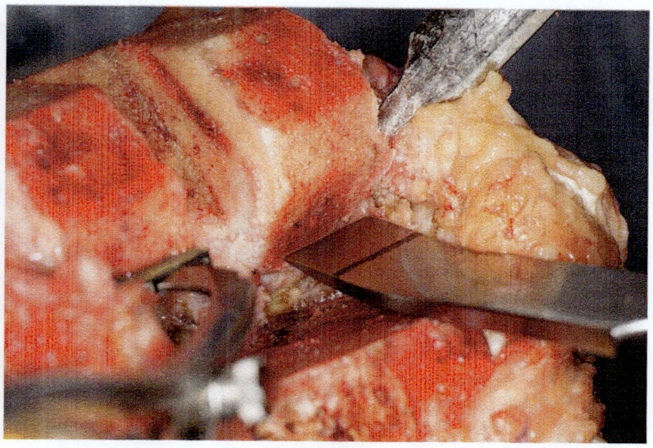

Figure 55.12 | Intraoperative photograph of a scored osteotome utilized to remove posterior femoral osteophytes.

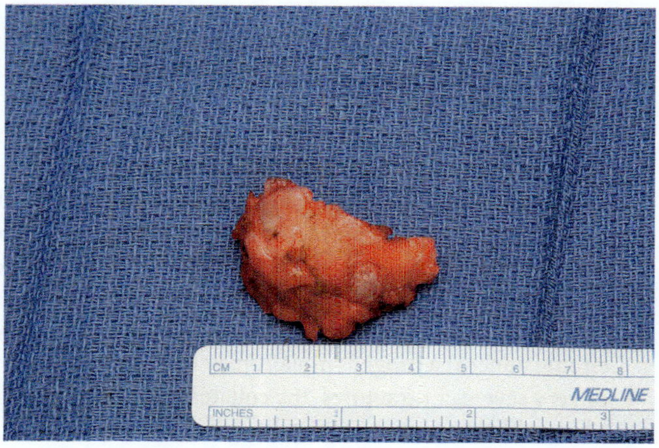

Figure 55.13 | An intraoperative picture of a large posterior osteophyte that was tenting the posterior capsule and preventing full extension at the time of TKA. This was removed with the careful use of an osteotome.

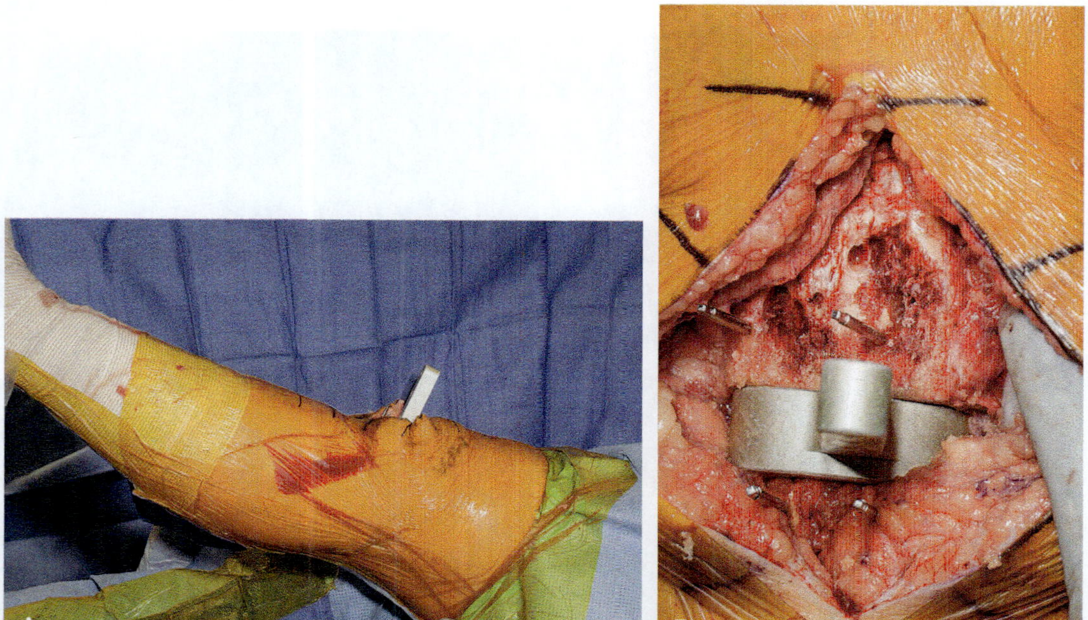

Figure 55.14 | A, By placing a spacer block in the knee after the distal femoral and proximal resections are completed, the surgeon is able to determine if additional distal femoral resection is needed in patients without significant posterior osteophytes or loose bodies. In this particular scenario, an additional 2 mm of distal femoral bone was resected to allow for full extension before moving forward through the use of the distal femoral pins, which were maintained (B).

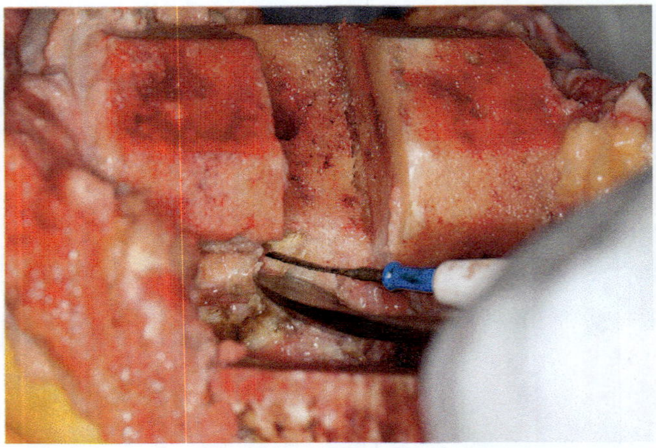

Figure 55.15 | A Cobb elevator and cautery are utilized to remove soft tissues directly off the posterior aspect of the femur.

- Laminar spreaders with the knee in extension can help identify posterior structures that contribute to flexion contractures. Coronal plane (varus-valgus) balance in extension should be achieved next via selective releases.
  - Varus knee—deep medial collateral ligament, semimembranosus insertion, posteromedial capsule
  - Valgus knee—posterolateral capsule, popliteus, lateral collateral ligament, iliotibial band
- If a persistent flexion contracture exists, careful subperiosteal release of the posterior capsule off the posterior femur can be performed with a Cobb elevator or electrocautery (Figure 55.15).
- Depending on the severity of the deformity and releases required, further distal femoral resection may be required. This may result in midflexion instability, and a varus-valgus constrained or (in rare circumstances) a hinged implant may be required (Figure 55.16A and B).
- In very severe contractures, the collateral ligaments may require complete release, which necessitates a hinged knee (Figure 55.17A-F).
- At the end of each case, consider obtaining an intraoperative lateral radiograph (Figure 55.18A) and photograph (Figure 55.18B) confirming that the limb is in full extension.

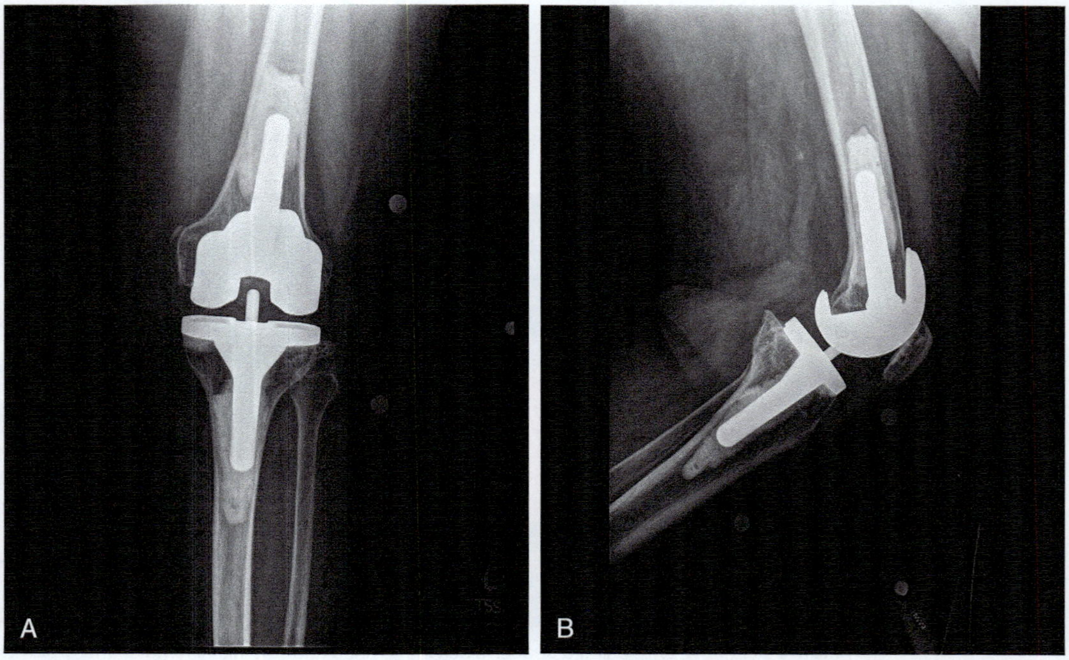

Figure 55.16 | The patient from Figures 55.1-55.5 required further distal femoral resection, resulting in midflexion laxity, and thus the use of a varus-valgus constrained device as noted on these AP (A) and lateral (B) radiographs.

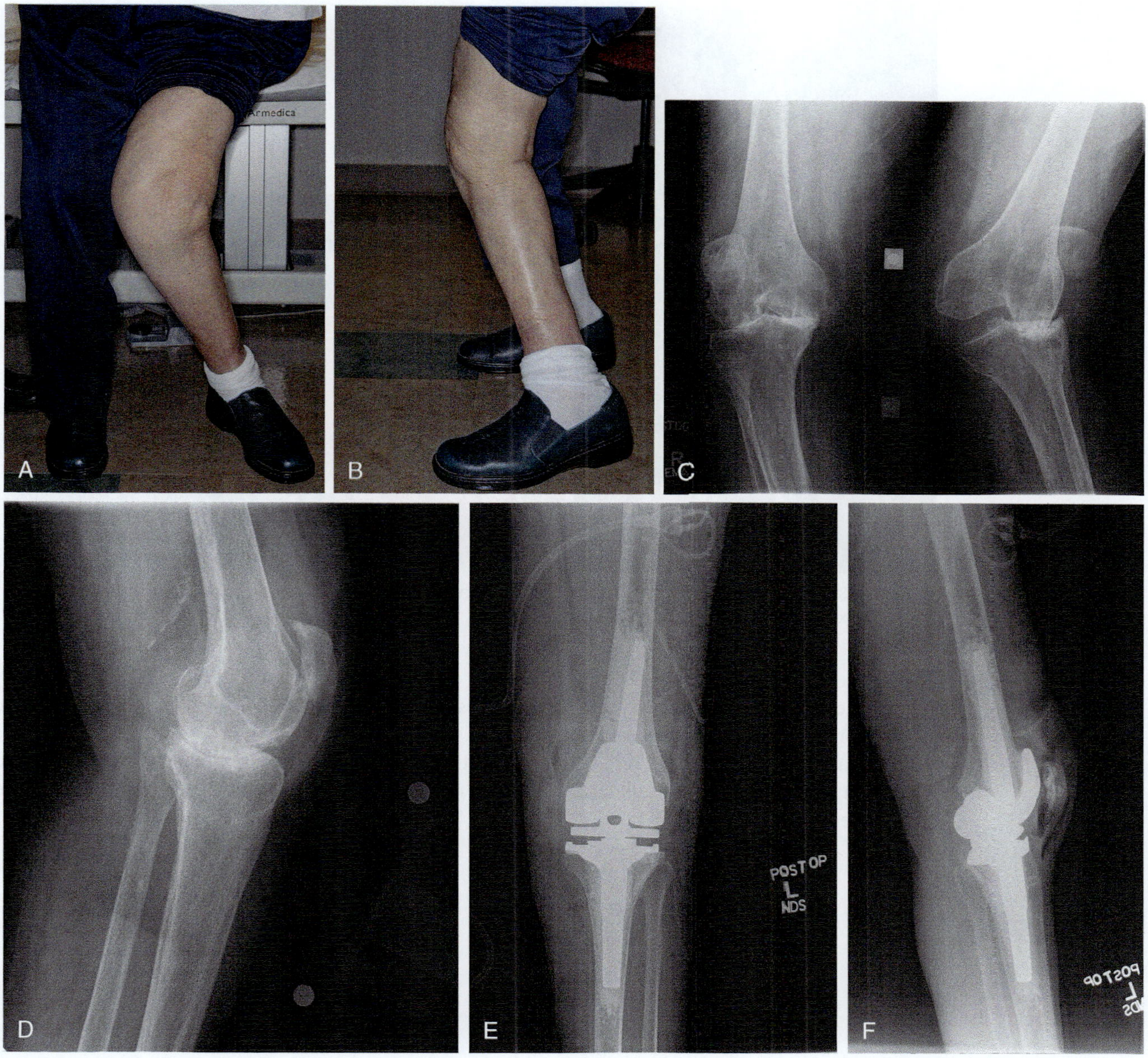

Figure 55.17 | Clinical AP (A) and lateral (B) pictures of this 92-year-old woman reveal a 45° valgus deformity and fixed 40° flexion contracture, which were also appreciated on AP (C) and lateral (D) knee radiographs. Given the large combined deformities and absolute lack of MCL integrity, a rotating hinge TKA was selected, allowing for correction of the patient's coronal (E) and sagittal (F) deformities.

Postoperative Care

- Patients are permitted to range and weight bear as tolerated, with physical therapy focusing on terminal knee extension during the early recovery after TKA. The one exception is in patients with combined fixed flexion and valgus deformities who are at risk for peroneal nerve palsies. In these patients the knee is maintained in 45° of flexion overnight in a loose dressing and gently extended on the morning after surgery as long as there is full peroneal nerve function.
- Extended treatment with an oral anti-inflammatory medication should be considered postoperatively to reduce the recurrence of severe flexion contractures.

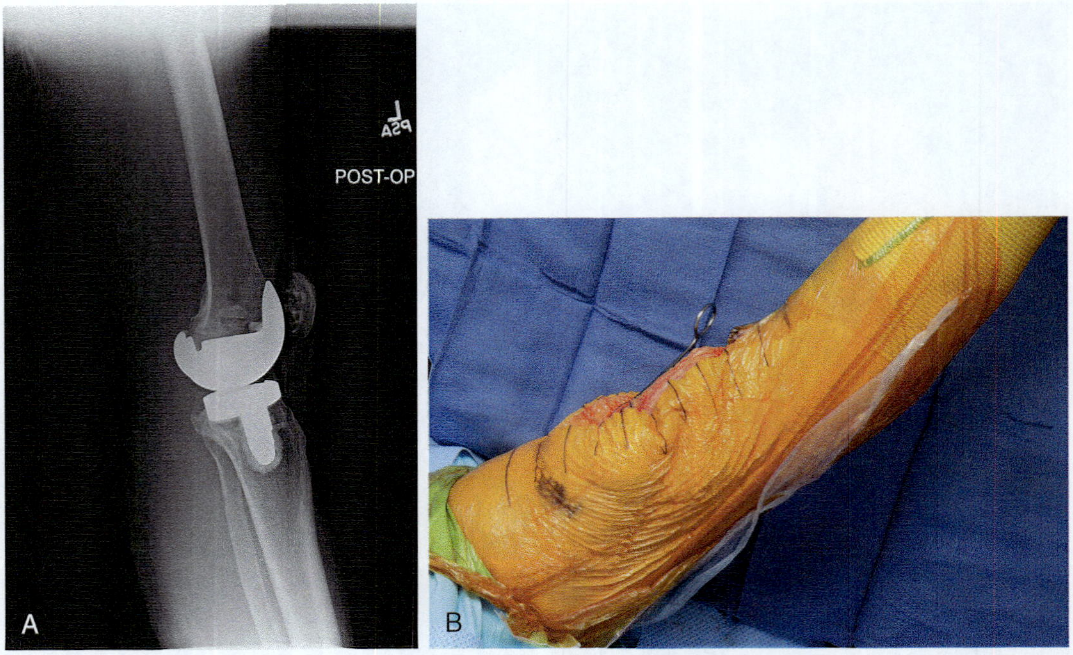

Figure 55.18 | It is often helpful to obtain an intraoperative lateral radiograph (A) and a clinical photograph (B) of the knee in full extension before leaving the operating room.

- For patients with significant posterior osteophytes or history of heterotopic ossification, prophylactic radiation (750 cGy) can be considered.
- If the patient has a contralateral flexion contracture that will be addressed in a staged fashion, the surgeon may consider a contralateral shoe lift to minimize the recurrence of the flexion contracture in the recently completed TKA.

Chapter 56
Previous High Tibial Osteotomy

BRIAN P. CHALMERS
TAD M. MABRY

Key Concepts

- Total knee arthroplasty (TKA) after high tibial osteotomy (HTO) is made challenging by prior skin incisions, patella baja, retained hardware, altered tibial anatomy, and altered knee kinematics.
- Careful planning of the incision must be done to avoid necrosis between prior incisions while also facilitating exposure and allowing selective hardware removal.
- In knees with patella baja or stiffness, a stepwise approach to surgical exposure is important to have in mind before surgery.
- Painful hardware should be removed; otherwise, partial in situ removal of only the hardware that impedes implant placement is preferred.
- Lateral tibial bone loss and distortion of proximal tibial anatomy causing an offset tibial canal after closing wedge HTO requires preoperative planning of the tibial cut and implant placement; the use of custom implants or corrective osteotomy may be necessary in severe deformities.
- Altered knee joint kinematics requires attention and appropriate ligament balancing to achieve symmetric gaps; the use of a posterior-stabilized implant is recommended to facilitate this.

Sterile Instruments and Implants

Basic Knee Instruments

- Cemented knee implant system (surgeon's choice); a prior HTO is a relative contraindication for a cementless TKA implant design; furthermore, even if not the surgeon's routine, strongly consider a posterior-stabilized implant; constrained and stemmed options should be available.
- Implant-specific screwdrivers, extraction devices, metal-cutting burr for hardware removal.

Surgical Approaches

- Careful assessment of previous skin incisions and planning of the operative skin incision is paramount for successful wound healing. Avoid far lateral incisions.
- Because many prior HTOs are laterally based closing-wedge osteotomies, make a slightly more medial skin incision to leave a skin bridge of at least 6 cm between previous lateral incisions; in prior medially based osteotomies, the old medial incision is typically acceptable.
- Cross transverse incisions perpendicularly, and for S-shaped or inverted L-shaped incisions, the vertical limb of the incision can be extended proximally.
- For stiff knees or knees with patella baja (Figure 56.1), a stepwise approach is necessary to achieve adequate surgical exposure:
  - Extended medial parapatellar arthrotomy
  - Free the medial and lateral gutters of scar tissue
  - Quadriceps snip if necessary
  - Tibial tubercle osteotomy rarely needed but utilized if necessary in the most severe cases

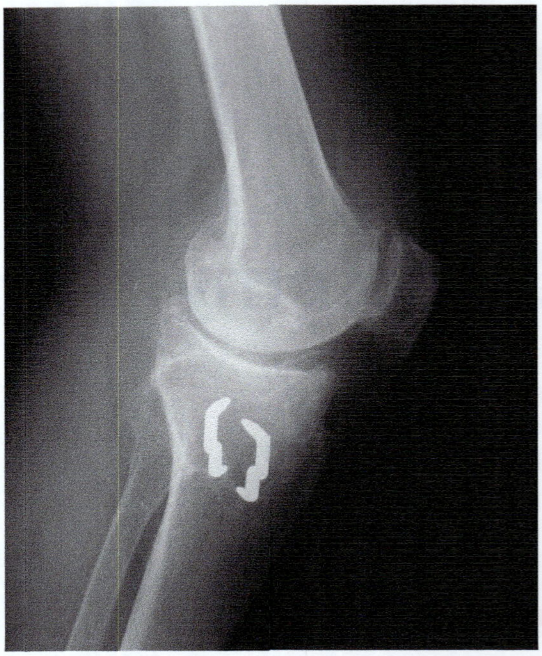

Figure 56.1 | A lateral radiograph of a patient status post high tibial osteotomy with retained step-staple hardware. Note both patella baja and the posterior translation of the proximal tibia.

Preoperative Planning

- A baseline infection evaluation with a C-reactive protein and erythrocyte sedimentation rate along with a detailed history of postoperative wound healing should be standard in these patients with previous open knee surgery and retained hardware; a knee aspiration should be considered in any patient with abnormal inflammatory markers, a history of wound drainage, or a history of infection.
- Assess the patient's knee range of motion preoperatively; stiff knees will be more challenging to obtain safe surgical exposure, as described previously.
- A careful varus-valgus ligamentous examination should be performed to ensure the prior surgery did not result in ligamentous insufficiency; if concerned, a varus-valgus constrained implant should be available.
- Standard anteroposterior, lateral, and standing hip to ankle radiographs should be obtained to assess for retained hardware, patella baja, tibiofemoral deformity, and a medially offset tibial canal.
- Patella baja or a posteriorly offset tibial plateau should alert the surgeon that adequate exposure may be more challenging.
- Lateral tibial plateau deficiency (Figure 56.2) is often present; preoperative planning of the proximal tibial cut is necessary to avoid overresection of the medial tibial plateau.
- A medially offset tibial canal (Figure 56.3) will make the use of a stem more challenging; if a tibial stem is desired, an offset or custom stem may be necessary.
- Note the location of retained hardware and determine if the retained hardware is symptomatic.

Bone, Implant, and Soft Tissue Techniques

- The senior author's routine is to first prepare the femur for a posterior-stabilized component.
- Attention is then turned to the tibial side. Avoid removal of the medial tibial osteophytes if present until appropriate tibial component positioning is determined.
- The proximal tibia is cut perpendicular to the anatomic axis of the tibia using an extramedullary cutting guide, with adjustments made based on the preoperative plan and the patient's anatomy.
- Start with placing the tibial resection guide at 2 to 3 mm off the arthritic/worn medial tibial plateau in a varus knee or 7 to 8 mm off a nonarthritic medial tibial plateau in a valgus knee.
- If there is mild lateral tibial plateau deficiency, an extra 2 to 4 mm of proximal tibia can be resected to compensate for the bone loss and obtain a bleeding surface on the lateral side.
- If the lateral tibial bone loss is more substantial, bone grafting or a lateral wedge (Figure 56.4) can be utilized but is rarely necessary in contemporary practice.

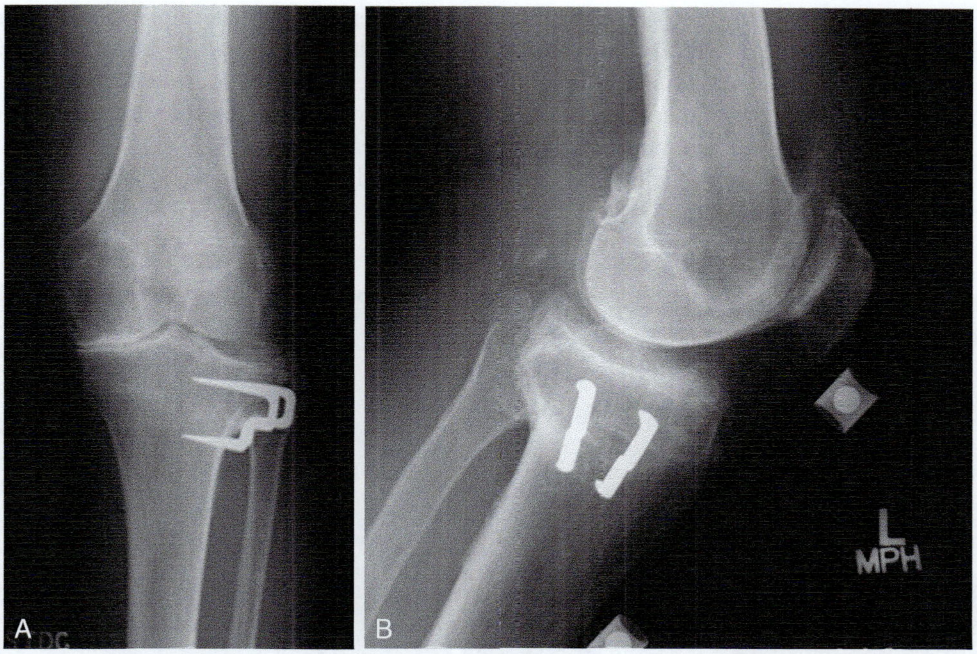

Figure 56.2 | Anteroposterior (A) and lateral (B) radiographs of a patient status post lateral closing-wedge high tibial osteotomy with varus gonarthrosis and concomitant lateral tibial bone deficiency.

- Before preparing the proximal tibia, the alignment of the tibial cut should be checked with a drop rod referencing the anatomic tibial axis and adjusted if in unacceptable varus or valgus.
- Trial components are placed and the knee is balanced in flexion and extension to obtain symmetric medial and lateral gaps.

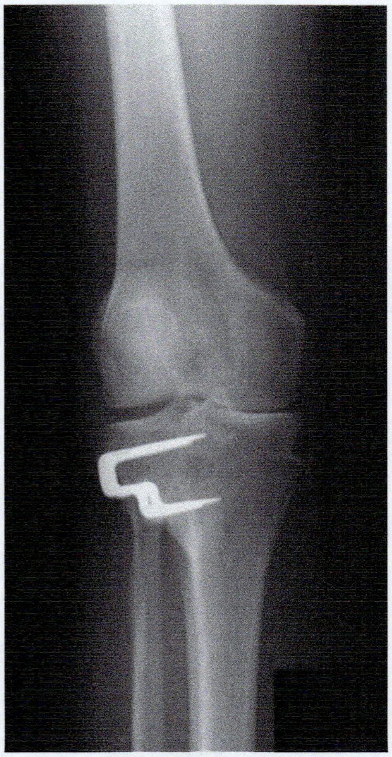

Figure 56.3 | An anteroposterior radiograph of a patient status post lateral closing-wedge high tibial osteotomy (HTO) with a medially offset tibial canal relative to the proximal tibia.

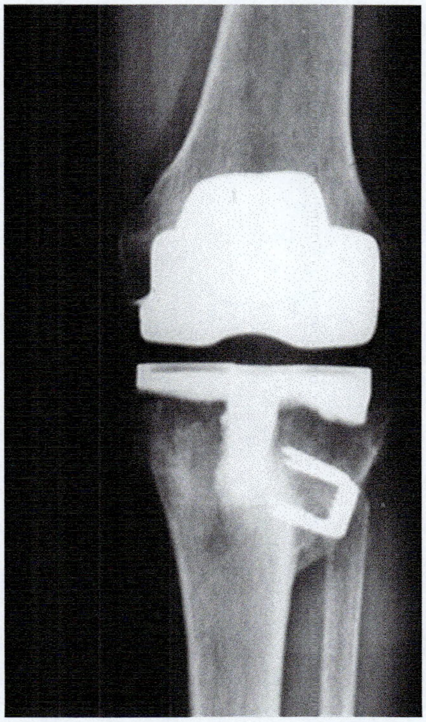

Figure 56.4 | An anteroposterior radiograph of a patient status post lateral closing-wedge high tibial osteotomy with a lateral wedge utilized to compensate for moderate lateral tibial bone loss.

- Retained hardware can be removed externally (before preparing the proximal tibia) (Figure 56.5) through the incision or internally (while preparing the proximal tibia); if the patient's hardware is asymptomatic, the senior author prefers to leave hardware in place and only partially remove hardware internally as necessary to prevent creating a stress riser in the proximal tibia and/or cement extrusion through prior hardware sites (Figure 56.6).
- Once the tibial cut has been made and the knee balanced, the proximal tibia is prepared.

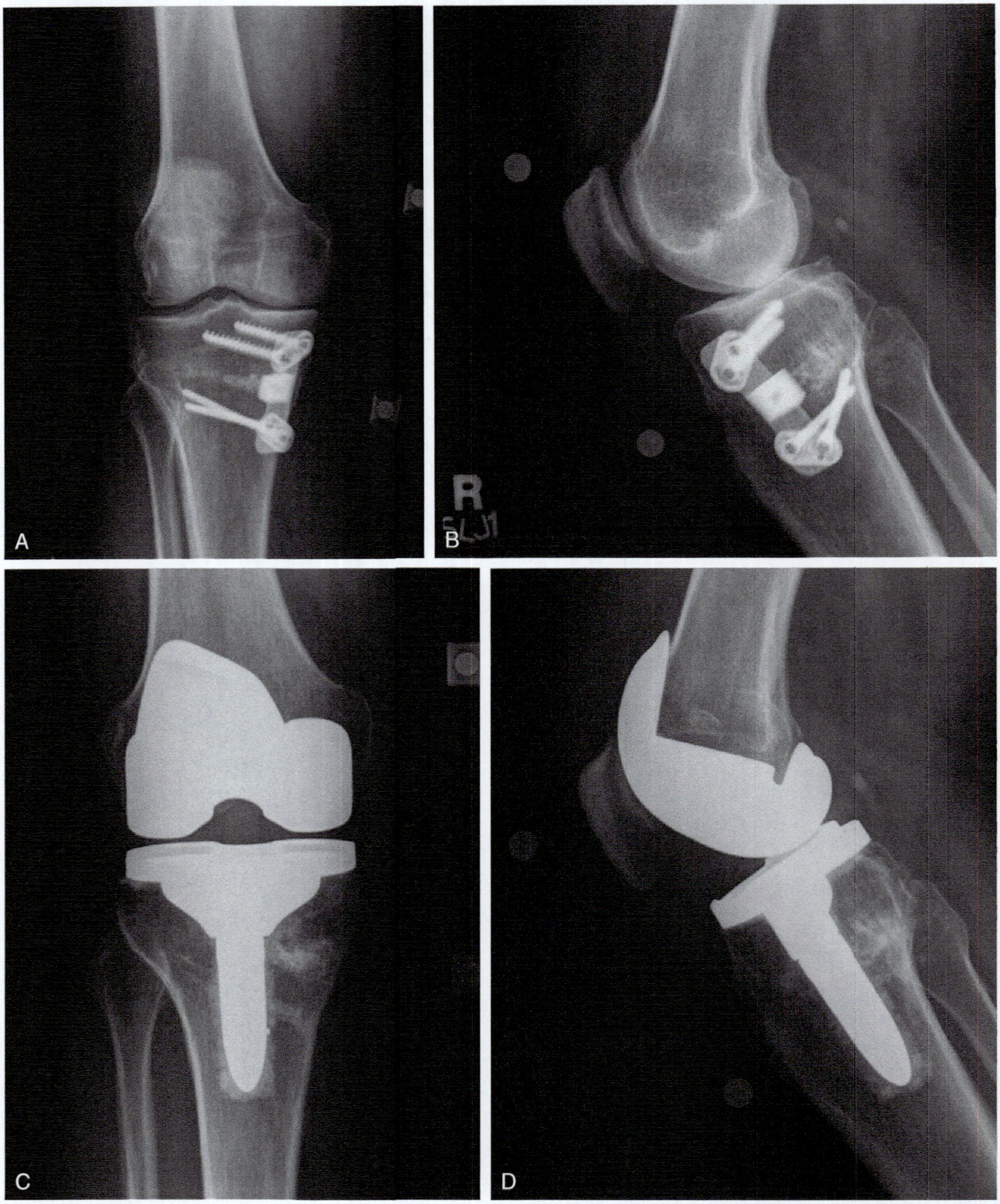

Figure 56.5 | Anteroposterior (A) and lateral (B) radiographs of a patient status post medial opening-wedge high tibial osteotomy with symptomatic hardware. Complete hardware removal was done through the prior medial incision, which was extended proximally and distally to perform the TKA, and a tibial stem was used to bypass the most distal screw holes, as seen on the postoperative AP (C) and lateral (D) radiographs.

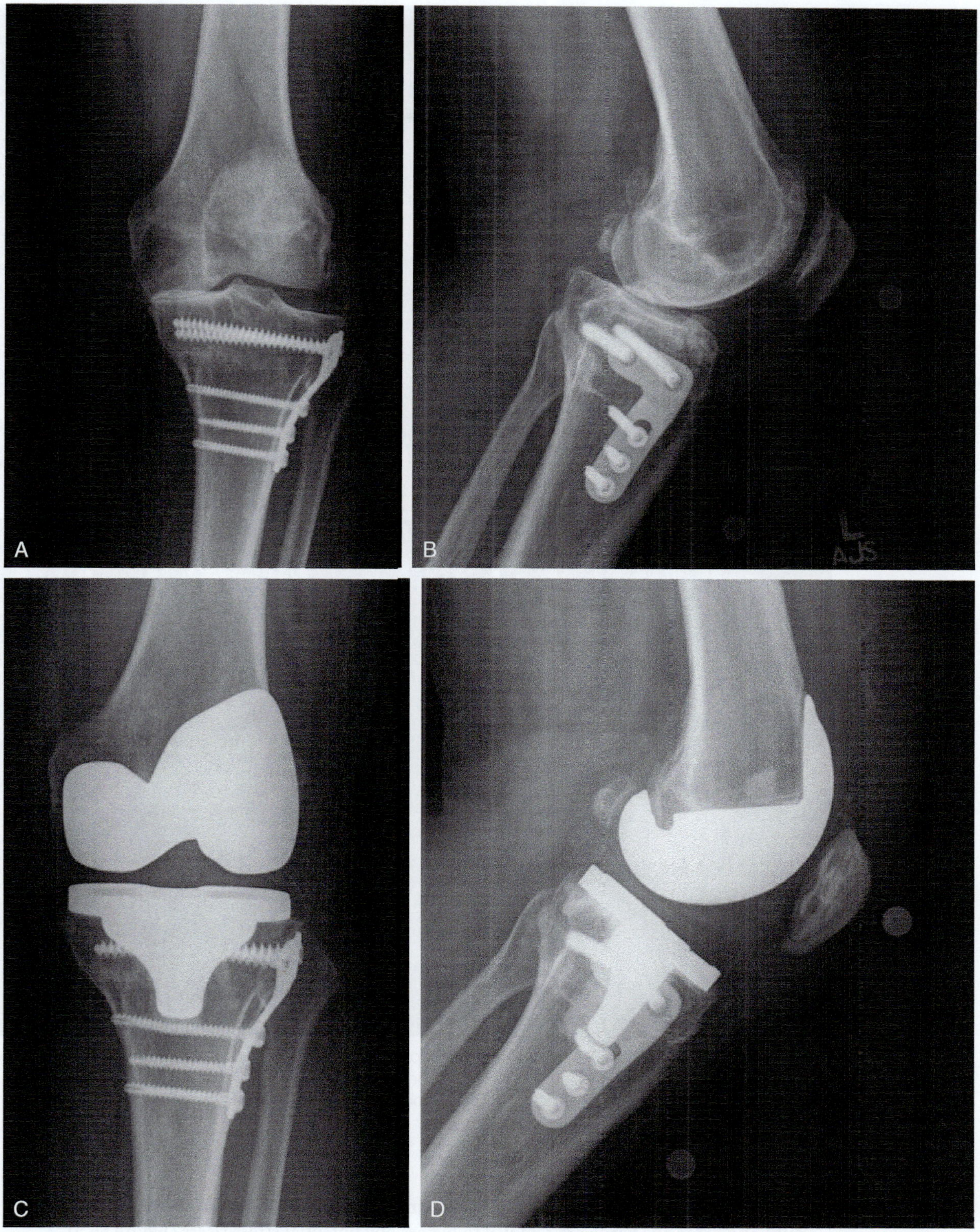

Figure 56.6 | Anteroposterior (A) and lateral (B) radiographs of a patient status post lateral closing-wedge high tibial osteotomy with plate fixation with end-stage varus gonarthrosis. The patient underwent a posterior-stabilized total knee arthroplasty with partial in situ hardware removal at the time of keel preparation using a metal-cutting burr as seen on postoperative radiographs (C and D).

- The tibial implant can be medialized to compensate for lateral bone loss and to avoid lateral hardware; once accomplished, pin the tibial tray in place.
- Anticipate based on preoperative radiographs before drilling for the tibial keel whether to expect retained hardware to interfere with keel preparation.
- If metal hardware is encountered, utilize a metal-cutting burr through the tibial tray to burr away any prominent hardware that will interfere with keel preparation (Figure 56.6).

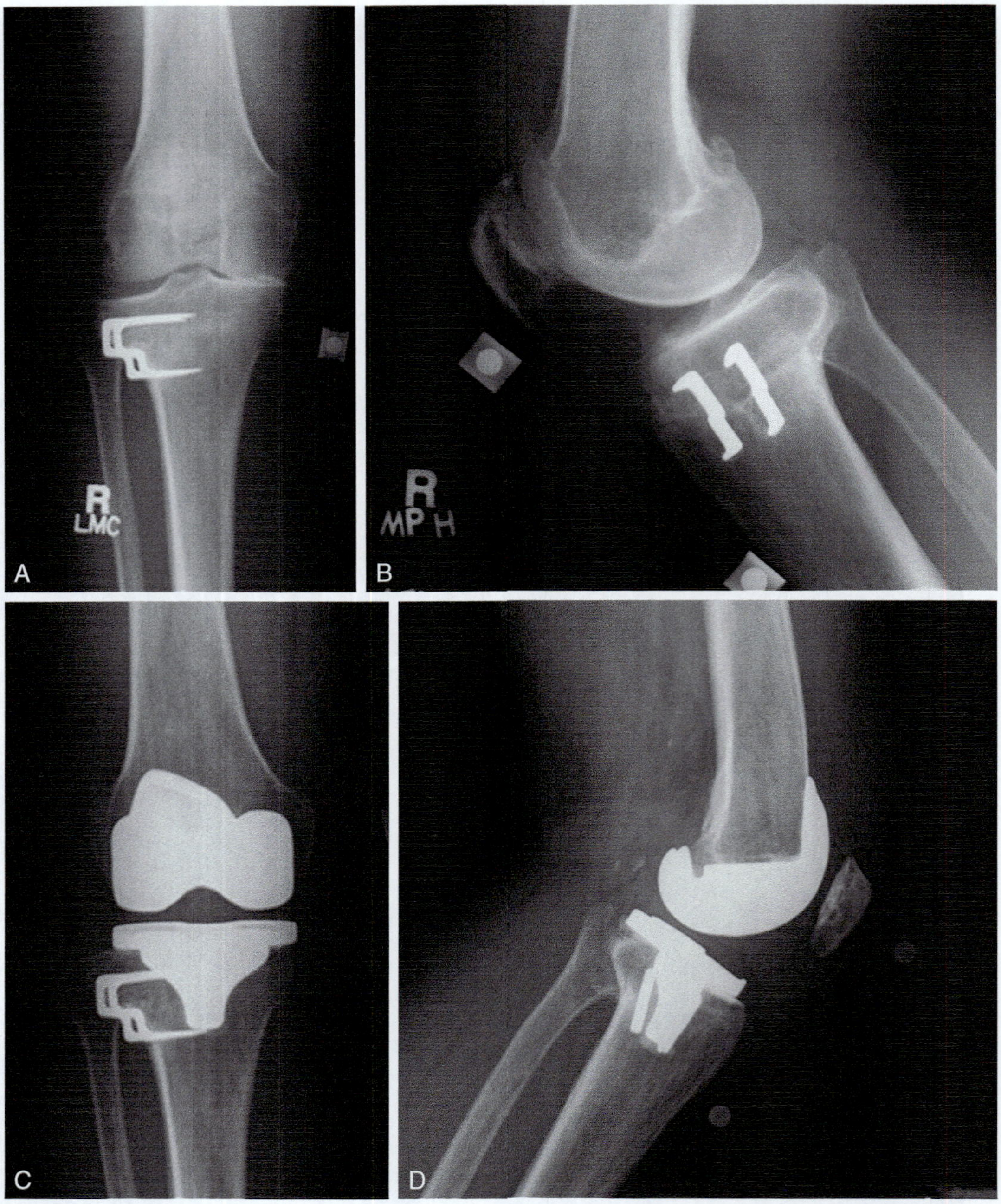

Figure 56.7 I Anteroposterior (A) and lateral (B) radiographs of a patient status post lateral closing-wedge high tibial osteotomy with lateral tibial plateau bone deficiency. During total knee arthroplasty, the tibial component was medialized to bypass the retained hardware and compensate for lateral tibial bone loss as seen on postoperative radiographs (C and D).

- A tibial stem should be considered in many circumstances including morbid obesity, marked deformity, and extensive hardware removal to bypass any potential stress risers (Figure 56.5).
- If the tibia canal is in line with the proximal tibia, the stem can be prepared in the normal fashion.
- If there is a medially offset tibial canal, consider using an offset tibial stem, a tibial component without a stem or with a smaller keel, or a custom TKA implant.
- With the approach of internal, partial removal of hardware and medialization of the tibial implant, standard nonstemmed implants can be utilized in the vast majority of cases, even in those with lateral bone deficiency (Figure 56.7) or offset tibial canals (Figure 56.8).
- Once the tibia is fully prepared and the knee balanced appropriately, cementation of the total knee components is done in the standard fashion. It is wise to use antibiotic-containing bone cement in these patients.

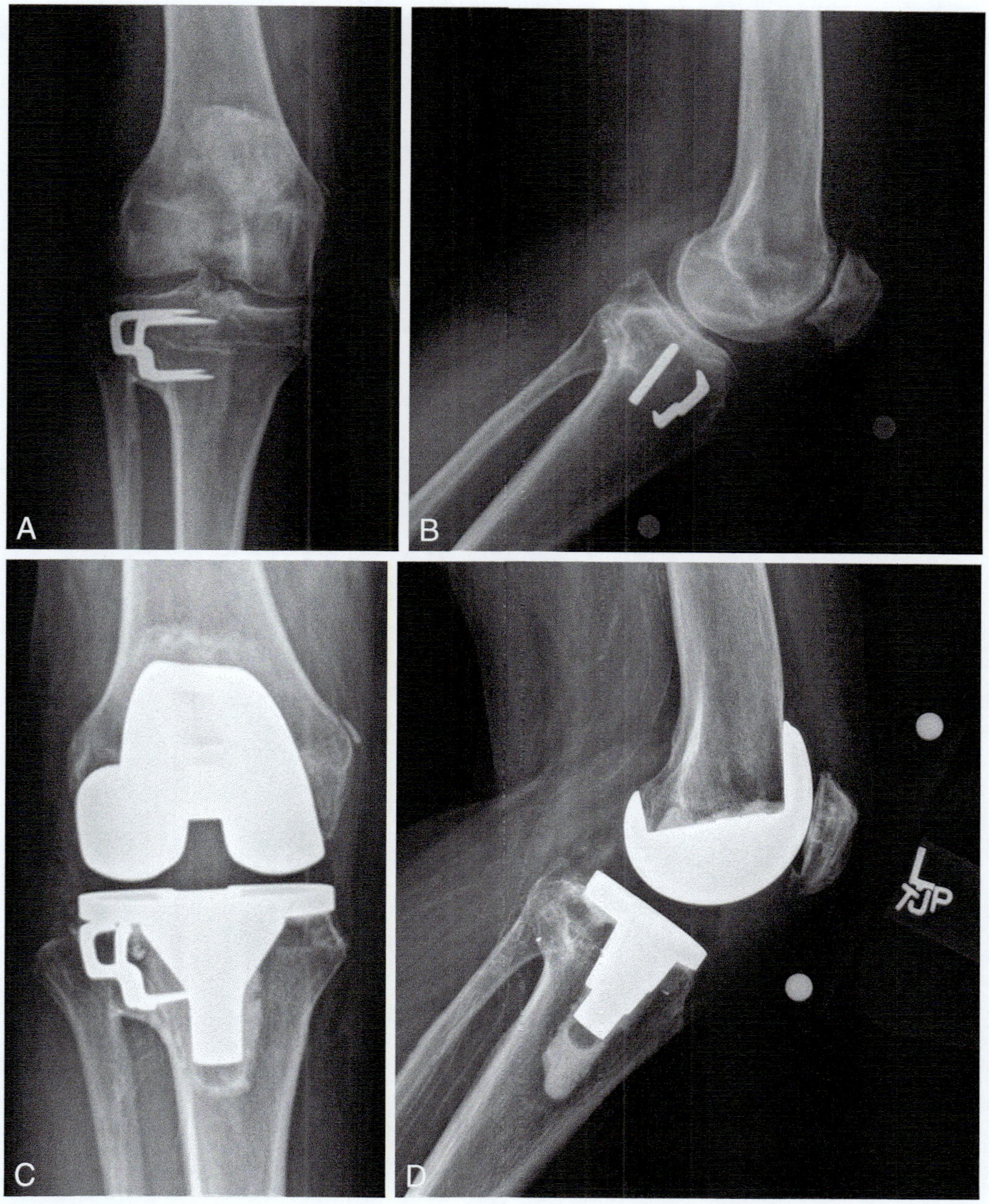

Figure 56.8 I Anteroposterior (A) and lateral (B) radiographs of a patient status post lateral closing-wedge high tibial osteotomy with a medially offset tibial canal in relation to the tibial plateau. A standard posterior-stabilized total knee implant was used, and the tibial component was placed without a stem to compensate for the offset canal as seen on postoperative radiographs (C and D).

- The real tibial polyethylene component is implanted once the cement has hardened and the balance remains appropriate.
- Meticulous layered closure is done per the surgeon's routine.

Postoperative Care

- Routine TKA postoperative care (weight bearing as tolerated, progressive range of motion protocol, etc.) per the surgeon's routine is appropriate for most patients. In some cases in which the wound is at risk or extensive dissection has been done for exposure or hardware removal, it is prudent to prioritize wound healing over early range of motion. In such circumstances the patient may be immobilized in full extension for a variable amount of time from 48 hours to 10 days to minimize swelling and promote wound healing.

Chapter 57
Extra-articular Deformity

ALAN K. SUTAK
MATTHEW P. ABDEL

Key Concepts

- Deformities at the knee can either be intra-articular or extra-articular in nature.
- Extra-articular deformities can be on either the femoral side (Figure 57.1A) or tibial side (Figure 57.1B). Moreover, they can be near the joint (Figure 57.2A) or far from the joint (Figure 57.2B). In general, deformities that are further from the joint are less likely to impact total knee surgical technique.
- Preoperative planning with a long-leg standing film (Figure 57.3) is critical to understanding the deformity and type of correction needed (intra-articular correction versus osteotomy versus use of hinged total knee arthroplasty [TKA]).
- If planned resection would damage the collateral ligaments on the distal femur (Figure 57.4A) or the tibial diaphyseal line (Figure 57.4B) passes outside of the tibial plateau, an extra-articular osteotomy is indicated in younger or more active patients. In elderly patients who are low demand, sacrificing the collateral ligaments and using a hinged TKA (Figure 57.5) without an osteotomy can be considered.

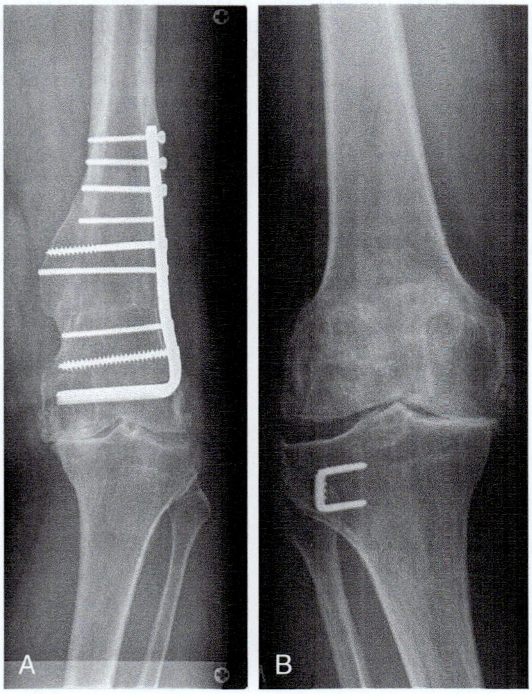

Figure 57.1 A, Anteroposterior (AP) knee radiograph of a 55-year-old man with a left distal femoral deformity secondary to a distal femur fracture with subsequent nonunion treated with revision open reduction and internal fixation. B, AP knee radiograph of a 51-year-old man with a right proximal tibial deformity secondary to a high tibial osteotomy completed 18 years previously.

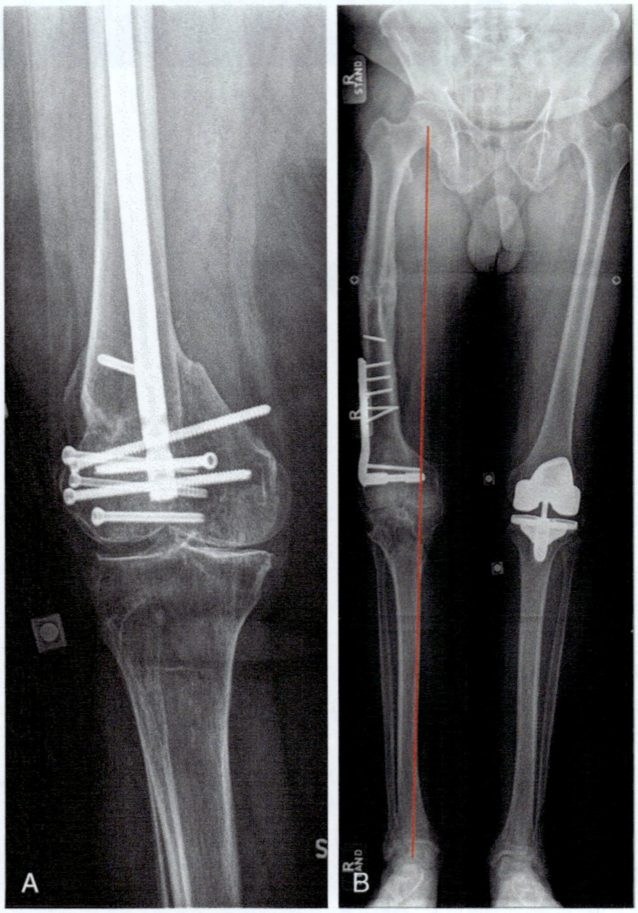

Figure 57.2 I A, AP radiograph of an 81-year-old woman with a right distal femoral deformity near the joint secondary to a distal femur fracture. B, This long-leg standing hip-knee-ankle radiograph shows a 62-year-old woman with 2 extra-articular deformities in the right femur (one far from the joint and one near the joint) secondary to spondyepiphyseal dysplasia.

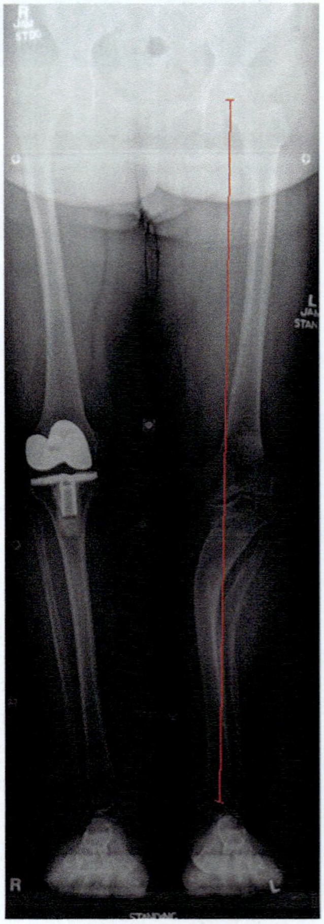

Figure 57.3 I This long-leg standing hip-knee-ankle radiograph reveals a significant left tibial deformity near the joint secondary to Blount disease in a 53-year-old woman. However, the overall mechanical alignment is near neutral.

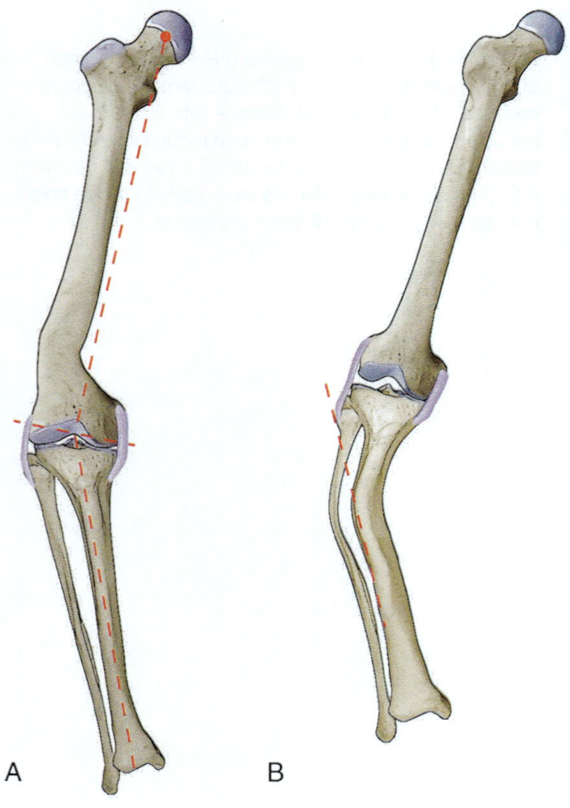

Figure 57.4 I If templating on standing long-leg hip-knee-ankle radiograph indicates compromise of the collateral ligaments on the femoral side (A) or the tibial diaphyseal line does not intersect the tibial plateau (B), then an osteotomy should be considered. (Redrawn with permission from Wang JW, Wang CJ. Total knee arthroplasty for arthritis of the knee with extra-articular deformity. *J Bone Joint Surg Am*. 2002;84-A(10):1769-1774.)

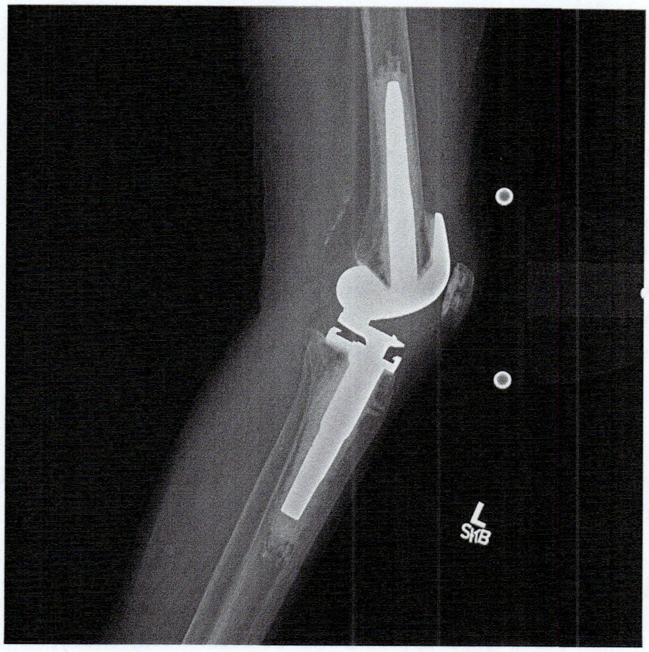

Figure 57.5 | This left lateral radiograph depicts a primary hinge TKA completed in a 91-year-old woman with a significant deformity that would have required an osteotomy.

- Regardless of technique, component position should be correct in all planes, and the joint line should be perpendicular to the mechanical axis (Figure 57.6).
  The focus of this chapter will be on nonosteotomy solutions.

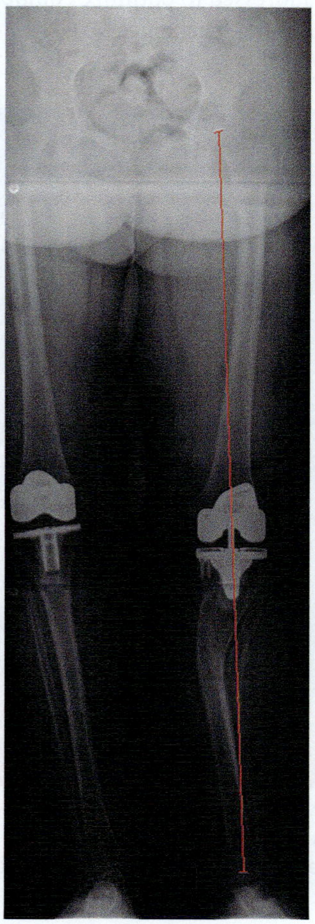

Figure 57.6 | With adequate planning and use of extramedullary alignment and intraoperative fluoroscopy, the patient from Figure 57.3 underwent an unremarkable left primary TKA without an osteotomy. The postoperative long-leg standing hip-knee-ankle radiograph reveals a neutral mechanical alignment with a joint line that is perpendicular to the mechanical axis.

Sterile Instruments and Implants

Instruments

- Standard TKA instrumentation
- Appropriate tools and instruments to remove prior hardware and/or implants, including diamond-cutting burrs and wheels and broken screw removal set
- Intraoperative radiographs or fluoroscopy to verify alignment
- Consider use of the following:
  - Extramedullary guide rods for alignment (Figure 57.7)
  - Handheld navigation (Figure 57.8)
  - Computer-assisted/robotically assisted surgery (Figure 57.9)

Implants

- Implants with varying levels of constraint should be available during all cases, from posterior-stabilized to varus-valgus constraint to rotating-hinge constructs.

Surgical Approaches

- In most cases, a medial parapatellar approach can be used. Occasionally, an extensile exposure such as a quadriceps snip may be required (Figure 57.10).

Preoperative Planning

- In patients with extra-articular deformities, a detailed preoperative planning is imperative for 3 reasons:
  - Previous skin incisions and compromised soft-tissue flaps will need to be addressed in many cases.
  - Previous hardware and/or instruments may need to be removed.
  - The extra-articular deformity will have to be addressed to optimize component positioning in all planes while having a joint line perpendicular to the mechanical axis.

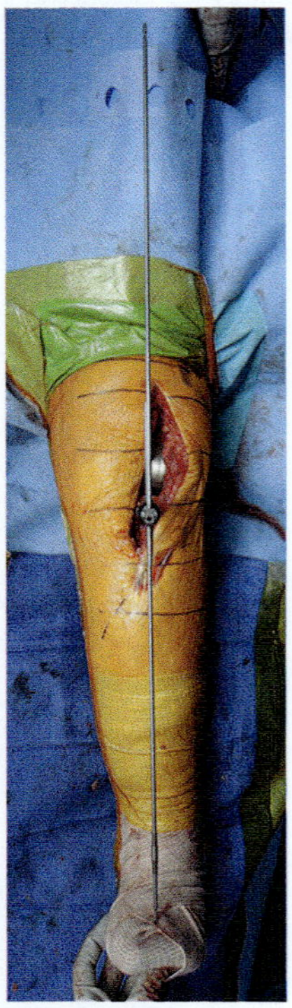

Figure 57.7 | Intraoperative picture of the patient from Figures 57.3 and 57.6 depicting the use of extramedullary alignment to obtain a neutral mechanical axis irrespective of the tibial deformity.

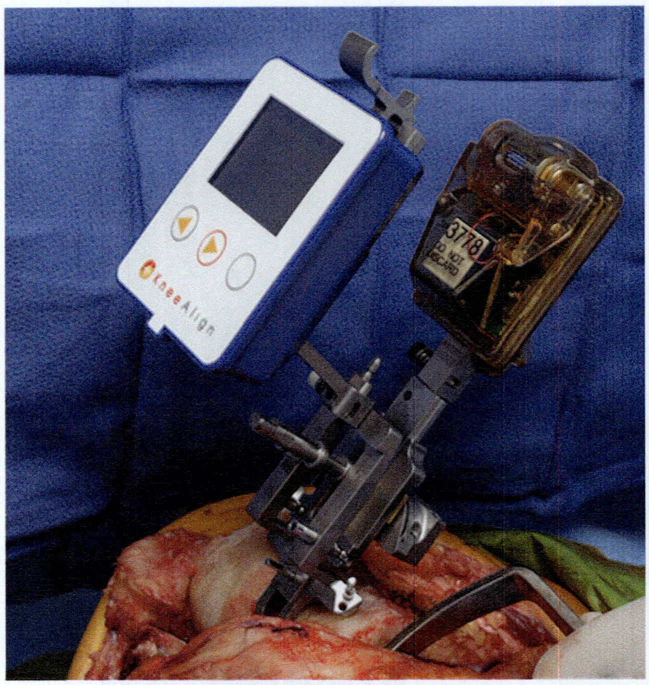

Figure 57.8 | This intraoperative picture depicts the use of handheld navigation on the femur for a patient with an extra-articular distal femoral deformity with in situ femoral hardware.

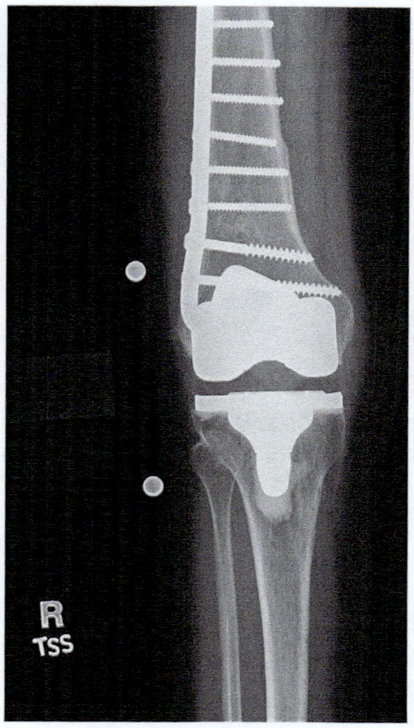

Figure 57.9 | The patient from Figure 57.2B with spondyepiphyseal dysplasia and 2 extra-articular femoral deformities underwent an uncomplicated right primary TKA utilizing robotically assisted surgery.

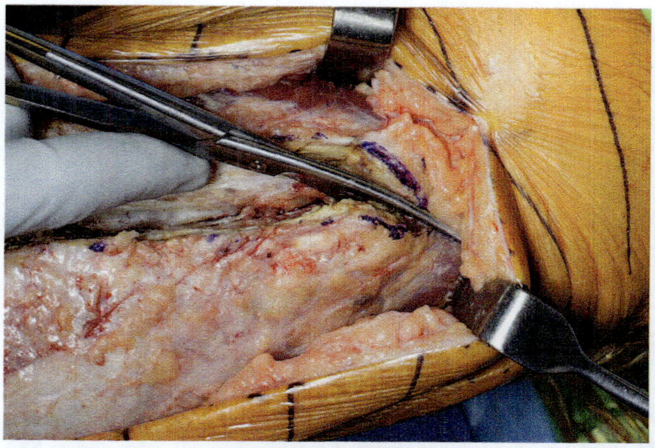

Figure 57.10 | This intraoperative picture depicts a quadriceps snip at the superior aspect of the quadriceps tendon at a 45° angle laterally toward the muscle fibers.

- Oftentimes, these patients may have acquired the deformity as a result of trauma and may have had previous surgery or skin damage (Figure 57.11A). Although the most laterally based incision often should be selected, a preoperative consultation with a plastic surgeon should be considered (Figure 57.11B).
- In addition, many patients with extra-articular deformities have hardware or implants from previous interventions (Figure 57.12). Careful planning is required to determine if partial (Figure 57.13) or complete hardware removal is required.

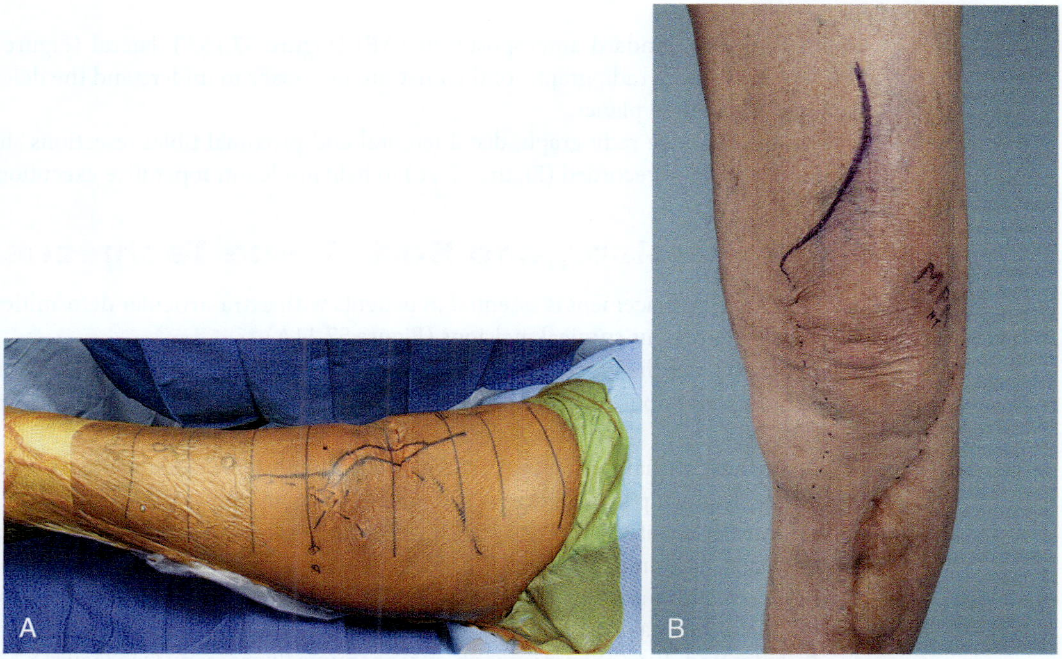

Figure 57.11 | A, Oftentimes, patients with extra-articular deformities have multiple incisions that must be appropriately managed at the time of TKA. B, In general, the most laterally based incision should be utilized if reasonable to complete the TKA. If the laterally based incision is not reasonable (as in this case), a plastic surgeon should be consulted.

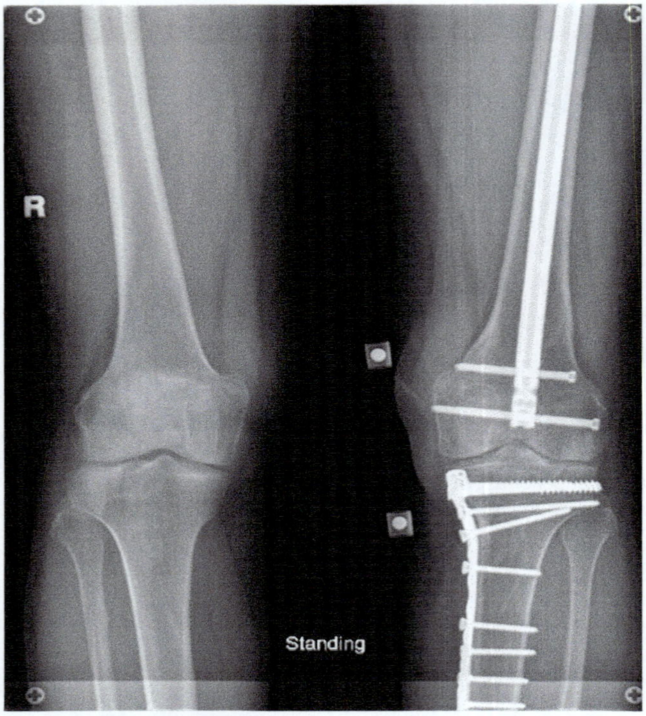

Figure 57.12 | The surgeon must be prepared to remove hardware on both the femoral and tibial sides.

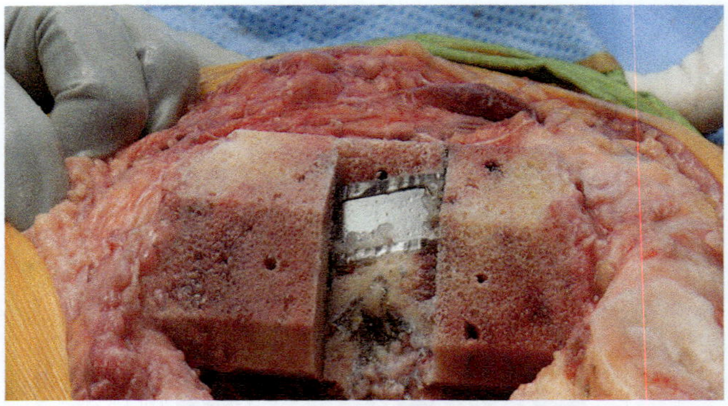

Figure 57.13 | In this intraoperative picture, the obstructive portion of the distal femoral blade plate is removed with a diamond-cutting burr. The senior author's preference is to only remove hardware that directly interferes with the TKA.

- If hardware removal is necessary, the surgeon may consider removing the hardware at the time of TKA (preferred technique) or in a staged fashion.
- When templating bony cuts and prostheses, plan for resections that place the joint line perpendicular to the mechanical axis (see Figure 57.6).
- Long-leg standing hip-knee-ankle radiographs allow the surgeon to identify the coronal deformity (Figure 57.14) and determine if intra-articular correction will sacrifice the collaterals or if the tibial diaphyseal line will pass outside the plateau. If that is the case, an osteotomy or hinged TKA is required.
- In addition, standard anteroposterior (AP) (Figure 57.15A), lateral (Figure 57.15B), and patellar (Figure 57.15C) radiographs of the knee are necessary to understand the deformity in both the coronal and sagittal planes.
- On the AP knee radiograph, distal femoral and proximal tibial resections should be measured via templating and recorded (Figure 57.16) to help guide intraoperative execution.

Bone, Implant, and Soft Tissue Techniques

- Skin incision placement is essential in patients with extra-articular deformities as many patients will have had previous surgical incisions (Figure 57.11A).
- In general, use the most lateral incision to preserve perfusion to the skin flap (Figure 57.11B).
- Cross any previous incisions at a 90° angle if possible. During the exposure, maintain full-thickness skin flaps.
- A standard medial parapatellar arthrotomy is often used. Occasionally, an extensile exposure such as a quadriceps snip (see Figure 57.10) will be required.
- Protect the collateral ligaments with well-placed retractors and keep the tibia externally rotated to minimize tension on the extensor mechanism.
- Bone resections are performed using one of several techniques to align the joint line perpendicular to the mechanical axis:
  - Extramedullary alignment with intraoperative fluoroscopy (see Figure 57.7)
  - Handheld navigation (see Figure 57.8)
  - Computer-assisted/robotically assisted surgery (see Figure 57.9)
- Determine if retained femoral and/or tibial hardware (Figure 57.17) needs to be removed.

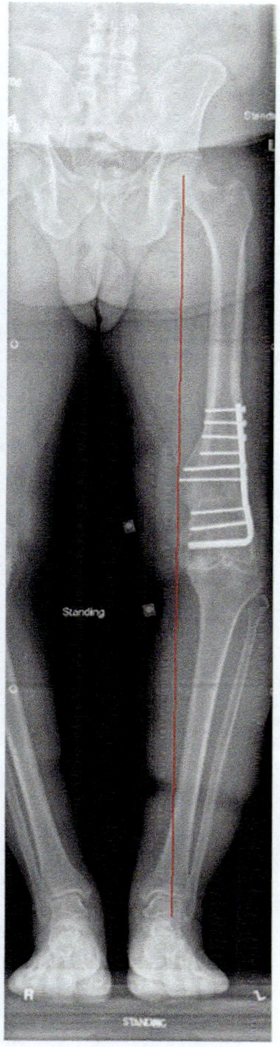

Figure 57.14 | The long-leg standing hip-knee-ankle radiograph of the 55-year-old man from Figure 57.1A with the left distal femoral deformity secondary to the distal femur fracture with subsequent nonunion is helpful in planning.

Extramedullary Alignment

- The distal femoral and proximal tibial cuts can be completed with a measured resection technique based on preoperative templating (see Figure 57.16).
- After the preliminary distal femur and proximal tibia cuts are completed, an appropriately sized spacer block and alignment rods can then be placed in the extension space to assess overall alignment (Figure 57.18).
- Intraoperative fluoroscopic images are then taken at the hip (Figure 57.19A) and ankle (Figure 57.19B). Additional distal femoral bone is resected on the medial side to increase the femoral varus or on the lateral side to increase the femoral valgus until the rod is in the center of the hip (Figure 57.19A).
- Additional proximal tibial bone is resected on the medial side to increase the tibial varus or on the lateral side to increase the tibial valgus until the rod is in the center of the talus (see Figure 57.19B).
- Alternatively, the surgeon may use intraoperative fluoroscopy and extramedullary rods to cut the distal femur and proximal tibia perpendicular to the mechanical axis of the femur and tibia without making preliminary cuts.

Handheld Navigation

- Advanced technologies such as handheld navigation may be utilized instead of extramedullary rods and intraoperative fluoroscopy.
- The senior author's preference is to utilize an accelerometer-based system (i.e., OrthAlign; Aliso Viejo, CA, USA) that captures the patient's hip center and ankle malleoli for registration of the femoral and tibial mechanical axes, respectively.

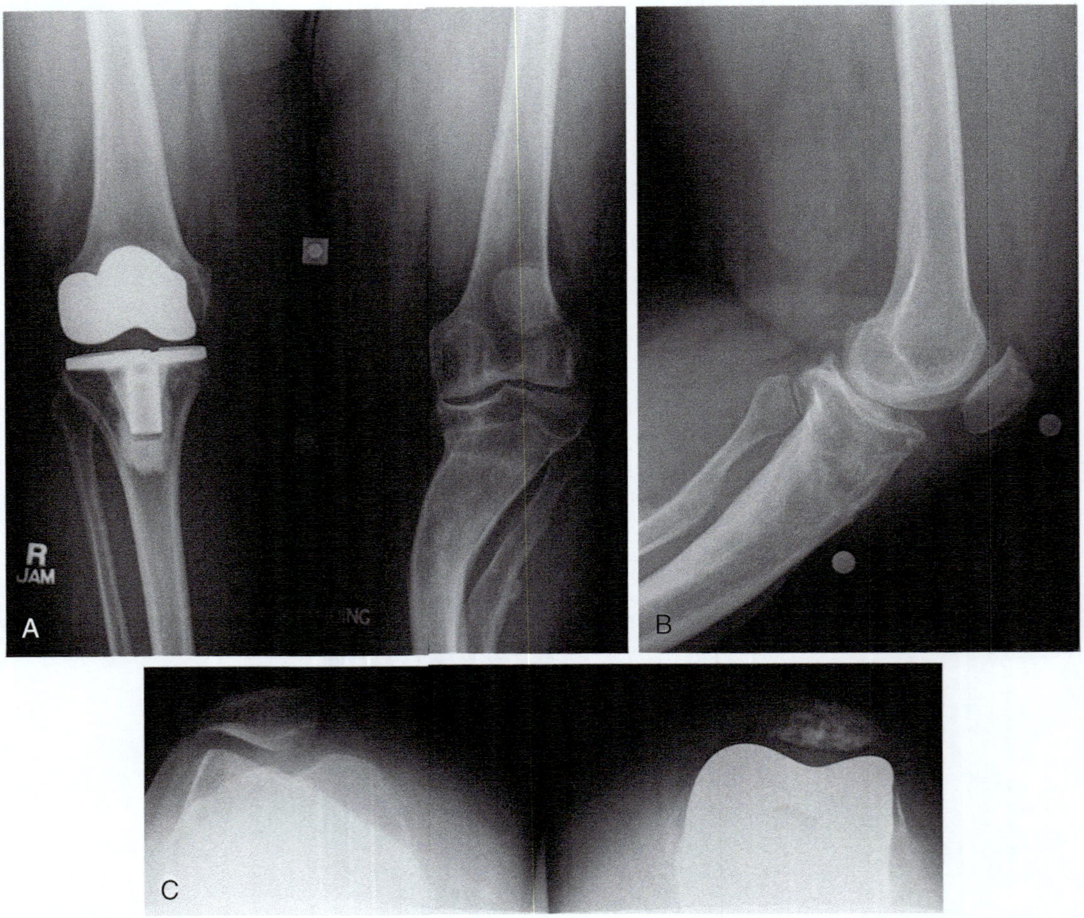

Figure 57.15 | The remaining AP (A) lateral (B) and patellar (C) radiographs for the 53-year-old woman with Blount disease of the left tibia from Figures 57.3 and 57.6 are helpful for preoperative planning.

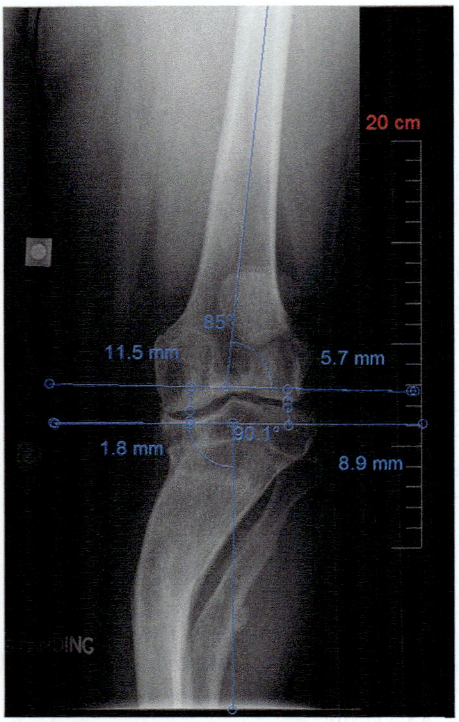

Figure 57.16 | In addition, planned distal femoral and proximal tibial resections aid in intraoperative execution.

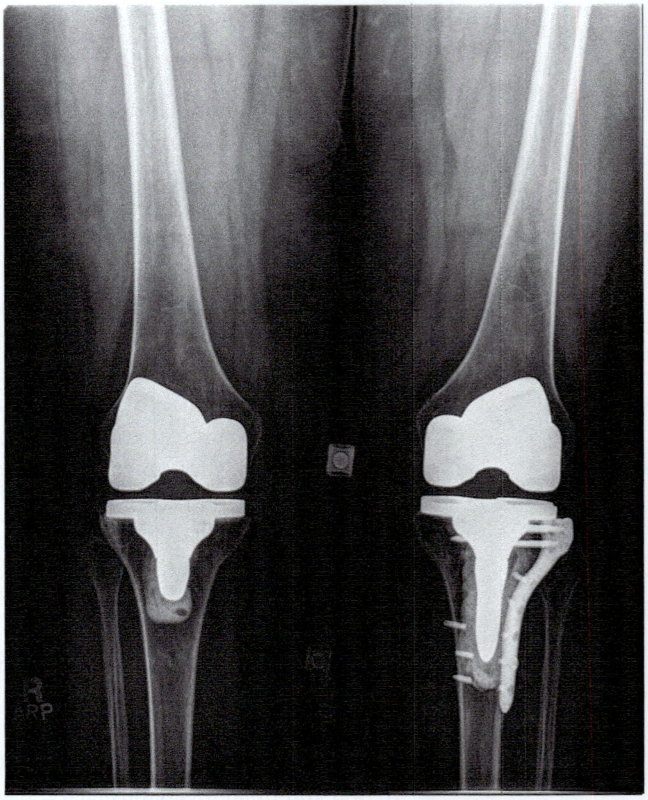

Figure 57.17 | In this case, only the tibial hardware interfering with the senior author's ability to complete the TKA was removed.

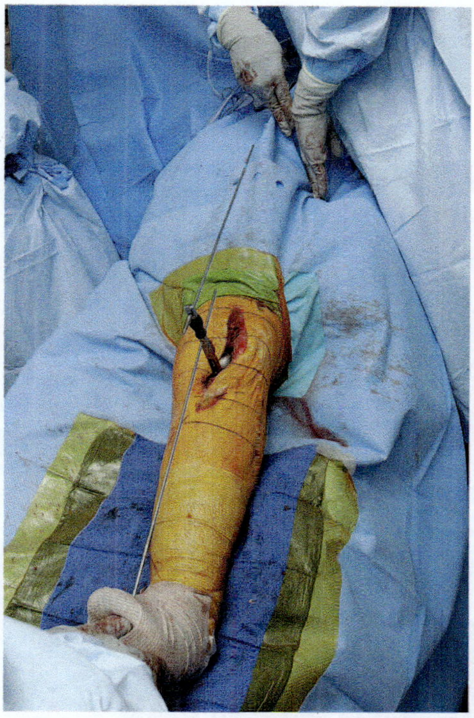

Figure 57.18 | An additional intraoperative picture of the patient from Figures 57.3, 57.6 and 57.15 depicting the use of extramedullary alignment to obtain a neutral mechanical axis irrespective of the tibial deformity.

- The handheld navigation then allows for correction of femoral coronal alignment (varus and valgus) and sagittal alignment (flexion and extension) at the surgeon's discretion (Figure 57.20A).
- The handheld navigation allows for correction of tibial coronal alignment (varus and valgus) and sagittal alignment (posterior slope) at the surgeon's discretion (Figure 57.20B). This allows for a neutral mechanical alignment and a joint line perpendicular to the mechanical axis.

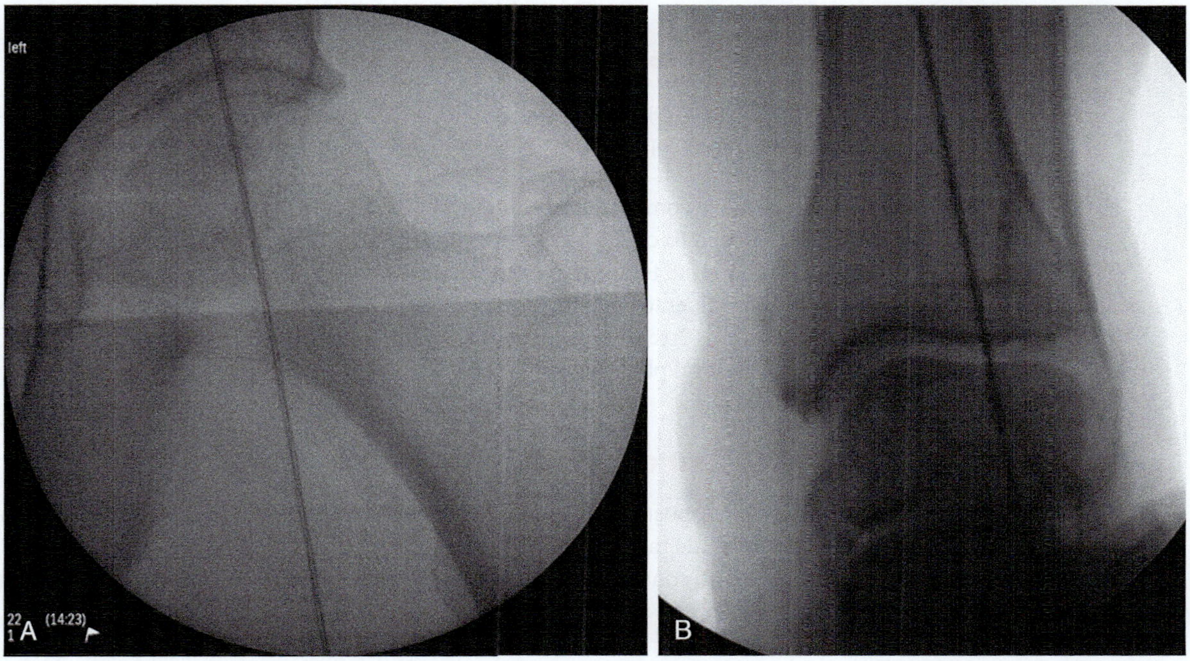

Figure 57.19 | A, An intraoperative fluoroscopic image with an electrocautery cord at the center of femoral head indicates neutral mechanical alignment of the femoral component. B, An intraoperative fluoroscopic image with an electrocautery cord at the center of the talus indicates neutral mechanical alignment of the tibial component.

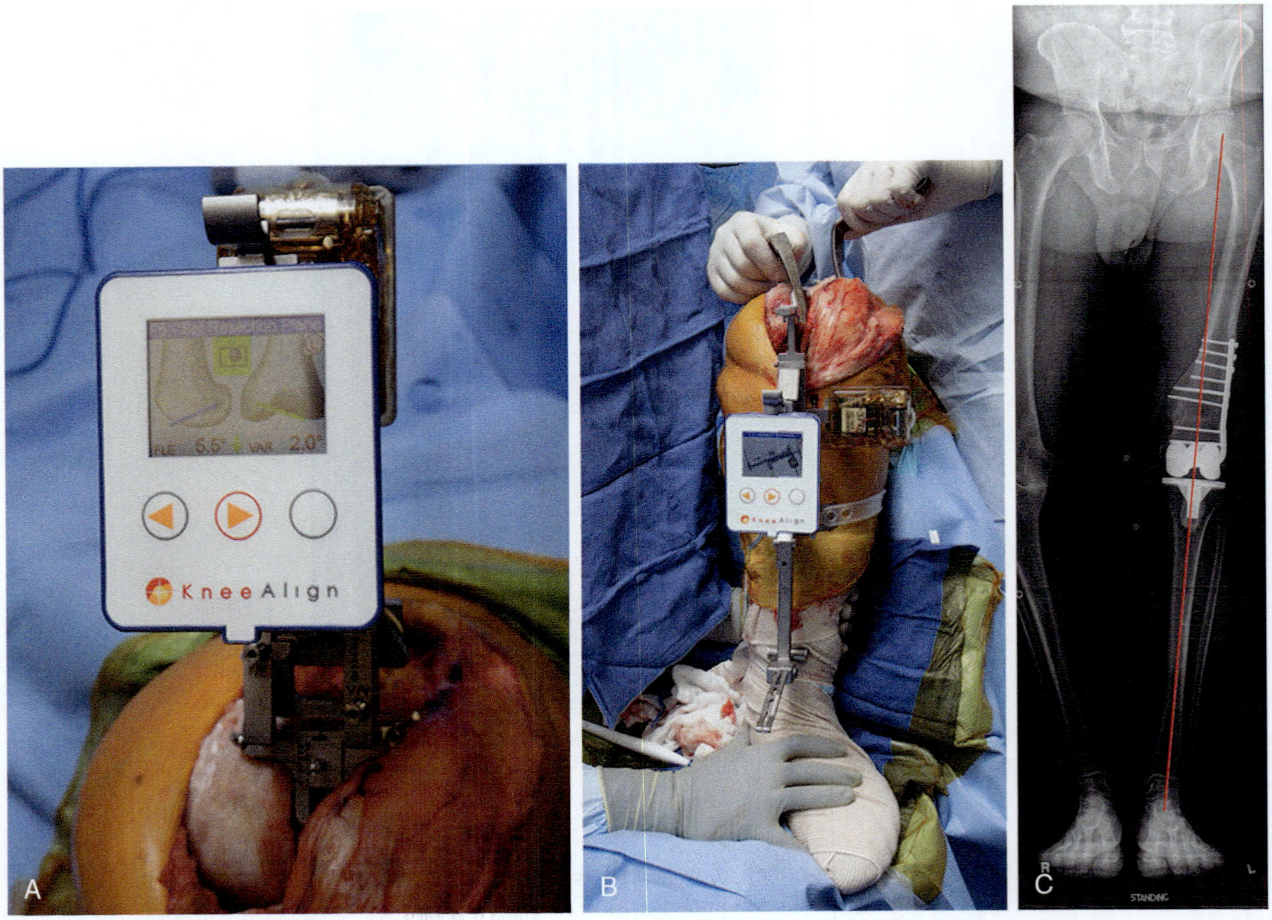

Figure 57.20 | A, Intraoperative picture of handheld navigation utilized for the 55-year-old man from Figures 57.1A and 57.14 to determine appropriate coronal and sagittal alignment of the femoral component. B, Similarly, handheld navigation is utilized to determine appropriate coronal alignment and slope of the tibial component. C, The resulting long-leg standing hip-knee-ankle radiograph indicated neutral mechanical alignment with a joint line perpendicular to the mechanical axis.

Computer-Assisted/Robotically Assisted Surgery

- An excellent indication for computer-assisted/robotically assisted surgery are femoral and/or tibial deformities. The senior author's preference is to utilize the MAKO system (Stryker; Mahwah, NJ, USA).
- In this system, a preoperative computerized tomography (CT) scan is obtained of the hip, knee, and ankle. The CT scan is utilized to create a customized plan for coronal, sagittal, and rotational alignment for the patient on both the femur and tibia.
- The robot is registered intraoperatively after adequate exposure. The robotic-arm assists the surgeon in completing all of the cuts irrespective of femoral and/or tibial deformities with precision and accuracy relative to the surgical plan (Figure 57.21A-C).

Postoperative Care

- In most cases, standard TKA postoperative protocols may be used, including patients being weight bearing as tolerated with gentle range of motion.
- If an osteotomy is performed, consider protected weight bearing for 6 to 8 weeks to allow for healing of the osteotomy site.

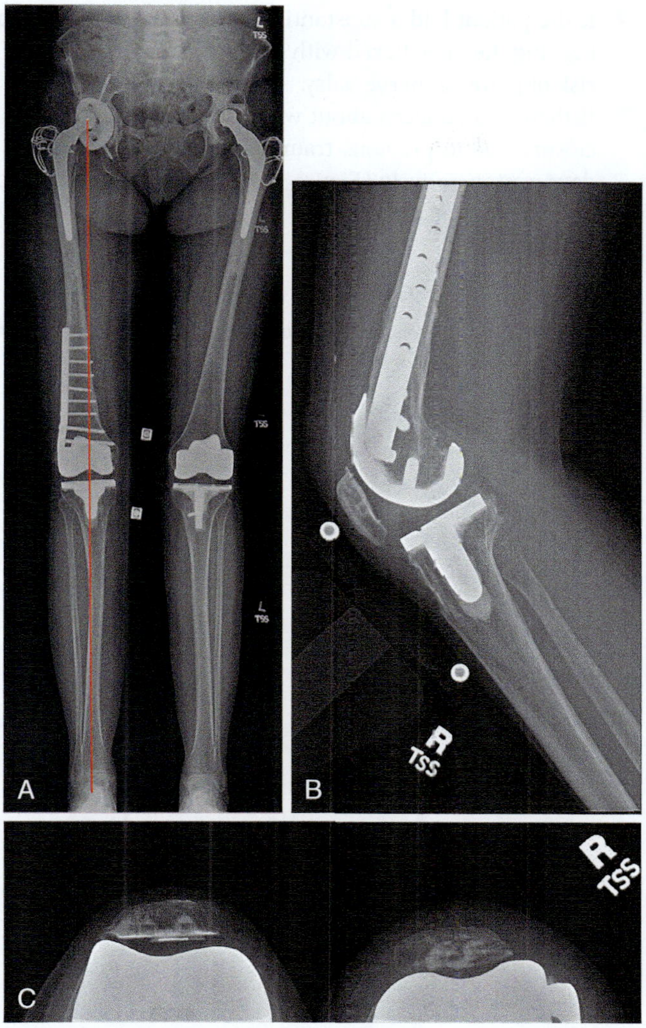

Figure 57.21 | A, Postoperative long-leg standing hip-knee-ankle, (B) lateral, and (C) patellar radiographs of the 62-year-old woman with spondyepiphyseal dysplasia from Figures 57.2B and 57.9 who underwent a complex TKA with robotically assisted surgery.

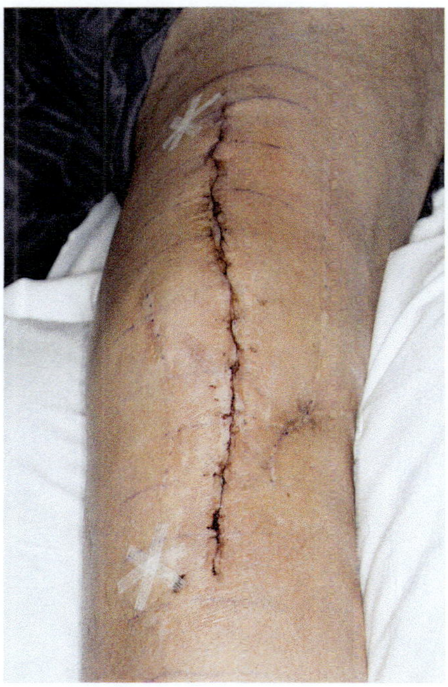

Figure 57.22 | A well-healing surgical incision after several days of immobilization after a TKA in a patient with extra-articular femoral and tibial deformities, prior trauma, and multiple prior surgical interventions (and thus incisions).

- If the patient had a substantial preoperative valgus deformity and/or flexion contracture, consider keeping the knee flexed with a nonconstrictive dressing for 1 to 2 days postoperatively to minimize risk of peroneal nerve palsy.
- If there is a concern about would healing (e.g., patient with multiple prior incisions and taut skin closure due to previous trauma), consider keeping the knee immobilized in extension for several days postoperatively (Figure 57.22), avoid ice to the knee, and give supplemental oxygen while the patient is hospitalized.

Suggested Reading

1. Wang JW, Wang CJ. Total knee arthroplasty for arthritis of the knee with extra-articular deformity. *J Bone Joint Surg Am.* 2002;84-A(10):1769-1774.

Part IV
Revision Total Knee Arthroplasty

Chapter 58
Preoperative Evaluation, Planning, and Templating for Revision Total Knee Arthroplasty

TIMOTHY S. BROWN
DANIEL J. BERRY

Preoperative Evaluation

- Establish a clear diagnosis. Understand what has failed and what you are trying to fix.
- Anticipate challenges related to exposure, implant removal, bone reconstruction, knee stability, and the extensor mechanism.
- The goal is to solve the patient's problem without creating new problems. A successful revision total knee arthroplasty (TKA) will be performed by gaining a well-fixed and durable, well-aligned, stable knee. At the same time, further bone loss should be minimized and soft tissues and the extensor mechanism protected.

History

- In addition to establishing a diagnosis for the cause of failure, learn more about the knee before TKA was performed: what was the grade of arthritis (prognostic value); what deformities or special circumstances were present?
- Obtain and review previous operative reports.
- Obtain "stickers" to confirm brand and size of implants in place.
- Determine if there is anything in the history to suggest infection.

Physical Examination

- Evaluate old incisions: Which one will you use? Most of the time the most lateral useable incision or the most recent longitudinal incision is chosen. If wound problems are anticipated, consider consultation with the plastic surgery team (Figure 58.1).
- Evaluate and document knee range of motion. If very stiff, anticipate need for an extensile exposure.
- Evaluate knee stability and ligament competence. If notably compromised, anticipate the need for more constrained implants, such as constrained condylar implants, or hinged implants.
- Evaluate and document neurovascular status. If good pulses are not present, consider vascular noninvasive studies and transcutaneous oxygen testing, and if appropriate, vascular specialist consultation.
- Evaluate extensor mechanism competence and tracking.
- Perform hip examination to make sure there is no coexistent hip pathology that could refer pain to knee.

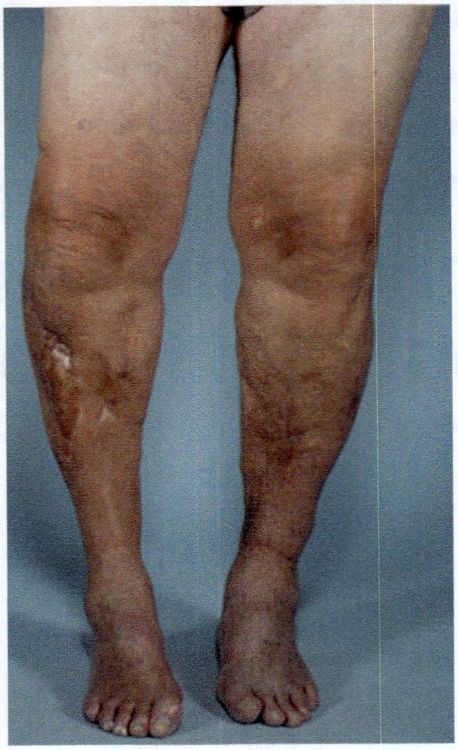

Figure 58.1 | Patient with previous serious soft tissue injury and multiple previous infections about the knee. Preoperative evaluation and coordination with plastic surgery team is valuable.

Radiographs

- Obtain anteroposterior, lateral, and patellar skyline views (Figure 58.2).
- A long-leg standing view provides information about extra-articular deformity and hip pathology (Figure 58.2).
- Fluoroscopically positioned views can provide images perfectly tangential to interfaces and are useful to look for loosening (Figure 58.3). Fluoroscopically positioned images are particularly valuable to look for radiolucent lines around uncemented implants.

Tests

- Routinely obtain erytrocyte sedimentation rate, C-reactive protein to look for infection.
- Aspirate most knees to evaluate for infection. Send fluid for culture and cell count with differential.
    - Nucleated cell count >1800; polymorphonuclear neutrophils (PMN) >80% → suggestive of chronic periprosthetic joint infection (PJI).
    - Nucleated cell count >10,000; PMN >90% → suggestive of acute PJI.
- Synovial fluid alpha defensin may provide further information about infection in equivocal circumstances.

Preoperative Planning

- Have a Plan A, Plan B, and Plan C for unexpected contingencies.
- Operative approach: routine medial parapatellar versus quadriceps snip versus tibial tubercle osteotomy.
- Implant removal: Will special instruments or exposure be needed?
    - Understand how to disengage the old polyethylene insert.
    - Evaluate whether special extraction instruments will be needed.
    - Anticipate any specific challenges in implant removal (well-fixed cement, well-fixed stems) (Figure 58.4). Will you need ultrasonic instruments, trephines, special saw blades, metal-cutting instruments?

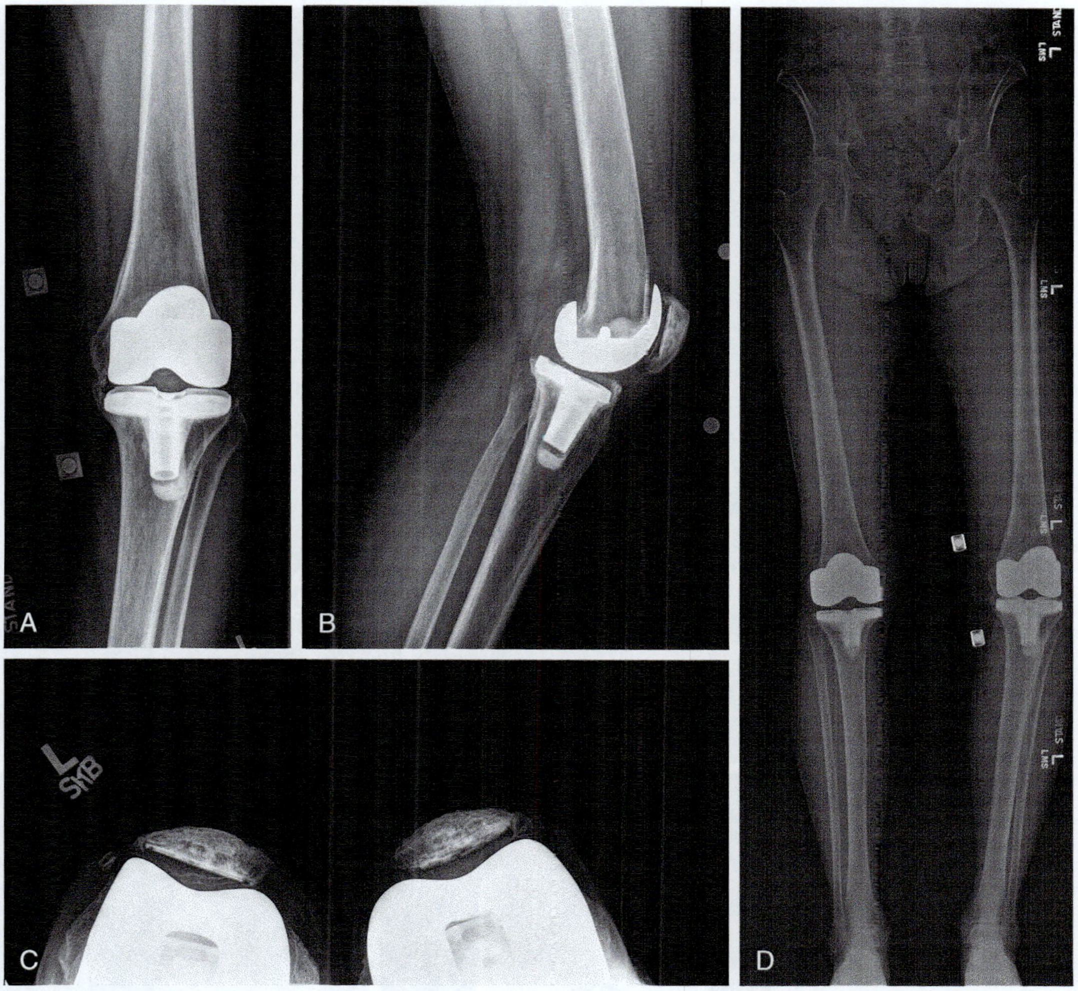

Figure 58.2 | Routine anteroposterior (A) lateral (B) patellar skyline (C) radiographs and (D) hip to ankle standing radiograph of failed left TKA.

Bone Reconstruction

- Plan to use stems to offload stress and/or gain fixation in almost all revisions. Revisions done with stems have lower failure rates than selective use of stems.
- Consider use of metaphyseal fixation with porous metal sleeves or cones, particularly if there is notable bone loss.
- If bone loss is present (and it usually is), determine how you will reconstruct (i.e., with bone graft or metaphyseal sleeves or cones). Cementing directly to deficient sclerotic bone usually does not provide good cement interdigitation for durable fixation.

Knee Stability

- Anticipate when there is likely a need for an increased level of constraint (varus-valgus constrained or hinged implants). Preoperative varus-valgus instability with known compromise of medial/lateral soft tissues or condyles and large deformities are circumstances when extra constraint probably will be needed.

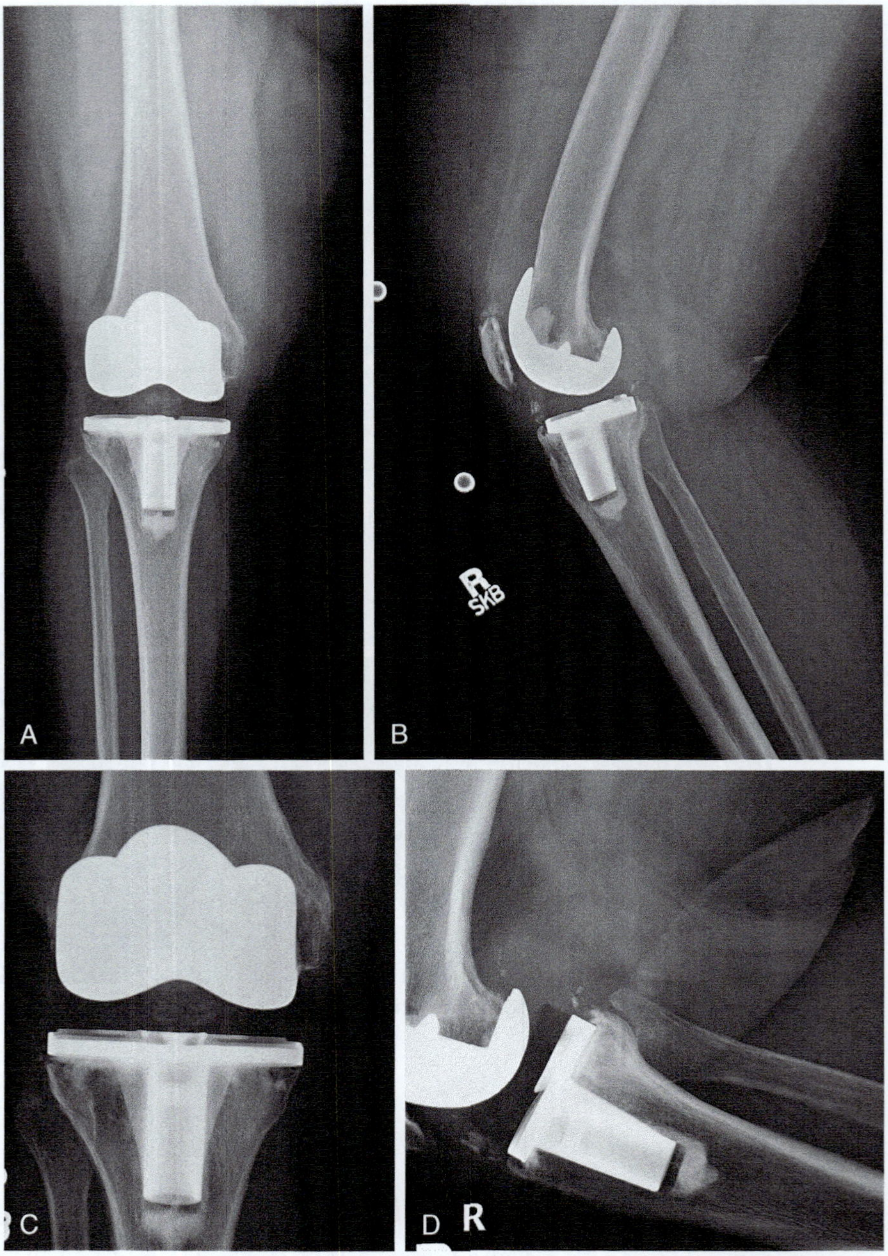

Figure 58.3 | Routine anteroposterior (A) and lateral (B) knee radiographs of patient with high level of clinical suspicion for tibial component loosening. These radiographs do not show definite component loosening. C and D, Fluoroscopically positioned anteroposterior lateral radiographs of the same knee. These radiographs, positioned with the beam exactly parallel to the tibial implant, show lysis beneath the tibial tray on the anteroposterior view and debonding of the tibial tray on the lateral view confirming implant loosening.

Extensor Mechanism

- Determine if the patella needs to be revised. Assess whether the patellar bone stock is good or deficient (in which case it may require special implants or reconstruction).
- Determine if extensor mechanism deficiency is present (quadriceps or patellar tendon). If so, be prepared for reconstruction with polymer mesh or extensor mechanism allograft.

Closure

- Are special closure methods or flaps anticipated? Does plastic surgery need to be involved?

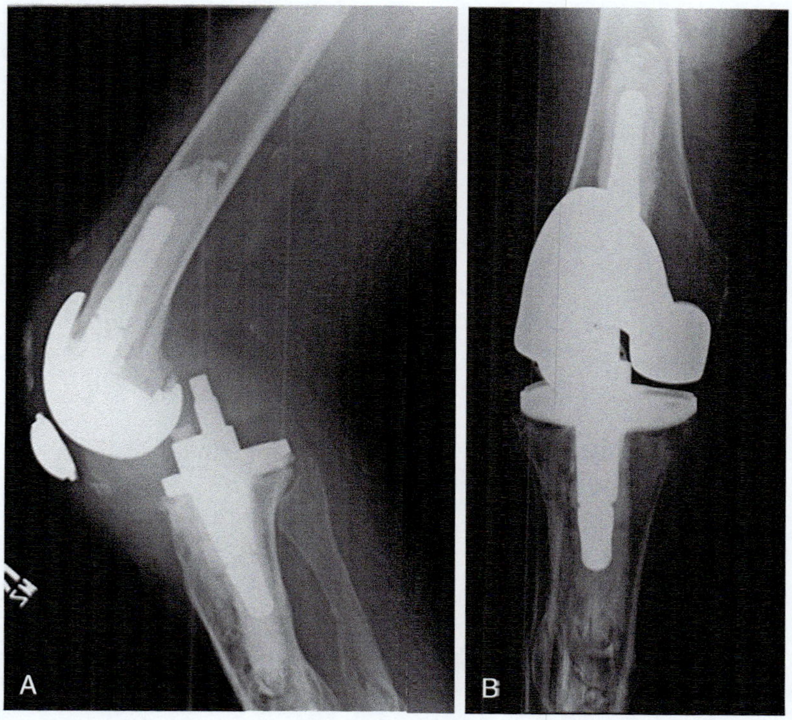

Figure 58.4 | Patient with (A) dislocated chronically infected TKA and (B) well-fixed cemented stemmed implants. In this case, anticipate the need for special techniques and implants to facilitate implant removal.

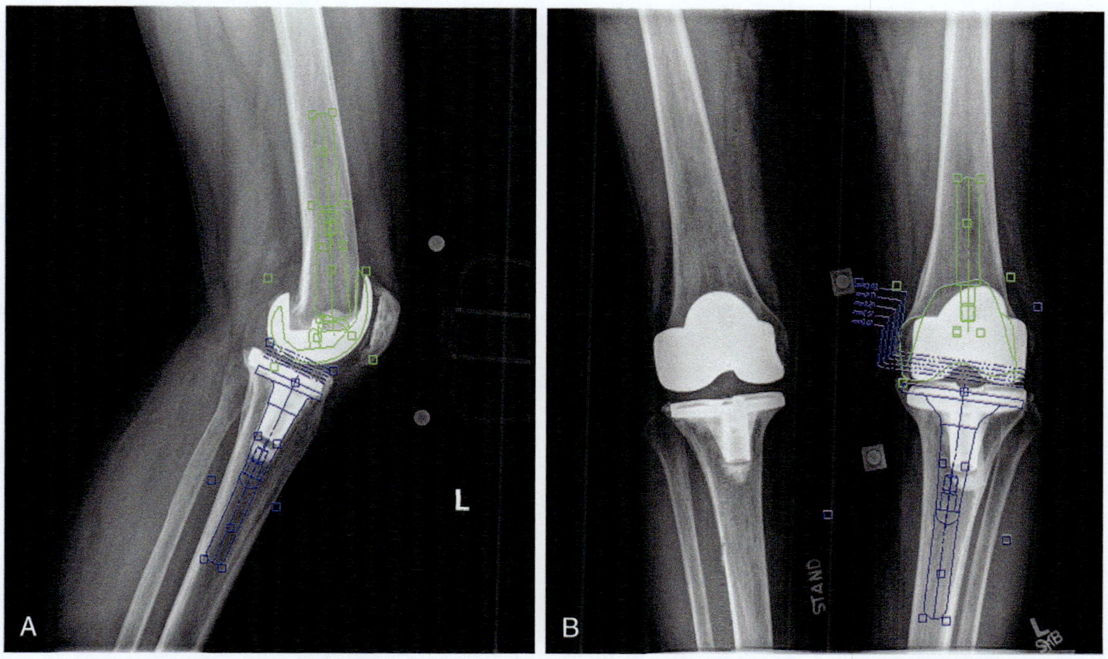

Figure 58.5 | Templating failed TKA for implant size, position, stem diameter, and length (A,B). In this case cemented stems were planned.

Templating

- Template anticipated design and size of tibial and femoral implants (Figure 58.5).
- Template anticipated length, diameter, and type of stem (cemented/uncemented). Are offset stems needed to center implants properly?
- Determine if any unique extra-articular geometry requires adjustments in implant selection or technique.

Section B
Revision TKA Implants

Chapter 59
Revision Total Knee Arthroplasty: Order of Attack

MARK W. PAGNANO

Key Concepts

- Having a coherent strategy in place before revision total knee arthroplasty (TKA) helps the surgeon order his or her thinking such that logical decisions can be made even if the unexpected is encountered.
- Preoperative planning identifies the need for nonstandard implants and major deformities that require osteotomy or an alternative surgical technique.
- Intraoperatively a methodical 3-step approach to revision TKA has proved reliable and reproducible over time: (1) reestablish the tibial platform, (2) restore balance in flexion by altering the anteroposterior (AP) size or offset of the femoral component, and (3) restore balance in extension by manipulating the joint line position proximally or distally.
- In certain very difficult revision TKA cases it is not possible to fill or "gain control of" the flexion gap owing to extreme laxity, and in such cases a hinged total knee design is required.

Sterile Instruments and Implants

- A complete set of the revision TKA instruments and implants from the surgeon's manufacturer of choice, including a full complement of tibial inserts. Do not get caught intraoperatively without the full range of sizes and constraint options.
- Appropriate range of augments, stems, porous metal cones, and/or metaphyseal sleeves to deal with a range of bone loss issues.
- Extraction instruments to safely and efficiently remove the failed TKA as outlined in the chapter on implant removal.
- Hinged total knee design available if this is a multiply revised TKA or the preoperative examination suggests marked ligamentous laxity or gross ligament incompetence.
- Intraoperative fluoroscopy or intraoperative radiograph to confirm trial component position.

Preoperative Planning

- Detailed medical history to identify risks for wound healing or neurovascular issues
  - Prior wound healing issues or history of infection after other procedures
  - Immunosuppressive medications
  - Smoking history
- Detailed surgical history focused on lower extremity
  - Prior difficulties in exposure, ligament balance, and bone quality as detailed in operative notes or per patient and family
  - Timing and mode of failure resulting in need for this revision TKA; are there lessons to be learned from the prior failed TKA?

Physical Examination

- Observe patient standing and walking
  - Identify and document gait abnormalities, coronal plane deformities, foot drop, pes planovalgus, knee hyperextension, etc.
- Examination of operative knee
  - Evaluate knee range of motion; identify and document preoperative contractures, coronal plane instability, and patellar stability.
  - Particular attention should be paid to ligamentous examination; look for clues to whether there is extreme laxity that might require hinged design; look for clues of excessive stiffness or woody/fibrotic tissue that will provide exposure challenges.
  - Examine the skin for open sores and prior incisions; treat or plan accordingly.
- Radiographic review
  - Determine fixation status of femur, tibia, and patella as a predictor of operative difficulty and time.
  - Predict the bone loss expected on the femoral, tibial, and patellar sides and prepare to encounter even more than predicted.
  - Assess the individual component position and determine if there are specific errors present that you deliberately wish to correct. For instance, if the tibia is in varus position with excessive posterior slope, then special effort should be made to address slope and to achieve neutral coronal alignment. If the femur is noted to be grossly undersized in the AP direction, then the revision femoral component should deliberately be sized 1 or 2 sizes larger.
  - Overall limb alignment can be assessed preoperatively to ensure there is not a substantial hip or foot/ankle abnormality that will cause gross malalignment if the standard revision TKA target of neutral mechanical alignment is chosen.

Bone, Implant, and Soft Tissue Techniques

Exposure

- A long incision that extends both slightly proximal and slightly distal to prior incisions is typically made (Figure 59.1). In most revision TKAs a long medial parapatellar arthrotomy with or without a quadriceps snip is used (Figure 59.2). The medial and lateral gutters are reestablished, and scar tissue is excised from the infrapatellar region to aid in exposure.
- The modular tibial liner is removed.
- The knee is typically flexed and the tibia externally rotated to deliver the tibia out from underneath the femur (Figure 59.3). The specifics of extensile exposure are presented in the following chapter.

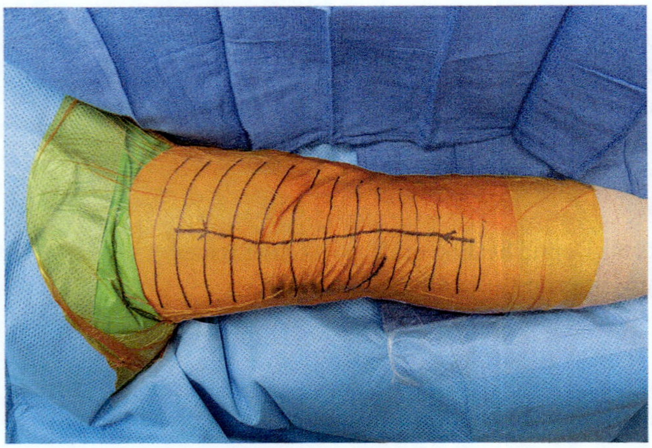

Figure 59.1 | Intraoperative photograph demonstrates the extent of prior incision (marked by arrowheads) and the typical extension of the incision proximally and distally to facilitate revision total knee replacement.

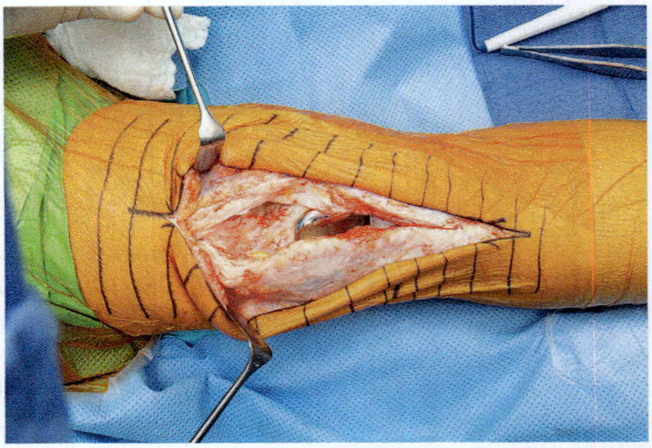

Figure 59.2 | Intraoperative photograph demonstrates the typical long, medial parapatellar arthrotomy used for revision TKA.

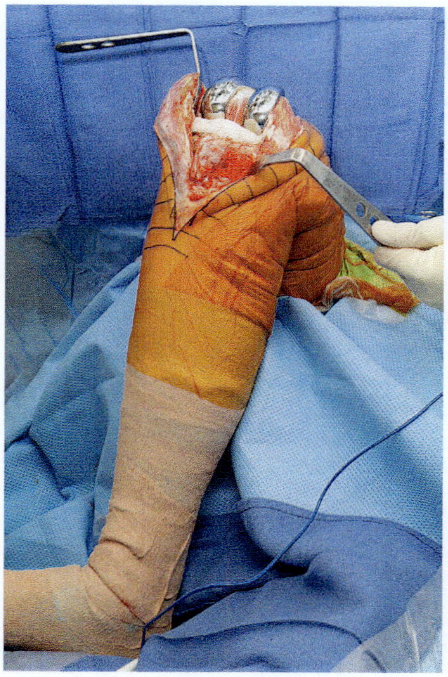

Figure 59.3 | Intraoperative photograph demonstrates the typical medial soft-tissue release and combined flexion of the knee and external rotation of the leg to obtain good exposure of the proximal tibia in revision TKA.

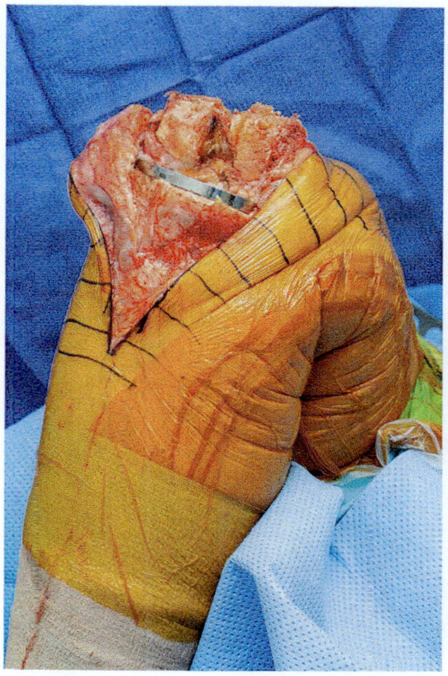

Figure 59.4 | Intraoperative photograph demonstrating the author's preference to remove the femoral component first, leaving the tibial tray in place to prevent femoral debris from falling into the tibial canal.

Femoral Component Removal

- It is the author's preference to typically remove the femoral component first, as the retained tibial component prevents cement and bone debris from falling into the tibial canal (Figure 59.4)
- The specifics of implant removal are outlined in a subsequent chapter, but a driving principle is to minimize iatrogenic bone loss. Preliminary preparation of the femur, including reaming, irrigating, and debriding the intramedullary canal, is carried out (Figure 59.5)

Tibial Component Removal

- The specifics of implant removal are outlined in a subsequent chapter, but a driving principle is to minimize iatrogenic bone loss. Wide exposure and access to the implant interfaces facilitates tibial component removal (Figure 59.6)

Patellar Component Assessment

- The vast majority of well-fixed patellar components can simply be left in place at the time of aseptic revision TKA.
- For loose or grossly malpositioned patellar components revision to a new component should be considered.

Reconstructive Step 1: Reestablish the Tibial Platform

- Conceptually, the tibia can be considered the foundation on which the remainder of the revision TKA is built. Having a solid, well-aligned foundation is then obviously important.
- Typically, only a minimal amount of bone is recut from the proximal tibia in contemporary revision TKA.
- Often it is useful to employ a combination of intramedullary (reamers) and extramedullary (drop rod) alignment techniques to ensure preparation of the tibia in neutral coronal alignment. In addition, an intraoperative radiograph with the trials in place is a helpful adjunct in the vast majority of cases.

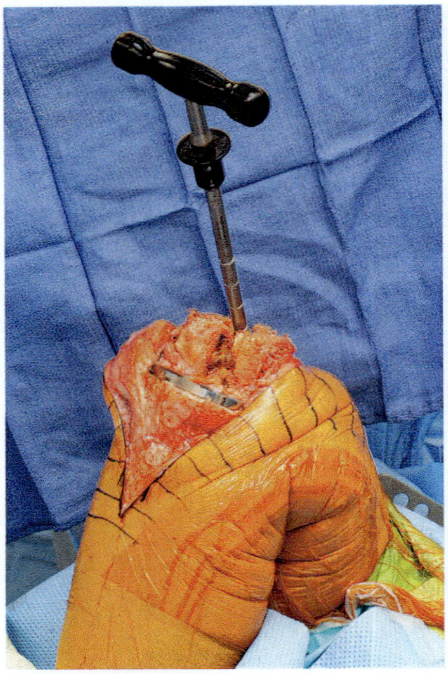

Figure 59.5 | Intraoperative photograph demonstrates reaming of the femoral canal for femoral stem preparation. Reaming is followed by thorough debridement and irrigation.

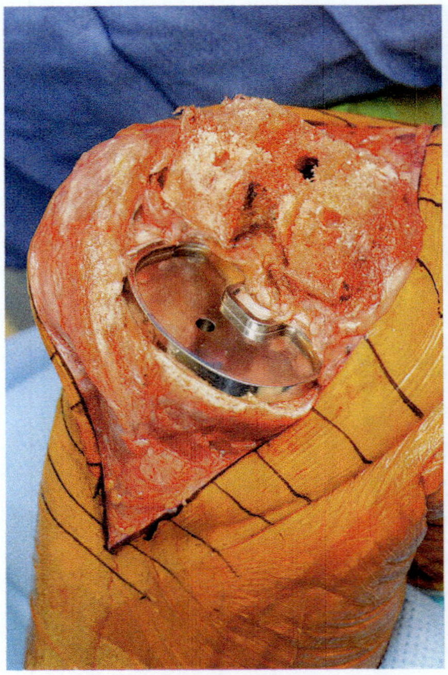

Figure 59.6 | Intraoperative photograph demonstrates good exposure of the entire periphery of the tibial tray before attempts at removal. Access to the cement-implant interfaces posteriorly is important to safely remove the tibia without excessive bone destruction.

- If intramedullary reamers are used for alignment or if press-fit stems are employed, the surgeons should be aware of 2 factors that can contribute to malalignment:
  - The center of the tibial canal is typically offset medially about 4 mm compared with the center of the articular surface.
  - The harder, sclerotic bone medially tends to push tibial reamers and broaches for metaphyseal sleeves into valgus.
  - To avoid valgus positioning of tibial stems and sleeves, specific attention often must be paid to deliberately ream more medially (Figure 59.7)
- Reestablish appropriate posterior tibial slope. In most, but not all, revision TKA systems the implants are designed for zero degrees of posterior slope. There is a strong tendency, however, to prepare the proximal tibia with excessive slope because there is often some posterior bone loss and the natural tendency is to let the implant tip posteriorly and help fill that space.
  - Reviewing the prerevision lateral radiograph can provide clues if the prior tibia was in excess slope and remind the surgeon to correct that.
  - Intraoperatively, tibial reamers often need to be deliberately moved slightly anterior and slightly medial to achieve both appropriate coronal and sagittal alignment.
  - Excessive posterior tibial slope selectively opens the flexion gap compared with the extension gap and that is seldom desired or useful in revision TKA.
- Address bone defects according to the surgeon's preferred method. The details on bone defect management are provided in a subsequent chapter but the chosen method must provide for neutral alignment of the tibial component in the coronal plane, zero posterior tibial slope in the sagittal plane, reestablishment of the tibial joint line proximal enough such that a range of tibial insert thicknesses are available, and reliable and durable mechanical fixation of the tibial implant (Figure 59.8)

Reconstructive Step 2: Reestablish Balance in Flexion

- Determine the appropriate femoral component rotation, which is typically parallel to the transepicondylar axis.
- Determine the appropriate femoral component size. Typically, this will be either the same AP size or 1 size larger from the femoral component that is being revised (Figure 59.9)
- Ensure the femoral component is not oversized in the mediolateral dimension.

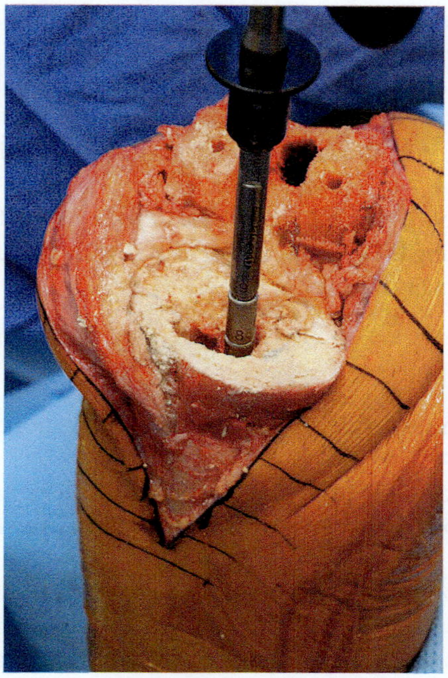

Figure 59.7 | Intraoperative photograph demonstrates the typical orientation of tibial reamers needed to ensure appropriate alignment. Note that the reamer is deliberately more medial and slightly more anterior than the center of the remaining proximal tibial articular surface.

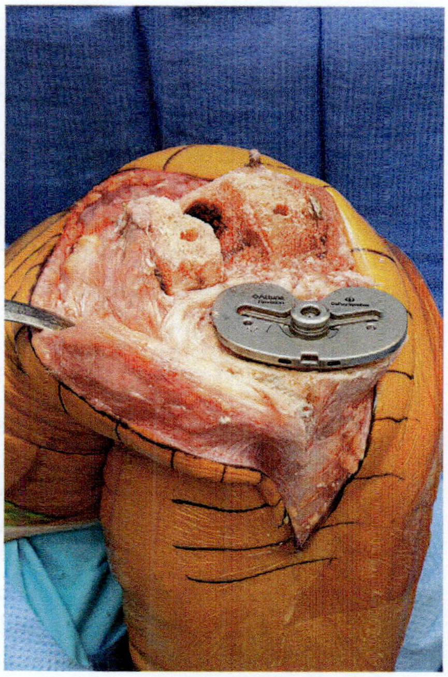

Figure 59.8 | Intraoperative photograph demonstrates reestablishment of the tibial platform perpendicular to the long axis of the tibia and with zero degrees posterior tibial slope. Note the slightly uncovered tibial bone laterally, which is typical when a straight tibial stem is used as the canal is offset slightly medial and anterior to the center of the proximal tibia.

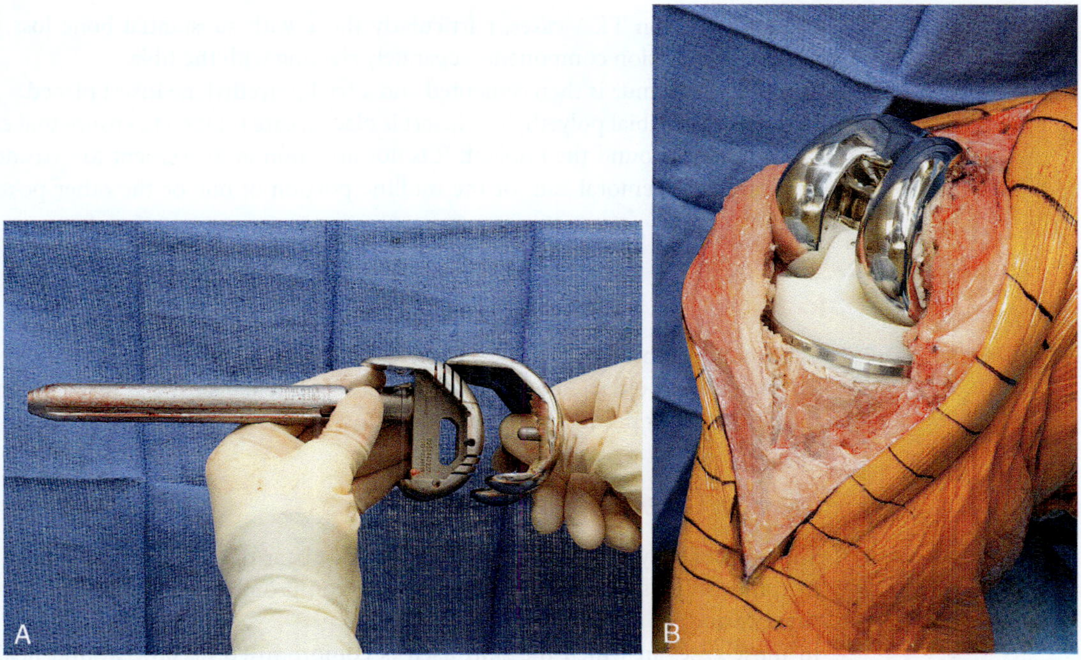

Figure 59.9 | Intraoperative photograph demonstrates that, when choosing the appropriate femoral component size in revision TKA, it is typically prudent to start with 1 size larger than that which was removed. A slightly larger femoral size helps the surgeon fill the flexion gap and restore stability in the revision TKA.

- Prepare the intramedullary canal of the femur for the surgeon's stem of choice.
- Address femoral bone defects at the articular surface with modular augments.
- Address cavitary or segmental femoral bone defects with porous metal cones or metaphyseal sleeves.
- Place trial femoral component, and assess stability in flexion with a trial tibial polyethylene insert.
- Fine tune the femoral component position in flexion if needed. Small adjustments to the flexion gap can be made with offset-stem adapters or by flexing the femoral component slightly and using a cemented femoral stem to achieve the desired flexion gap balance.

Reconstructive Step 3: Ensure Balance in Extension

- Determine if the extension space matches the flexion space just created by the chosen femoral component plus the tibial insert thickness.
- In some revision TKA cases the extension space is too loose or too big relative to the flexion space. In such circumstances, distal femoral augments can be added to move the joint line distally to restore balance.
- In many revision TKA cases, the extension space is too tight or too small relative to the flexion space. In such circumstances, additional distal femoral bone should be resected until the knee can fully extend. Although additional femoral resection does raise the joint, it is preferable to have a well-balanced knee than to become fixated upon maintaining the joint line.

Intraoperative Radiographs

- In most revision TKA cases, it is appropriate to check intraoperative radiographs with the trial components in place.
- On the AP radiograph the overall limb alignment, individual component varus-valgus alignment, and stem position are assessed.
- On the lateral radiograph the tibial slope, femoral offset, and stem position are assessed.

Cementing Components

- In many revision TKA cases, particularly those with substantial bone loss, it may be prudent to cement the revision components separately starting with the tibia.
- Typically, the femur is then cemented and a trial polyethylene insert placed.
- Before the real tibial polyethylene insert is placed, care is taken to ensure that excess cement has been cleaned from around the implant. It is not uncommon for cement to extrude posteriorly around a portion of the femoral cam or the midline portion of one or the other posterior femoral condyle (Figure 59.9)

Closure

- The wound is closed in multiple layers.
- The skin is most often closed with a running subcuticular suture as there is some evidence that allows the best vascular perfusion to the skin.

Postoperative Management

- The vast majority of patients are allowed weight bearing as tolerated (Figure 59.10)
- In some circumstances, bony or soft-tissue compromise will dictate protected weight bearing for some period.
- In those cases in which the skin itself is compromised or slow wound healing is anticipated the surgeon should prioritize wound healing over early range of motion and consider immobilizing the limb for a period.

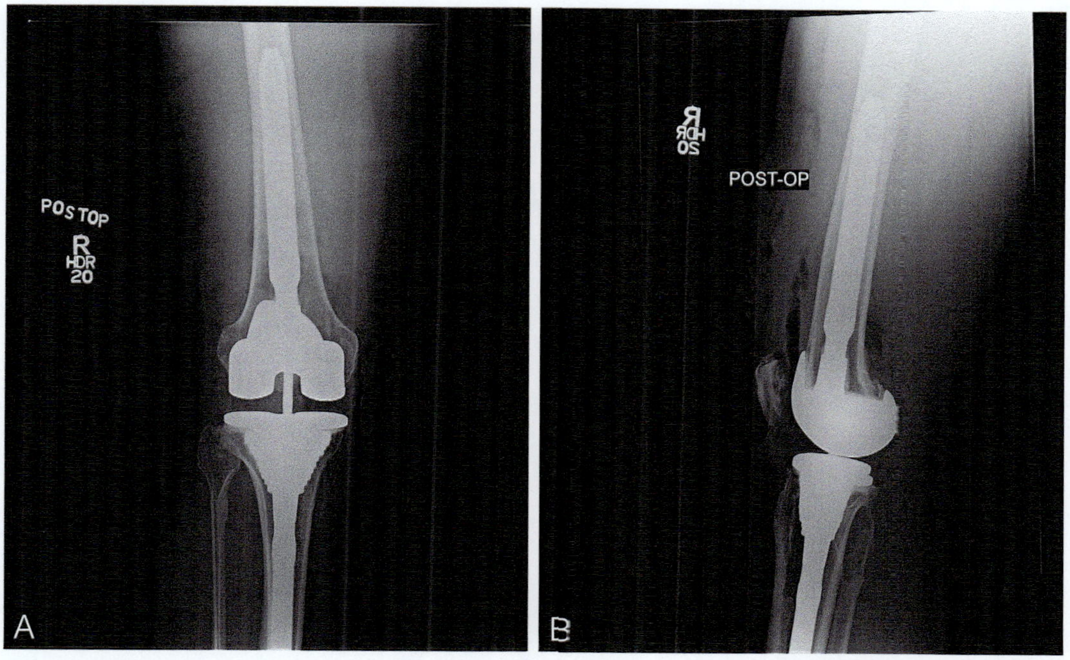

Figure 59.10 | Postoperative anteroposterior (A) and lateral (B) radiographs of a revision TKA that demonstrate appropriate reconstruction of the tibial platform in the sagittal and coronal planes, reestablishment of the flexion gap by restoring posterior femoral offset, and balance with full knee extension.

Summary

- An organized coherent strategy to revision TKA orders the surgeon's thinking such that logical decisions can be made even if the unexpected is encountered.
- The methodical 3-step approach to revision TKA has proved to be reliable, reproducible, and pragmatic: (1) reestablish the tibial platform, (2) restore balance in flexion by altering the AP size and offset of the femoral component, and (3) restore balance in extension by manipulating the joint line position proximally or distally.

Chapter 60
Extensile Exposures

ADAM HART
ROBERT T. TROUSDALE

Key Concepts

- Indications of a potentially difficult exposure (Figure 60.1) during revision surgery should be sought preoperatively by considering:
  - The superficial exposure—Evaluation of the skin and location of prior incisions, which may mandate the approach used at revision or prompt the opinion/help of a plastic surgeon.
  - The deep exposure—Evaluation for prior surgeries and implants, limited preoperative range of motion, significant obesity, and patella baja.
- Excellent exposure to the knee can be safely obtained by following a sequence of stepwise maneuvers described in this chapter, which consists of:
  - Skin and superficial dissection creating full-thickness skin flaps.
  - Medial arthrotomy and sequential soft tissue releases.
  - Removal of components.
  - Additional extensile exposures such as the quadriceps snip and tibial tubercle osteotomy.

Sterile Instruments and Implants

- Perioperative—Consider using intraoperative blood salvage systems, tranexamic acid, tourniquet, Foley catheterization, intraoperative fluoroscopy or x-rays.
- Extras—Consider a small blade saw, flexible osteotomes, and cerclage wires (for fixation of a tibial tubercle osteotomy).

Surgical Approaches

- A midline incision (unless contraindicated by prior surgeries) with a medial parapatellar arthrotomy with subluxation of the patella is most commonly used. The sub- or midvastus and lateral parapatellar approaches are less extensile and therefore avoided for revision surgeries.

Preoperative Planning

- Skin considerations—Careful evaluation of the skin for lesions, wounds, and prior incisions is mandatory. Generally, the cutaneous blood supply is from medial to lateral; therefore, the lateral-most acceptable longitudinal incision should be utilized. This also minimizes disruption of the lymphatic system, which drains from lateral to medial. A skin bridge of 7 cm is usually sufficient, and crossing incisions should be made at right angles (Figure 60.2). In complex cases, consultation with a plastic surgeon should be considered where soft tissue expanders or flaps may be necessary.
- Physical examination—Patients with notable stiffness are most likely to have a difficult exposure. Examination of passive range of motion as well as laxity in the coronal and sagittal planes and extensor mechanism function are paramount.

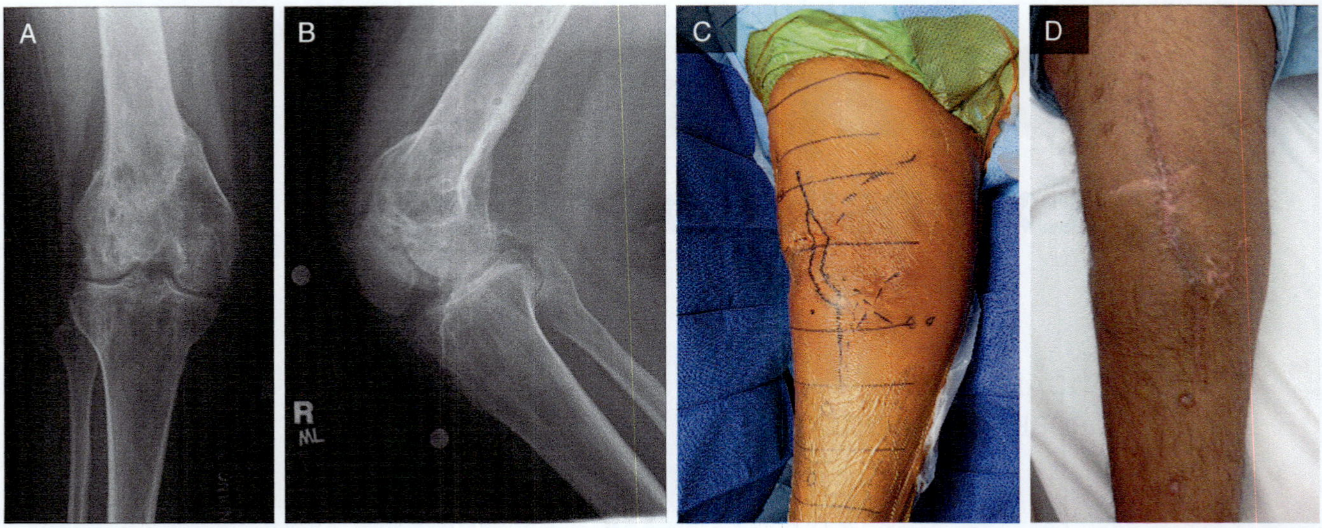

Figure 60.1 | A 20-year-old patient with posttraumatic arthritis of his right knee following a motor vehicle accident, traumatic arthrotomy, and subsequent open reduction and internal fixation (hardware removed). Preoperative radiographs (A and B), photograph of planed incision (solid lines) (C), and photograph of healed incision 6 weeks after total knee replacement (D).

- Radiographs—Evaluate the presence of deformity, bone quality, patella position, and current implanted components. A stemmed, cemented tibial component may prompt the use of a tibial tubercle osteotomy to facilitate implant and cement removal (Figure 60.3). Furthermore, review of prior operative reports is recommended to know exactly what components are implanted. Plan ahead to have the necessary instruments and parts needed during the revision surgery.

Bone, Implant, and Soft Tissue Techniques

- Place the patient in the supine position with supports according to surgeon preference, and drape a wider-than-usual field.
- Superficial exposure—Create full-thickness skin flaps through the planned incision. The correct plane of dissection can be found using the patella as a deep landmark, applying traction to the soft tissues during dissection with the knee in flexion, and extending the dissection proximal to the scar tissue to find the undisturbed soft tissue planes above the quadriceps muscle.

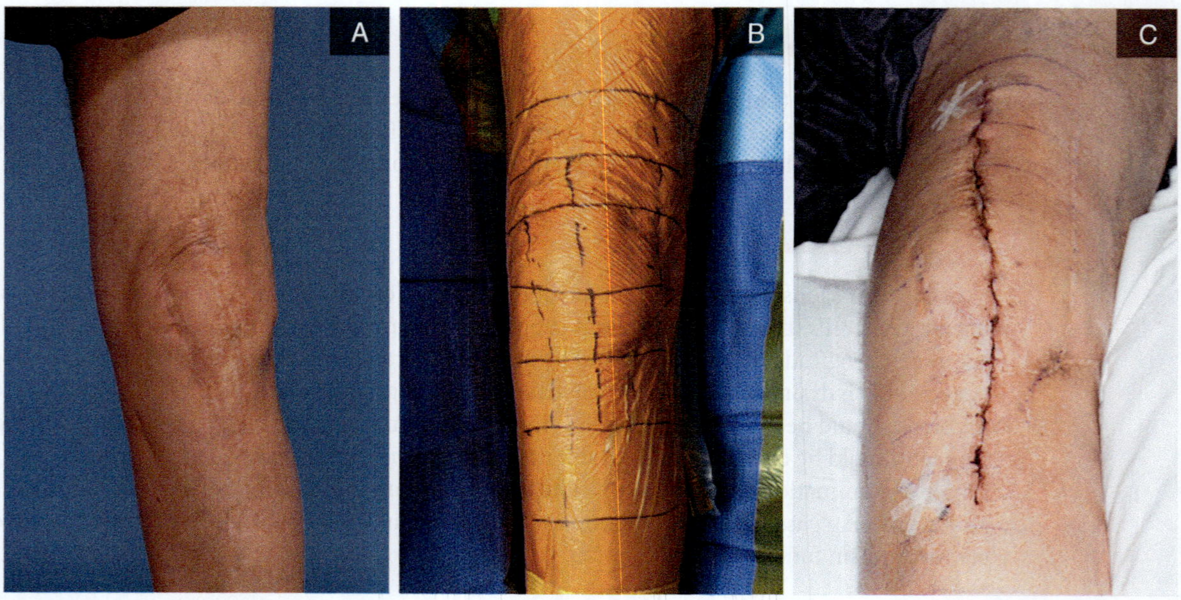

Figure 60.2 | Incision planning in a patient who has had multiple knee surgeries. Photograph preoperative (A), intraoperative (B), and postoperative (C).

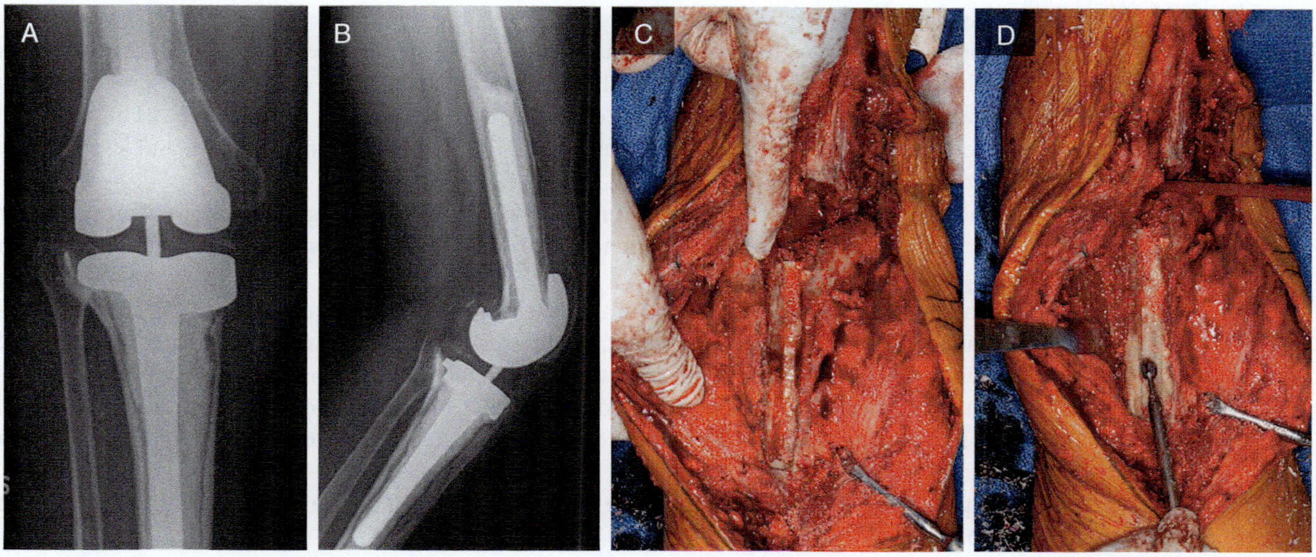

Figure 60.3 | A 59-year-old man with an infected total knee arthroplasty: preoperative radiographs (A and B) and intraoperative photographs of a tibial tubercle osteotomy to facilitate exposure and removal of the cemented tibial component (C and D).

- Medial parapatellar arthrotomy—Locate the medial aspect of the patella, patellar tendon, and tibial tubercle by palpation. Sutures from prior arthrotomy closure may help guide the trajectory of the arthrotomy. Sharp dissection may be used for the lower half of the arthrotomy followed by use of Mayo scissors to split the tendon proximally.
- Soft tissue releases—A systematic set of releases helps expose the knee:
  - Medial release (Figure 60.4A)—While placing medial traction on the soft tissues with a rake, release a full-thickness sleeve from the proximal medial tibia. This facilitates external rotation of the tibia and reduces tension over the extensor mechanism. The release may be extended all the way to the posteromedial tibial plateau. The insertion of the superficial medial collateral ligament must be carefully preserved 5 to 7 cm distal to the native joint line.
  - Femoral flange and gutters—With the knee in extension, scar and synovium should be released and excised from the anterior femur above the implanted component. Next, the medial and lateral gutters are released using a finger to palpate for bands of adhesions in need of release.
  - Retropatellar space (Figure 60.4B)—At the time of revision surgery, the extensor mechanism is often thickened and laden with scar tissue. With the knee still in extension, use a clamp to evert the patella and carefully excise scar/redundant soft tissues from the deep surface of the extensor mechanism taking care not to violate the tendon.

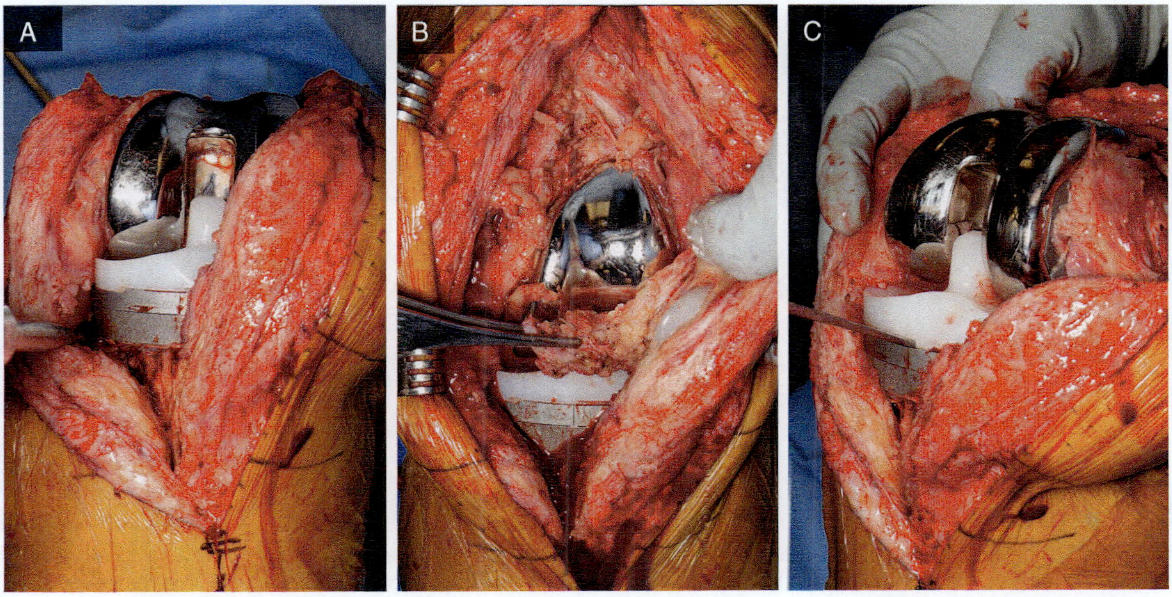

Figure 60.4 | Exposure with medial release (A), clearing of gutters and retropatellar scar (B), and removal of the polyethylene insert (C).

- Component removal
  - Before evaluating the need for an extensile exposure, the polyethylene should be removed, which will loosen the joint and facilitate mobilization of the patella. Many constrained inserts will have a screw or metal locking rod that needs to be removed before taking out the liner. A 1-inch curved osteotome is introduced between the insert and the metal tibial tray to unlock and lever out the polyethylene (Figure 60.4C).
  - If the patellar component requires removal (for example, during a resection arthroplasty for infection or a loose patellar component), this should be done now as it will help relieve tension along the extensor mechanism.
  - At this point, the ability to subluxate the patella should be assessed by placing a lateral retractor anchored on the tibial component, positioning the leg in maximum external rotation, and cautiously flexing the knee while assessing tension along the extensor mechanism. If the knee is still tight and exposure is compromised, an extensile maneuver should be considered (discussed later). In many revisions, lateral subluxation of the patella without patellar eversion is sufficient and most safe.
  - If exposure is sufficient, removal of the femoral and then tibial components will further improve exposure.
    - Femoral component: Use an oscillating saw with a thin blade to divide the interface on either side of the component (Figure 60.5A). A thin osteotome may be used to loosen the distal and posterior condyles. A square-tip impactor is then used to explant the component (Figure 60.5B).
    - Tibial component: In a similar fashion, use the oscillating saw to free the interface below the tibial tray. An osteotome may be inserted from medial to lateral posteriorly to free the interface behind the keel. A square-tip impactor is placed underneath the tray anteriorly to explant the component (Figure 60.5C).
- Extensile maneuvers
  - Quadriceps snip—This should be the first extensile maneuver to consider because it is fast and easy and can dramatically improve exposure by relieving tension over the extensor mechanism.
    - Following a standard medial parapatellar arthrotomy (Figure 60.6A and B), the tendon is divided at a 45° angle laterally using a knife or scissors approximately 10 cm proximal to the patella (Figure 60.6C and D).
    - Marking sutures may be placed on both sides of the snip's apex to facilitate anatomic repair during closure.
    - The authors use simple Vicryl sutures to repair the arthrotomy and include the snip portion of the arthrotomy in the repair.
  - Tibial tubercle osteotomy (Figure 60.7)—This method provides excellent exposure by allowing complete eversion of the extensor mechanism laterally. It may also be used to translate the tibial tubercle for patellar realignment or to improve access to a well-fixed tibial component for removal (Figure 60.3).

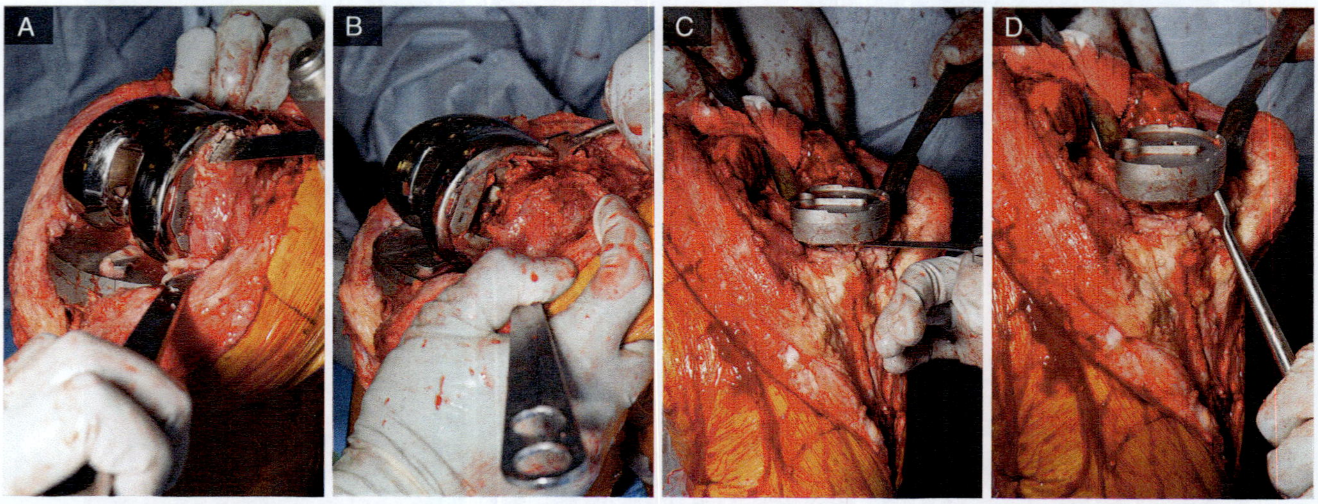

Figure 60.5 I Removal of implants using an oscillating saw to divide the implant-cement interface (A), square-tip impactor to explant the femoral component (B), oscillating saw to free the interface below the tibial tray (C), and square-tip impactor to explant the tibial component (D).

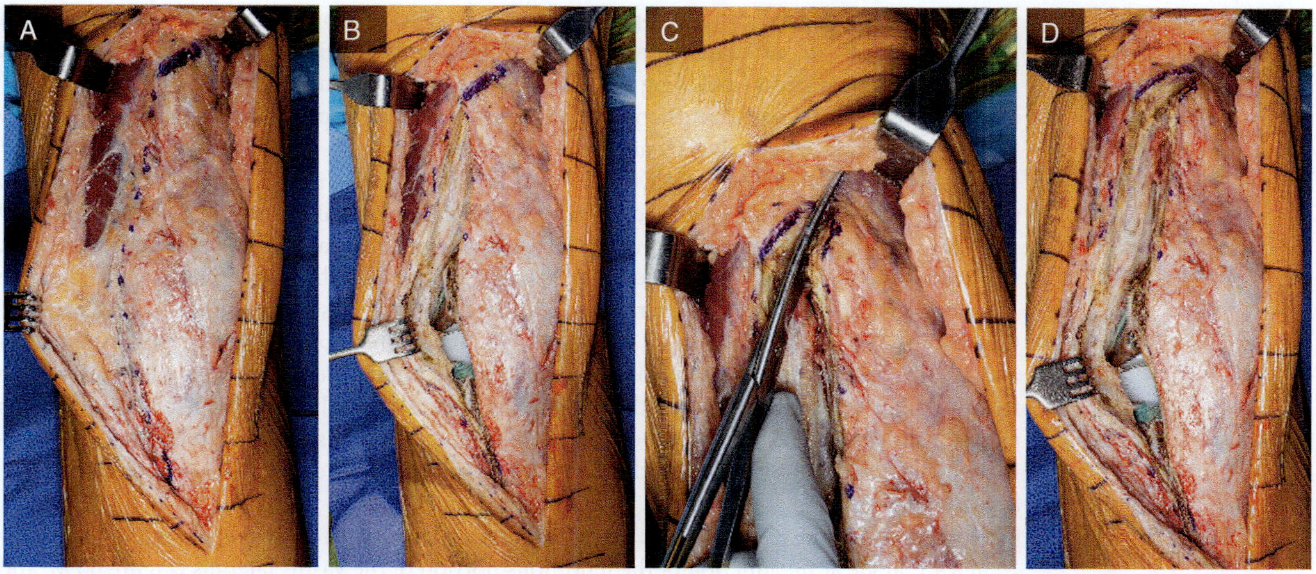

Figure 60.6 | Intraoperative photographs of a quadriceps snip during reimplantation of an infected knee replacement. Wide exposure is obtained in the appropriate plane above the tendon (A); the snip is performed approximately 10 cm above the patella at a 45° angle (B-D).

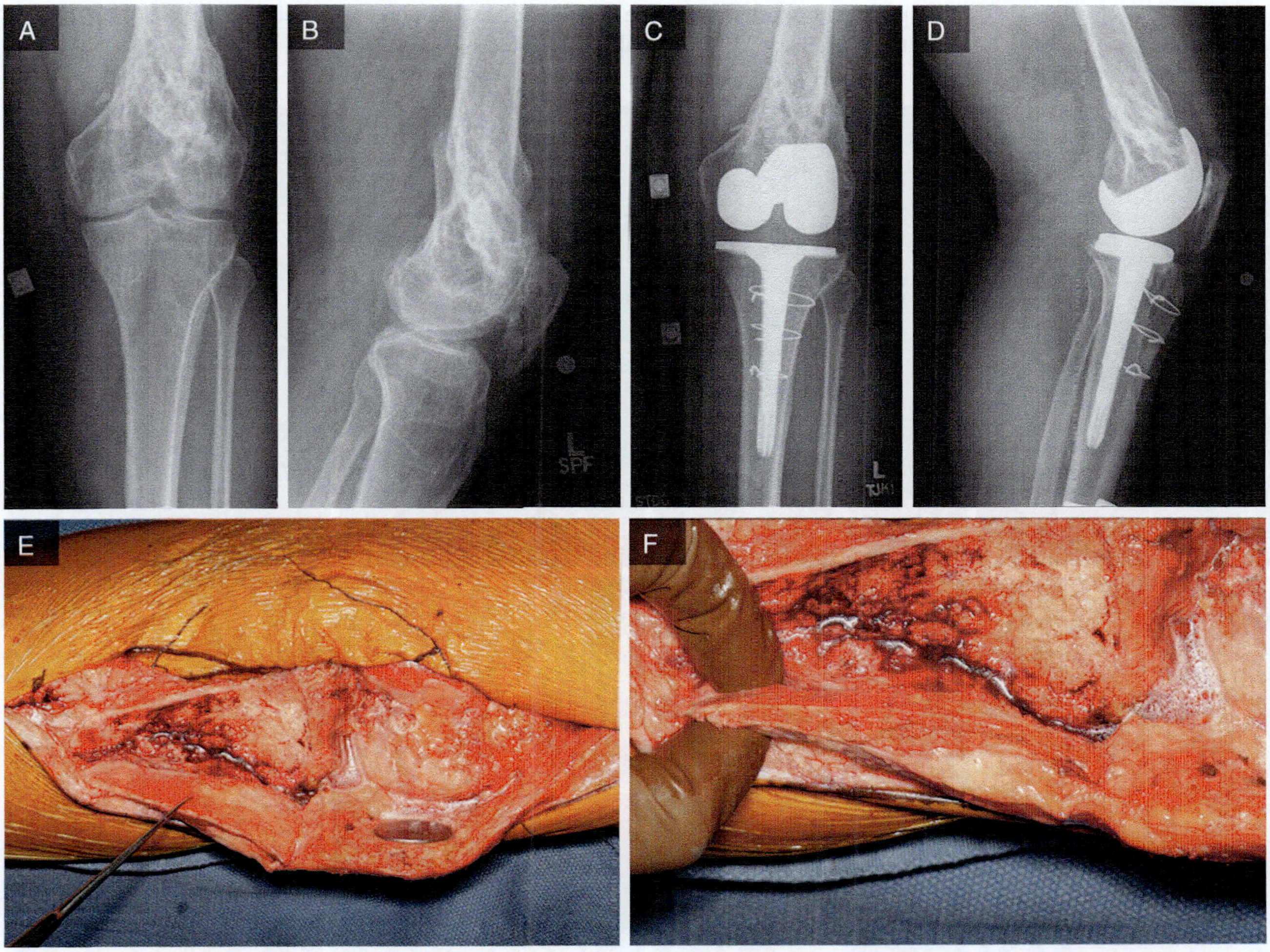

Figure 60.7 | Preoperative (A and B) and postoperative (C and D) radiographs of a primary total knee replacement in a patient with posttraumatic arthritis and a stiff knee. Intraoperative photographs (E and F) demonstrating use of a tibial tubercle osteotomy to facilitate exposure. A stemmed implant was used to bypass the osteotomy to protect against tibial fracture.

- Exposure is extended distally approximately 10 to 20 cm below the joint line. Using a small oscillating saw to cut along the anteromedial tibia (from medial to lateral), a long and thick segment of tibial crest (including the tibial tubercle) is osteotomized.
- Proximally, a flat transverse osteotomy surface is created to improve stability and resistance to proximal displacement after repair of the osteotomy.
- Distally, a tapered geometry is favored to avoid creating a stress riser at the tip of the osteotomy.
- The fragment is carefully wedged open from the anteromedial side using flat osteotomes by effectively hinging on the *preserved* periosteum and muscle attachments along the lateral side.
- Pass several 16-gauge wires through the intact anteromedial tibia to cerclage and stabilize the osteotomy. Screws or heavy sutures may also been used for this purpose.

- Quadriceps V-Y turndown (Figure 60.8)—provides excellent exposure by reflecting the patella and patellar tendon inferiorly. Although recovery and clinical results are generally inferior to those of other extensile exposures, the quadriceps turndown might rarely be used when a quads snip is insufficient and the tibial tubercle is compromised (e.g., has significant osteolysis precluding reliable healing of a tibial tubercle osteotomy). To repeat: this exposure is rarely required.
  - A standard medial arthrotomy is performed (Figure 60.8E).
  - Starting above the patella, the quadriceps tendon is divided laterally and extending inferiorly at a 45° angle at the junction of the tendinous portion of the vastus lateralis (Figure 60.8F and G). The lateral division may be carried inferiorly as far as the joint line to reflect the extensor mechanism inferiorly.
  - Repair of the tendon is performed on both medial and lateral arthrotomies. If the extensor mechanism is excessively tight and cannot be repaired anatomically, it may be lengthened at the junction proximally using a "V" to "Y" technique. Note that excessive lengthening may lead to an extensor lag and should be avoided.

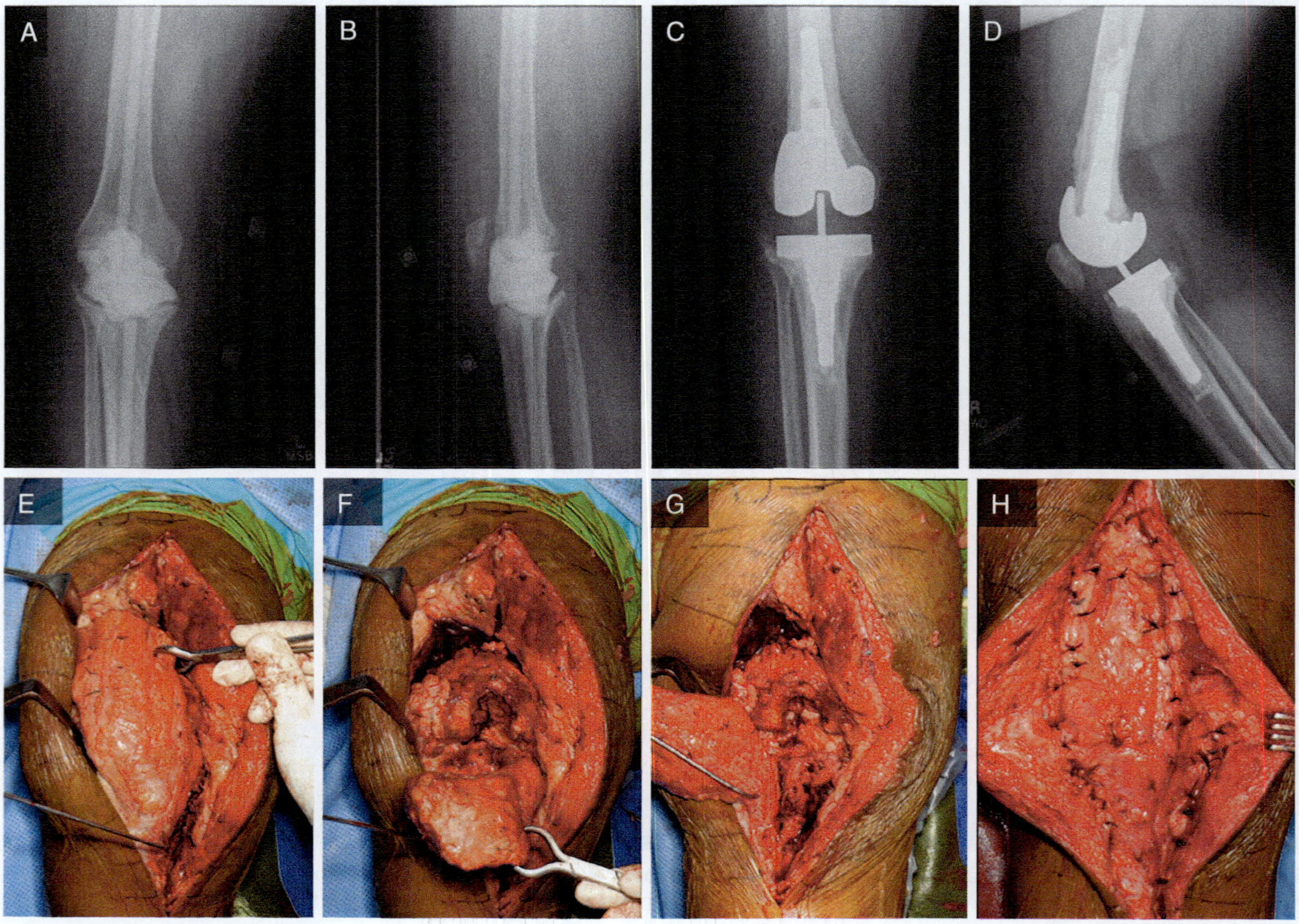

Figure 60.8 | Preoperative (A and B) and postoperative (C and D) radiographs of a reimplantation following resection arthroplasty for infection. A quadriceps V-Y turndown was utilized owing to significant scaring of the extensor mechanism and tenuous attachment at the tibial tubercle. Intraoperative photographs demonstrating scared extensor mechanism (E), exposure following turndown (F and G), and repair (H).

Postoperative Care

- Quadriceps snip—no change in postoperative care is needed. Unless otherwise contraindicated, we allow for full weight bearing and activity as tolerated.
- Tibial tubercle osteotomy—Assuming a relatively solid repair of the fragment, the authors allow unrestricted range of motion with protected weight bearing for 6 weeks.
- Quadriceps V-Y turndown—The repair is protected postoperatively by placing the knee in a cast or immobilizer in full extension and partial weight bearing for 6 weeks. A hinged brace is then applied to progress knee flexion in 30° intervals over the next 6 weeks.

Chapter 61
Implant Removal

ASHTON H. GOLDMAN
KEVIN I. PERRY

Key Concepts

- Bone preservation is critical to ensure host bone for uncemented metaphyseal fixation augmented with either uncemented or cemented diaphyseal fixation in the revision setting.
- For the removal of cemented implants, first define and delineate the implant/cement interface, then disrupt the implant/cement interface for a few millimeters with a saw, and then use osteotomes to complete interface disruption.
- Do not try to remove a component before complete interface disruption.
- Often the patellar component can be retained. Scenarios that require patella removal include significant patellar wear, patellar component loosening, or periprosthetic joint infection.
- The patellar tendon should be protected throughout the entirety of the case.

Sterile Instruments and Implants

- Standard knee retractors
- Sagittal saw
- Gigli saw for removal of uncemented implants
- Flexible and stiff osteotomes of multiple widths
- Moreland type osteotomes
- 6.5 mm and pencil-tip burrs
- Cerclage wires if osteotomy is performed
- Metal cutting burr (if needed)
- Diamond cutting wheel (if needed)

Surgical Approaches

- A standard extensile medial parapatellar approach is recommended.
- A quadriceps snip can be performed and is recommended for the stiff knee revision. No change in postoperative protocols is necessary when performed.
- A tibial tubercle osteotomy (TTO) can be useful in cases with severe patella baja or with a well-fixed long press fit or cemented stem to facilitate implant removal.
- Minimally invasive approaches are not recommended.

Preoperative Planning

- Anteroposterior and lateral radiographs of the entire implants aid with identification of current implants, fixation methods, as well as anatomical features that may increase difficulty in implant removal (i.e., patella baja).
- Certain implants have specific locking mechanisms on the polyethylene liner or have modular connections where implant-specific extraction devices are useful.

- Osteolysis is always underestimated on preoperative films and must be considered. A metal suppression computed tomography scan may sometimes be useful to more accurately assess bone loss.
- Plan for the specific implant that will be utilized at the time of revision and consider a backup plan. Often higher levels of constraint are needed. If substantial femoral osteolysis is present, then a hinge should be available in case either collateral ligaments is compromised.

Bone, Implant, and Soft Tissue Techniques

- Perform a standard approach to the knee.
- After medial parapatellar arthrotomy, clear the gutters and evaluate the need for a quadriceps snip or TTO to protect the extensor mechanism.

Polyethylene

- Remove the modular polyethylene insert with implant-specific tools that disrupt the locking mechanism, or it can be removed with an osteotome and mallet with relative ease. If removing a varus-valgus constrained insert, often the metal support post must be removed before removing the polyethylene insert.
- For an all-polyethylene component a saw can be utilized at the implant-cement interface to separate the keel and facilitate removal.

Femoral Component

- Define femoral interface and use a small saw blade at the implant-cement interface to initiate disruption. This is not possible for the posterior condyles of the femur. This can also be accomplished with a pencil-tip burr (Figures 61.1 and 61.2).
- Use flexible osteotomes in the implant-cement interface to connect the medial and lateral sides of the anterior flange. In the cruciate retaining component, small osteotomes can be used in the central cut out to further aid with bone preservation (Figures 61.3 and 61.4).
- While protecting the medial and lateral collateral ligaments, respectively, use narrow flexible osteotome to disrupt interface of the posterior condyles medially and laterally (Figure 61.5).
- Tamp the implant out. Be careful not to stress the extensor mechanism during this maneuver. External rotation of the tibia helps protect the patellar tendon insertion.

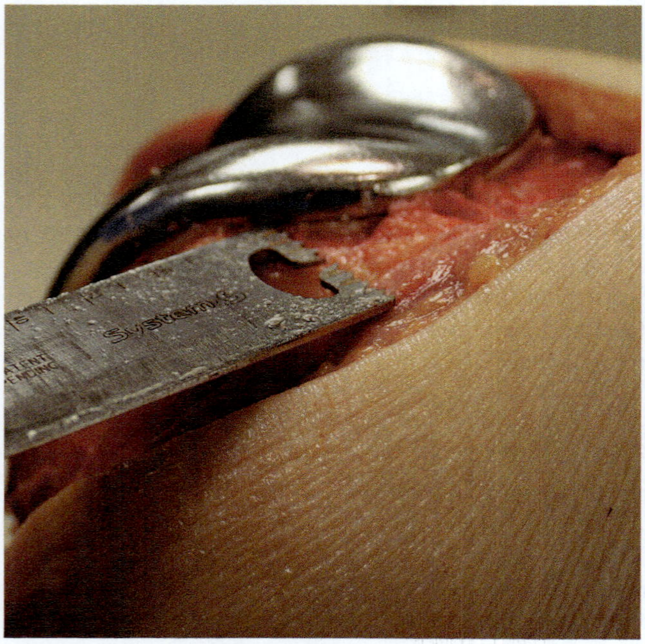

Figure 61.1 | Define the implant-cement interface with a sagittal saw.

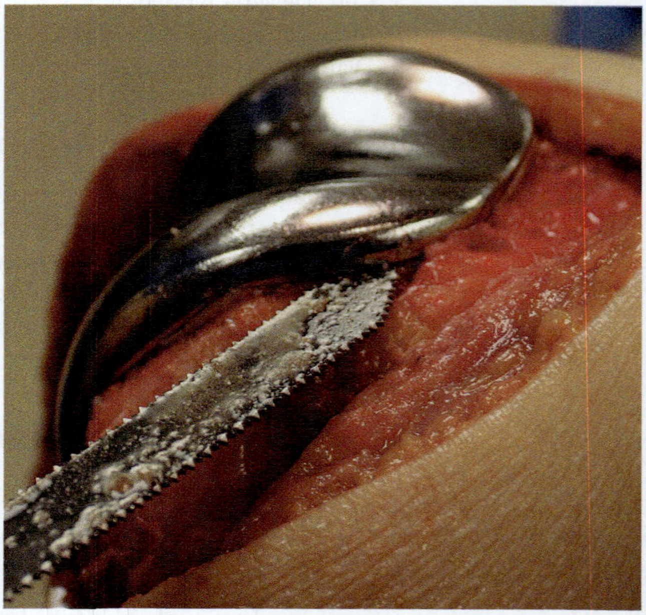

Figure 61.2 | Alternatively, define the implant-cement interface with a reciprocating saw.

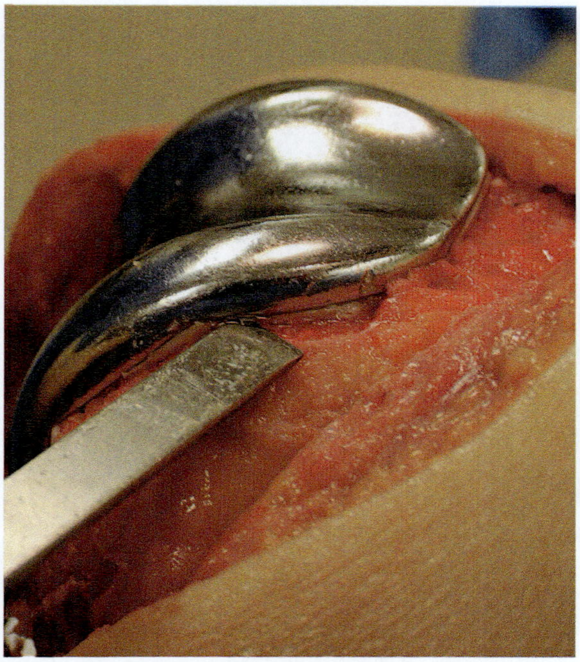

Figure 61.3 | Identify the correct plane of the interface after it has been disrupted with an osteotome.

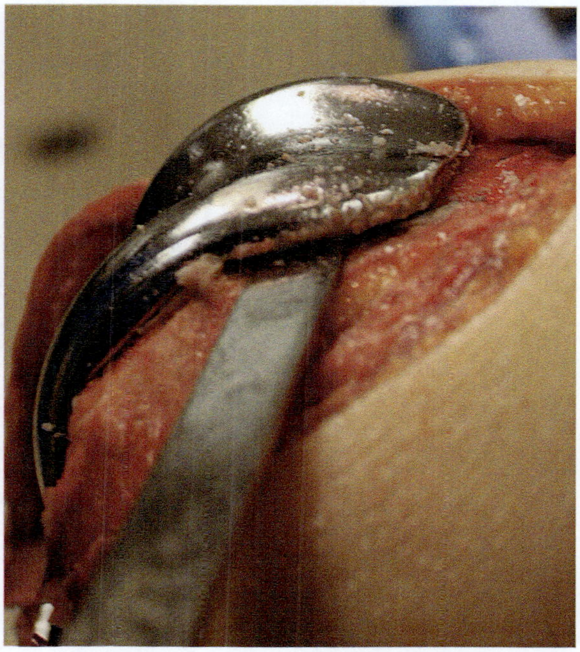

Figure 61.4 | Pass an osteotome to the midline from both sides ensuring a complete disruption of the anterior flange interface.

- Following implant removal, osteotomes can be used to create several cracks in the cement mantle. Removing cement in small sections minimizes bone loss.
- Cement in the canal can be removed with Moreland-type osteotomes: Several propagation cracks are created circumferentially followed by narrow osteotomes around the bone cement interface.
- If the cement mantle is robust, the use of an ultrasound device can facilitate cement removal.
- If a cement restrictor needs to be removed, use a drill to create a hole followed by back scratching canal debriders. If there is concern for perforation, as in the case of a long cemented stem, do this under fluoroscopic guidance.

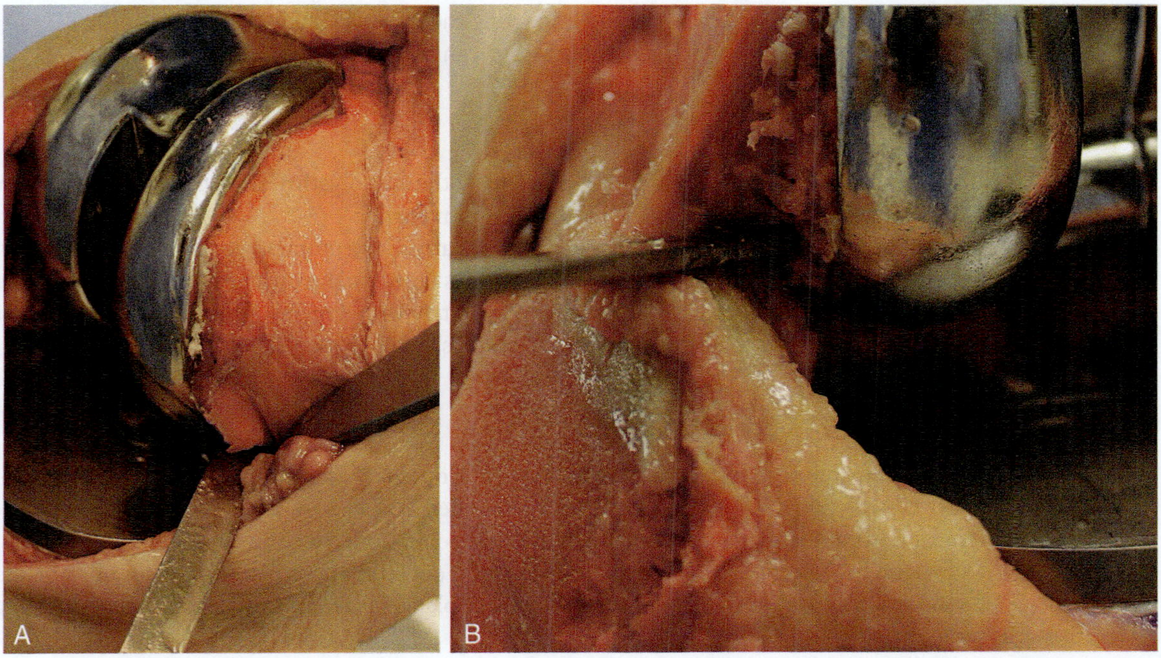

Figure 61.5 | On both the medial (A) and lateral sides (B) pass a small osteotome along the posterior femoral condyle to free this portion of the implant. If not done, marked posterior bone loss can occur making sizing and rotation of the revision construct more difficult.

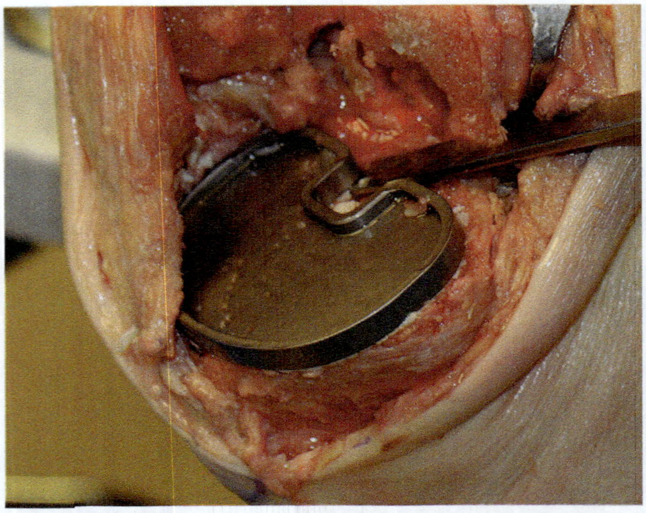

Figure 61.6 | A complete release medially to reach the posteromedial corner allows one to pass an osteotome to the posterolateral tibia behind a keeled implant.

Tibial Component

- Define implant-cement interface from as far laterally as the patellar tendon safely allows all the way to the posterior cruciate ligament insertion. This can be safely done without for 1 cm from the joint line.
- Flexion and external rotation allows access to the posteromedial corner of the tibia.
- Begin anteriorly and disrupt implant cement interface with a saw and osteotome.
- Work posteromedially to get a small, narrow osteotome from medial to lateral behind the keel to release the posterolateral corner of the tibial implant. This is the most difficult area for implant disruption and if not appropriately released can cause significant bone loss (Figure 61.6).
- Wide osteotomes and saws are not recommended for release of the posterolateral corner owing to the risk to neurovascular structures.
- An alternative method of tibial implant removal can be performed by placing a small metaphyseal perforation on the medial or lateral side of the tibia and placing a small round impactor against the metaphyseal side of the tibial tray and impacting the tray proximally (Figure 61.7).
- Be careful not to lever on the intact tibia as this can easily cause fracture (Figure 61.8).

Patella Component

- A saw at the implant cement interface can remove the all-polyethylene patella component. The pegs can be removed separately with the use of a 6.5-mm burr.
- Metal-backed components can be removed with narrow osteotomes between the pegs to loosen the implant. If it remains well fixed, a diamond wheel is useful to disrupt the bone-implant interface and transect the pegs. The pegs can be removed separately with a metal cutting burr if they remain well fixed or simply left in place during aseptic revisions.

Stemmed Components

- Most uncemented stemmed components are not designed for bone ingrowth and are commonly removed with standard techniques described earlier. Likewise, most cemented components can be removed from their cement mantle with the above-mentioned techniques.
- Occasionally, stemmed components do not come out with the articular portion of implants often because of the complex geometry at the stem-implant junction. If this occurs, the following steps can be utilized.
- First, disassemble modular connections and remove the articular portion of the implant. This should afford access to the stem and cement mantle.

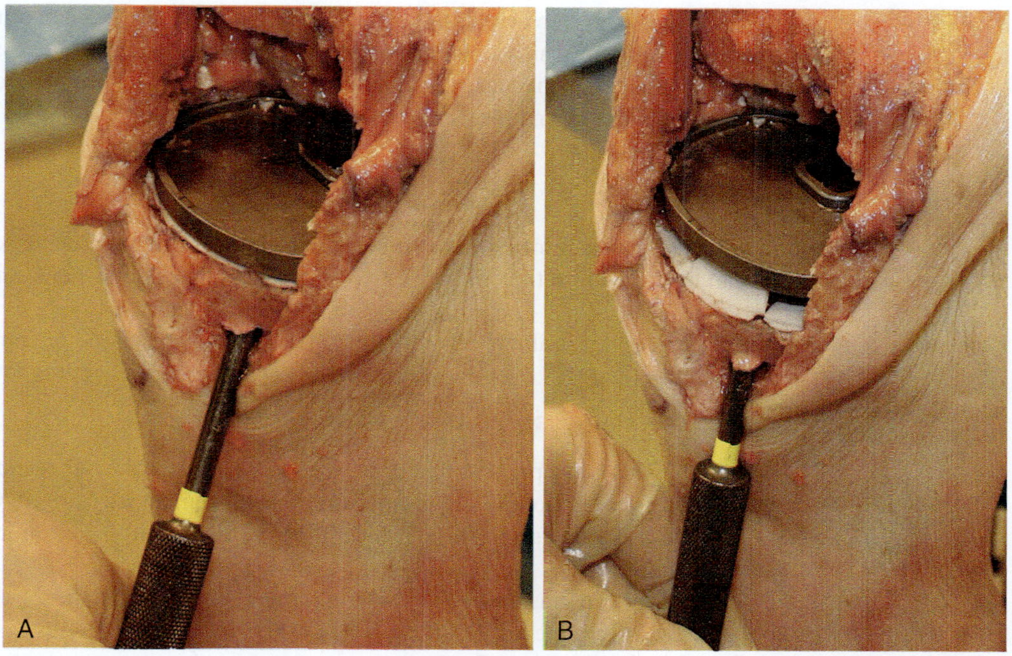

Figure 61.7 I A small round impactor can aid in removing the tibial component. A,B. A controlled metaphyseal perforation can be created that allows placement of a small round impactor against the metaphyseal side of the tibial tray to aid with removing the tibial component.

- In rare circumstances, diamond cutting wheel or metal cutting burr can be used to cut a box out of the tibial tray overlying the tibial stem to gain access to the stem. Likewise, on the femur, the stem can be cut at the most proximal aspect of the implant seen.
- An undercutting tool can create a trough in the stem to use an extraction back-slap hammer.
- Avoid the temptation to place osteotomes down the surface of the implant as this can cause fracture or perforation of the bone.
- If a femoral stem is well fixed proximally, a femoral episiotomy or anteriorly based osteotomy can be performed to aid in removal. If an osteotomy is done, the cortical piece should be kept vascular to allow healing.

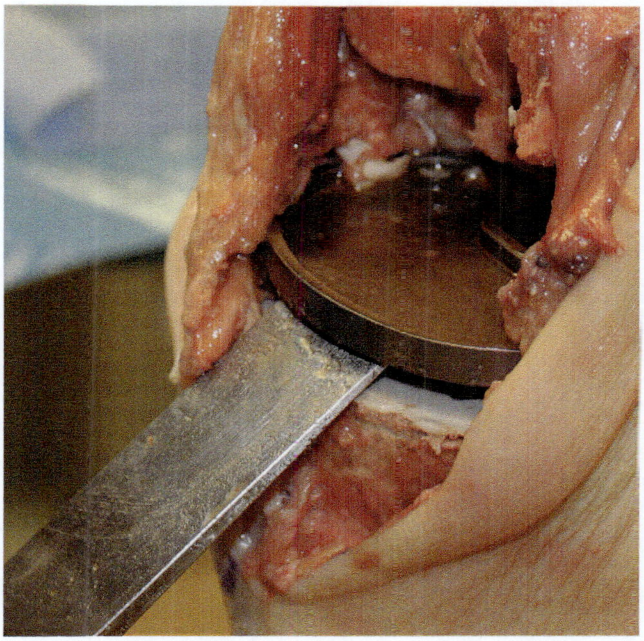

Figure 61.8 I When removing the tibial component with osteotomes do not lever on the already compromised bone as it is easy to create a fracture.

- A TTO can be used to gain access to the tibial canal for extraction or cement removal.
- In the rare scenario in which tibial osteotomy fails to provide enough access to remove the distal portion of the implant, a metal cutting burr can be used to transect the stem followed by the use of a trephine to remove the remaining stem.

Cement Columns

- Fluoroscopic guidance is important to prevent perforations when removing cement columns.
- A drill can be placed into the cement restrictor and canal back-scratchers can aid in the removal of cement.
- Ultrasonic devices can facilitate cement removal but are expensive and often not necessary.

Ingrown Metaphyseal Cones and Sleeves

- Narrow osteotomes and a pencil-tip burr can be used to disrupt the bone-implant interface.
- After all implants are removed, one must ensure that all cement is removed. Canal cement can disrupt alignment in the revision setting or be a nidus for recurrent infection in the case of periprosthetic joint infection.
- A thorough inspection must be done following cement removal. Sometimes it is necessary to change positions (i.e., move to the head of the table or other side of the table) to gain an adequate view of areas of cement that remains. The 3 most common areas for cement retention are the femoral lug holes, the patellar lug holes, and the tibial drill holes for the extramedullary cutting jig.

Postoperative Care

- In a revision for infection, critically analyze postoperative radiographs to ensure all cement was removed.
- In an aseptic revision with previous press-fit stems, understand that the canal is now polished and that diaphyseal cement fixation alone is inadequate for fixation.
- If a quadriceps snip or TTO is performed and adequately repaired, no change to the postoperative course is needed.
- Protected weight bearing is recommend if a further episiotomy or cortical window was established.

Chapter 62
Use of Stems: Cemented and Uncemented

GRAHAM D. PALLANTE
DANIEL J. BERRY

Key Concepts

- Stems are indicated in almost all revision total knee arthroplasty (TKA). Data show that routine use of stems in revision TKA leads to fewer failures than discretionary use of stems.
- Stems provide the benefit of enhanced mechanical fixation while distributing the load over a greater area, which is important in total knee arthroplasty revision (TKAR) because bone quality and quantity usually are compromised by failure of the previous implant, stress shielding, or bone loss related to implant removal.
- Conceptually, there are 3 main areas for implant fixation in TKAR: (1) the bone surfaces of the femur and tibia, (2) the metaphyses of the femur and tibia, and (3) the diaphysis of the femur and tibia. The bone surfaces typically are fixed with cement. Metaphyseal fixation may be with cement or with uncemented sleeves or cones. Diaphyseal fixation is with stems, which may be cemented or uncemented.
- Both cemented and uncemented stems can provide reliable, stable fixation in revision TKA. Each has advantages and disadvantages.
- Stem choice should be based on available implants, remaining bone stock, presence of bony deformity, and ease of extraction.
- Most uncemented stems obtain a press fit in the diaphysis but do not provide true biologic fixation because most do not have bone ingrowth or ongrowth surfaces. Uncemented stems may be easier to insert and extract than cemented stems. Final implant position is dictated by the diaphysis. This can sometimes be modified with offset stems. When bone deformity is present, uncemented stems allow less latitude to compensate than cemented stems. Pain at the stem tip has been reported in some patients with uncemented stems.
- Cemented stems provide immediate and long-term fixation. They provide more versatility in the presence of bone deformity than uncemented stems but in the presence of normal anatomy provide less alignment guidance. Cemented stems allow for local antibiotic delivery from the cement. Cemented stems typically are more difficult to extract than uncemented stems.
- Despite advantages and disadvantages of each method, cemented or uncemented stems can be used in most cases, depending on surgeon preference (Figures 62.1 and 62.2).
- Suggested indications for uncemented stems:
  - Good diaphyseal bone quality, favorable canal geometry, minimal or reconstructible metaphyseal bone loss that allows a good cement interface.
- Suggested indications for cemented stems:
  - Poor diaphyseal bone quality, unfavorable canal geometry for uncemented implant.

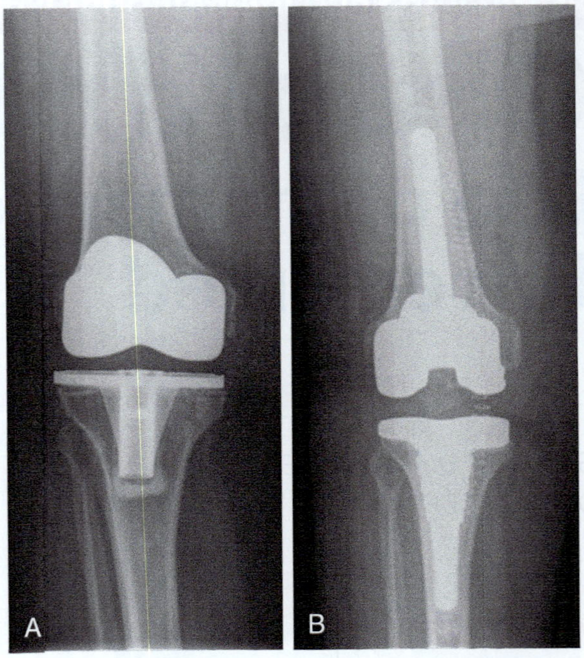

Figure 62.1 | A, Preoperative radiograph of patient with loose tibial component. B, Postoperative radiograph after revision with components with cemented stems.

Sterile Instruments and Implants

Instruments

- Revision TKA instrumentation
- Reamers for cemented or uncemented stems
- Trial implants for cemented or uncemented stems
- Power and hand reaming instruments for the stems
- Pulse lavage with femoral attachment for canal irrigation
- Metaphyseal cones, sleeves as needed
- Bone grafts as needed

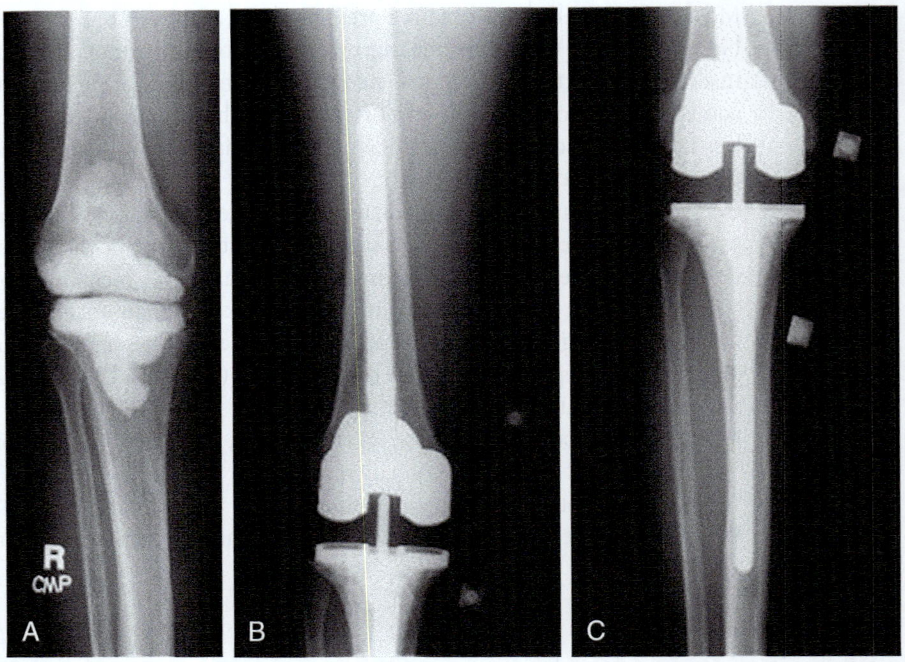

Figure 62.2 | A, Radiograph of patient after resection arthroplasty for infection with static antibiotic-loaded cement spacer in place. B and C, Radiographs after reconstruction with uncemented stems.

- Intraoperative radiography capability
- For cemented stems: cement gun, cement restrictor, vacuum cement mixer

Implants

- Uncemented stems (with instrumentation) in multiple lengths and diameters, with offset options if desired
- Cemented stems (with instrumentation) in multiple lengths and diameters

Positioning

- Revision TKA: femoral and tibial implants
- Supine
- Nonsterile tourniquet

Surgical Approaches

- Standard, midline approach with median parapatellar arthrotomy is preferred. Considerations should be made for previous skin incisions or soft tissue defects.
- Extensile knee approaches such as quadriceps snip or tibial tubercle osteotomy may be required. See Section IV-B, Chapter 2 for details.

Preoperative Planning

- Obtain previous operative reports and implant records.
- Obtain full-length hip-to-ankle radiograph. Determine the desired mechanical alignment and determine which stem configurations can help achieve this.
- If the tibial or femoral component will be retained, review the manufacturer's revision instrumentation options. Custom or seldom used implants may require shipment from the device company.
- Template femoral and tibial stem length, diameter, and component position. Anticipate use of uncemented or cemented stems.

Bone, Implant, and Soft Tissue Techniques

- Perform the desired approach to the knee, employing an extensile approach if needed. If possible, it is preferable to use the previous incision. If multiple incisions are present, utilizing the most lateral incision possible is desirable.
- Remove implants, being careful to preserve as much bone as possible (see Section IV-B, Chapter 3).
- After implant removal, there is often a thin membrane of fibrous tissue within the canal that requires removal. Use reverse or uterine curettes to extract this layer.
- Remove cement from host bone using a combination of osteotomes, curettes, high-speed burrs, and ultrasonic cement extraction set as needed. If planning for an uncemented stem, it is important to meticulously extract cement in the diaphysis, where a concentric press fit is required.
- After debridement, perform thorough irrigation of the intramedullary canal and metaphyseal bone.

Bone Preparation

- Assess bone loss and deformity to determine need for augmentation, sleeves, or cones.
- Utilize landmarks such as the tibial tubercle, femoral condyles, fibular head, and meniscal remnant to estimate the level of the joint line.
- Based on preoperative templating, ream the tibia and/or femur to the desired diameter. Depth can be approximated based on markings found on the reamer.
- When reaming the femur, utilize preoperative AP and lateral radiographs to set the starting point.
- While reaming, make sure the reamer remains centralized within the canal to avoid eccentric reaming. This is particularly important on the femoral side, where anterior bow can lead to flexion of the component if reamer is not in line with the axis of the femur.

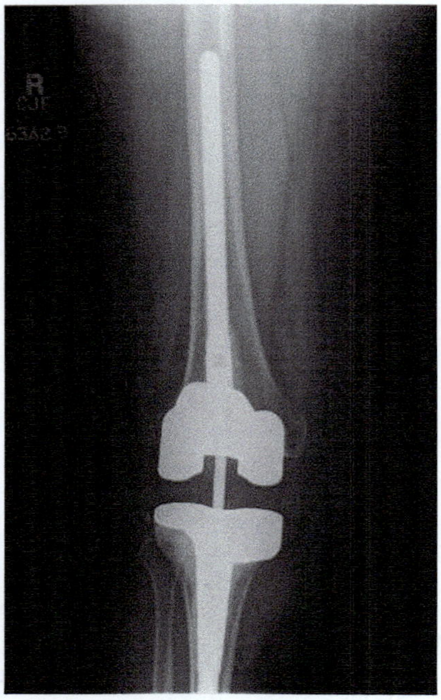

Figure 62.3 | Radiograph of uncemented femoral stem engaging the distal femoral diaphysis following line-to-line reaming.

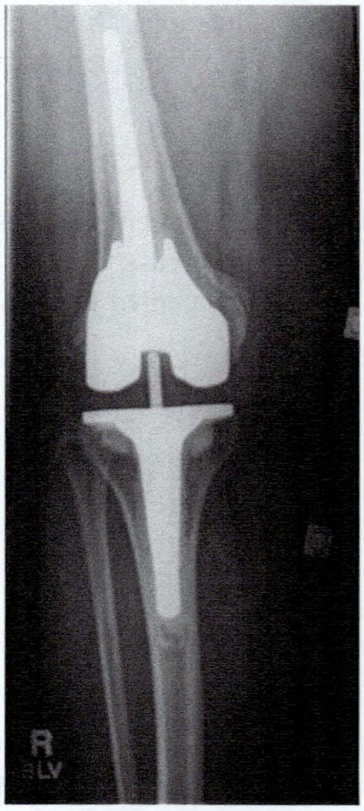

Figure 62.4 | Reconstruction of a knee with cemented stems and a femoral metaphyseal cone. Note the good cement interdigitation provided by maintenance of the cancellous bone and good cement pressurization.

- For uncemented stems, ream until firm, cortical contact is established. Diaphyseal engagement is critical for stability (Figure 62.3). Particular attention should be paid while reaming osteopenic bone to ensure an iatrogenic fracture or perforation does not occur. Hand reamers can be utilized to allow direct tactile feedback to the surgeon during reaming. Flexible reamers may decrease the risk of perforating an especially thin cortex but usually are used only when a curved stem will be used. Line-to-line reaming is often preferred. However, stem geometry may necessitate slight overreaming or underreaming.
- For cemented stems, the canal should be slightly overreamed to accommodate the stem and a cement mantle (utilize a reamer approximately 2 mm larger in diameter than the stem). Care should be taken not to ream more than necessary to avoid removing valuable cancellous bone needed for cement interdigitation (Figure 62.4). Additionally, excessive reaming leaves a larger bone envelope, which increases the chance of implant malalignment.
- If metaphyseal sleeves or cones will be utilized, ream/mill/broach to prepare for these implants at this stage.
- Trial components should then be assembled and inserted with augments as appropriate. If needed, offset stems can be chosen to optimize position of the femoral and tibial components on the distal femur and proximal tibia.
- Evaluate flexion/extension gaps. Determine if adjustments are required to achieve good soft tissue balance in flexion and extension.
- Obtain an intraoperative radiograph after trial implants are placed to assess alignment. This is particularly important for uncemented stems to assess stem sizing and alignment (Figure 62.5) and for cemented stems to assess alignment.

Component Implantation

Uncemented Stems

- Use pulse lavage to thoroughly clear bony surfaces of debris. Dry exposed surfaces while cement is mixed on the back table. Cover the surface of bone with cement and push cement well into the cancellous metaphyseal bone of the distal femoral canal and proximal tibial canal (Figure 62.6). This step is important because it provides metaphyseal cement fixation of the implant in addition to the modest cement fixation provided by surface cementation to the prepared surfaces of the femur and tibia. Avoid putting cement into the center of the canal that could be carried all the way into the canal by the stem tip (Figure 62.7).

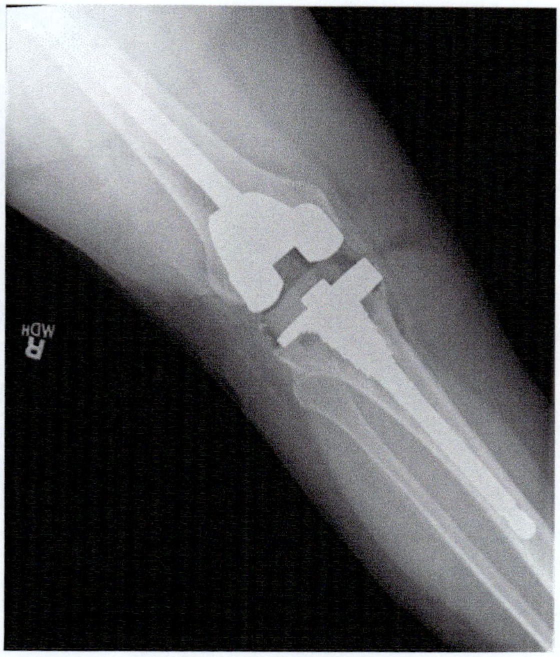

Figure 62.5 | Intraoperative radiograph to check implant alignment and stem fit for TKA revision with uncemented stems.

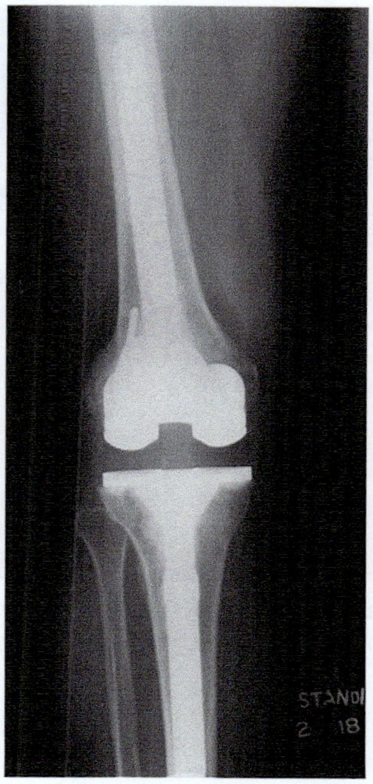

Figure 62.6 | When using uncemented stems, pressurize cement well into the metaphysis.

- Coat the distal femoral and proximal tibial implants with cement, including about 5 to 8 cm of the metaphyseal portion of the implant (Figure 62.8). Next, generously impact the implant in position. As the uncemented stem engages in the diaphysis, make sure the implant rotation is correct, because flutes (if present) will guide rotation once they are engaged.
- Remove excess cement around the periphery of the component and posteriorly.

Cemented Stems

- A cement restrictor should be placed no more than 1 cm beyond the planned stem tip. While holding the trial component with stem attached next to the cement restrictor implantation tool, use a marking pen to set the depth (Figure 62.9).
- Once the cement restrictor is in place, use pulse lavage with both standard and femoral attachments to thoroughly irrigate the canal and cut femoral and tibial surfaces to clear all debris at the cement-bone interface (Figure 62.10). Dry the canal with suction and dry sponges making sure the sponge is completely extracted.

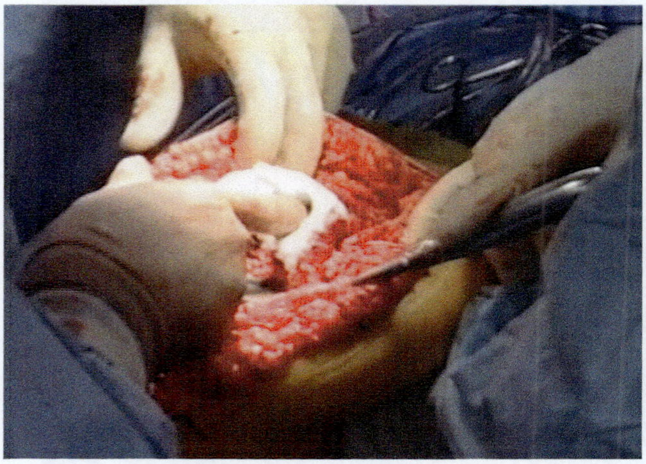

Figure 62.7 | Pressurization of cement well into the femoral metaphyseal bone in preparation for a revision component with a stem that is uncemented in the diaphysis.

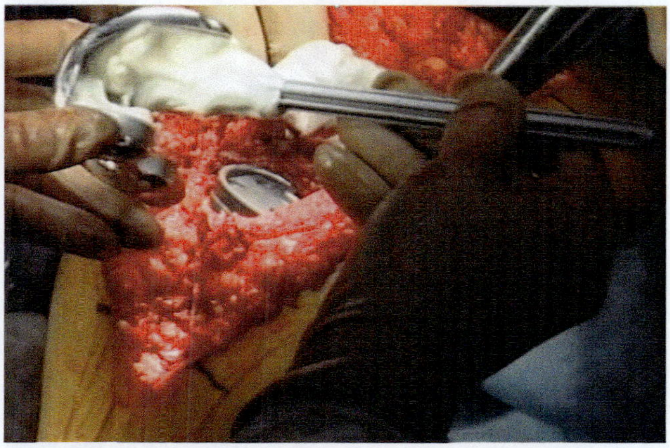

Figure 62.8 | Placement of cement onto the metaphyseal portion of the implant when using an uncemented stem.

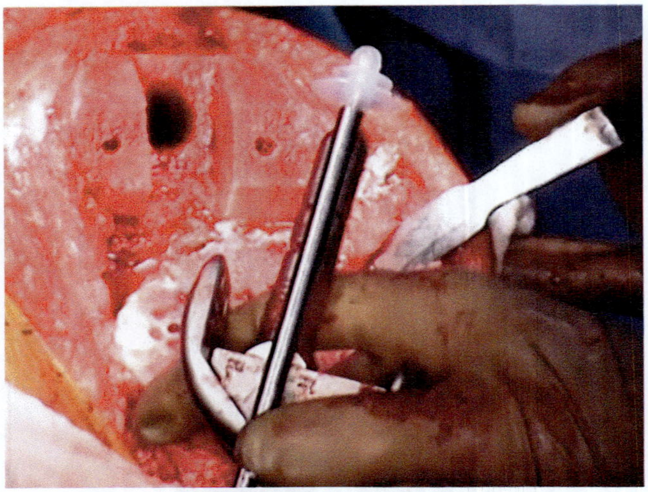

Figure 62.9 | Measuring for depth of insertion of cement restrictor. Mark the depth on the insertion rod with a marking pen.

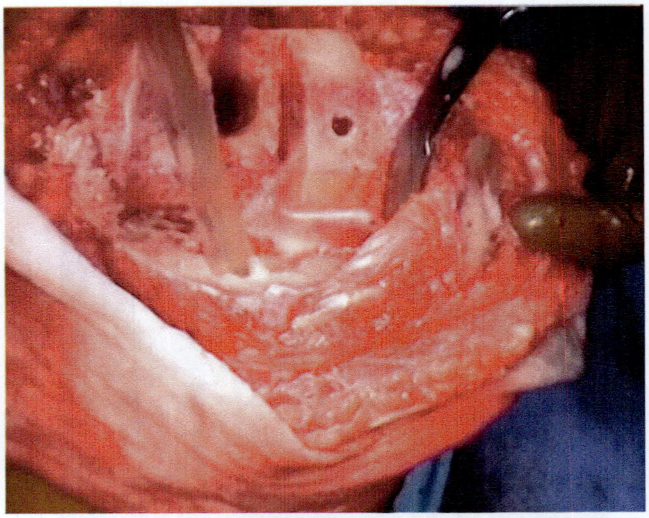

Figure 62.10 | Remove all fibrous tissue from exposed bone where cement will be placed and optimize conditions for cement interdigitation with pulsatile lavage followed by meticulous drying of the bone surfaces.

- Prepare/assemble final implants on the back table before cement mixing. Ensure instrumentation required for implant insertion is immediately available.
- Begin mixing the cement utilizing a vacuum mixing cement gun system. Often, antibiotics are added to the cement at this stage to provide site-specific antimicrobial prophylaxis.

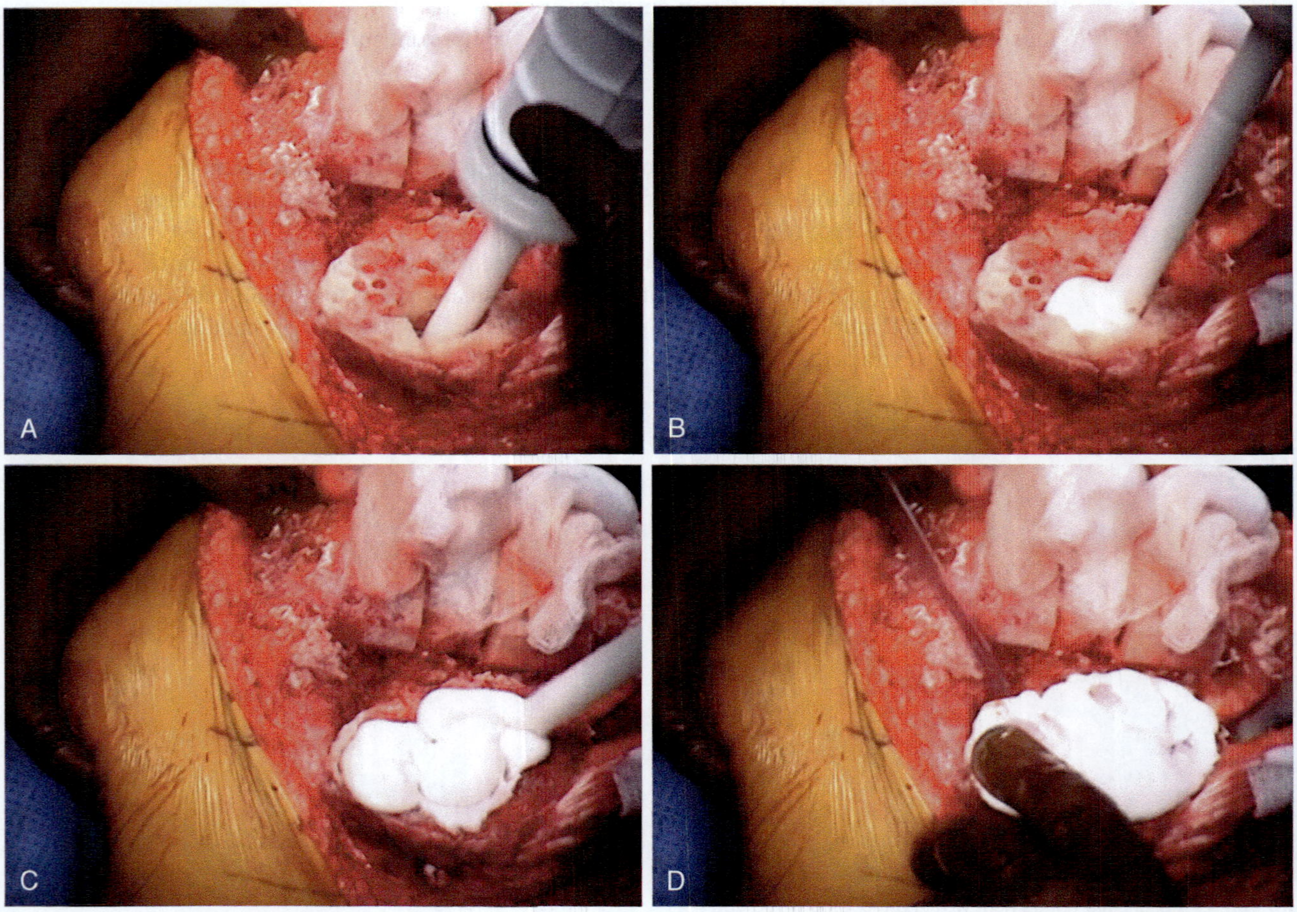

Figure 62.11 | A-D, Inject cement into the canal with a cement gun and pressurize the cement into the surface of the bone and into the canal with thumb pressure.

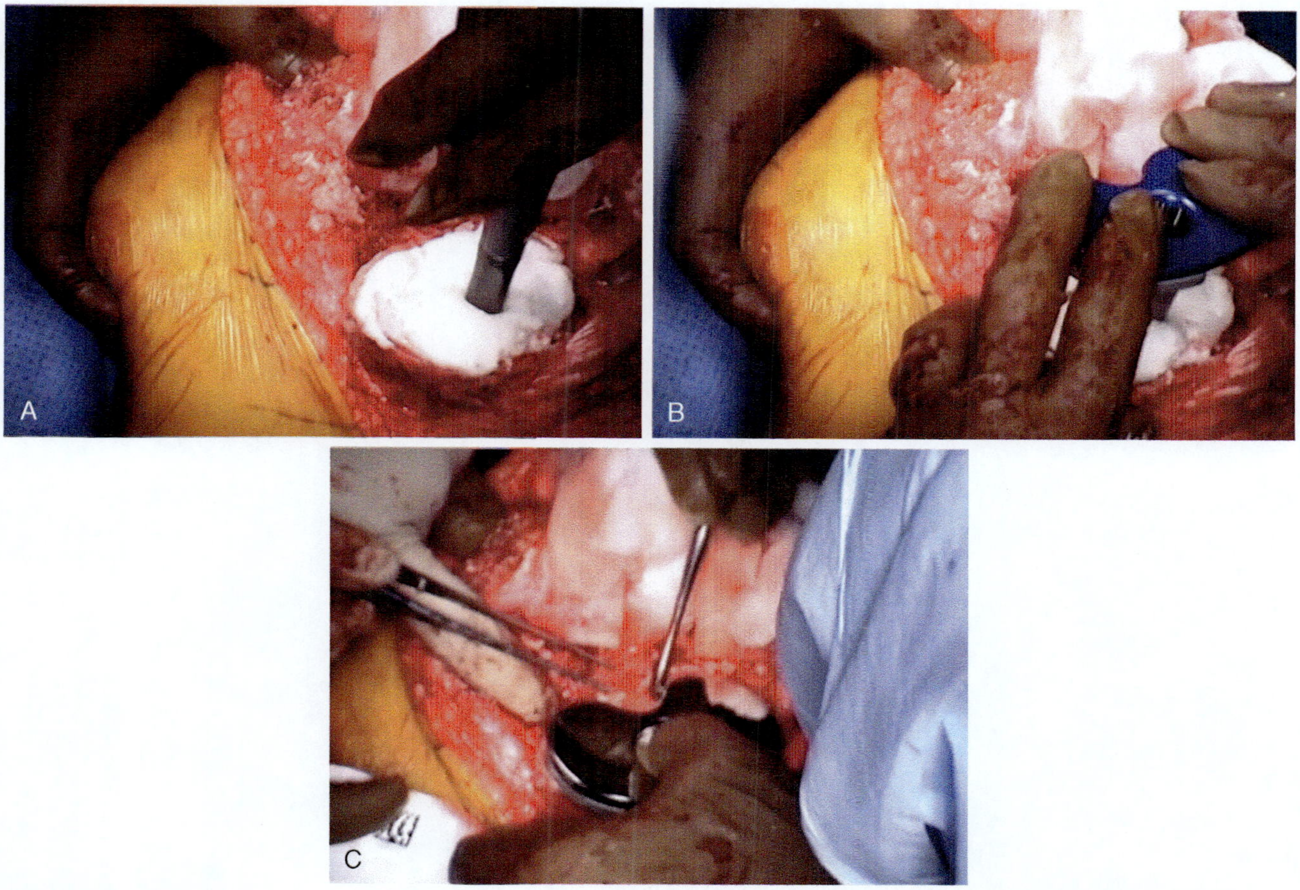

Figure 62.12 | A and B, Implant insertion into cement. C, Meticulous removal of excess cement while stabilizing the implant securely.

- If both the femur and tibia are being revised, one may cement in 2 stages or by first mixing for the tibia and then shortly thereafter mixing for the femur, using 2 cement guns. Two packs of cement usually are needed for the tibia, and at least 2 packs of cement usually are needed for the femur.
- Once the canal and exposed bone is as clean and dry as possible, begin cementation with the cement gun. Insert the cement gun nozzle until the tip touches the cement restrictor. Gradually pull outward to allow even fill of the canal while avoiding air pockets. However, be careful not to bury the cement gun nozzle by removing it too slowly. Pressurize the cement in the canal with thumb pressure, and pressurize the cement into the exposed bone surfaces manually (Figure 62.11A-D).
- Before inserting the component, align it so as to minimize movement of the stem within the canal. Insert the implant slowly and deliberately. Once the stem and cement are in contact, anything more than minor adjustments will pull cement away for the implant or bone and disrupt the interface (Figure 62.12A and B).
- Remove excess cement from the periphery of the implant and posteriorly (Figure 62.12C).

Final trialing and polyethylene insertion

- Once the cement has completely hardened, perform the final trial reduction.
- Once satisfied, place the final polyethylene insert.

Postoperative Care

- Weight bearing is individualized based on the specifics of the reconstruction. In cases of mild bone loss and good soft tissue quality, weight bearing may be as tolerated, whereas in cases of more severe bone loss or compromised soft tissues, weight bearing often will be partial for 8 weeks.

Chapter 63
Metaphyseal Fixation: Sleeves and Cones

BRIAN P. CHALMERS
DAVID G. LEWALLEN

Key Concepts

- Reestablish metaphyseal support for revision total knee arthroplasty (TKA) implants with ingrowth porous-metal metaphyseal cones or porous-coated metaphyseal sleeves.
- Ensure long-term component stability with synergistic hybrid fixation.
  - Cemented components and stems (cemented or uncemented) to provide immediate stability that promotes subsequent biologic ingrowth of the metaphyseal cone or sleeve.
  - Porous ingrowth cones or sleeves to achieve bone ingrowth and thus provide long-term stability and diminish stress on cemented interfaces.

Sterile Instruments and Implants

- Basic revision TKA retractors
- Metaphyseal cones and trials (with implant-specific instrumentation) and/or metaphyseal sleeves and trials (with implant-specific instrumentation)
- Revision TKA implant system of surgeon's choice (with instrumentation) with higher levels of constraint (typically at least a varus-valgus constrained design in those revision TKAs requiring adjunctive metaphyseal fixation)
- Standard and metal-cutting burrs
- Saw

Surgical Approaches

- Standard medial parapatellar arthrotomy with a generous medial release on tibial side.
- Extensile approaches as necessary—quadriceps snip or tibial tubercle osteotomy.

Preoperative Planning

- Obtain the prior operative reports for better knowledge of the current implants and any notations that indicate unique aspects of the patient's anatomy or intraoperative challenges.
- Template a revision TKA implant system for both the femur and the tibia.
- Assess likely bone defects (location, size, segmental versus cavitary) to aid in planning benefits of bone graft, sleeves, or cones and potential benefit of any combinations of these to ensure availability at surgery. Remember, radiographs tend to underestimate the extent of bone loss.

Bone, Implant, and Soft Tissue Techniques

- Perform the skin incision, medial parapatellar arthrotomy, generous medial release, and medial and lateral gutter release; use an extensile exposure with a quadriceps snip as necessary to safely expose the knee.
- Longer incisions and more generous soft tissue releases are the standard.
- Carefully remove the polyethylene insert to relax the extensor mechanism and soft tissue tension.
- Remove scar tissue to expose the cement interface of the femoral and tibial components circumferentially with electrocautery or a small rongeur.
- Minimize host bone removal and/or damage during implant removal: use a saw or pencil-tip burr to divide the cemented interface of the femoral component.
- Try to divide all femoral interfaces (anterior and posterior condyles and chamfers).
- Thin flexible osteotomes can be useful to ensure as complete a division of cement-implant bond as possible.
- Use a square-tip impactor on the anterior flange and a mallet for gentle disimpaction of the femoral component. If unable to disimpact, revisit the above-mentioned steps.
- After femoral component removal, hyperflex and externally rotate the leg to expose the tibia. Again, use a saw or pencil-tip burr to divide the cemented interface under the tibial component. Access the underside of the posterior portion of the tray (behind the keel) by using a narrow saw at the posteromedial corner of the tibia and advancing it parallel to the posterior aspect of the tibial cortex from medial to lateral staying under the implant.
- The posterolateral corner and the anterolateral aspect just behind the patellar tendon are the most difficult areas to access: try to ensure that a thin osteotome passes underneath as much of the undersurface of component as possible especially in these areas laterally.
- Hyperflex the knee and disimpact the tibial component using a narrow square-tip impactor placed under the tray anteromedially or through a vertical slit lateral to the patellar tendon. Ensure that the tibial component clears the posterior condyle of the femur laterally. The biggest risk of iatrogenic bone damage is a posterolateral tibial fracture if that cement-implant interface has not been adequately freed before tibial disimpaction.
- If the femoral or tibial component is not freed rather easily with this method, repeat each step from the beginning and try again.
- After implant removal, assess bone defects intraoperatively and estimate appropriate size of cone (Figure 63.1) or sleeve (Figure 63.2) that will be necessary.
- Clean the cement debris left on the femur and tibia with a high-speed burr or rongeur.
- Recut the proximal tibia ***removing minimal bone*** to reestablish a neutral mechanical alignment and slope. Some residual defects are usual to minimize bone removal.
- Remove some central metaphyseal bone from the femur and tibia (if still present) with a large curette to allow reamer placement. Save this bone for use as autograft.
- Sequentially ream the tibial canal to 14 or 15 mm for an intermediate-length cemented stem or until stable reamer with diaphyseal engagement for a longer cementless stem.
  - Recognize that the dense medial bone of the tibia tends to push tibial reamers and broaches into valgus, and thus a deliberate effort to avoid this should be made particularly when broaching for porous-coated metaphyseal sleeves.
- For bone preparation for cone or sleeve placement, leave the final reamer or a trial stem with rod extension in place as an intramedullary guide for broaching/reaming (depending on the instrumentation system) (Figure 63.3).
- Sequentially broach (or ream), starting from the smallest size.
- Attempt to prepare the bone so as to minimize bone removed while also maximizing cone or sleeve contact on host bone.
- Align the tibial cone/sleeve in appropriate rotation, in-line with the medial edge of the tibial tubercle and anterior crest of the tibia (Figure 63.4).
- Broach or ream sequentially larger until both the metaphyseal defect is filled and the metaphyseal implant is both axially and rotationally stable.
- Some cone systems have oblong or stepped cones that may fill certain shaped defects better; it is important to be aware of these options intraoperatively when assessing the size and shapes of tibial and femoral bone defects (Figure 63.5).
- Place the trial tibial cone (Figure 63.3).
- Recut the tibia, making any prominent bone flush with the superior margin of the cone/sleeve.

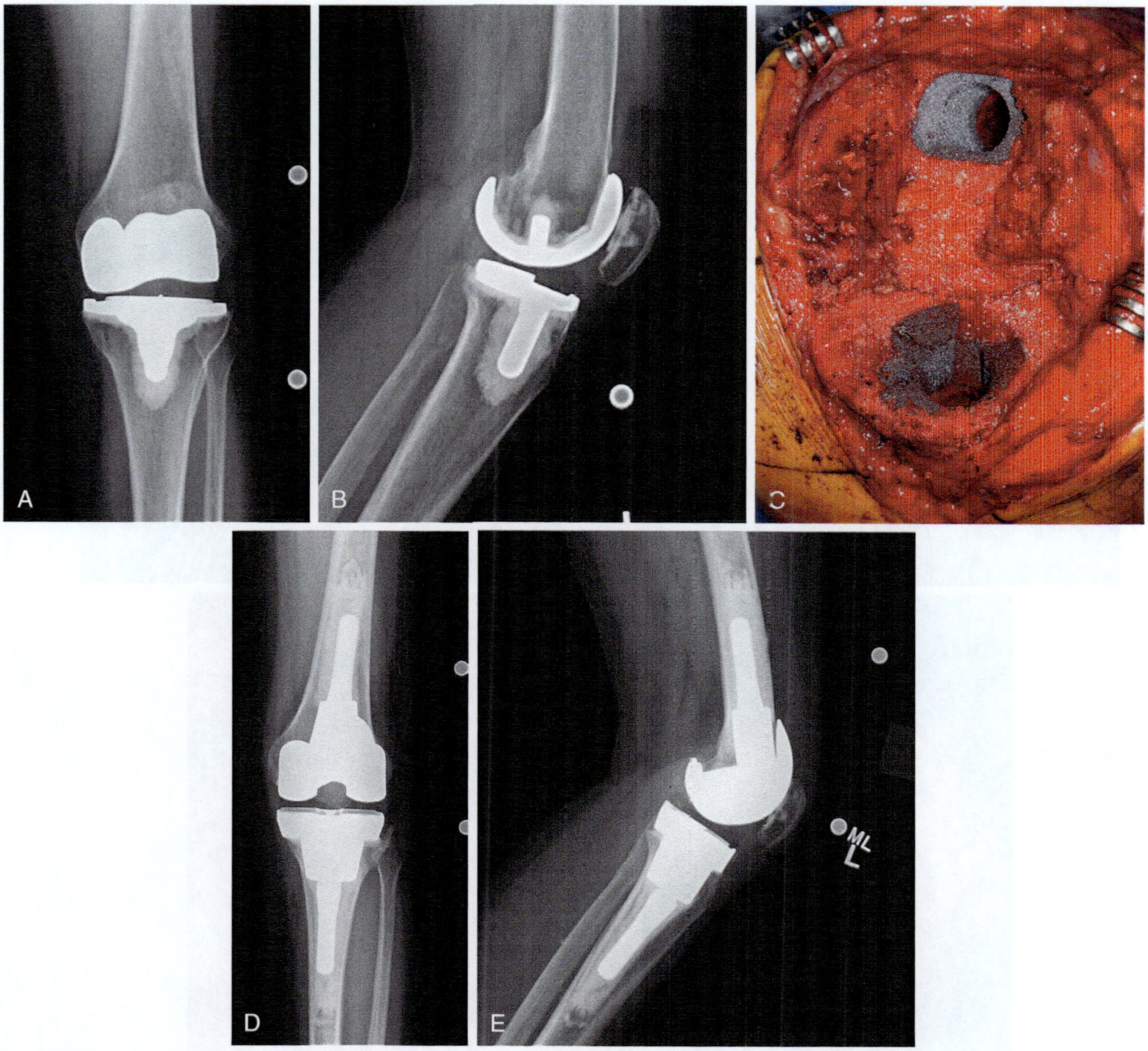

Figure 63.1 | A 69-year-old man who underwent both component revision total knee arthroplasty for flexion instability (A and B). To fill these type IIb bone defects porous metal femoral and tibial cones were utilized (C) and combined with intermediate-length cemented stems (D and E).

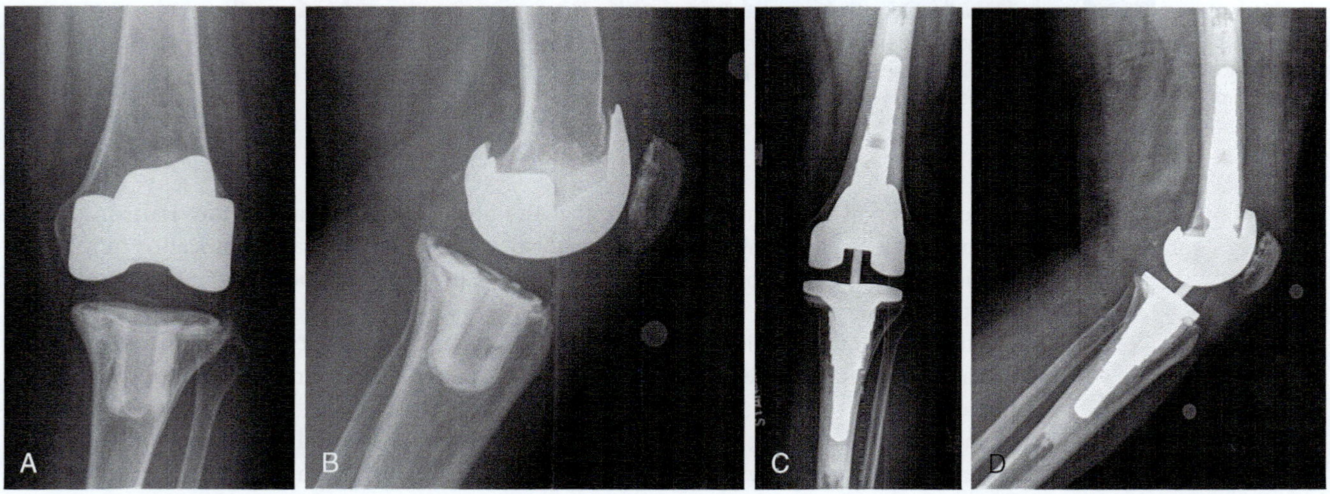

Figure 63.2 | A 76-year-old woman who underwent a both-component revision total knee arthroplasty for aseptic loosening (A and B). To fill these type II tibial and femoral defects porous coated metaphyseal sleeves with cemented stems were utilized (C and D).

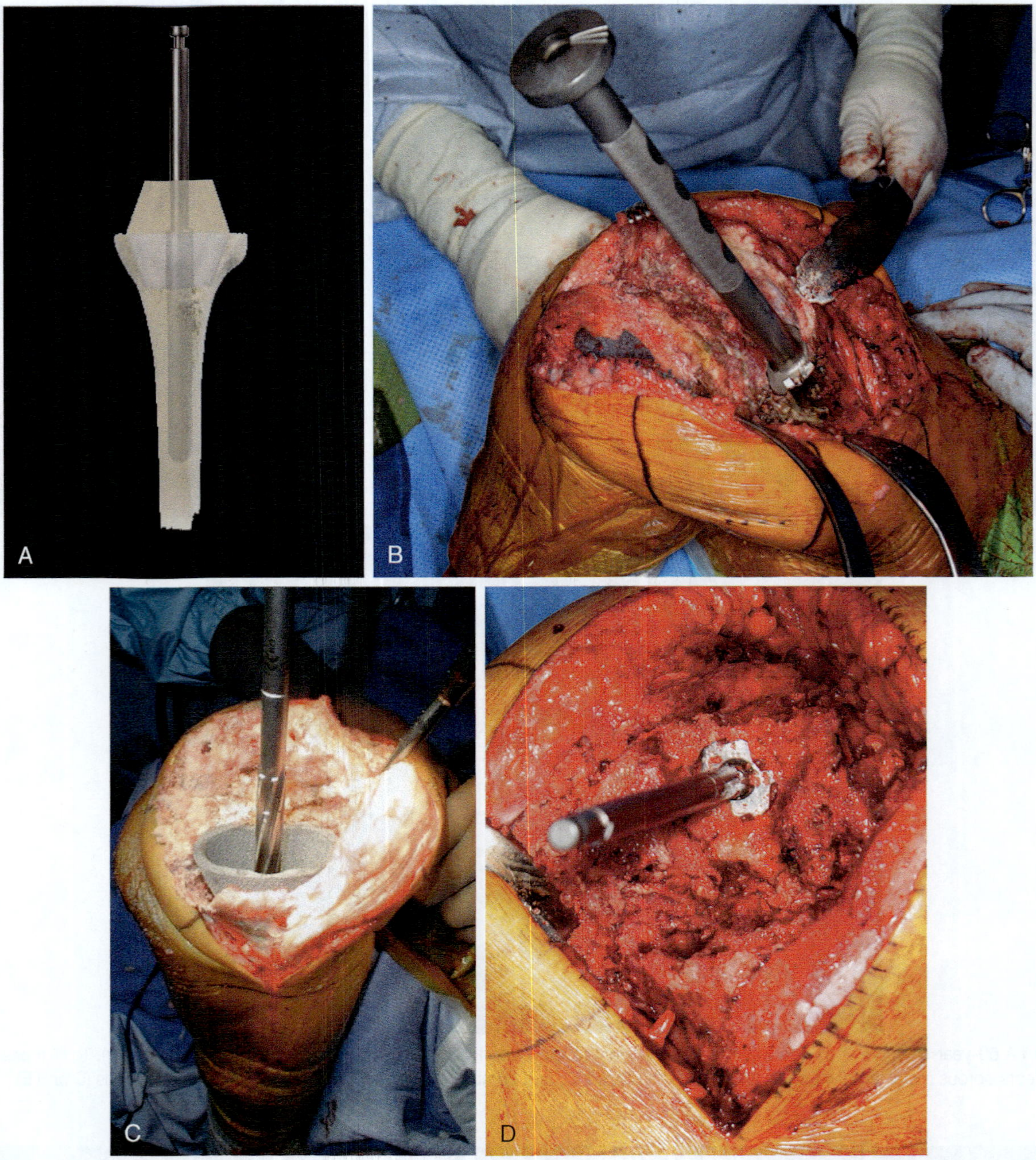

Figure 63.3 | Schematic drawing (A) and intraoperative photographs demonstrate the use of long intramedullary reamers as intramedullary guides (A) for metaphyseal cone broaching (B) and final implant placement (C). An intramedullary reamer used as a guide before broaching for a femoral porous-coated metaphyseal sleeve (D).

- Place the trial tibial component to ensure that the tibial tray fully seats on the trial cone/sleeve. Adjust the position if the bony preparation or position of cone/sleeve tray is not seating fully.
  - Consider getting an intraoperative x-ray if there are any concerns about alignment, stem size, or stem position exist.
- Once satisfied with the position, place the real tibial cone, impacting it into final position with the trial tibial component (Figure 63.6) and the desired intramedullary stem in the proper position and orientation.
- Sleeves are nonmodular (i.e., mated with the real tibial and/or femoral component and stem) and therefore must be impacted with the final components; therefore, the trials are generally kept in place until final implant placement; cones are modular (i.e., not mated with the real tibial and/or femoral component and stem) and therefore can be placed before final implant placement (Figure 63.7).

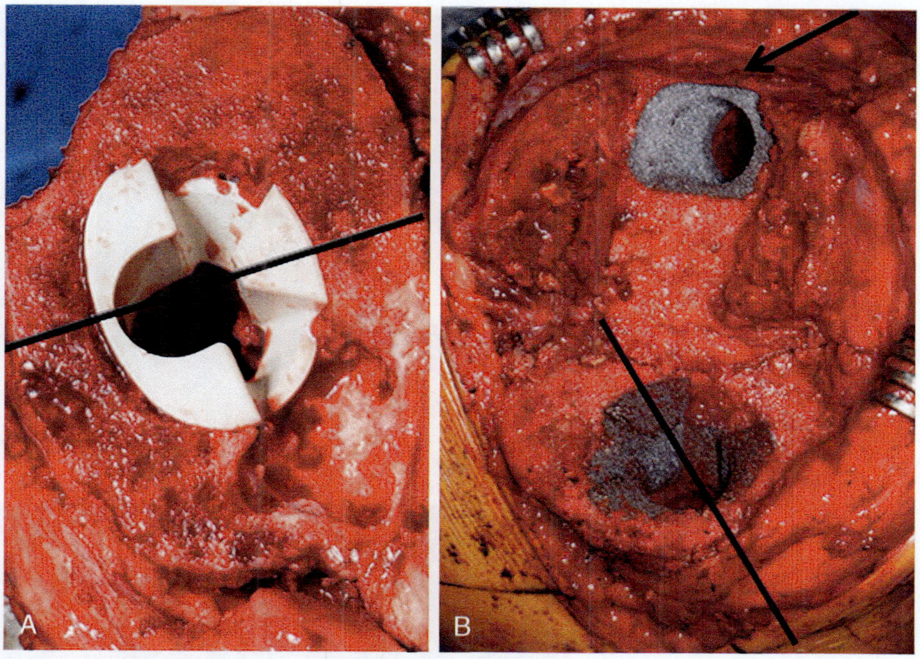

Figure 63.4 | Intraoperative photographs showing proper external rotation of the tibial trial cone (A and B) as indicated by the black line in relation to the tibial tubercle. The black arrow (B) also shows the position of the femoral cone in relation to the anterior cortex to prevent flexion of the cone; care should be taken while broaching/reaming as the anterior cortex thins during cone placement.

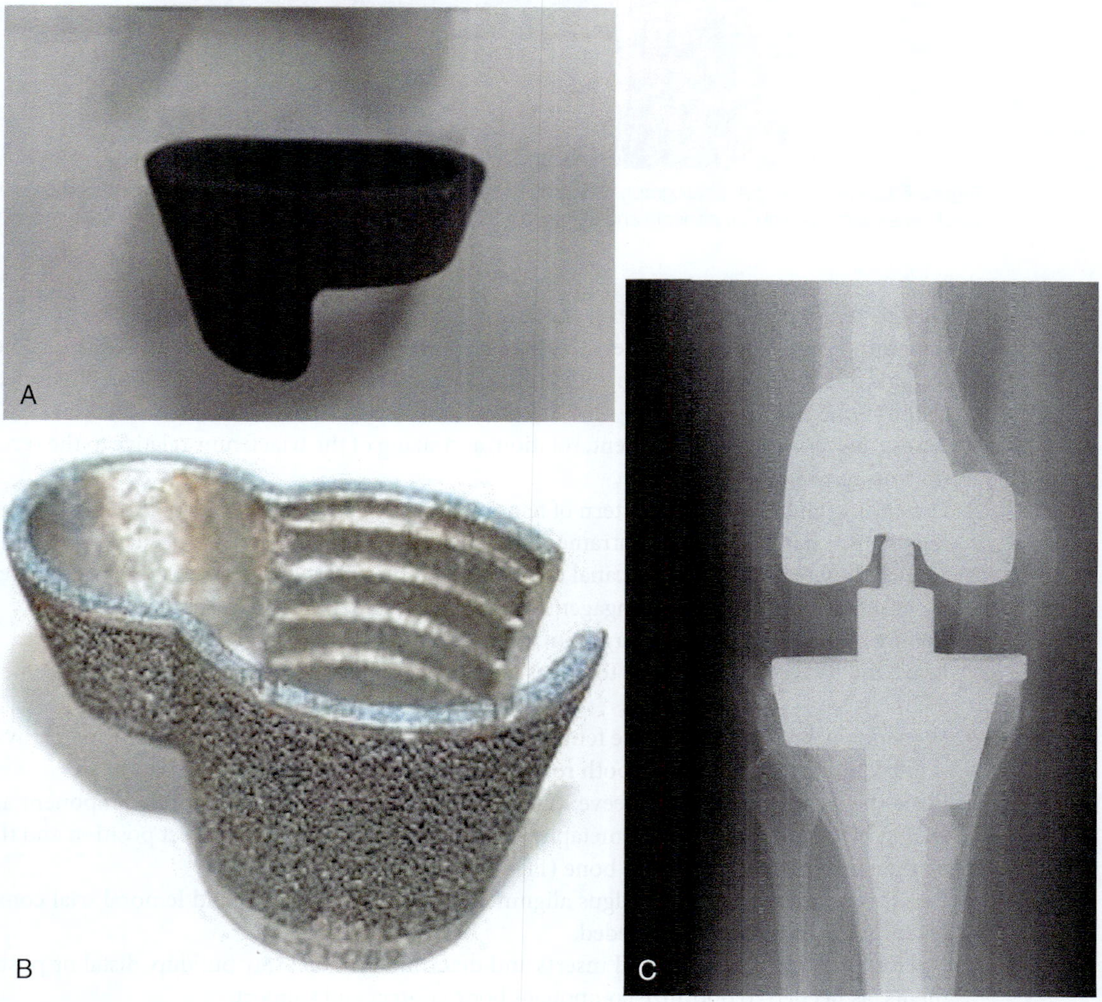

Figure 63.5 | Photographs of a stepped porous metal cone (A) and an oblong porous metal cone (B) utilized to fill irregularly shaped metaphyseal defects. A radiograph depicting one of those porous metal cones in situ is also shown (C).

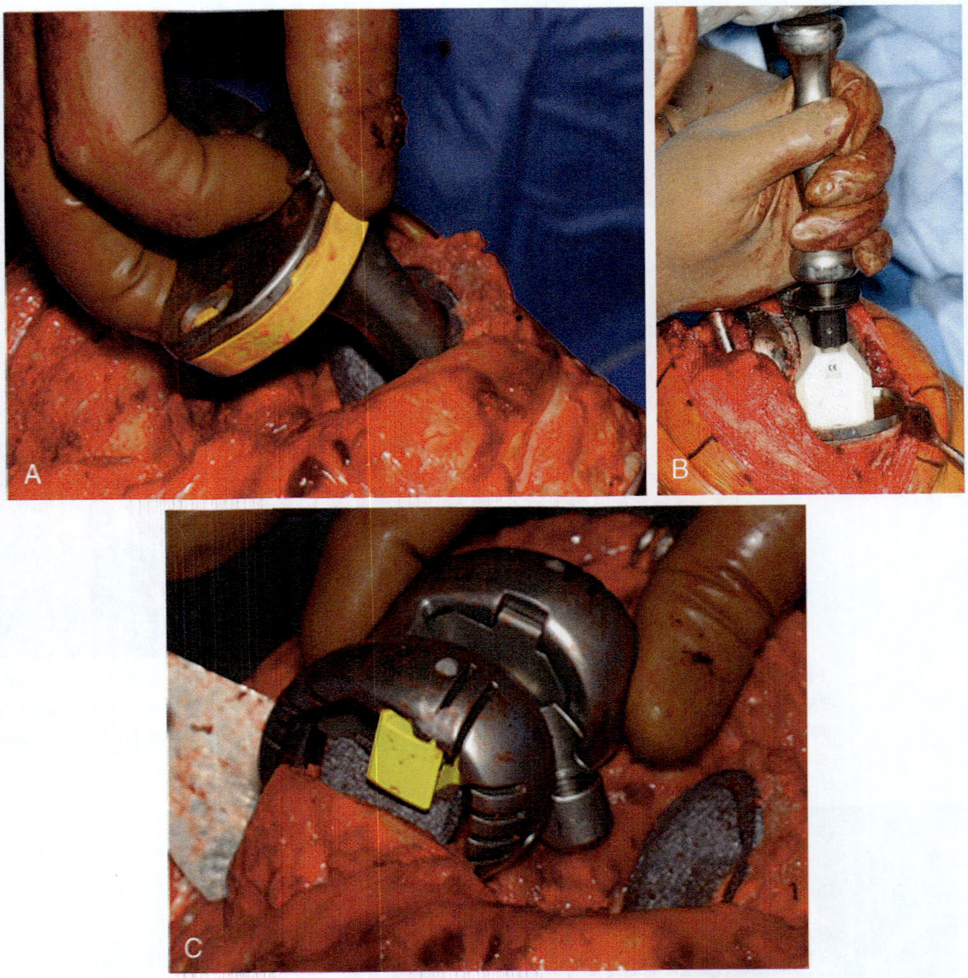

Figure 63.6 | Intraoperative photographs showing impaction of the tibial (A and B) and femoral (C) porous metal metaphyseal cones with the trial components and stems to ensure full seating of the cones and proper implant positioning.

- On the femoral side remove excess cement from the femur; assess bone deficiency; remove any remaining posterior osteophytes. In aseptic revisions, it is not necessary to remove cement that is well fixed to the underlying bone and often leaving that cement will protect the otherwise soft cancellous bone that remains.
- Assess the varus/valgus alignment, rotation, and sizing of the trial femur relative to the reconstructed tibia using trial inserts.
- Depending on location and pattern of femoral bone defects: small recuts of the distal femur, anterior femur, and chamfers with an intramedullary jig or freehand are done as needed.
- Sequentially ream the femoral canal to 14 or 15 mm if a short or intermediate-length cemented stem is chosen or until diaphyseal engagement if a longer cementless stem is intended.
- Remove reamed bone with a large curette.
- Leave the final reamer in place to use as an intramedullary guide for cone/sleeve placement (Figure 63.3).
- Sequentially broach or ream the femur for the metaphyseal sleeve/cone until the metaphyseal defect is filled and the sleeve/cone is both rotationally and axially stable (Figure 63.4).
- Place the trial femoral cone/sleeve; this can be impacted with the femoral component and a stem trial in place to ensure that the metaphyseal cone/sleeve seats in the correct position and the femoral component fully seats onto the bone (Figure 63.6)
- Reassess rotation and varus/valgus alignment with the cone/sleeve and femoral trial component in place; make adjustments as needed.
- Place a trial femoral, tibial, and inserts and determine if tibial tray buildup, distal or posterior augments, as needed to optimize component bone contact and support.
- Balance the soft tissues in flexion and extension and determine the level of constraint needed.

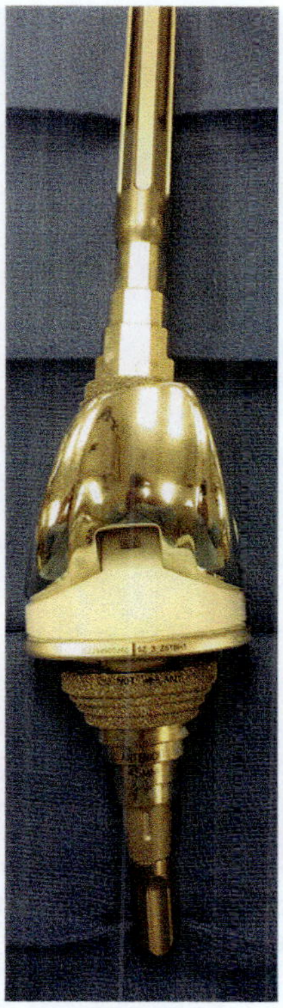

Figure 63.7 I Photograph depicting fully assembled femoral and tibial porous coated metaphyseal sleeves coupled with the respective femoral and tibial components and stems before implantation.

- Once satisfied with the stability and range of motion, obtain an anteroposterior and lateral intraoperative radiograph to assess for TKA alignment and sizing, then make adjustments as needed.
- Place saved bone autograft and/or allograft putty or chips into any gaps between the bone and the metaphyseal sleeve/cone to protect the bone-ingrowth interface from bone cement access and to aid biologic bone ingrowth potential (Figure 63.8).
- Finalize choice of cemented versus cementless stems and assemble the real components.
- Use cement restrictors if fully cemented stems are used to aid in cement pressurization and limit cement fill of the canal.
- Cemented stems are 2 to 4 mm smaller in diameter than the final reamer and usually 30 to 60 mm in length (rarely longer) giving a composite or total length of 50 to 100 mm for the tibia and 100 to 150 mm for the femur (Figures 63.1 and 63.2). Cementless stems must be longer to completely engage the diaphysis.
- Assemble the femoral and tibial components/stems on the back table; insert them into the knee without cement first, making sure that they fully seat into the cone.
- Depending on the system used, and the size of the cone and implant used, there can be conflict between the fins of the tibial keel or the femoral housing, which may require adjustment or modification of one of the implants with a metal cutting burr (Figure 63.8).
- Metaphyseal sleeves are assembled to the knee components on the back table; therefore, any conflict will occur at the bone-implant interface during insertion; the surgeon should be cognizant of this as it may require additional bone preparation when inserting the nonmodular sleeved knee component (Figure 63.7).
- Inflate the tourniquet if not done so already; water pick the bone surfaces and thoroughly dry them; mix 2-3 batches of cement with 2 to 2.4 g of powdered antibiotic and a few drops of methylene blue per batch of cement.
- Cement components into position. In many circumstances it is best to cement the tibia and femur separately. That is particularly true in cases with substantial bone loss, and most surgeons choose to cement the tibia first, allow the cement to harden, and then cement the femur.
- Place a trial polyethylene insert and hold axial pressure on the knee in full extension until the cement fully hardens.

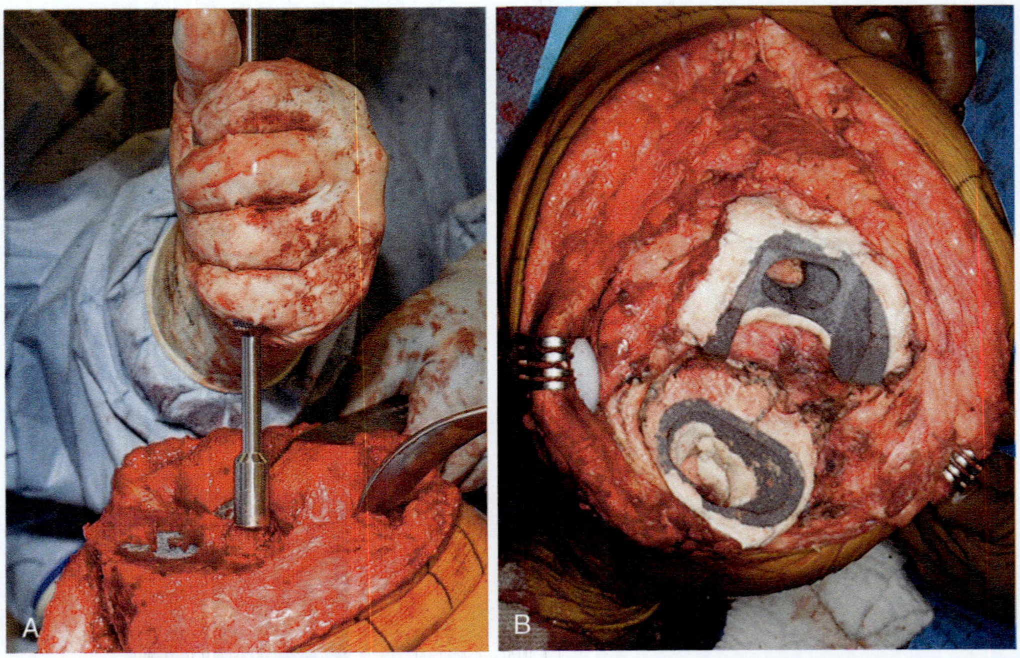

Figure 63.8 | A and B, Intraoperative photographs demonstrating impaction of locally harvested autograft and allograft to fill the porous-metal metaphyseal-cone-to-bone interface to limit cement interposition and to thus promote biologic fixation.

- Use trial polyethylene inserts to optimize range of motion and stability in all planes and ensure proper patellar tracking.
- Remove excess cement at the back of the knee and around the interfaces.
- Once satisfied, place the final tibial polyethylene insert.
- Irrigate the knee.
- Perform a layered closure in the typical fashion.

Postoperative Management

- Management is similar to any revision TKA and is dictated by soft tissue status and prioritizes initial wound healing over range of motion or activity. Typically, however, range of motion exercises and ambulation with partial weight bearing can be started immediately.
- After 6 weeks, weight bearing is typically advanced as tolerated, but these milestones may be individualized and delayed if substantial bony or soft tissue problems were encountered.

Chapter 64
Distal Femoral Replacement

GRAHAM D. PALLANTE
RAFAEL J. SIERRA

Key Concepts

- Distal femoral replacement most commonly is used as a salvage procedure in revision total knee arthroplasty (TKA) involving severe bone loss, following oncologic resection, or in supracondylar periprosthetic femur fracture with poor bone quality and loose/malpositioned implants.
- Resection of the distal femur involves removal of the collateral ligaments, and constructs are therefore highly constrained designs. Rotating-hinge prostheses usually are preferred to decrease stress transfer to the bone-implant interface.
- Distal femoral replacement allows immediate, stable fixation, and thus immediate weight bearing.
- Distal femoral replacement may be considered in selected revision TKA in which bone loss cannot be managed with metal augments, sleeves, or cones in isolation.
- Uncemented or cemented stems may be used for fixation. Cemented stems are preferred in patients with poor diaphyseal bone or host factors that may limit bony ingrowth potential.
- Soft tissue management is important. Often, the soft tissue envelope is deficient. In this scenario, use the smallest possible implant to minimize the need for local or free soft tissue transfer.
- Implant design improvements have decreased rates of aseptic loosening. However, distal femoral replacement still incurs elevated risks of infection, periprosthetic fracture, and mechanical failure.

Sterile Instruments and Implants

- Routine knee retractors
- Small and large oscillating saw
- Straight, thin osteotomes
- High-speed burr
- Cement extraction tools, trephines if removing a well-fixed stemmed implant. See Chapter 61 for details regarding implant removal
- Pulse lavage with femoral adapter for canal irrigation
- Metaphyseal cones, sleeves
- Reamers, manual and/or power; straight and/or flexible. Consider the quality of the diaphyseal bone to be reamed and deformity
- Intraoperative radiographs
- For cemented stems: cement gun, cement restrictor, vacuum cement mixer

Implants

- Uncemented stems (with instrumentation)

  or
- Cemented stems (with instrumentation)

Positioning

- Supine
- Wide prep
- Nonsterile tourniquet preferred

Surgical Approaches

- Standard, midline approach with medial parapatellar arthrotomy is preferred. Considerations should be made for previous skin incisions or soft tissue defects.
- Extensile knee approaches such as quadriceps snip or tibial tubercle osteotomy may be required. See Chapter 60 for details.

Preoperative Planning

- Obtain previous operative reports and implant records if this is a revision case.
- Full-length films preoperatively can aid in the assessment of overall alignment and leg length. Dedicated full-length femur and/or tibia films may also be useful in templating.
- Determine femoral resection level, and template based on this. The knee joint line can be used as a guide for femoral length.
- Measure the femoral canal diameter to obtain an estimate of stem extension size. This will vary based on whether a cemented or uncemented implant is desired.
- Review implant-specific requirements for bony resection, as the femoral resection level may need to be altered to accommodate different implant construct lengths.
- Carefully assess the soft tissues. Often, patients have undergone multiple surgeries, and wound closure/healing may be a concern. Skin grafting, local, or free flap coverage may be necessary.

Bone, Implant, and Soft Tissue Techniques

- Perform the desired approach to the knee, if necessary, employing an extensile approach to expose the distal femur and proximal tibia. In the revision setting, it is preferable to use the most lateral usable previous incision.
- With the knee extended, use a straight-edged ruler or Bovie cord to place a longitudinal line on the anterior cortex of the femur in line with the linea aspera above the level of resection. Next, make a corresponding vertical line on the proximal tibia. These marks will be used to guide implant rotation, which is difficult to judge after distal femoral resection. If either of the femoral condyles are present, they can also be used for reference. Careful attention to rotation is important to avoid patellar maltracking.
- Based on preoperative templating, measure and mark the distal femoral resection level before any bony resection or implant removal.
- If previous orthopedic hardware is present at the level of planned femoral or tibial osteotomy, remove as necessary, preserving as much host bone as possible (see Chapter 61).

Femoral Resection

- The distal femur is resected/excised first to aid in tibial exposure. Take care to keep the dissection plane against the bone to protect neurovascular structures.
- Clear all soft tissue circumferentially around the femur at the level of planned femoral osteotomy.
- Assess leg length clinically by comparing the operative and contralateral extremities with the knee extended. If length is preserved, use a ruler to measure the total length of the resection. This distance can be used as a guide when building the implant to calculate the approximate length (Figure 64.1).
- Use an oscillating saw to cut the femur 1 to 2 mm distal to planned final femoral osteotomy level. Depending on the implant design, a small rim of bone should be left distally to accommodate a facing reamer. One or more curved, smooth retractors can be used to protect the soft tissues and femoral neurovascular bundle posteromedially during the bone cut.
- Remove soft tissue attachments from the distal femur from proximal to distal. It is important to support the femur after it has been osteotomized to avoid injury to nearby neurovascular structures (Figure 64.2). Also take care to keep the dissection plane against the bone to protect neurovascular structures.
- The distal femur is then removed, allowing for exposure of the proximal tibia.
- The tourniquet may be let down temporarily to ensure adequate hemostasis.
- During revision of previously cemented implants, any remaining bone cement should be removed from host bone using a combination of osteotomes, curettes, high-speed burr, and ultrasonic cement extraction set as needed. If planning for an uncemented implant, it is important to meticulously extract cement in the diaphysis, where a concentric press fit is required.

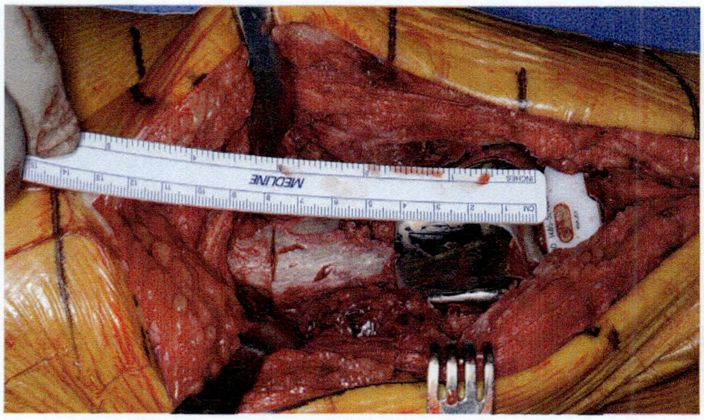

Figure 64.1 | A ruler is used to measure and record the planned resection. This should correspond with preoperative templating. After inserting trial components, one can repeat this measurement as a secondary check to ensure that length will be restored with the knee prosthesis.

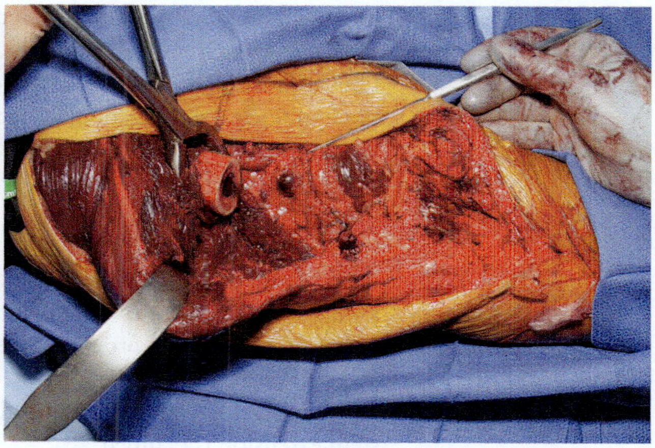

Figure 64.2 | The distal femur has been resected and is held in place with a large clamp. Note the proximity of the femoral neurovascular bundle (probe).

Tibial Preparation

- If performing revision TKA, use desired technique for removal of tibial implants. If present, remove excess cement as earlier.
- In oncologic cases, perform standard tibial resection and prepare the canal for a stemmed tibial component.
- A series of straight reamers is introduced into the tibial canal to the predetermined depth and diameter based on templating. Continue to incrementally increase the reamer diameter until firm endosteal contact is obtained. Avoid eccentric reaming.
- In severely osteopenic bone, hand reamers can be utilized to allow direct tactile feedback to the surgeon during reaming.
- Metal augments, metaphyseal sleeves, or porous cones often are required for management of bone defects. When possible, adjunctive fixation with cones or sleeves is used to mitigate the elevated aseptic loosening risk associated with megaprostheses. Ream, mill, or broach to accommodate cones or sleeves that may provide supplemental uncemented fixation at this stage (Figure 64.3A and B).

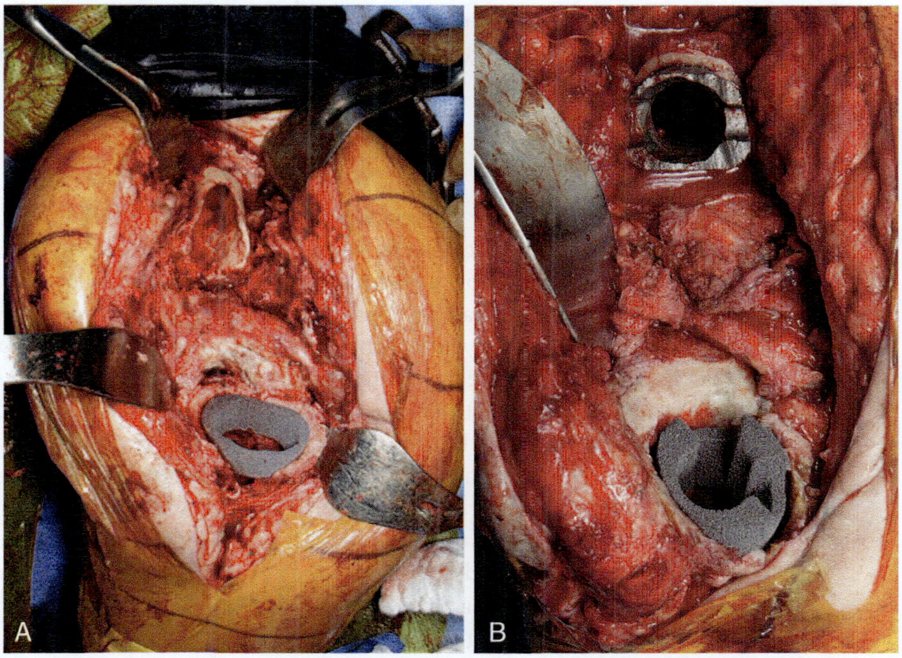

Figure 64.3 | Porous metal augments can provide additional fixation where bone is deficient, thus increasing stability at the bone-implant interface of the femur, tibia (A), or both (B).

- The tibial resection jig is then assembled using an intramedullary guide. Depending on the system, the jig may be assembled off of the last (largest) reamer or may have a separate guide. Cut and size the tibia at the desired level, with the goal of reestablishing the joint line. Utilize landmarks such as the tibial tubercle, femoral condyles, fibular head, and meniscal remnant and the patella to estimate the level of the joint line. If a sleeve or cone is utilized, it can be used to guide bony resection.

Femoral Preparation

- Assess bone loss and deformity to determine the need for augmentation of fixation with metal augments, sleeves, or cones on the femoral side. As on the tibial side, augmentation with uncemented cones or sleeves can provide uncemented fixation, which may improve durability of these constrained implants.
- The femur is then prepared with either straight or flexible reamers, depending on if bowed or straight stem extension is planned.
- Based on preoperative templating, ream the femur to the desired diameter. A flexible reamer may be used over a guidewire to accommodate femoral bow. A prophylactic wire or cable may be placed around the femur proximally to mitigate the risk of iatrogenic fracture. This is particularly important when reaming osteopenic bone, as in treatment of a periprosthetic fracture.
- If placing a cemented stem, ream to 2 mm greater than the stem diameter to accommodate a cement mantle. Depth can be approximated based on attachments or markings on the reamer.
- When using cemented stems, care should be taken not to ream more than necessary to avoid removing valuable cancellous bone needed for cement interdigitation.
- For uncemented stems, ream until firm, endosteal cortical contact is established. Diaphyseal engagement is critical for stability. Use caution while reaming osteopenic bone to ensure that an iatrogenic fracture or perforation does not occur. Line-to-line or slight underreaming is often preferred to obtain press fit. However, stem and/or host bone geometry may necessitate slight overreaming or underreaming.
- Some stems have a taper. A second, tapered reamer is utilized if necessary. Alternatively, a cone or sleeve may be used at the site of the femoral osteotomy to augment stability. Ream or broach at this stage.

Patellar Preparation

- A stable, intact patella or patellar component may be left unresurfaced/unrevised, provided tracking is appropriate.
- If these conditions are not met, remove previous patellar component, if present. Debride nonviable tissue and resurface the patella.
- Patellar bone loss or extensor mechanism deficiency may be present. See Chapters 72 and 73 for management strategies.

Trial Reduction

- Assemble and insert the femoral and tibial trials (Figure 64.4).
- Use previous markings on the femur and tibia to ensure appropriate rotation during trial insertion. Local landmarks may not be present. The linea aspera may be used to guide femoral rotation, but this can sometimes be misleading; therefore, marking rotation preresection is important.
- Reduce the knee. Assess the length and soft tissue tension. Grossly approximate skin and subcutaneous tissues to ensure the size of the implant will not impede wound closure, realizing overall length can affect the tension of the soft tissue envelope. Using a smaller-sized femoral component may facilitate soft tissue closure. Despite careful attention and implantation of appropriately sized implants, adjunctive techniques such as local muscle flap coverage may be required.
- Put the knee through a range of motion. Pay close attention to patellar height and alignment, as well as extensor mechanism tension and tracking. Perform soft tissue releases, and adjust polyethylene trial thickness as needed. Patellar tracking problems are a common complication of this procedure, so attention to this step is important.
- Fine adjustments in length not corrected by soft tissue release may require additional bony resection from the femur or tibia. Rereaming may be needed if this strategy is employed.
- Punch the tibia at this stage if using a baseplate with a keel.

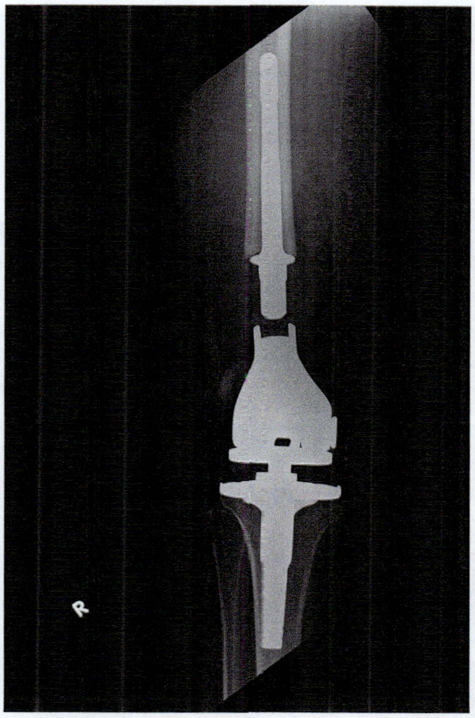

Figure 64.4 | Radiographs obtained after insertion of trial components are used to evaluate length, alignment, and rotation of the prosthesis.

Final Implantation

- Assemble final implants on the back table.
- Use pulse lavage to thoroughly clear bony surfaces of debris. Insert final tibial or femoral cones/sleeves. Retrial before final component implantation.
- The tibial component is implanted first. If placing a cemented femoral component, it is preferable to cement in 2 stages.
- The patellar component is cemented last.

Uncemented Femoral Stem Insertion

- Impact the uncemented stem in the correct rotation using a mallet based on previous femoral markings. To avoid fracture during impaction, use multiple taps with the mallet of moderate force. Make sure the stem is continuously advancing. If there is significant resistance, it may be necessary to remove the component and geream.

Cemented Femoral Stem Insertion

- A cement restrictor should be placed no more than 1 cm proximal to the planned stem tip location. While holding the trial component with stem attached next to the cement restrictor implantation tool, use a marking pen to set the depth.
- Once the cement restrictor is in place, use pulse lavage with the femoral adapter to thoroughly irrigate the canal to clear all debris at the bone-cement interface.
- Prepare/assemble final implants on the back table before cement mixing. Ensure instrumentation required for implant insertion is immediately available.
- Begin mixing polymethyl methacrylate cement utilizing a vacuum mixed cement gun system. Antibiotics are often added to the cement at this stage to provide site-specific antimicrobial prophylaxis, or premixed antibiotic cement may be used.
- Once the canal is as clean and dry as possible, begin cementation with the cement gun. Insert the cement gun nozzle until the tip touches the cement restrictor. Begin filling the canal by squeezing the cement gun trigger hard to pressurize the cement into any remaining cancellous bone and aid in interdigitation. Gradually pull outward to allow even fill of the canal while avoiding air pockets. However, be careful not to bury the cement gun nozzle by removing it too slowly.

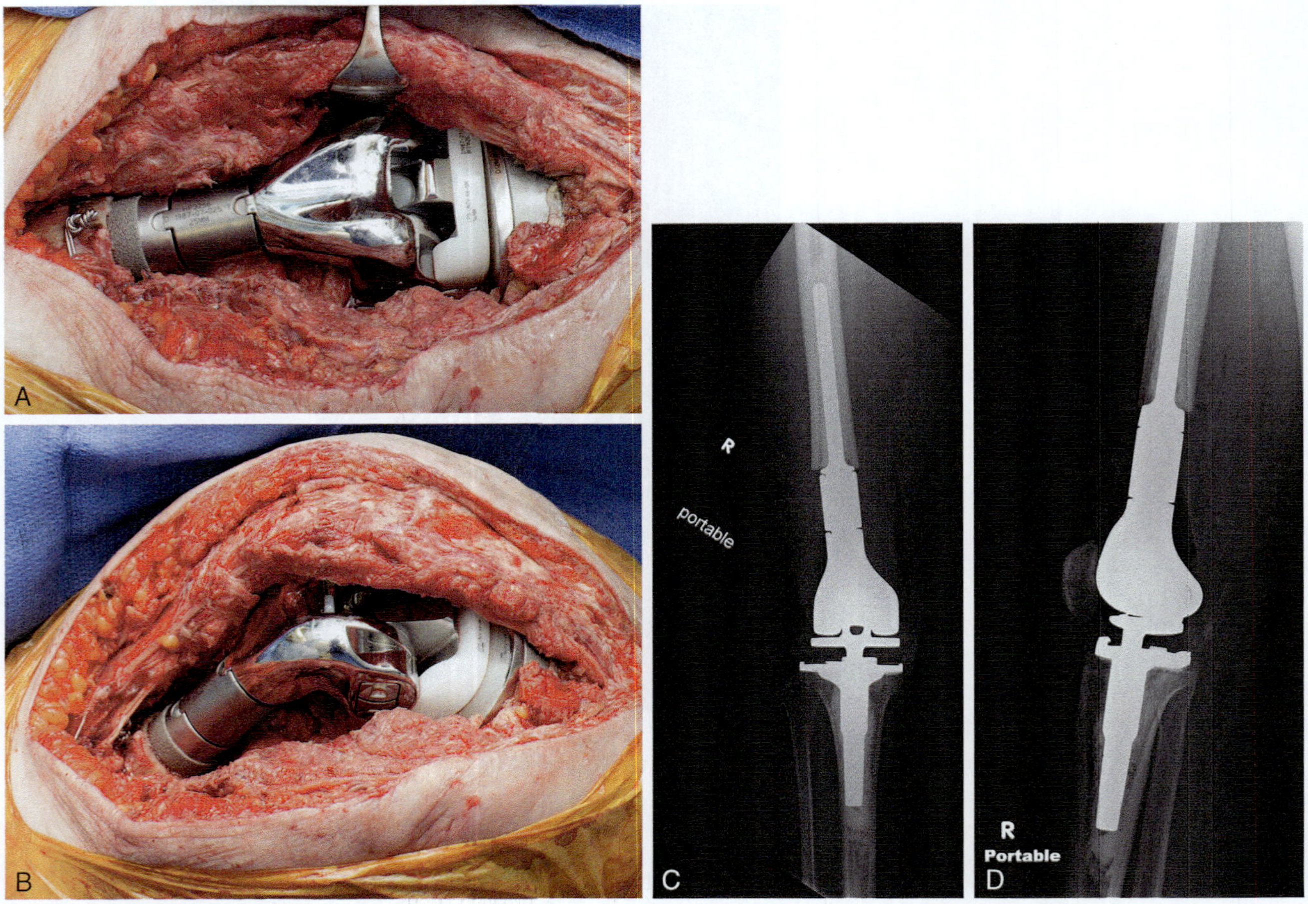

Figure 64.5 | Clinical photographs (A and B) and final radiographs (C and D) after components are cemented in place.

- Before inserting the component, align it so as to minimize movement of the stem within the canal. Insert the stem slowly and deliberately. Once the stem and cement are in contact, anything more than minor adjustments will pull cement away for the implant or bone and disrupt the interface.
- Use a nerve hook periosteal elevator and small forceps to remove excess cement.
- After all components are securely placed, a final trial reduction is performed. Again, pay particular attention to stability, patellar tracking, and height. Adjust polyethylene thickness as needed.
- Once satisfied, secure the final polyethylene insert (Figure 64.5A-D) and complete assembly of the hinged implant.
- Close the wound in layers, being mindful of soft tissue tension.

Postoperative Care

- Patients are generally made weight bearing as tolerated. In cases of extensive bone loss, or when the soft tissues require additional protection, weight-bearing or range-of-motion restrictions may be employed.
- In patients with a femoral nerve block or nerve catheter a knee immobilizer may be utilized initially until quadriceps function has returned.

Chapter 65
Bone Grafting Methods and Allograft Prosthetic Replacement

ROBERT T. TROUSDALE

Key Concepts

- Cancellous bone grafts and structural allografts remain an excellent choice for bone loss issues in selective cases during revision total knee arthroplasty (TKA).
- Cancellous graft is a good choice when irregular defects are present or in ectatic bone when sleeves or cones are unlikely to get stability (Figure 65.1).
- Intussusception allografts are a good choice in massive defects when sleeves or cones are unlikely to get stability (Figure 65.2).

Sterile Instruments and Implants

- Routine revision knee components.
- Press-fit or cemented stems to bypass bone defects.
- High-speed burrs to prepare host bone and shape bulk allograft.

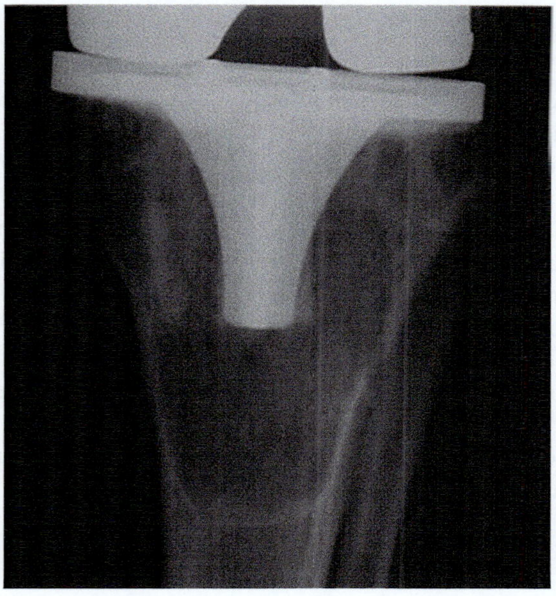

Figure 65.1 | Anteroposterior radiograph showing marked osteolysis with periprosthetic fracture. A sleeve or cone would have difficulty getting good stability in such bone.

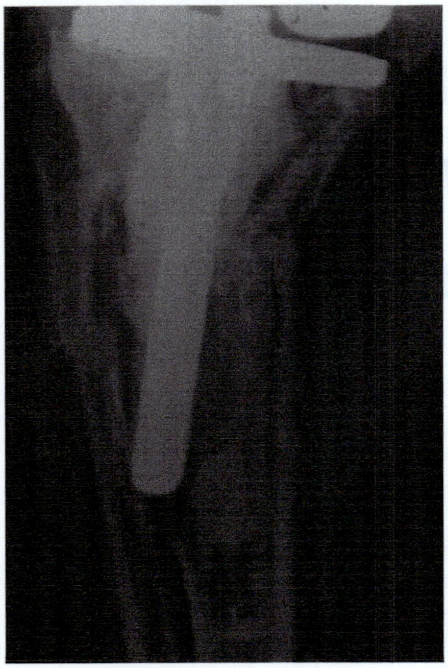

Figure 65.2 | Anteroposterior radiograph showing marked tibial bone loss subsequently treated with intussusception allograft (See Figure 65.7).

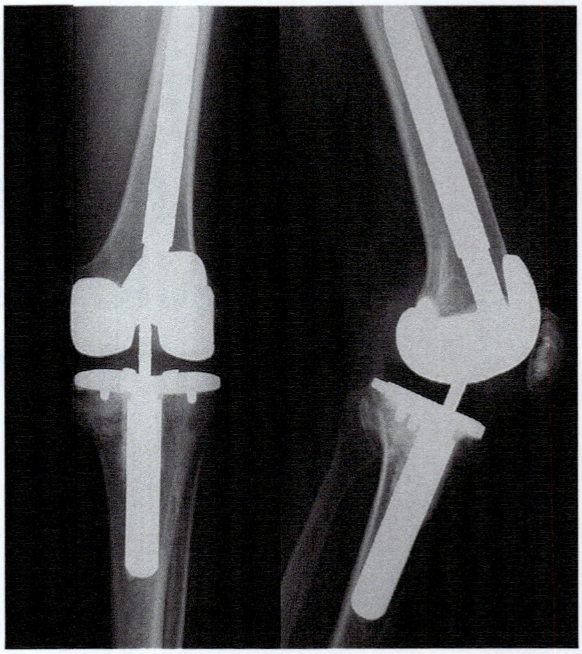

Figure 65.3 | Anteroposterior and lateral radiographs of a young patient anticipated to have substantial cavitary bone defects following implant removal.

Surgical Approaches

- By surgeon preference. Medial parapatellar arthrotomy is adequate for the majority.
- More extensive approaches (i.e., quadriceps snip or tibial tubercle osteotomy) may be utilized.
- Drape majority of femur and tibia.
- Be prepared to utilize an intraoperative radiograph if desired.

Preoperative Planning

- Template size and position of femur and tibial components as well as approximate stem diameter and length.
- Have available morselized cancellous allograft or structural allografts.

Bone/Implant/Soft Tissue Techniques

For cancellous impaction grafting:

- Routine exposure
- Remove failed implants. Use of thin-blade oscillating saw facilitates implant removal while minimizing host bone damage (Figure 65.3).
- Use a curet and high-speed burr to facilitate complete removal of membranous tissue, cement, and necrotic bone.
- Place a "trial stem" down the intramedullary canal. If doing impaction grafting along the diaphysis, place a small trial stem and impact bone densely around the stem after placing a restrictor. If performing impaction grafting only at the meta-diaphyseal portion of the distal femur or proximal tibia, a more canal filling trial may be utilized (Figure 65.4).
- Be sure to densely pack bone into defects (Figure 65.5).
- Cement components into place with antibiotic cement, pressurizing the cement into the cancellous bone (Figure 65.6).
- Trial reduction, then selection and insertion of real polyethylene followed by routine closure.
- Obtain a postoperative radiograph in the operating room or recovery room.

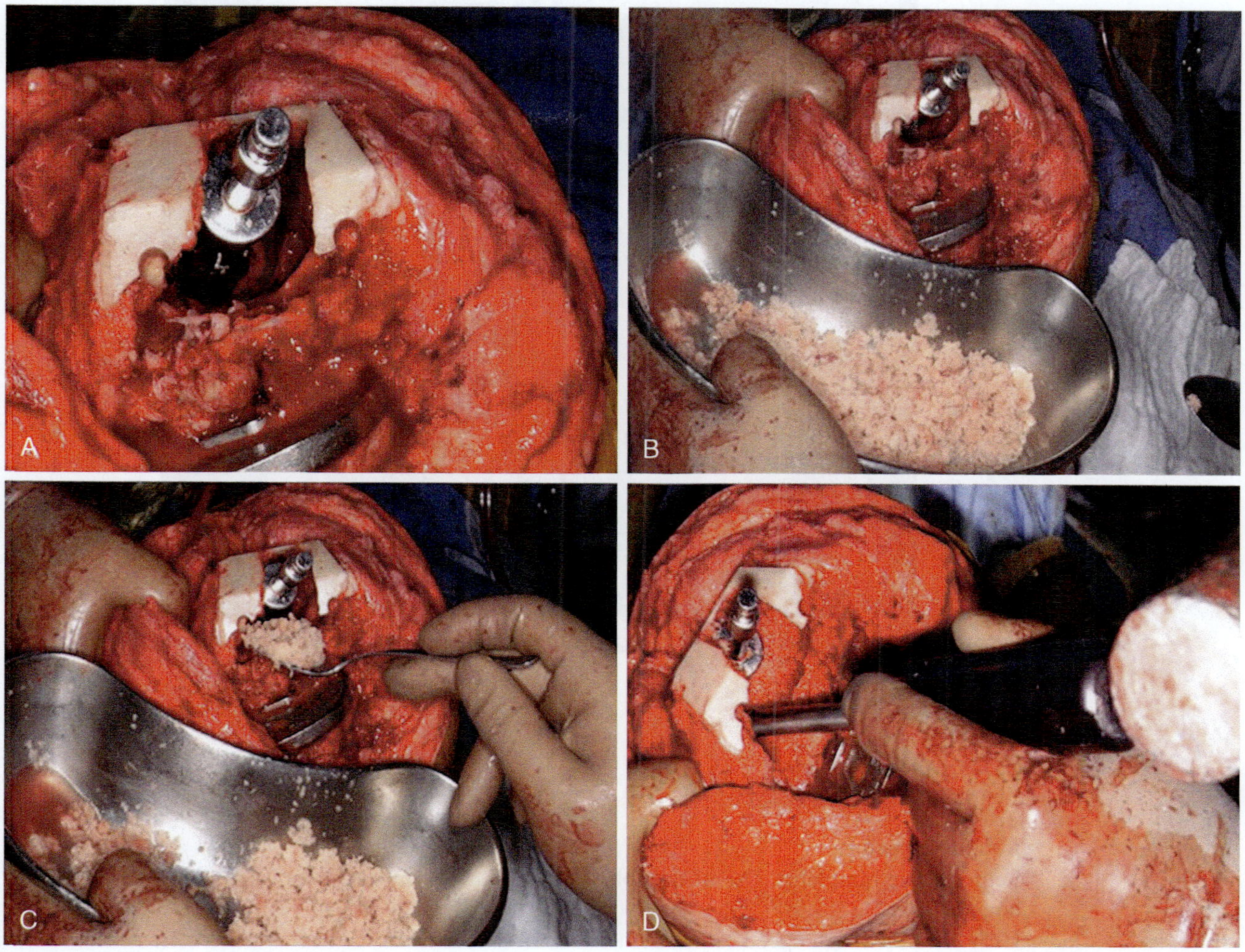

Figure 65.4 | A-D. Steps involved in tightly impacting morselized cancellous bone graft around a trial stem.

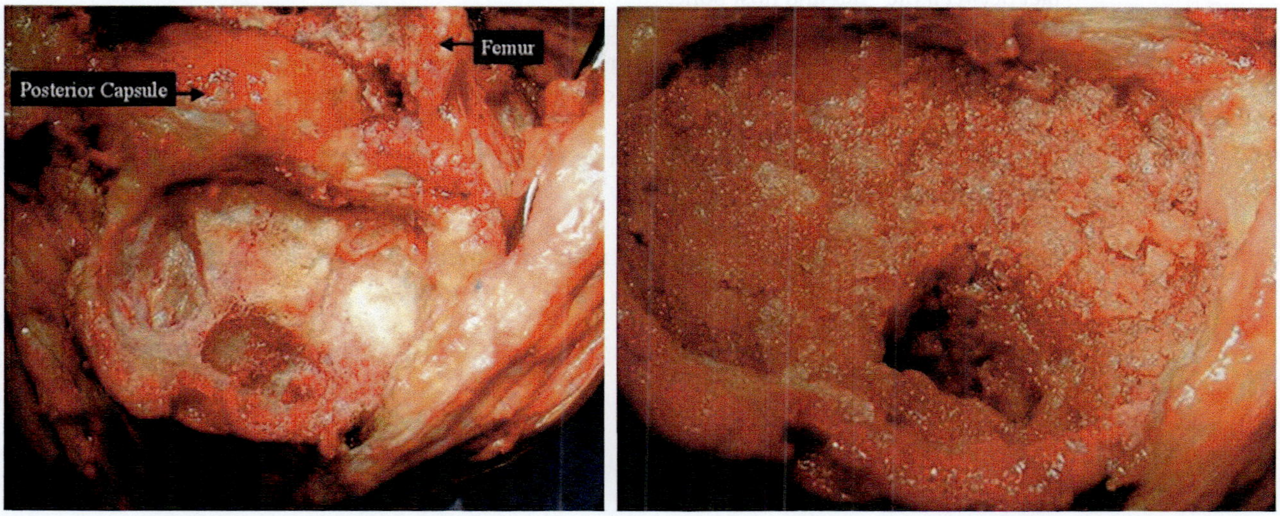

Figure 65.5 | Photograph showing cavitary defects and reconstruction with tightly packed morselized allograft.

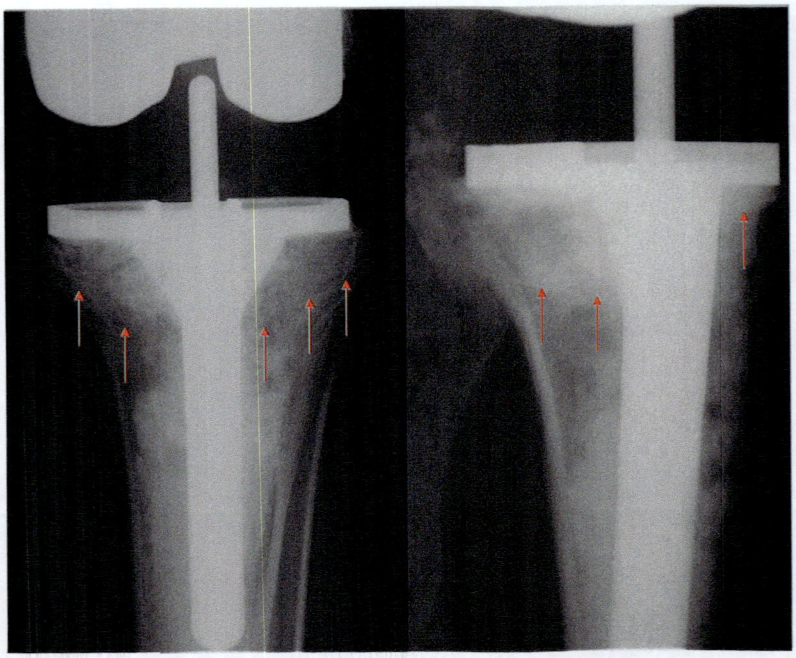

Figure 65.6 | Postoperative radiographs showing tibial metaphyseal allograft reconstruction and antibiotic cement interdigitation into allograft.

For Intussusception Allografts

- Routine exposure.
- Remove failed implants. Use of thin-blade saw facilitates implant removal while minimizing host bone damage.
- Use a curet and high-speed burr to remove membranous tissue, cement, and necrotic bone.
- If tibial tubercle is involved, can incorporate tubercle osteotomy and then fix the native tubercle segment to the allograft after implantation.
- Pick allograft that is an appropriate size and shape to fill defect. I prefer to select anatomically similar tissue, using a femoral allograft for a femoral defect and tibial bone for a tibial defect.
- Shape the external aspect of the graft to fill defect. Ideally, one should maximize the amount of contact between the graft and host bone.
- Prepare the inner aspect of graft to allow appropriate placement of a cemented component.
- Plan on bypassing the proximal (femur) or distal (tibia) portion of the graft with a stem.
- Cement implant into graft with antibiotic cement.
- Impact allograft prosthesis into host bone.
- Occasionally one will have to cement stem into host bone. Be careful to minimize cement interdigitation between graft and host bone.
- Routine closure.
- Postoperative radiograph in the operating room or recovery area (Figure 65.7).

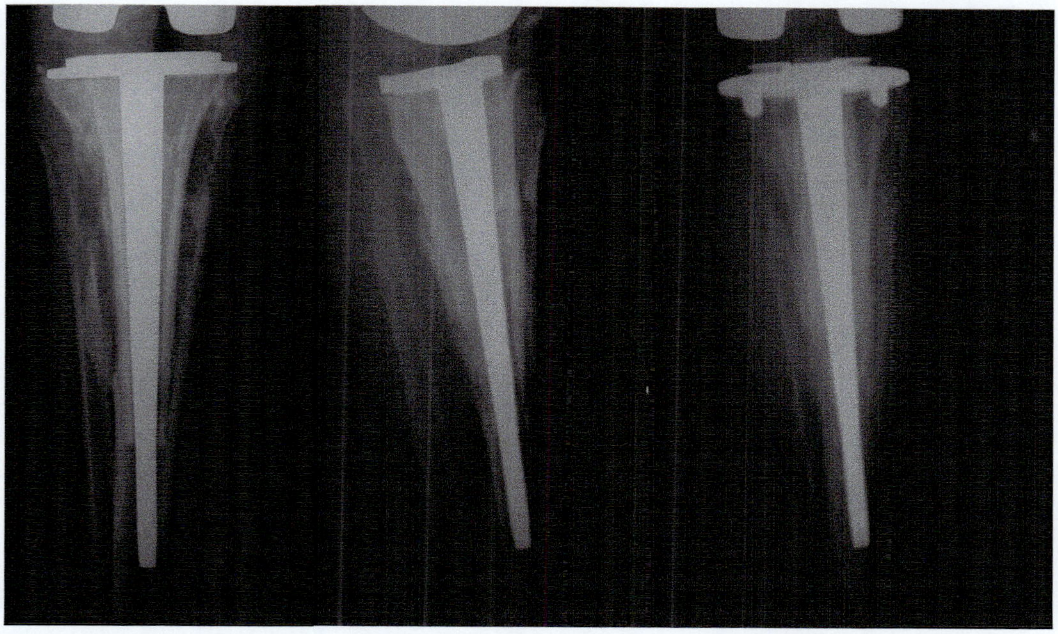

Figure 65.7 | Postoperative radiographs showing intussusception allograft tibial reconstruction.

Postoperative Management

- Touch weight bearing for 6 to 8 weeks. Progressive weight bearing thereafter.
- Range of motion started within 48 hours.
- Routine DVT prophylaxis.

Chapter 66
Constrained Implants

KEVIN I. PERRY

Key Concepts

- Instability is equal to infection as the most common cause of revision in the first 5 years after total knee arthroplasty (TKA).
- Additionally, instability accounts for one-fifth of TKAs revised after 5 years.
- The spectrum of implant constraint in the revision setting typically includes posterior stabilized (PS) implants, varus-valgus constrained (VVC) implants, and hinged implants.
- Remember that constraint varies between different implant designs and between manufacturers. Not all PS or VVC implants offer the same inherent knee stability.
- With increasing constraint there is a theoretical trade-off between reducing instability of the knee and increasing forces at the implant-cement-bone interfaces.
- VVC implants should be considered when deformity exists but the collateral ligaments are intact, when there is substantial ligament imbalance between the medial and lateral structures, or if there is an intraoperative medial collateral ligament (MCL) injury that can be repaired.
- Indications for rotating-hinge TKA implants include true ligament incompetence from major bone loss (from infection (Figure 66.1), trauma, osteolysis (Figure 66.2), or iatrogenic (Figure 66.3) damaged, uncorrectable severe flexion/extension space mismatch, oncologic cases that violate the collateral ligaments, distal femur fractures that are not amenable to fixation (Figures 66.4 and 66.5), and uncorrectable recurvatum.
- With all constrained implants it is wise to add stems and/or metaphyseal cones or sleeves to offload the implant-cement-bone interfaces.

Sterile Instruments and Implants

Instruments

- Standard TKA retractors and instruments
- Sagittal saw
- Flexible and stiff osteotomes of multiple widths
- Moreland-type osteotomes
- 6.5-mm and pencil-tip burrs (for implant removal)
- Metal cutting burr (if needed for implant removal)

Implants

- Varying levels of constrained implants should be available (PS, VVC, and rotating hinge) if stability concerns exist.

Positioning

- Supine position

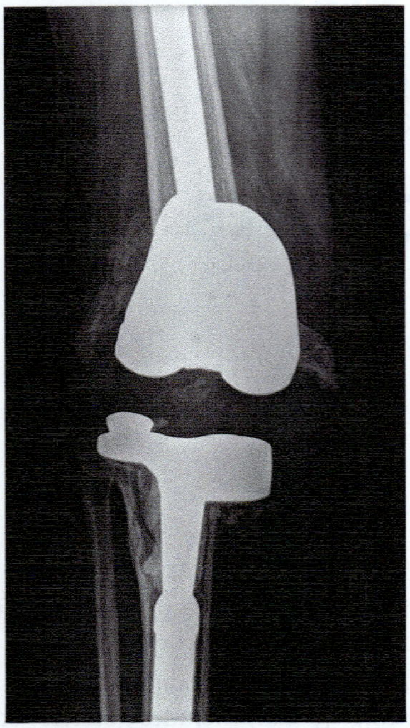

Figure 66.1 | AP radiograph demonstrating major bone loss from infection.

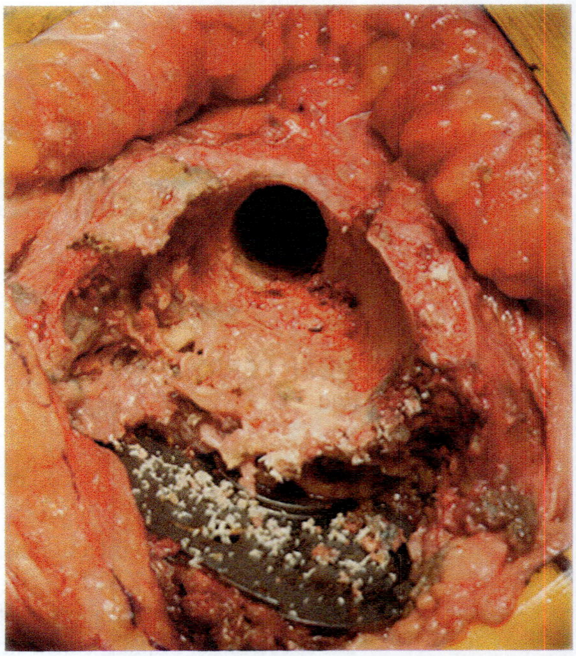

Figure 66.2 | Intraoperative photograph demonstrating extensive osteolysis involving both femoral condyles.

Surgical Approaches

- A standard median parapatellar approach is most often used in the revision TKA setting.
- A quadriceps snip can be added and often is required in the sniff knee.
- A tibial tubercle osteotomy can be used in rare cases with severe patella baja or with a well-fixed long press fit or cemented stem to simplify implant removal.
- If extensile exposure is needed, this can be carried out according to the descriptions in Chapter 61.

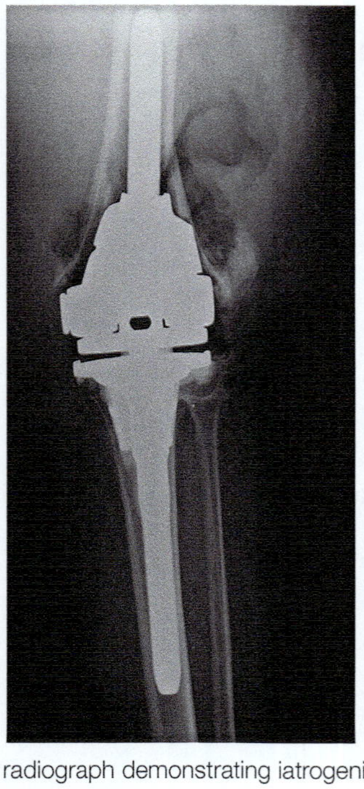

Figure 66.3 | AP radiograph demonstrating iatrogenic femoral condyle fracture.

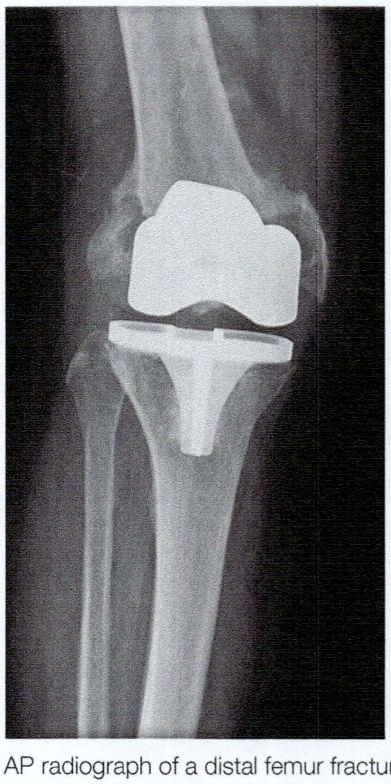

Figure 66.4 | AP radiograph of a distal femur fracture that was not amenable to open reduction and internal fixation.

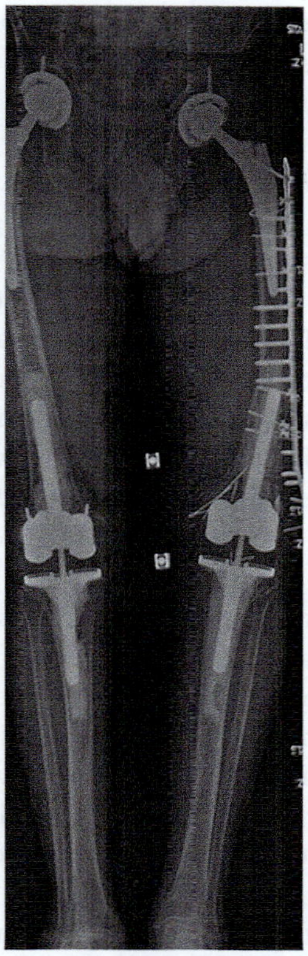

Figure 66.5 I AP radiograph of a distal femur fracture that was not amenable to fixation.

Preoperative Planning

- Preoperatively determine the varying levels of constraint and types of implants to have available at the time of surgery. Nearly all revisions need a VVC implant available, and some should have a hinged implant available.
- Anteroposterior (AP) and lateral radiographs are examined to identify the brand and fixation methods of the current implants. Radiographs should also be scrutinized for the extent and location of osteolysis. If the femoral condyles are severely compromised, a hinged construct should be available.
- A preoperative physical examination is done to assess the competence of the collateral ligaments and level of deformity. Increasing level of deformity and/or collateral incompetence suggest that fully constrained implants should be available at the time of revision surgery.

Bone, Implant, and Soft Tissue Techniques

- A standard approach to the knee should be done.
- Alternative extended exposure techniques are described in Section IV-B, Chapter 2.
- If utilizing a hinged TKA implant, particularly in the setting of a very stiff knee, it can be helpful early in the case to dissect the origins of the collateral ligaments off the femur for better exposure.
- Implant removal should be carried out according to the techniques described in Section IV-B, Chapter 3.
- Multiple cultures should be sent from predictable, reproducible parts of the exposure:
  - Suprapatellar pouch synovium
  - Femoral canal
  - Tibial canal
- The femoral and tibial canals are then prepared for cemented or cementless fixation as per surgeon preference as described in Chapter 62.
- The tibia is prepared at 90° to the intramedullary reamer and prepared for cementless metaphyseal fixation (cone/sleeve) if needed for fixation or if constrained implants will be utilized.
- The femur is prepared with a new distal cut off an intramedullary reamer followed by new 4-in-1 cuts and the femoral box cut. The need for augments is judged off of the distal femoral cutting jig and the 4-in-1 cutting block in each system. If there is substantial bone loss or it is judged that increased TKA constraint may be necessary, then the femur is prepared for cementless metaphyseal fixation (either a metaphyseal cone/sleeve).

- When both the femur and tibia have been prepared, trial components are built on the back table and placed into the knee.
- A trial PS polyethylene is placed, and the soft tissue balance in both flexion and extension is examined. Intraoperative assessment of the collateral ligaments is done to determine the integrity of both the medial and lateral collateral ligaments. If either has been fully compromised, consideration should be given to a hinged TKA design.
- VVC implants should be used when severe deformity exists but the collateral ligaments are intact, there is severe ligament imbalance between the medial and lateral structures, or if there is an intraoperative MCL injury that can be repaired at the time of surgery.
- Indications for rotating hinge TKA implants can include iatrogenic femoral condyle fracture, uncorrectable flexion/extension space mismatch and recurvatum.
- When constrained implants are used, we typically add stems along with metaphyseal cones or sleeves to improve metaphyseal fixation and offload bone-cement-implant forces (described in Chapter 64).
- Intraoperative radiographs are obtained with the trials in place to ensure appropriate positioning of the implants.
- When appropriate positioning of the implants and the stability of the knee has been achieved, the trials can be removed and the real femoral and tibial components can be cemented into place. In cases with marked bone deficiency we sometimes cement the tibia and femur separately.
- After cementing both components, stability can once again be assessed with trialing of different polyethylene inserts and the final polyethylene insert can be inserted.
- If a hinged construct is utilized, the hinge mechanism should be assembled at this time.
- The wound is thoroughly irrigated and closed in layers.
- Postoperative radiographs should be obtained. Figure 66.6A and B demonstrates AP and lateral radiographs of a VVC implant, whereas Figure 66.7A and B demonstrates AP and lateral radiographs of a hinged TKA construct.

Postoperative Care

- If intraoperative injury to the medial collateral or lateral collateral ligaments occurred and a hinged construct was not used, patients should be protected in a brace for 6 weeks postoperatively.
- Patients are typically allowed to be weight bearing as tolerated.
- Gentle range-of-motion exercises are encouraged and started on postoperative day 1.

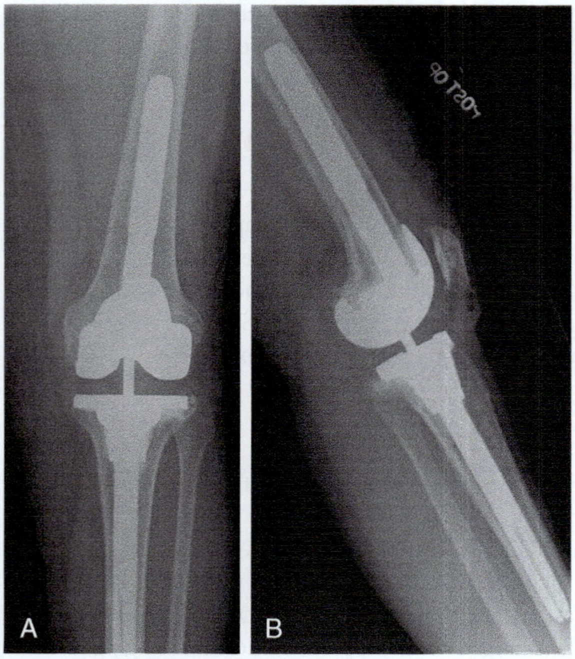

Figure 66.6 | AP (A) and lateral (B) radiographs of a varus-valgus constrained implant after revision TKA.

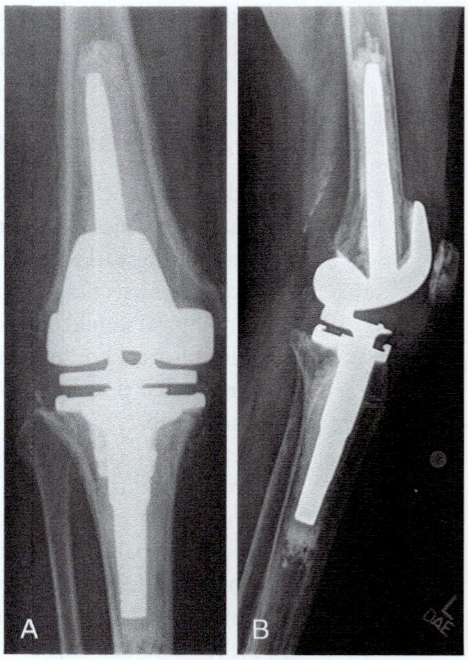

Figure 66.7 | AP (A) and lateral (B) radiographs of a hinged knee design for revision TKA.

Section D
Revision TKA for Specific Conditions

Chapter 67
Tibiofemoral Instability

TIMOTHY S. BROWN
MATTHEW P. ABDEL

Key Concepts

- Instability accounts for approximately 10 to 25% of revision total knee arthroplasties (TKAs).
- Types of tibiofemoral instability include:
  - Sagittal (anteroposterior) instability (Figure 67.1) due to flexion-extension mismatch such as flexion instability (Figure 67.2).
  - Coronal (varus-valgus) instability
    - Iatrogenic from
      - Ligamentous release
      - Condylar fracture (Figure 67.3)
    - Attritional damage to ligaments, such as from
      - Polyethylene wear synovitis (Figure 67.4)
      - Cement synovitis from debonded tibial component (Figure 67.5A and B)
      - Periprosthetic joint infection
  - Midflexion instability
  - Global instability (Figure 67.6)
  - Hyperextension (recurvatum) instability (Figure 67.7)
- Accurate diagnosis of the etiology causing instability is essential to appropriately manage this complication.

Sterile Instruments and Implants

Instruments

- Routine revision TKA instruments
- Large and small sagittal saws
- Large and small flexible osteotomes
- High-speed 6.5-mm and pencil-tip burrs
- Square tip impactor

Implants

- Implants with varying levels of constraint should be available during all cases, from posterior-stabilized to varus-valgus constraint (VVC) to rotating-hinge constructs.

Surgical Approaches

- In most cases, a medial parapatellar approach can be used. Occasionally, an extensile exposure may be required, such as a quadriceps snip.

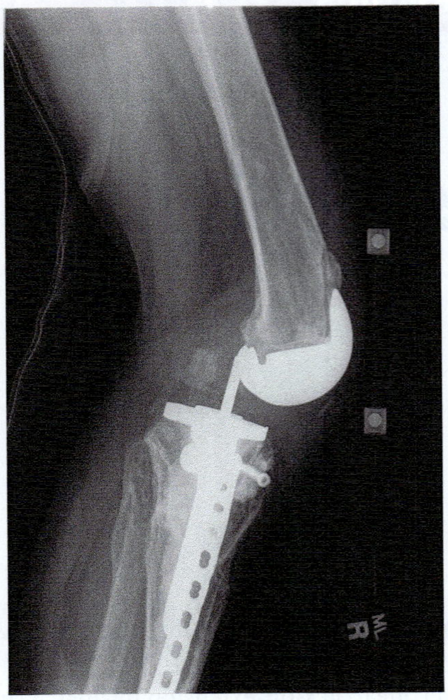

Figure 67.1 | Lateral radiograph of a 55-year-old man with a dislocated knee after a revision TKA completed at an outside institution.

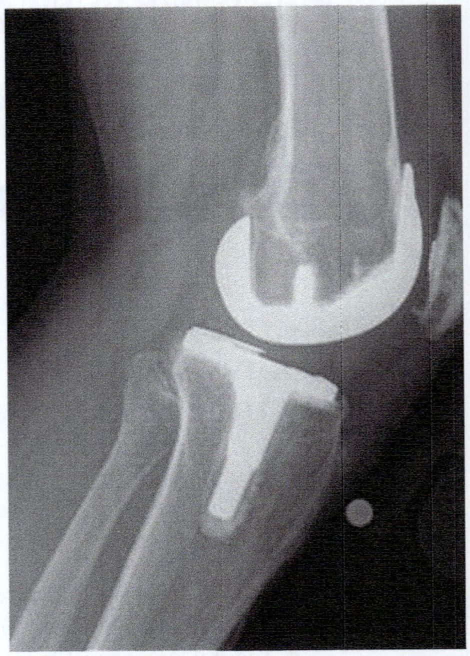

Figure 67.2 | Lateral radiograph of a 69-year-old woman with radiographic findings concerning for flexion instability including excessive posterior tibial slope and decreased condylar offset.

Preoperative Planning

- A full complement of knee radiographs are recommended, including a long-leg hip-knee-ankle radiograph, standing anteroposterior (AP) radiograph, standing posteroanterior flexion radiograph, lateral radiograph, and patellar view.
- Prior radiographs for comparison are often very helpful.
- As with any revision TKA, periprosthetic joint infection (PJI) should be excluded with inflammatory markers (erythrocyte sedimentation rate and C-reactive protein) and a joint aspiration.

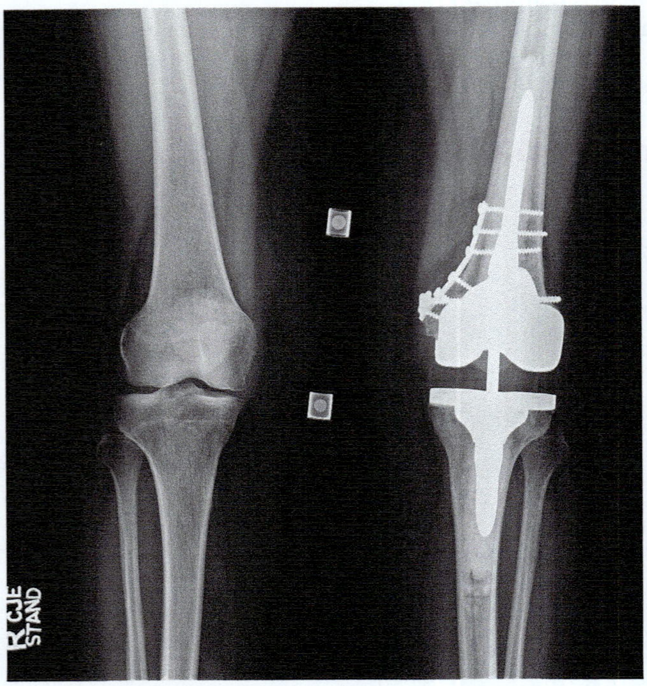

Figure 67.3 | Anteroposterior radiograph of an 89-year-old woman with an intraoperative medial femoral condyle fracture at the time of reimplantation treated with open reduction and internal fixation. Lack of adequate treatment would result in coronal instability.

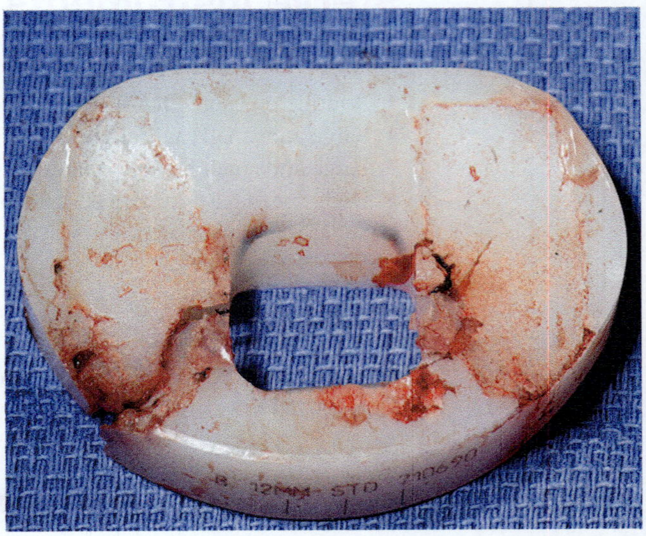

Figure 67.4 | Intraoperative picture of a 25-year-old man with marked polyethylene wear 8 years after a distal femoral replacement for oncologic purposes. Even with a hinged construct, this resulted in instability.

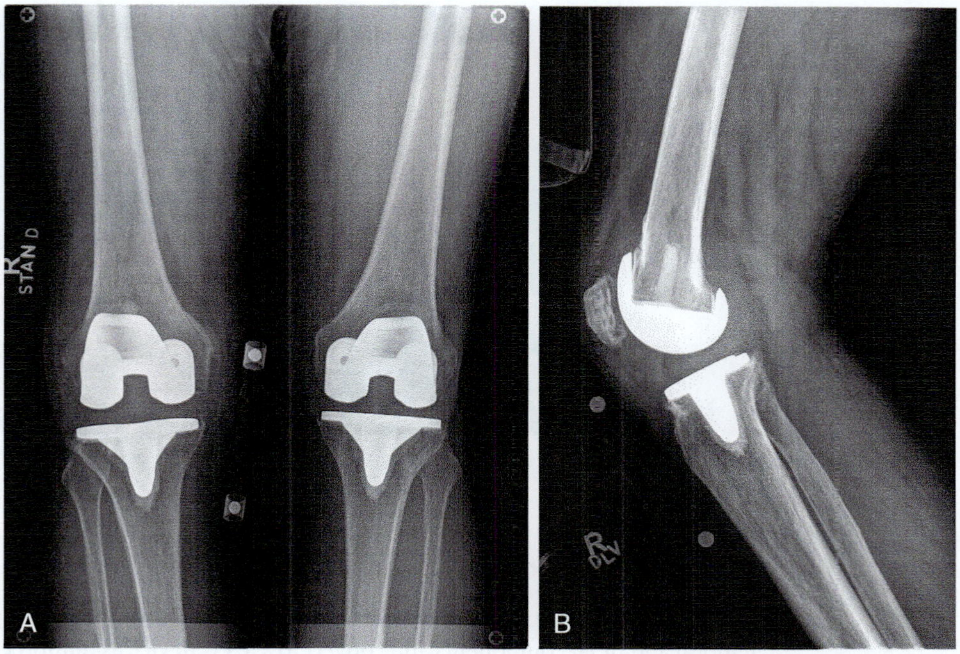

Figure 67.5 | Anteroposterior (A) and lateral (B) radiographs of a 60-year-old man revealing asymmetric gaps, indicative of coronal instability.

Bone, Implant, and Soft Tissue Techniques

- The patient should be positioned supine.
- The knee should be examined under anesthesia to determine the true form and extent of instability (Figure 67.8).

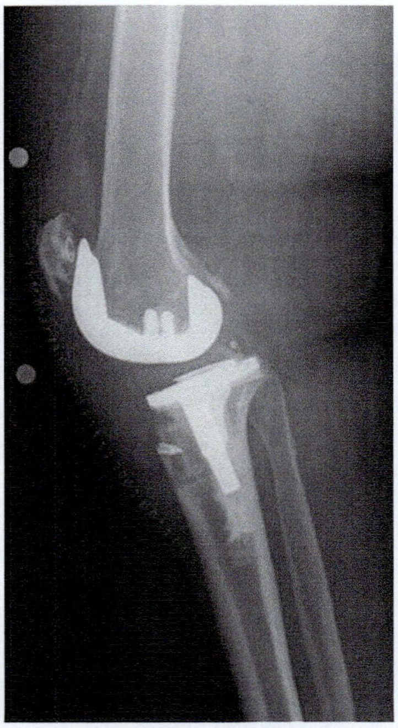

Figure 67.6 | Lateral radiograph of a 61-year-old woman with global instability related to her extensor mechanism disruption.

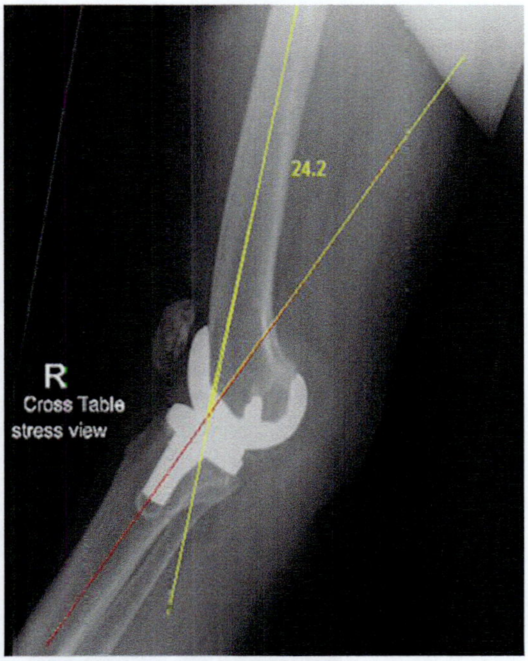

Figure 67.7 | Lateral radiograph of an 84-year-old man with 24° of hyperextension (recurvatum) instability.

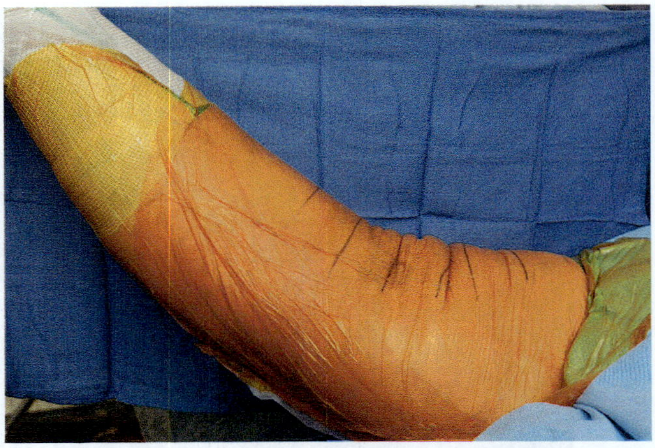

Figure 67.8 | Intraoperative picture of the patient from Figure 67.7 demonstrating marked recurvatum while under anesthesia.

Sagittal (Anteroposterior) Instability

- If flexion instability exists (Figure 67.9A and B), it is the senior author's preference to revise both the femoral and tibial components and convert to a VVC device as reinforcement, and not as a substitute for poor surgical technique or inadequate soft tissue balancing.
  Surgical correction includes the following stepwise approach (Figure 67.10):
  - Correction of any excessive posterior tibial slope to neutral slope.
  - Correction of any tibial component malrotation by placing the revision tibial component in line with the tibial crest.
  - Correction of any rotational malalignment of the femoral component so that it is colinear with the surgical transepicondylar axis.
  - Upsize the femoral component to increase condylar offset. This will often require posterior augments. Because external rotation often is deliberately increased, the posterior-lateral augment (e.g., 10 mm) is frequently larger than the posterior-medial augment (e.g., 5 mm).

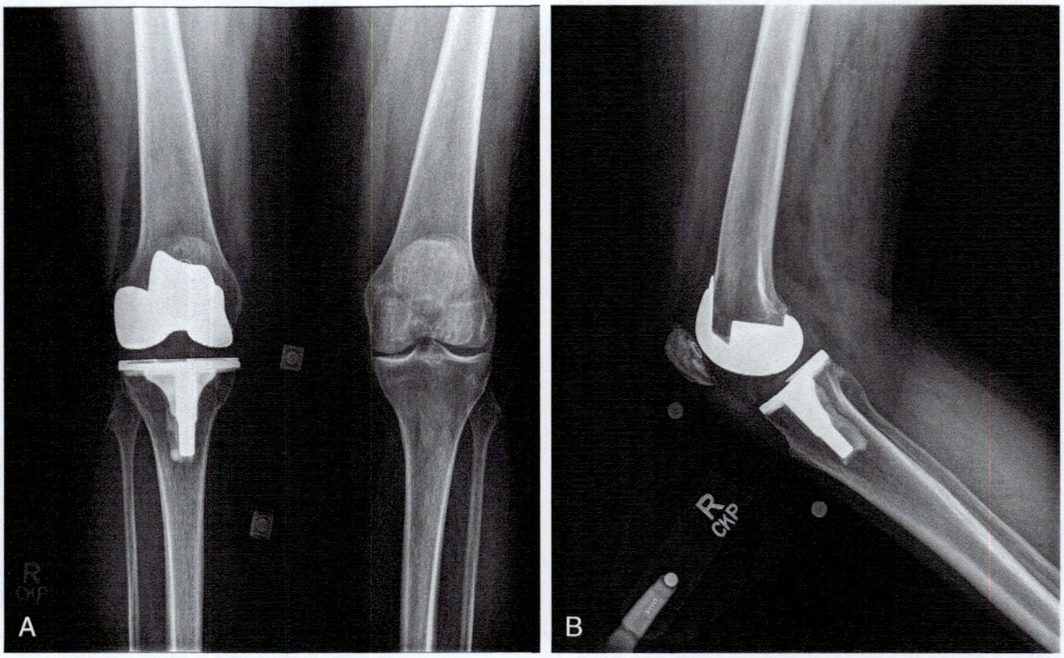

Figure 67.9 | Anteroposterior (A) and lateral (B) radiographs of a 71-year-old woman with radiographic findings concerning for flexion instability, including excessive posterior tibial slope, decreased condylar offset, coronal malalignment, and distalization of the femoral component.

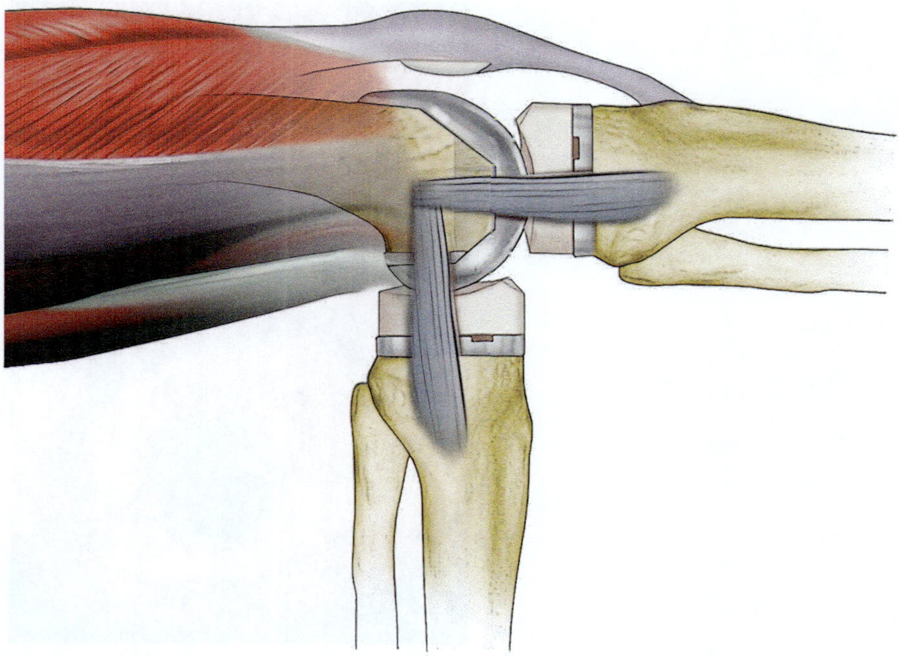

Figure 67.10 | Illustration of the maneuvers required to correct flexion instability, including a neutral posterior tibial slope, upsizing the femoral component, adding posterior augments, additional distal femoral resection, and a thicker polyethylene. (Used with permission of Mayo Foundation for Medical Education and Research. All rights reserved.)

- If the flexion gap remains looser than the extension gap, additional distal femoral bone is resected in 2-mm increments until the flexion and extension gaps are equivalent.
- A thicker polyethylene is selected to match the now equivalent flexion and extension gaps. It is the senior author's preference to utilize a VVC polyethylene as reinforcement in most revision TKA situations (Figure 67.11A and B).

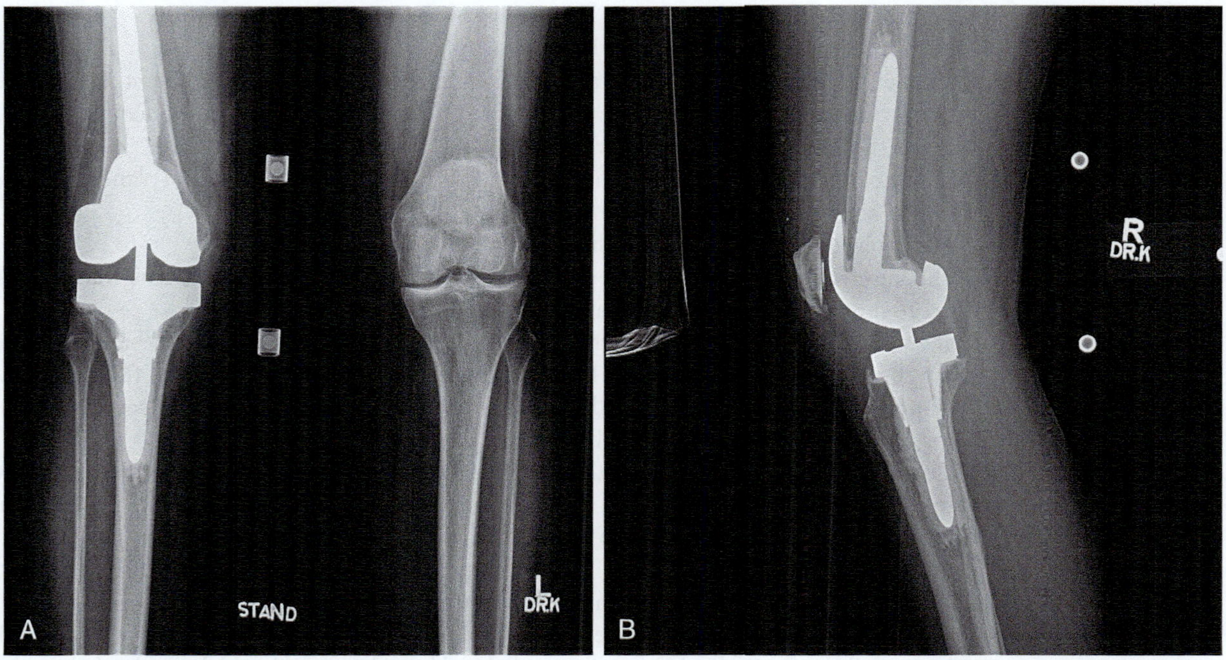

Figure 67.11 | Anteroposterior (A) and lateral (B) radiographs of the patient from Figure 67.9 after revision TKA for flexion instability with correction of posterior tibial slope, increased condylar offset with posterior augments, correction of coronal malalignment, proximalization of the femoral component, and a thicker polyethylene with varus-valgus constraint.

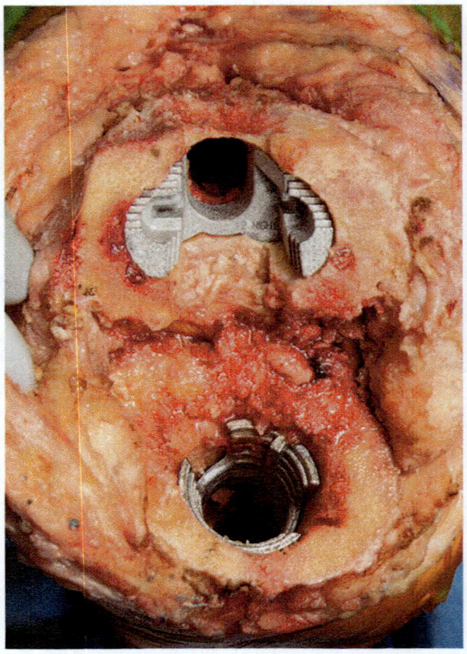

Figure 67.12 | Intraoperative picture depicting the use of uncemented femoral and tibial cones while revising the patient in Figure 67.5 with marked bone loss.

Coronal (Varus-Valgus) Instability

- Various etiologies may contribute to coronal instability, including iatrogenic injury (see Figure 67.3), PJI, polyethylene wear and subsequent osteolysis, and third-body cement debris from debonded components resulting in osteolysis (see Figure 67.5A and B).
- As in the case of sagittal instability, it is the senior author's preference to revise both components and utilize a VVC device in most revision situations.
- As with sagittal instability, a step-wise surgical approach is required that includes:
  - Correction of any tibial slope malalignment to neutral, correction of any tibial coronal malalignment to neutral, and correction of any tibial rotational malalignment so that rotation is in line with the tibial crest.
  - At first, tibial augments should not be utilized until trialing is performed.
  - Bone defects should be addressed according to the location, depth, and extent. It is the senior author's preference to often utilize uncemented porous tibial cones on the femur and tibia to address substantial bone loss (Figure 67.12).
  - Any femoral component malalignment in the coronal, sagittal, and rotational planes is addressed. Femoral augments are not typically utilized until trialing is performed.
  - A trial polyethylene is placed and the stability of the knee is assessed.
  - If the knee is loose in both flexion and extension equally, but the polyethylene thickness is less than 20 mm, then tibial augments are not needed.
  - If the knee is loose in both flexion and extension equally, but the polyethylene thickness is greater than 20 mm, augments (e.g., 5 or 10 mm) should be placed underneath the tibial baseplate to minimize utilizing a polyethylene thickness at the extreme of modularity. In some revision systems a specific thick tibial tray can be used.
  - If flexion is looser than extension, then the femoral component should be upsized and posterior femoral augments added. If flexion laxity persists, then additional distal femoral resection and a thicker polyethylene can be used to balance the knee.
  - If extension is looser than flexion, then distal femoral augments should be utilized (e.g., 5 or 10 mm) to selectively move the joint line distally and fill the loose extension space.
  - At this point, the surgeon must carefully evaluate the soft tissue balance. Occasionally, additional releases will be required to balance the medial and lateral gaps and a thicker polyethylene may be required. If that is the case, the surgeon should reevaluate if additional tibial augments are needed to mitigate the risk of being at the extreme of modularity.

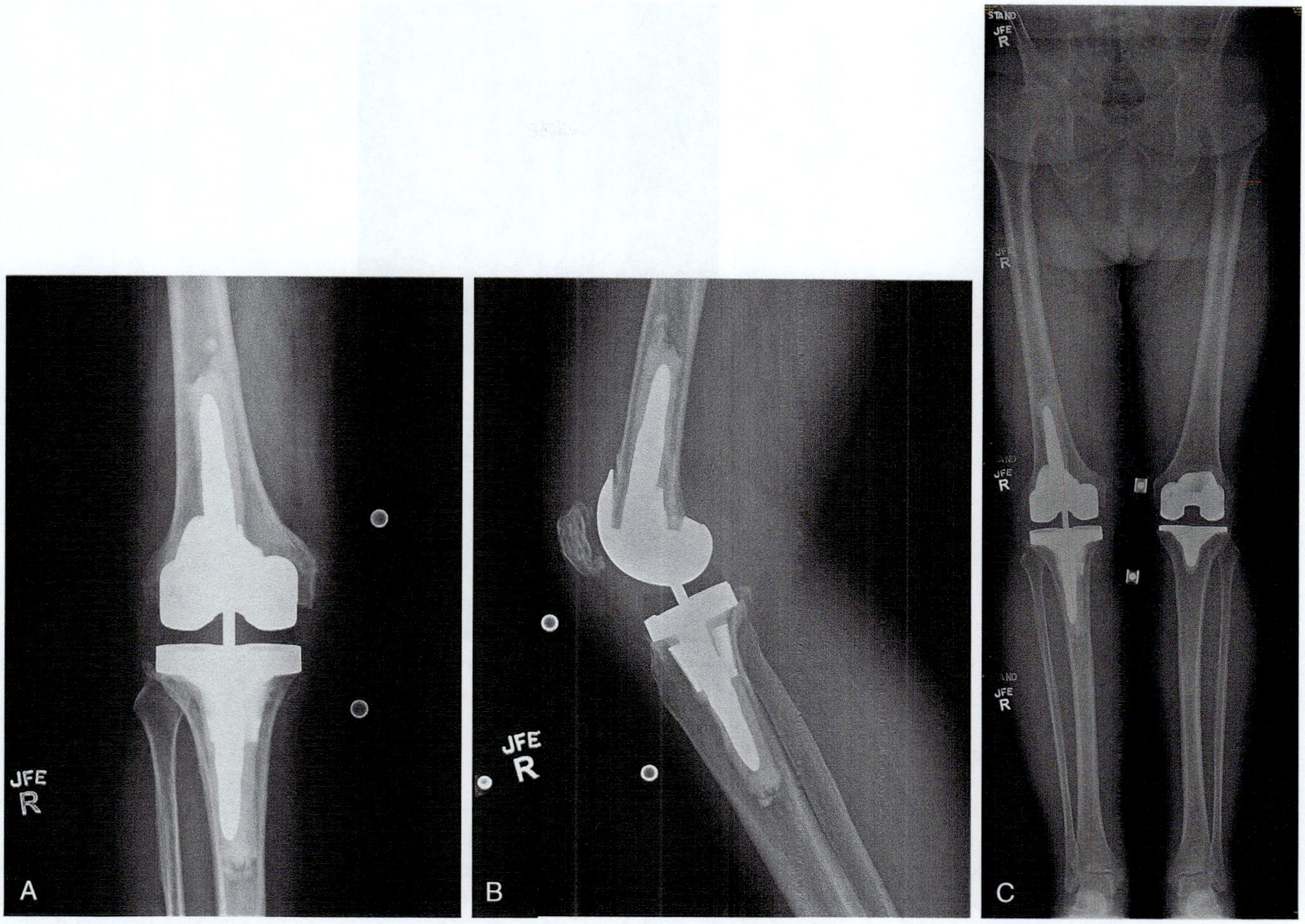

Figure 67.13 | Anteroposterior (A), lateral (B), and long-leg hip-knee-ankle (C) radiographs of the patient from Figures 67.5 and 67.12 depicting correction of the coronal instability with revision of the femoral and tibial components utilizing a large femoral component with 5-mm posterior augments on both the medial and lateral sides, a tibial component with 5-mm medial and lateral augments, cemented femoral and tibial stems, uncemented femoral and tibial cones, and thicker polyethylene with varus-valgus constraint.

- Once the gaps are well balanced on the medial and lateral sides in both flexion and extension, it is the senior author's preference to utilize a VVC polyethylene as reinforcement, and not as compensation for poor surgical technique and inadequate soft tissue balancing (Figure 67.13A-C).
- Note if there is complete incompetence of the medial collateral ligament (MCL), complete loss of the flexion gap, or recurvatum, then a hinged total knee implant is required (see later discussion).

Global Instability

- Similar management to coronal instability, except when there is complete incompetence of the MCL, complete loss of the flexion gap, or severe recurvatum that is not correctable. In those cases, a hinged total knee implant is required (see later discussion).

Hyperextension (Recurvatum) Instability

- True recurvatum (Figure 67.14) should be addressed with a hinged TKA.
- Surgeons should be aware that not all contemporary rotating-hinge devices on the market prevent and/or treat recurvatum. As such, it is important to pick a device that accommodates for not only coronal instability but also hyperextension instability (Figure 67.15A and B).

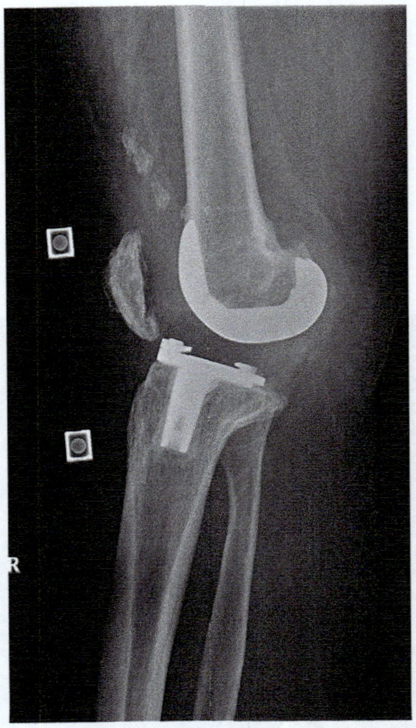

Figure 67.14 | Preoperative lateral radiograph of a 74-year-old man with post-polio syndrome and marked recurvatum mandating a rotating hinge TKA.

Postoperative Care

- Often standard TKA postoperative protocols may be used, including weight bearing as tolerated with gentle range of motion, but this is sometimes modified.
- One exception is when the tibiofemoral instability is secondary to a condylar fracture that has undergone open reduction and internal fixation (see Figure 67.3). In those cases, the weight-bearing and range-of-motion protocols are limited for the first 6 weeks to toe-touch weight bearing and flexion limited to 60°.
- If the patient had a significant preoperative valgus deformity and/or flexion contracture, consider keeping the knee partially flexed with a nonconstrictive dressing for 1 to 2 days postoperatively to minimize risk of peroneal nerve palsy.

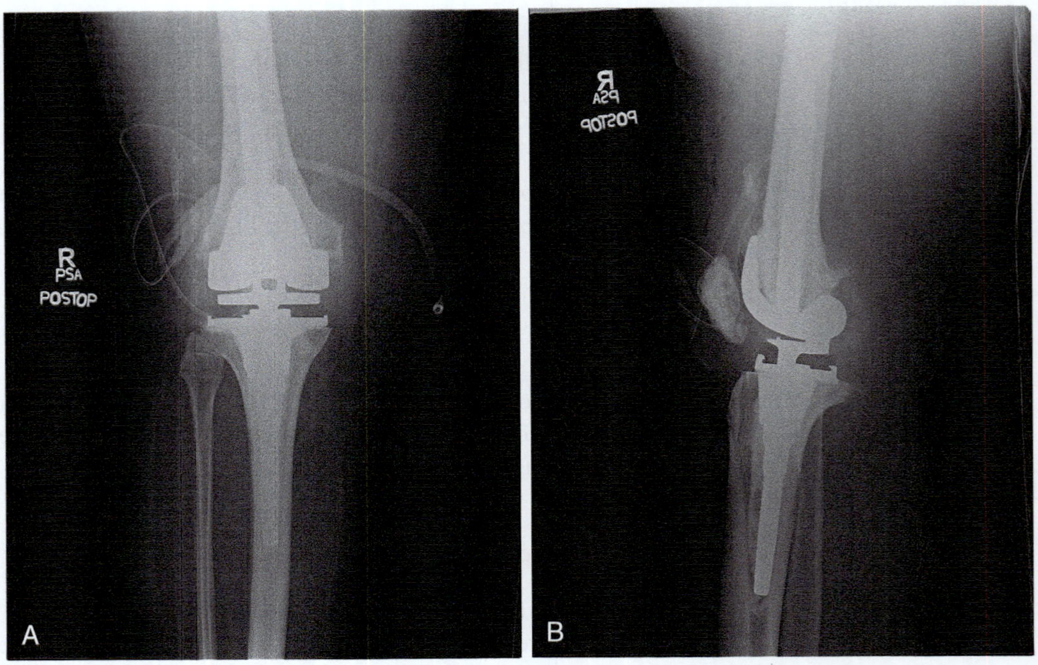

Figure 67.15 | Postoperative anteroposterior (A) and lateral (B) radiographs of the patient from Figure 67.14 after a revision to a rotating hinge TKA.

Suggested Reading

1. Abdel MP, Ledford CK, Kobic A, Taunton MJ, Hanssen AD. Contemporary failure aetiologies of the primary, posterior-stabilised total knee arthroplasty. *Bone Joint J*. 2017;99-B(5):647-652.
2. Cottino U, Abdel MP, Perry KI, Mara KC, Lewallen DG, Hanssen AD. Long-term results after total knee arthroplasty with contemporary rotating-hinge prostheses. *J Bone Joint Surg Am*. 2017;99(4):324-330.
3. Abdel MP, Pulido L, Severson EP, Hanssen AD. Stepwise surgical correction of instability in flexion after total knee replacement. *Bone Joint J*. 2014;96-B(12):1644-1648.

Chapter 68
Knee Stiffness

STEPHEN M. PETIS
MARK W. PAGNANO

Key Concepts

Stiffness after total knee arthroplasty (TKA) is a frustrating problem for patient and surgeon alike. Few patients with substantial limitation of knee range of motion are satisfied with the result of their TKA. Depending on the definition of stiffness, somewhere between 1.5 and 3% of contemporary TKAs have limited postoperative range of motion. Although specific effort must be made to determine the reason for the stiffness following TKA, the fact remains that the precise cause remains poorly understood in the majority of cases (Figure 68.1A and B).

Select subgroups of patients do have a clear etiology for their postoperative stiffness, and it is critical to identify those patients as the results of treatment are predictably better. There are a multitude of small series that implicate one small technical factor or another as a cause of stiffness after TKA. Those include overstuffing the patella, a tight posterior cruciate ligament, flexion gap mismatch, component malposition, joint line elevation, poor postoperative pain control, and inadequate postoperative rehabilitation. Surgeons should be cautious about recommending revision surgery for stiffness if only one small problem is identifiable, as the results of additional surgery in such cases are likely to be modest.

One pragmatic approach to the painful TKA is to methodically look for extrinsic causes, intrinsic causes, and patient-specific causes for stiffness and pain. To do this most predictably it is useful to have a preset routine in which every patient with a stiff or painful TKA gets (1) a full-length hip-knee-ankle radiograph, (2) fluoroscopically positioned radiographs of the knee, and (3) serum erythrocyte sedimentation rate and C-reactive protein, and plan for (4) knee aspiration for cell count and culture.

Extrinsic causes for stiffness are those outside the knee joint itself and primarily focus on the hip and spine. It is not uncommon to get tunnel vision and keep thinking knee, knee, knee and in doing so overlook advanced hip arthritis or lumbar radiculopathy as the cause of knee pain and disability. The hip-knee-ankle radiograph builds in a reminder to check the hip in all of these cases.

Intrinsic causes for stiffness include infection, aseptic loosening or failure of ingrowth, and surgical technical errors. Infection is assessed with the sedimentation rate and C-reactive protein tests followed by knee aspiration. Infection presents a good news/bad news scenario where the good news is a clear cause for the stiffness and pain, whereas the bad news is the additional surgical intervention needed. Loosening of cemented components or failed ingrowth of uncemented components is most readily assessed with high-quality serial radiographs.

Patient-specific causes of stiffness include secondary gain problems (workers compensation, disability claims), poor pain tolerance, and arthrofibrosis related to an abnormal inflammatory response. Separate strategies must be developed if one chooses to reoperate on one of these patients with a presumed patient-specific cause of stiffness so as to not simply repeat the prior events that led to stiffness.

Document previous interventions or procedures that have been used to treat stiffness (i.e., manipulation under anesthesia, arthrolysis, polyethylene liner exchange, component revision).

A detailed preoperative assessment and critical appraisal of radiographs will determine whether one or both components need to be revised to address stiffness. Variables to consider include:

- Implant position—coronal, sagittal, and axial plane alignment
- Sizing of implants—retropatellar and femoral condylar offset

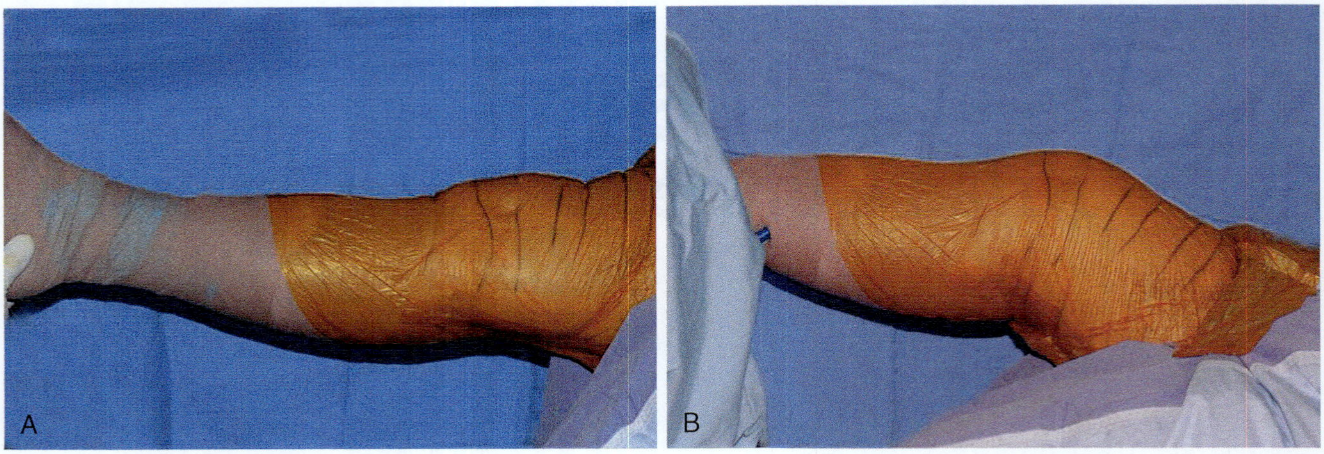

Figure 68.1 | The knee may be stiff in extension, flexion, or both. In this example (A) the knee still extends well but (B) has marked limitation of flexion.

- Joint line position
- Retained osteophytes, loose bodies, or heterotopic ossification

Acquiring operative reports and implant stickers is paramount if there is a plan to retain one or both implants to ensure modular options, and appropriate extraction tools are available if required.

The results of revision TKA for stiffness are unpredictable; however, most studies report a modest improvement in range of motion and patient-reported outcome measures.

Manipulation under anesthesia done either closed or arthroscopically is often useful for the patient who presents with early postoperative stiffness and occasionally useful for the patient with stiffness who presents late. Manipulation is typically done under a brief general anesthetic, and it is useful to have full muscle relaxation through pharmacologic paralysis during the manipulation. Care must be taken to gradually flex the knee and to avoid sudden forceful motions that could cause a femoral or patellar fracture. By holding the leg close to the tibial tubercle, as opposed to at the ankle, one minimizes the lever-arm and decreases the risk of iatrogenic fracture (Figure 68.2A and B). Typically, the knee is flexed over a 2- to 5-minute time period and it is helpful to listen carefully for the sound of intra-articular scar tissue slowly breaking. As long as one can hear scar tissue continuing to break free it is safe to continue applying pressure and pursuing additional flexion. If one chooses to manipulate a knee at more than 1 year postoperatively, then it is wise to consider doing that arthroscopically or at least assisted with arthroscopic instruments. For these very stiff knees one can make 2 or 3 arthroscopic portals around the knee and insert a standard knee scope sheath and trocar together. The sheath and trocar are then used to physically disrupt scar tissue by methodically re-establishing the suprapatellar pouch, the medial

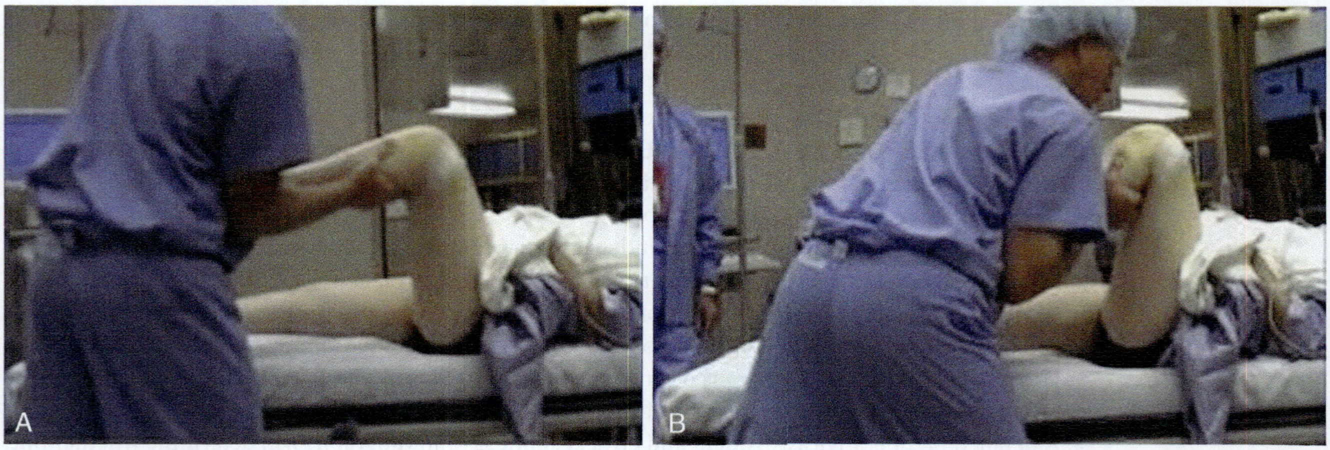

Figure 68.2 | Closed manipulation under anesthesia is most safely performed by (A) flexing the ipsilateral hip to 90° and then grasping the leg proximally, close to the tibial tubercle, to minimize the lever arm and (B) gradually leaning into the patient while listening for the characteristic crunching sound of scar tissue giving way. To avoid iatrogenic fracture of the femur or disruption of the extensor mechanism it is wise to stop flexing once the audible cues of progress have ceased.

and lateral gutters adjacent to the femur, and the retropatellar space behind the patellar tendon. Those maneuvers can be easily performed blindly without actually inserting the arthroscopic camera. Once the scar tissue has been freed bluntly with the sheath and trocar, the knee is progressively manipulated under anesthesia. Manipulation under anesthesia is predictably useful in regaining flexion but is both unpredictable and somewhat risky when attempting to regain extension. Although it may be useful in certain circumstances, manipulating a stiff knee in extension puts the distal femur at particular risk of fracture.

Sterile Instruments and Implants

Instruments

- Typical instruments for revision TKA

Implants

- Cruciate-retaining or posterior-stabilized TKA system
- Varus-valgus constrained, and hinged knee options for severe stiffness
- Femoral and tibial stems

Positioning

- Supine

Surgical Approaches

A midline incision with a medial parapatellar arthrotomy is performed in almost every instance.

The surgeon should have familiarity with the typical extensile approaches to prevent damage to the extensor mechanism. A quadriceps snip is used in many revision TKAs done for stiffness, whereas a tibial tubercle osteotomy occasionally may be required in the very, very stiff TKA.

Preoperative Planning

A full complement of knee radiographs is recommended—standing anteroposterior (AP), standing posteroanterior flexion view, standing lateral, skyline, and 3-foot standing films.

The radiographs are used to identify signs of loosening and assess implant positioning.

Joint arthrocentesis and synovial fluid analysis should be used to rule out infection.

A physical examination should document stiffness in flexion and/or extension. As well, the flexion and extension gaps should be assessed for concomitant instability that may have to be revised at the time of surgery.

Bone/Implant/Soft Tissue Techniques

While the patient is under anesthesia, assess and document knee range of motion.

Perform a midline incision with a medial parapatellar arthrotomy. It is critical to excise excess scar tissue from the following areas to both gain exposure during the revision and to mitigate the risk of postoperative stiffness:

- Suprapatellar pouch extending up and under the quadriceps tendon proximally
- Medial and lateral gutters
- Infrapatellar area/fat pad
- Adhesions along femoral metadiaphysis

The patella is laterally subluxated to avoid injury to the extensor mechanism. If it is difficult to mobilize the extensor mechanism, there should be a low threshold to perform a quadriceps snip. Typically, the exposure on the tibial side extends both distally and posteriorly such that the knee can be concomitantly flexed and externally rotated to bring the tibia out from underneath the femur (Figure 68.3).

The coronal, sagittal, and axial positions of the components should be critically assessed. Substantial component malposition should be corrected by revising the components. A resurfaced patella also

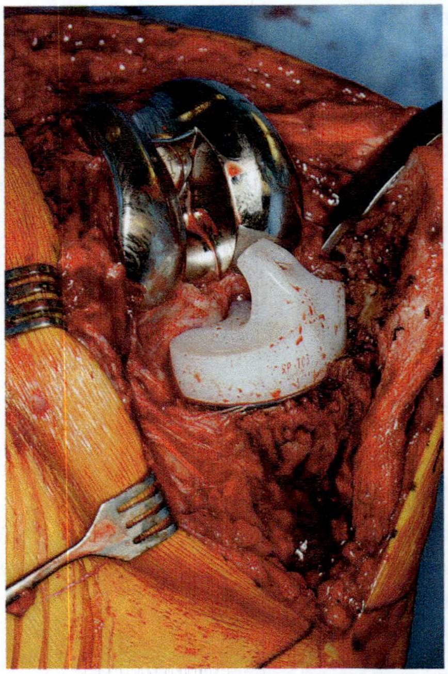

Figure 68.3 I This clinical photograph illustrates the typical exposure of a stiff TKA at the time of revision. A moderate to extensive medial release that extends distally and posteriorly to allow combined flexion and external rotation of the leg to deliver the tibial component out from underneath the femur is demonstrated.

requires assessment to ensure that the patellofemoral compartment is not overstuffed. If the posterior cruciate ligament (PCL) was retained and the flexion space is tight, it is most prudent to excise the PCL and convert to a posterior-stabilized design.

The implants that require revision are removed using previously described techniques, minimizing further bone loss.

Osteophytes, excess cement, and heterotopic bone should be removed, as these can tether soft tissues contributing to stiffness (Figure 68.4A-C).

The tibial cut is revised to ensure it is perpendicular to the mechanical axis. It is critical not to cut excess posterior slope with the tibial cut, as this can cause relative tightness in extension and open the flexion space. The initial amount of bone resected should be minimal to start.

The femoral cuts are revised to ensure optimal coronal, sagittal, and axial plane alignment. If the knee is particularly tight in extension, then the go-to move is typically to resect additional distal femoral bone until full extension has been obtained. It is foolhardy to revise a knee for stiffness and leave the operating room with anything less than full extension.

Femoral rotation should be assessed using the transepicondylar axis and re-creation of a rectangular flexion space. If there was excessive tightness in flexion, one solution is to downsize the femoral component.

After the femoral and tibial osteotomies are completed, flexion-extension blocks can help identify areas of tightness that require releasing for optimal coronal and sagittal plane balancing.

Laminar spreaders with the knee in extension can help identify posterior structures that contribute to stiffness in extension. A posterior capsular release is often necessary in this case. No matter which method is used to release the posterior capsule (i.e., electrocautery, blunt dissection with elevators), it is imperative to dissect along the posterior femoral cortex to avoid neurovascular injury.

In rare instances with very severe stiffness the collateral ligaments may require complete release or so much distal femur is resected that the origin of the collaterals is compromised. In such cases a hinged knee design is the implant of choice.

Postoperative Care

Patients are encouraged to pursue range-of-motion exercises and to weight bear as tolerated. Most of these patients are best served with supervised physical therapy for the first 6 weeks postoperatively, and all of these patients should be closely monitored by the surgical team to ensure progress. We do not

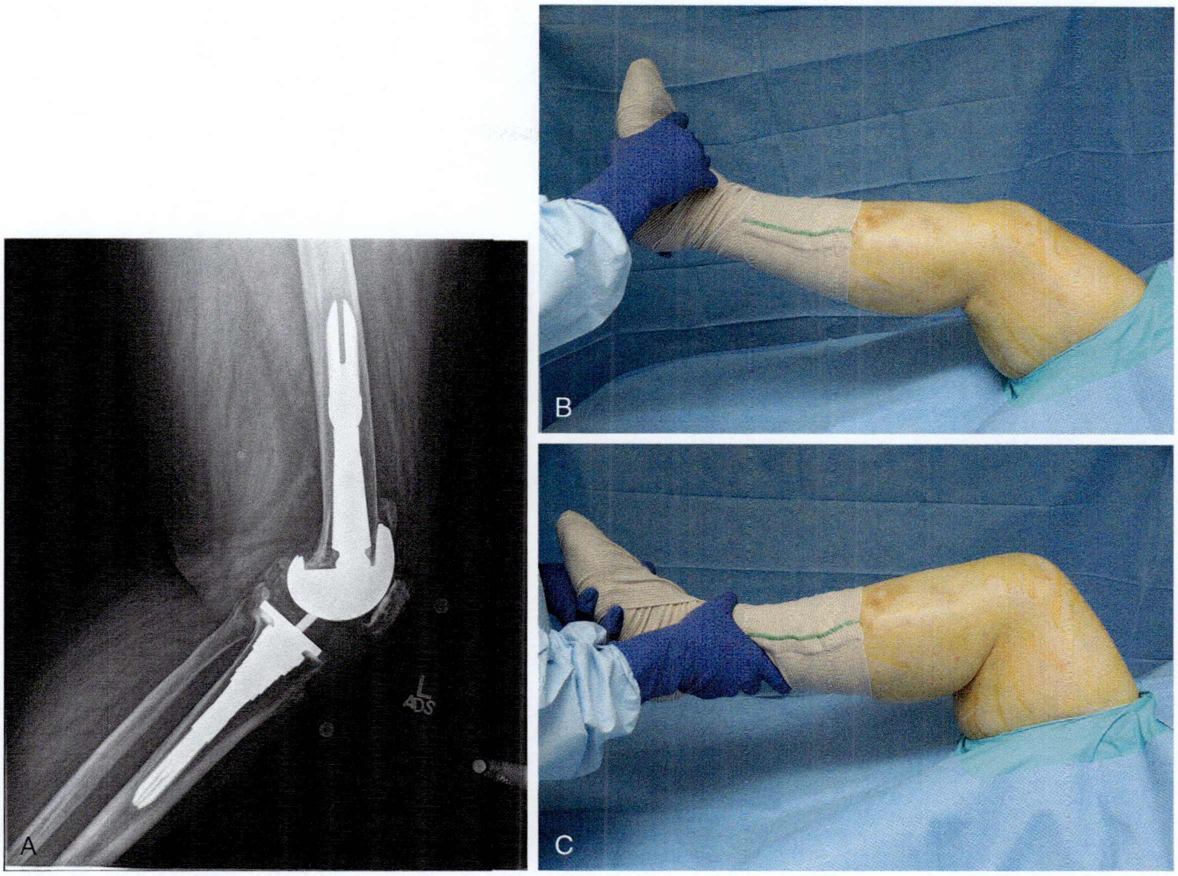

Figure 68.4 | Preoperative lateral radiograph (A) and clinical photographs demonstrating marked limitation of extension (B) and flexion (C) in a patient with both heterotopic bone and arthrofibrosis after a revision TKA.

typically employ either continuous passive motion machines nor do we employ long-term indwelling epidural catheters for these patients (Figure 68.5A and B).

Nonsteroidal anti-inflammatory medication should be routinely used postoperatively to reduce the recurrence of arthrofibrosis. In many circumstances, it is entirely appropriate to consider the use of oral prednisone for a period of 3 to 6 weeks after either manipulation or revision TKA for marked stiffness.

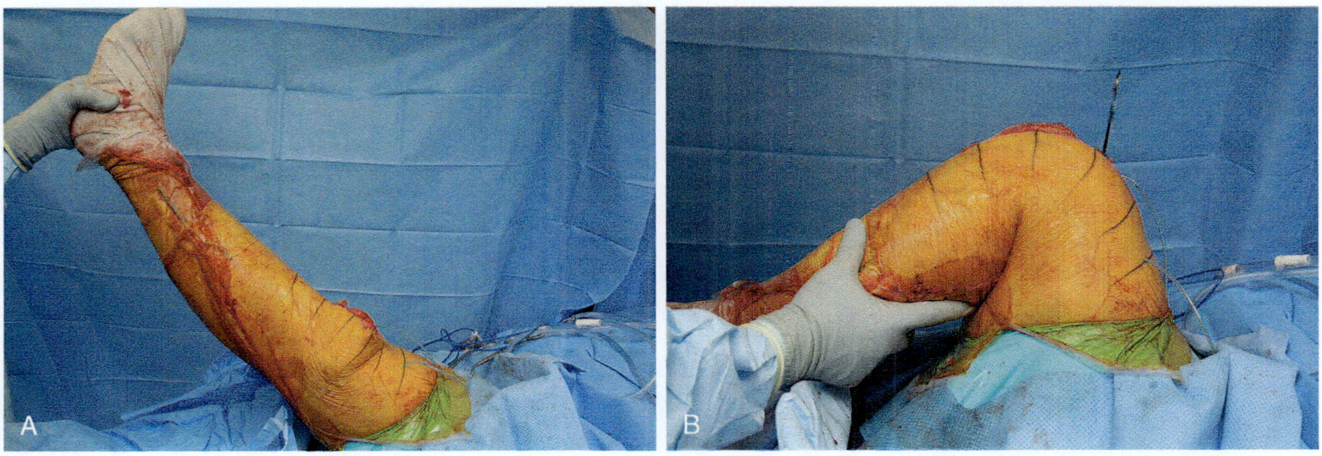

Figure 68.5 | Intraoperative photographs after re-revision surgery of the patient with marked stiffness from heterotopic bone and arthrofibrosis demonstrating (A) full knee extension and (B) a marked improvement in knee flexion.

Chapter 69
Infection: Two-Stage Methods

TIMOTHY S. BROWN
KEVIN I. PERRY

Key Concepts

- Successful treatment of knee chronic periprosthetic infection begins with complete removal of implants, cement, and foreign material and includes an extensive debridement.
- Identification of the causative organism is critical to the success of the treatment.
- The antibiotic spacer type is chosen to fit the needs of the individual patient.
- The decision to proceed with reimplantation is carefully considered and comes after a complete treatment course with intravenous antibiotics followed by an antibiotic holiday.
- At the time of reimplantation the absence of acute inflammation is confirmed, the joint is thoroughly debrided, and a well-balanced knee with rigid implant fixation is obtained with a combination of cementless metaphyseal cones or sleeves and cemented or cementless stems.

Sterile Instruments and Implants

- Rigid and flexible osteotomes
- Cement osteotomes
- Small sagittal saw
- Large Steinmann pins (for static spacer)
- Cement gun (for static spacer dowel construction)
- Luque wires (for static spacer)
- Large external fixation set

Preoperative Planning

- Important keys for successful removal of implants in total knee arthroplasty (TKA):
  - Adequate surgical exposure:
    - How many operations have been performed on this joint? Have there been prior soft tissue complications? Is there a sinus tract that must be excised (Figure 69.1)?
    - What is the preoperative range of motion? Will a quadriceps snip be likely?
    - Will a more extensile exposure such as tibial tubercle osteotomy be necessary to remove components or cement (Figure 69.2A and B)?
  - Obtain implant records from prior operations if at all possible.
  - Specific implant extraction tools are sometimes available for removal of components.
  - Some constructs should involve more planning:
    - Broken modular components (Figure 69.3A and B).
    - Components with offset stems
    - Components next to other hardware (plates, screws, staples)
    - Prior extensor mechanism reconstruction

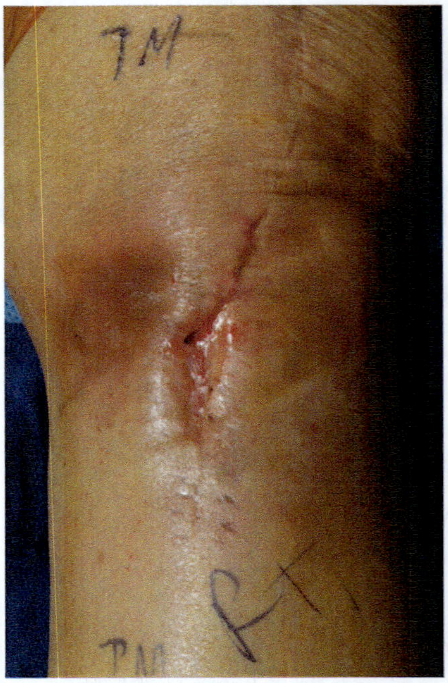

Figure 69.1 | Photograph of the knee demonstrating an anterior sinus tract.

- Radiography
  - Long leg
    - Important for understanding overall limb alignment.
  - Knee
    - Anteroposterior (AP), lateral, merchant, posteroanterior flexion. Used to assess implant interfaces, areas of bone loss, osteolysis. Also helpful in planning for the type of spacer and for the areas that will need augmentation during the spacer construction (Figure 69.4).
- Know the previous operations
  - Get operative reports
    - Surgical approach.
    - Any complications?

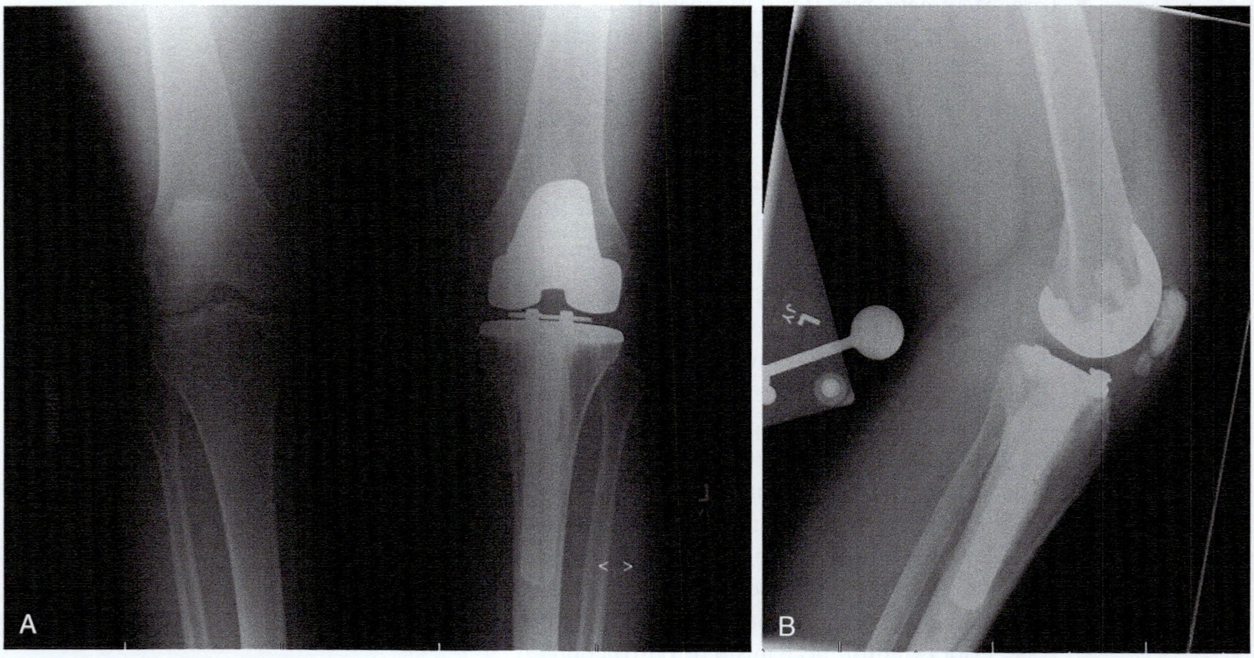

Figure 69.2 | A and B, Cemented, offset stem with multiple prosthetic modular junctions within the cement mantle.

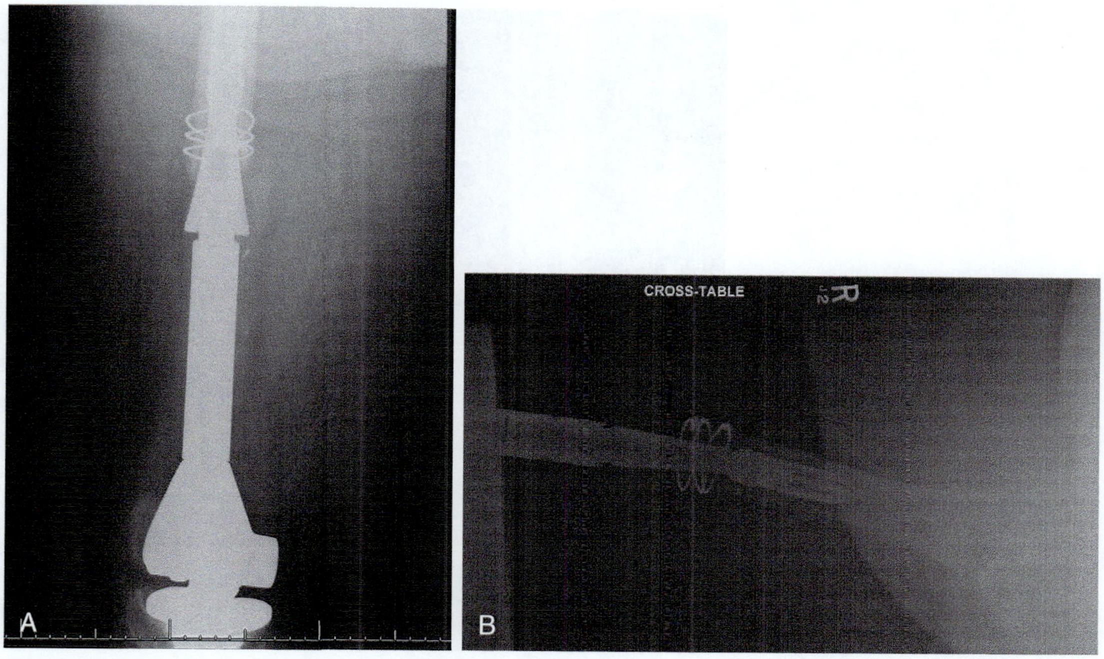

Figure 69.3 | A and B, Broken modular junction in an infected distal femoral replacing total knee arthroplasty.

- Plan for the type of antibiotic spacer
  - No spacer (resection alone)
    - Used rarely
    - Predominately for patients who are very sick, who ar immunocompromised, with poor soft tissue envelope, or who have already failed treatment with antibiotic spacers.
  - Static spacer
    - Extensive bone loss (Anderson Orthopedic Research Institute [AORI] types 2B, 3) (Figure 69.5A-D).
    - Lack of collateral ligament integrity
    - Lack of extensor mechanism
    - Need for soft tissue reconstruction procedure (flap or graft)

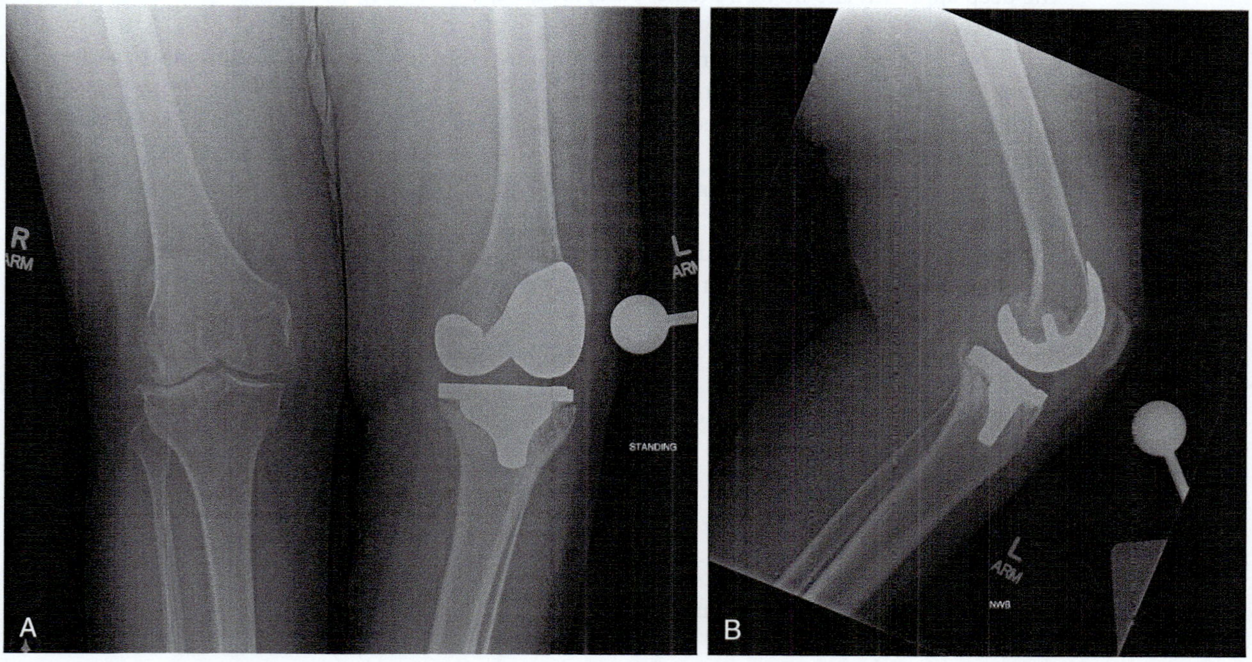

Figure 69.4 | A and B, Infected, loose total knee arthroplasty with extensive bone loss on the medial tibial plateau.

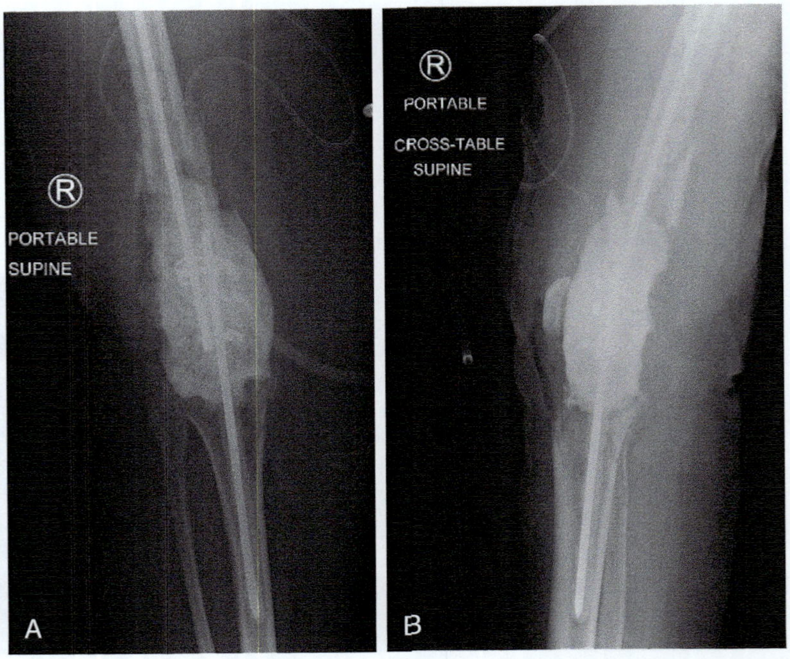

Figure 69.5 | A,B. AP and lateral radiographs of an infected periprosthetic femur fracture and the static spacer used at the time of resection.

- Articulating spacer
  - Minimal bone loss (AORI 1, 2A)
  - Intact collateral ligaments
  - Intact extensor mechanism
  - Good soft tissue envelope
  - Reliable patient

Bone, Implant, and Soft Tissue Techniques

- The skin incision used should be the most lateral usable prior incision to protect the blood supply to the anterior skin. Sinus tracts and avascular, wide scars should be excised to promote healing.
- The deep approach should be a medial parapatellar approach with possible extension via a quadriceps snip or a tibial tubercle osteotomy.
- The femoral, tibial, and patellar components are removed using the techniques described in Chapter 61: Removal of TKA Components
- Multiple deep cultures are obtained from all aspects of the joint: femoral canal, tibial canal, posterior synovium.
- A thorough debridement is performed, removing all cement, scar tissue, synovium, and fibrinous tissue from within the joint.
- The femoral and tibial canals are debrided with pituitary rongeur, back scrapers, and rigid reamers.
- An irrigation is performed using the following solutions in sequence:
  - 3 L normal saline, pulse lavage
  - 15 mL sterile povidone-iodine in 500 mL normal saline
  - 3 L normal saline, pulse lavage
  - 500 mL Dakin solution, H_2O_2, or Hibiclens
  - 3 L normal saline, pulse lavage

Static Spacer

- High-dose antibiotic cement recipe:
  - One batch simplex bone cement
  - 3 g vancomycin
  - 3.6 g tobramycin

    - 300 mg amphotericin B
    - 1 to 2 drops methylene blue
    - Mix the cement monomer and polymer together first until they react and create a liquid
    - Add the 2 drops of methylene blue
    - Slowly mix in the powdered antibiotics until dough is formed
- Create 2 dowels for the intramedullary canals:
    - One batch high-dose cement, mixed and placed into gun.
    - Push cement to tip of gun and unscrew the barrel.
    - Allow the cement to harden, then remove the dowel from the barrel (Figure 69.6). If the dowel gets stuck, use a sagittal saw to disrupt the plastic at one end and then remove with a rongeur.
    - Create one dowel for implantation into the femur and one for implantation into the tibia.
    - If a large defect is being bridged with the static spacer, we will use either a 3/16 inches Steinmann pin as the central core for the dowel (Figure 69.7) or a large external fixator bar.
    - Place the dowels into the femoral and tibial canals, ensuring that the canal is adequately prepared to accept their diameter and length.
- Create the spacer:
    - Mix 2 to 3 batches (or more depending on the size of the defect) of high-dose antibiotic cement using prior formula. Note that other bone cements such as Palacos elute antibiotics more quickly, and a reduction in total antibiotic load may be needed to avoid systemic complications.
    - Place the knee in full extension and neutral coronal alignment. Place the doughy cement into the knee, and mold into a shape that fills the defect and contacts both the tibia and femur. Bring the patella and extensor mechanism over the cement while still soft to ensure the soft tissues will close. Allow the cement to harden.
    - If a large defect is being bridged with Steinmann pins:
        - Bring the pins together at the joint, place the joint in full extension and neutral coronal alignment, and use Luque wires to connect the 2 dowels (Figure 69.8).
        - Place the doughy cement into the knee, and mold into a shape that fills the defect and covers the Luque wire and Steinmann pins and contacts both the tibia and femur. Bring the patella and extensor mechanism over the cement while still soft to ensure the soft tissues will close. Allow the cement to harden.
    - If a large defect is being bridged with an external fixator:
        - Bring the 2 bars together with a bar-to-bar clamp at the level of the knee. Place the knee in full extension and neutral coronal alignment and tighten the clamp.
        - Place the doughy cement into the knee and mold into a shape that fills the defect, covers the ends of the bars and the clamp, and contacts both the tibia and femur. Bring the patella and extensor mechanism over the cement while still soft to ensure the soft tissues will close. Allow the cement to harden.

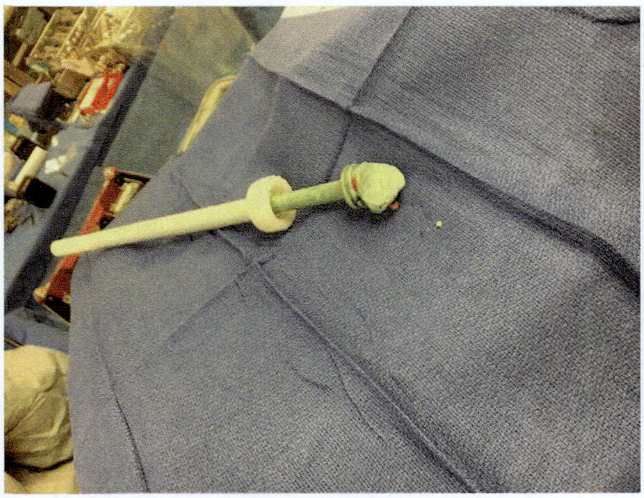

Figure 69.6 | High-dose antibiotic cement dowel.

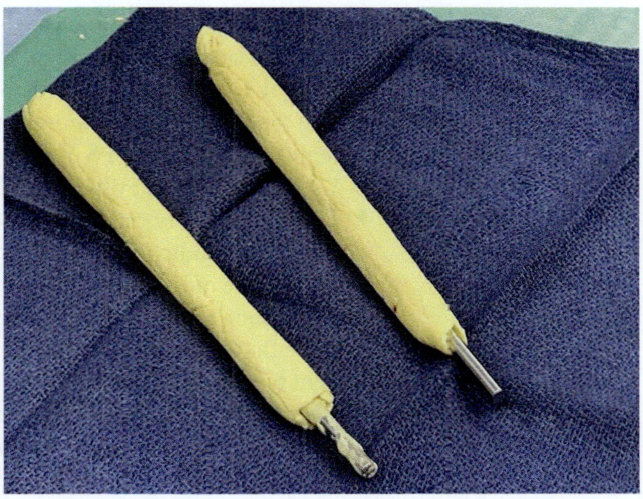

Figure 69.7 | High-dose antibiotic cement dowel with Steinmann pin core, with large defect static spacer.

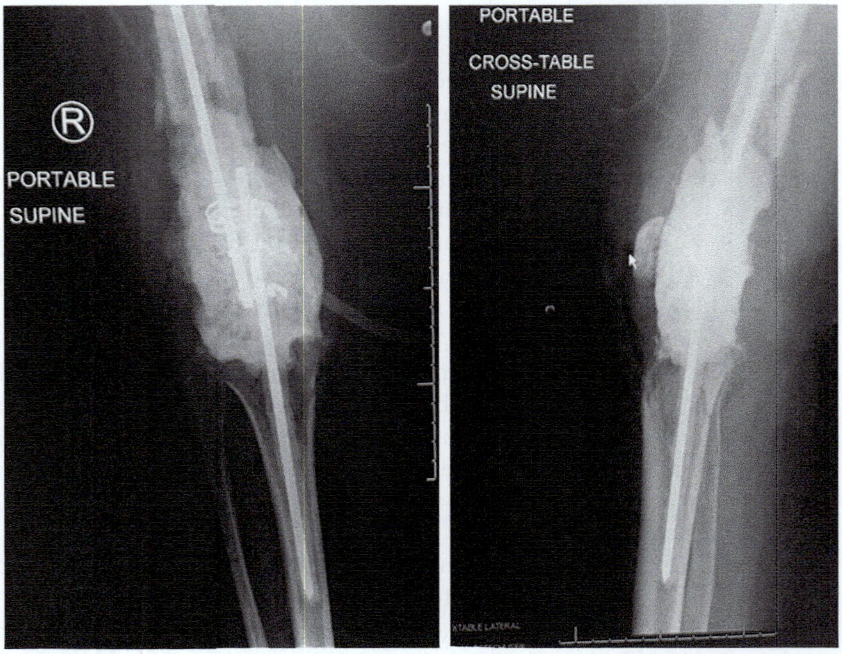

Figure 69.8 I AP and lateral radiographs demonstrating a large defect with a static antibiotic spacer in place.

- Choose a method of immobilization:
  - Prolonged treatment with a static spacer requires external immobilization as a prophylactic against bone loss and soft tissue injury.
  - Depending on the size of the patient, defect, and other medical comorbidities (diabetic neuropathy), we will use a knee immobilizer, hinged knee brace locked in extension, or a long leg cast
  - If a cast is used, we will have q3 week cast room visits with exchange of the cast and inspection of the wound.

Dynamic Spacer

- Create dowels:
  - One batch high-dose cement, mixed and placed into gun.
  - Push cement to tip of gun and unscrew the barrel.
  - Allow the cement to harden, then remove the dowel from the barrel. If the dowel gets stuck, use a sagittal saw to disrupt the plastic at one end and then remove with a rongeur.
  - Create one dowel for implantation into the femur and one for implantation into the tibia.
  - Place the dowels into the femoral and tibial canals, ensuring that the canal is adequately prepared to accept their diameter and that the length is appropriate.
- Create the tibial and femoral caps.
  - Put the leg into extension and measure the extension gap.
  - Place the leg in 90° of flexion and measure the flexion gap.
  - Size the femur with a femoral component trial. Size the tibia with a tibial tray trial. Open the real femoral component (PS or CR).
  - Use 2 batches (1 for tibia and 1 for femur) of high-dose antibiotic cement.
  - Place the doughy cement onto the tibia, filling metaphyseal defects and creating a level surface that is perpendicular to the shaft of the tibia. Large, asymmetric defects can be buttressed with a small piece of hardened dowel as shown in Figure 69.9A and B.
  - Place doughy cement onto the femur, filling metaphyseal defects. While the cement is doughy, place the real femoral component over the cement to shape it. Remove the real femoral component before cement hardening.
- Cement the dynamic spacer in place.
  - Place the trial femoral component in place and then trial different size polyethylene inserts. A size is needed that will allow adequate cement mantle while also balancing soft tissues.
  - Open the real polyethylene insert for the appropriate femur (PS or CR). Use a 5-mm burr to place shallow holes on the underside of the polyethylene insert (Figure 69.10A and B).

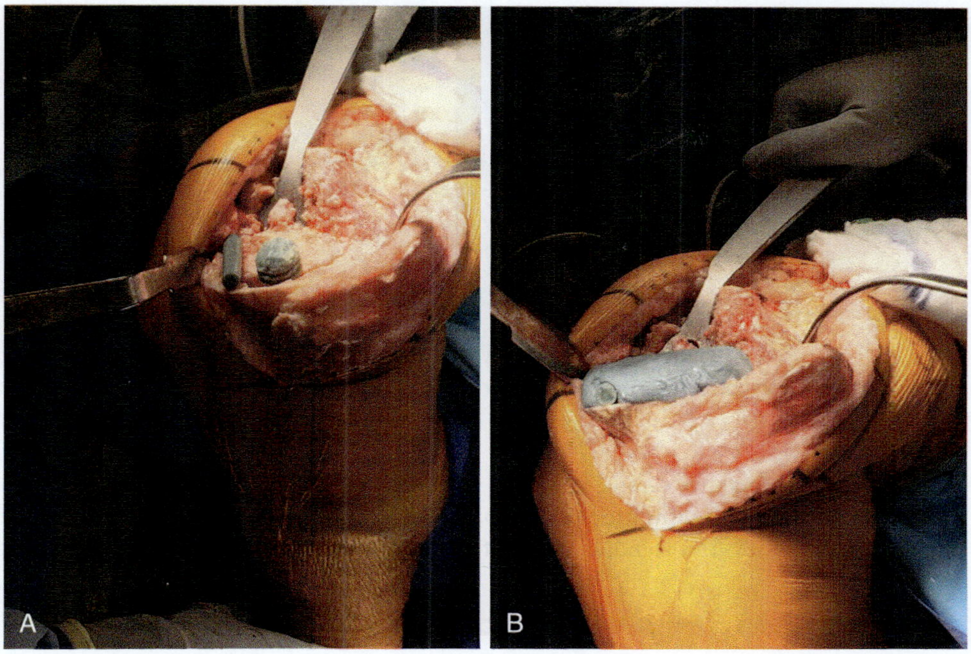

Figure 69.9 | A and B, Creation of an antibiotic cap for the tibia.

- Cement the femoral component in place (Figure 69.11).
- Cement the tibial polyethylene on top of the tibial cement cap (Figure 69.12), and cement the femoral component onto the femoral cement cap. Place the knee into full extension while the cement hardens.
- After the cement has fully hardened, flex the knee to 90° and check the joint for sharp pieces of cement that can cause irritation to the soft tissues. Use the burr to smooth these rough edges. Remove any loose pieces of cement from the joint (Figure 69.13A and B)

- Closure:
    - Close the capsule with interrupted monofilament #1 PDS.
    - Close the soft tissues with 0 PDS, 2 to 0 PDS, and 3 to 0 Monocryl.
    - Closure of the skin depends on the integrity of the soft tissues. We prefer running Monocryl closure for maintenance of blood supply, but occasionally use 2 to 0 or 3 to 0 nylon/prolene mattress sutures for a stronger closure.

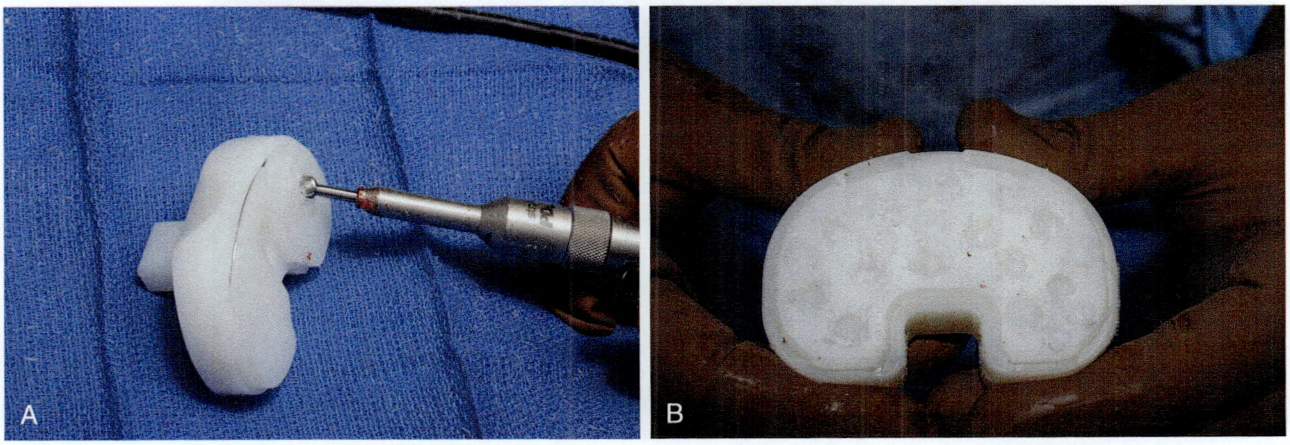

Figure 69.10 | Burring the undersurface of the tibial insert (A) and what the undersurface looks like after completion (B).

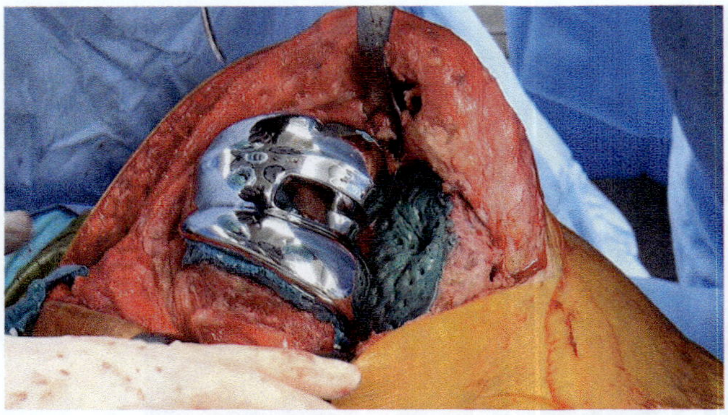

Figure 69.11 | Intraoperative photograph of the femoral component after it has been cemented into place.

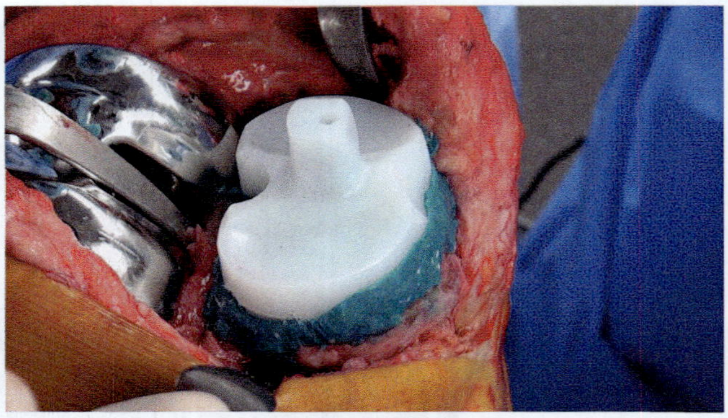

Figure 69.12 | Intraoperative photograph after final cementation of the tibial insert.

- Postoperative care:
  - We will allow articulating spacers to bear weight as tolerated, with full range of motion in most cases. This is individualized to ensure wound healing first and then range of motion.

Treatment With Spacer in Place

- Intravenous antibiotics for at least 6 weeks.
- Antibiotic holiday for at least 2 weeks.
- Follow-up with laboratory tests, clinical examination, and possible aspiration of the joint at 8 weeks.
- Decision made to proceed with reimplantation once laboratory tests have normalized and clinical examination is not concerning. We do not hesitate to extend the period with a spacer in place and will return to the operating room for a repeat irrigation and debridement with spacer exchange if the examination and serum laboratory tests are not improving.

Reimplantation

- If the soft tissue will allow it, we excise the previous scar during reimplantation.
- An extensile exposure is done, using a quadriceps snip if needed for safe exposure.

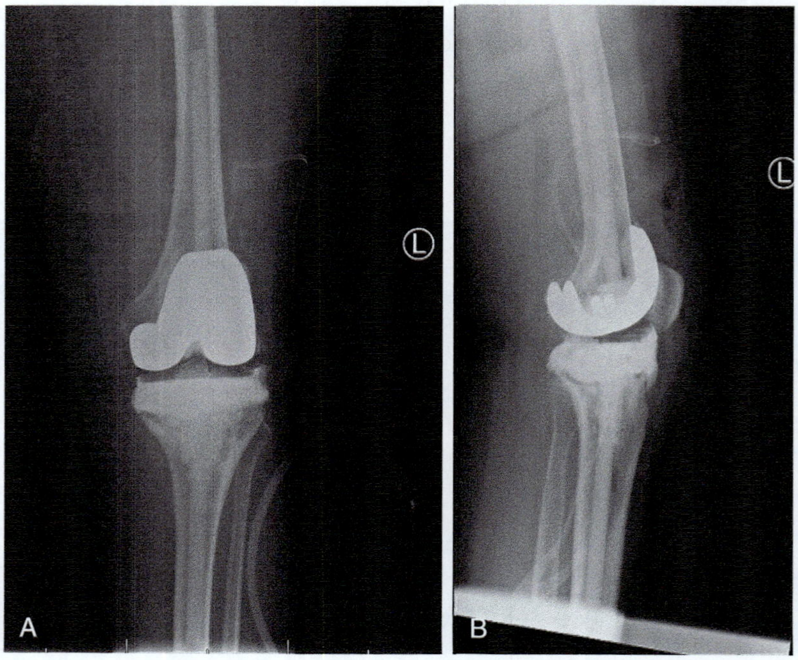

Figure 69.13 | A and B, AP and lateral radiographs demonstrating the final articulating antibiotic spacer.

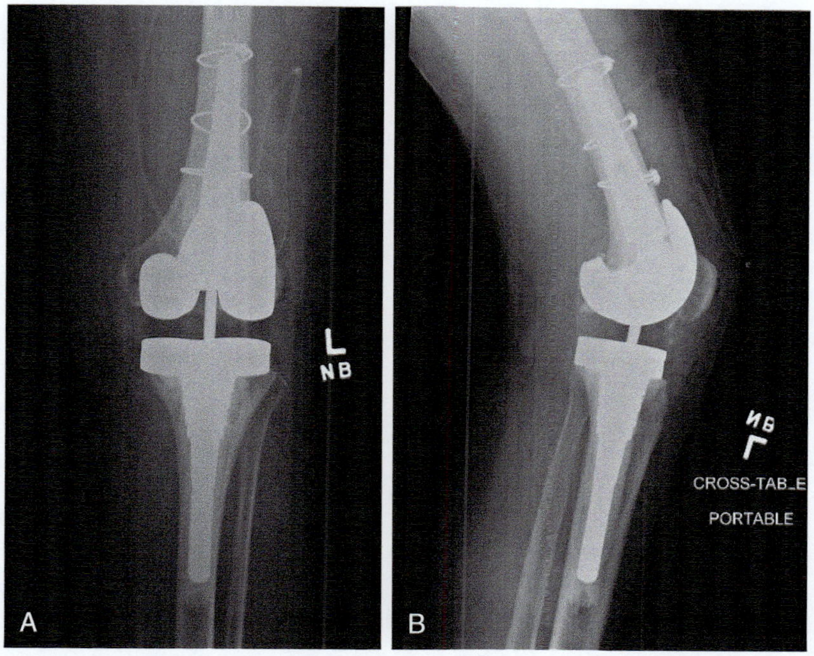

Figure 69.14 | A and B, AP and lateral radiographs demonstrating the revision TKA following reimplantation.

- The spacer is carefully removed using techniques described in Chapter IVB3: Implant Removal.
- Multiple cultures are sent from predictable, reproducible parts of the exposure:
  - Suprapatellar pouch synovium
  - Femoral canal
  - Tibial canal
- The femoral and tibial canals are debrided with a back scraper and pituitary rongeur.
- The wound should be thoroughly irrigated with 3 L of normal saline before preparation of the femur and the tibia.
- The femoral and tibial canals are then reamed until a fit is obtained.
- The tibia is cut at 90° to the intramedullary reamer and prepared for cementless metaphyseal fixation (cone/sleeve).
- The femur is prepared with a new distal cut off the intramedullary reamer followed by new 4-in-1 cuts and a new box cut. The need for augments is judged off of the 4-in-1 block. If there is enough bone loss, then the femur is prepared for cementless metaphyseal fixation (cone/sleeve).
- Trial components are built on the back table and placed into the knee.
- A trial PS polyethylene is placed, and the soft tissue balance in both flexion and extension is examined.
- Real components are cemented into place, and again a trial polyethylene is placed.
- The real polyethylene is inserted, and the soft tissues are closed over a drain (Figure 69.14A and B).
- The patient is kept on oral antibiotics directed against the prior organism until the final intraoperative cultures come back at 14 days postoperatively.

Conclusion

- Successful treatment of knee chronic periprosthetic infection begins with complete removal of implants, cement, and all foreign material and a thorough stepwise irrigation.
- Identification of the causative organism is critical to the success of the treatment and ideally occurs preoperatively.
- Dynamic versus static spacer is chosen on the basis of bone loss and patient characteristics.
- Reimplantation should come after infection has been successfully treated.
- The goals of reimplantation are to obtain a well-balanced knee with rigid implant fixation through a combination of cementless metaphyseal cones or sleeves and cemented or cementless stems.

Chapter 70
Periprosthetic Fracture

MATTHEW W. TETREAULT
BRANDON J. YUAN
MATTHEW P. ABDEL

Key Concepts

- Periprosthetic fractures around the knee are relatively uncommon.
- Management considerations include fracture location and displacement, stability of the prosthesis, bone quality, and patient health.
- Classification systems help categorize and guide the treatment of periprosthetic femur, tibia, and patella fractures.
- Goals of operative treatment include:
  - A stable and well-aligned construct that allows early motion and weight bearing
  - Maximizing implant longevity while mitigating further complications
- Supracondylar femur fractures continue to be the most common periprosthetic fractures around a total knee arthroplasty (TKA).
- The evolution of locked plating and retrograde intramedullary nailing techniques decreased surgical morbidity and improved union rates in the setting of well-fixed implants.
- Revision TKA with diaphyseal-engaging stems or distal femoral replacement may be indicated when the prosthesis is compromised, when adequate fixation and bony union is unlikely, or when a previous attempt at internal fixation has failed.
- Nonoperative treatment is rarely indicated given a strong predisposition to stiffness.
- Intraoperative periprosthetic tibia fractures are treated according to fracture location and pattern. Postoperative periprosthetic tibia fractures are rare and often associated with loose tibial components; the preferred management in this scenario is revision TKA.
- Operative treatment of periprosthetic patellar fractures is associated with a high rate of complications and should be reserved for cases of extensor mechanism disruption and patellar component loosening. That topic is discussed in another chapter.

Sterile Instruments and Implants

Instruments

Open Reduction Internal Fixation (ORIF)/Intramedullary Nail (IMN)

- Routine knee retractors
- Fracture reduction instruments (e.g., bone hooks, reduction clamps, Kirschner wires)
- Femoral distractor versus sterile external fixator versus sterile skeletal traction to aid in provisional reduction
- Metal-cutting, high-speed burr if the need to expand femoral box for IMN is anticipated

Revision TKA

- Routine knee retractors
- A full set of revision TKA instruments to remove well-fixed implants while preserving bone, including:
  - Reciprocating and oscillating saws
  - High-speed burrs (e.g., short and long pencil-tip burrs, 6.5-mm round burr)
  - Flexible osteotomes
  - Cement removal instruments to clean out intramedullary canal
  - Trephines may be required if stemmed components are in place
- Cerclage cables or wires and wire passers
- Diaphyseal and metaphyseal reamers and revision TKA cutting jigs

Implants

ORIF/Retrograde IMN of the Femur

- Periarticular distal femoral locking plates and retrograde intramedullary nails are commonly utilized for fixation of these fractures.
- Locking plates amenable to "hybrid" constructs (with locked and unlocked screws) and polyaxial locking screws are favored over fixed-angle locking plates for these often complex fractures with deficient distal bone stock.
- Have compatible polyethylene liners (and trials) available when a retrograde IMN is planned, as polyethylene liner removal can facilitate nail placement.

ORIF of the Tibia

- Metaphyseal plates, buttress plates, and/or periarticular locking plates (preferred)
- Stainless steel wire if fixation of tibial tubercle fracture is planned

Revision TKA

- Revision TKA system, including:
  - Tibial and femoral components with cemented stems
  - Increasing degrees of implant constraint, including varus-valgus constrained implants and rotating-hinge options
  - Not infrequently, a distal femoral replacement with a rotating-hinge construct is required
  - Metal augments, sleeves, and/or porous metal cones based on assessment of bone loss
  - Appropriate polyethylene liners
  - Patellar component from compatible manufacturer
- Cerclage cables and/or Luque wires
- Bone cement and cement plugs
- Allograft bone

Positioning

ORIF/Retrograde IMN of the Femur

- Supine on a radiolucent operative table. Of note, ORIF can also be performed in a lateral position.
- In the case of fractures that show significant shortening preoperatively, it may be difficult to restore length off the fracture table. Before preparing the limb, consider the following:
  - With the patient under anesthesia with full muscle paralysis, an attempted reduction should be performed under fluoroscopy before preparing the limb. If length is difficult to restore manually, a femoral distractor, spanning external fixator, or sterile traction device should be used for the procedure.
  - The contralateral extremity should be examined to verify normal leg length and rotation. Femoral length can be evaluated using a radiographic ruler and fluoroscopy. Rotational profile can be gauged preoperatively by checking the internal and external rotation of the uninjured hip and by examining the normal resting position of the foot.

- For ORIF, a bump under the ipsilateral hip aids in internal rotation of the limb and a sterile thigh tourniquet ensures access to the proximal thigh if needed. The extremity should be draped free from the anterior superior iliac spine to the ankle, with the entire hip included.
- A radiolucent triangle, sterile towels, or sheets under the distal metadiaphyseal region of the femur create a bump to aid in reduction and facilitate imaging of the knee.
- At least 40° of knee flexion is needed for intramedullary nailing.
- One may consider preparing the well leg and including it in the operative field so that it may be elevated during lateral imaging of the operative femur.
- Intraoperative fluoroscopy should come in from the uninjured side.

ORIF of the Tibia

- Supine on a radiolucent operative table
- Bump under ipsilateral hip to aid in internal rotation of limb
- Sterile thigh tourniquet
- Stack of towels or Bone Foam Ramp under the distal leg can facilitate imaging
- Intraoperative fluoroscopy should come in from the uninjured side

Revision TKA

- Supine on a standard operative table
- Nonsterile tourniquet placed high on upper thigh
- Intraoperative radiographs in orthogonal planes should be obtained intraoperatively with trials in place. The x-ray machine will come in from the well side.

Surgical Approaches

ORIF of the Femur

- Exposure of the distal femur for ORIF is typically achieved through a lateral approach.
- The exposure should be consistent with the planned reduction and fixation method. For comminuted fractures, the goal is a functional, indirect reduction and no direct exposure of the fracture site is necessary. As long as an acceptable reduction is obtained, only the distal aspect of the lateral exposure need be performed, and proximal screws may be placed percutaneously. For relatively simple fractures when direct reduction is planned, an extensile lateral incision with a subvastus approach to the femur is performed.
  - The distal aspect of the incision is curvilinear and centered over the lateral femoral epicondyle to Gerdy tubercle.
  - The incision can be extended proximally along the posterior aspect of the femur.
  - Effort should be made to maximize the skin bridge between the lateral incision and the anterior TKA incision.
  - Superficial dissection proceeds through the subcutaneous fat, and the iliotibial band is incised in line with its fibers and the skin incision.
  - The vastus lateralis is reflected anteriorly off the intermuscular septum to provide direct visualization of the periosteum.
    - The extent of dissection depends on the fracture pattern, the components in place, and the surgeon's comfort level with percutaneous fixation techniques.
    - Minimization of soft tissue and periosteal stripping is paramount.
    - Perforating vessels that cross the field are coagulated or ligated; deliberate dissection is advised as transection of the perforating vessels can cause them to retract, making hemostasis difficult and blood loss substantial.
- Exposure of the medial aspect of the distal femur is occasionally needed and can be achieved through an anteromedial approach.
  - A longitudinal incision is made over the interval between the vastus medialis and the rectus femoris.
  - Distally, the extensor mechanism is incised using a medial parapatellar arthrotomy.

- This approach can be extended proximally as needed.
  - With proximal dissection, the vastus intermedius is incised in line with its fibers and elevated to expose the femoral shaft.
  - Care is required in the distal one-third of the medial thigh given the proximity of the femoral vessels within the adductor hiatus.

Retrograde IMN of the Femur

- The starting point for a retrograde IMN can be accessed through the prior anterior knee incision.
- A medial parapatellar arthrotomy is advised to allow subluxation of the patella and removal of the polyethylene liner (if a replacement liner is available) to facilitate access to the intercondylar notch.

ORIF of the Tibia

- The proximal tibia can be accessed through an anterior exposure by extending a prior longitudinal TKA incision distally or through a separate medial or lateral approach (depending on fracture location).
- Be mindful of spacing if using a separate incision given the potential for skin bridge necrosis.
- Incisions should be medial or lateral to the tibial tubercle and not directly over this bony prominence.

Revision TKA

- An extensile longitudinal incision over the anterior knee that incorporates a prior TKA incision is favored for revision TKAs.
  - If several scars are present, incorporation of the most laterally based incision that will allow extensile exposure proximally and distally is preferred to preserve blood supply to the overlying skin.
- Conservative, full-thickness skin flaps also help to minimize the insult to skin perfusion.
- A medial parapatellar arthrotomy is most often utilized.
- Mobilization of the patella can be difficult in the revision setting owing to scarring and patella baja.
  - Fastidious release of scar tissue in the suprapatellar pouch, the medial and lateral gutters, and behind the patellar tendon can help to mobilize the patella.
  - Mobilization of the patella can be further aided by proximal extension of the incision, lateral retinacular release, and a quadriceps snip. A low threshold to utilize a quadriceps snip in this setting is recommended given the exposure benefits and lack of need to modify postoperative rehabilitation.[1]
  - Removing the polyethylene insert helps relax the extensor mechanism.
  - Extensile exposures such as a tibial tubercle osteotomy or a V-Y quadriceps turndown are very rarely, if ever, utilized.
  - Exposure is facilitated by avoiding patella eversion with knee flexion. After the patella component is addressed in knee extension, the patella can be translated into the lateral gutter and retracted safely.

Preoperative Planning

- Key factors in determining the appropriate management of periprosthetic fractures around the knee include fracture location and displacement, stability and alignment of the current prosthesis, bone quality, associated functional deficits, and patient health. As such, a thorough clinical history, physical examination and radiographic review are paramount.

Clinical History

- Mechanism and timing of injury
- Antecedent pain
- Functional level
- Medical comorbidities

Physical Examination

- Soft-tissue envelope, including prior incisions or open wounds
- Gross deformity
- Competence of extensor mechanism
- Neurovascular examination
- Status of compartments
    - Avoid missing compartment syndrome, particularly with higher energy mechanisms of injury or in patients found down.

Radiographic Review

- Orthogonal full-length radiographs of the injured extremity are needed.
    - Radiographs should include a complete knee series (anteroposterior [AP], lateral, and patellar views) and full-length AP and lateral views of the femur and tibia to evaluate the joint above and below the fracture.
    - Evaluation of the stability of the TKA components is key. In particular, the surgeon should evaluate for:
        - Subsidence
        - Radiolucency around implants
        - Change in component positioning or alignment
        - Fractured cement mantle
        - Comparison to preinjury radiographs
    - Make note of patellar height as this can provide insight regarding the integrity of the extensor mechanism.
    - Observe bone loss and quality of remaining host bone.
    - Note alignment and rotation of the implants, overall mechanical alignment of the limb, and other hardware or deformity that may affect operative planning.
    - Take care to screen for contributory pathologic lesions in this often older patient population, particularly in the setting of low-energy fractures (Figure 70.1A and B).
- A computerized tomography scan may be warranted for periprosthetic fractures when the fracture pattern is poorly understood, to better assess bone stock around the implants, or when component stability remains in question after plain radiographs. This study can have the added benefit of providing insight into the rotation of components.

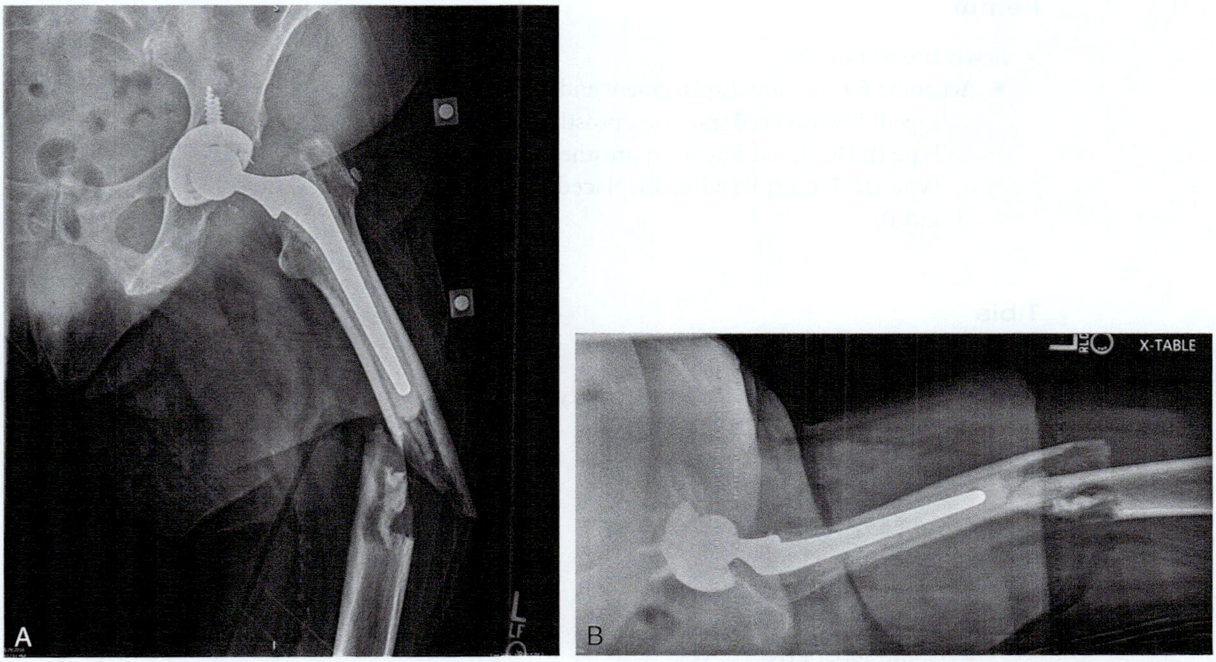

Figure 70.1 I Anteroposterior (A) and lateral (B) hip radiographs of an interprosthetic fracture (knee replacement not pictured) revealing a moth-eaten cortex at the fracture site, which proved to be metastatic carcinoma on biopsy.

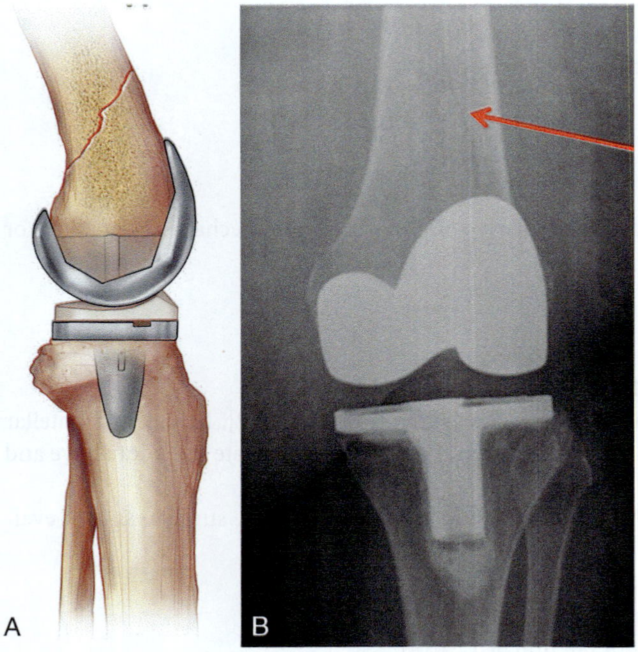

Figure 70.2 | Illustration (A) and anteroposterior radiograph (B) of a Lewis and Rorabeck type I periprosthetic femur fracture (arrow). (Used with permission of Mayo Foundation for Medical Education and Research. All rights reserved.)

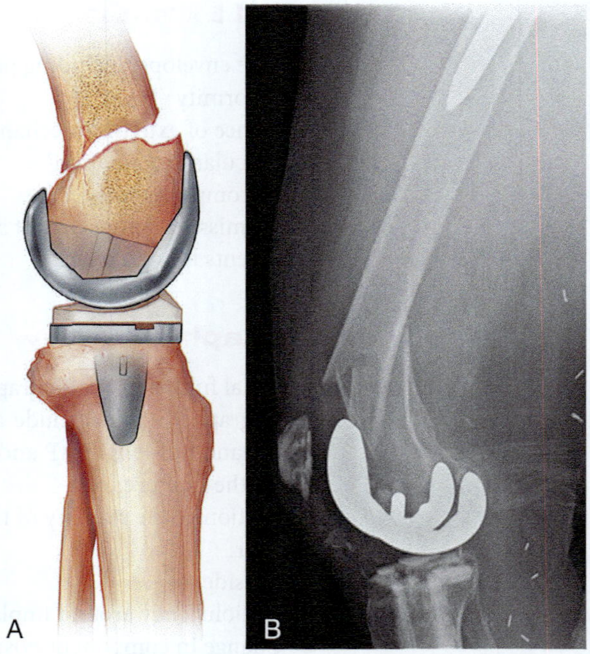

Figure 70.3 | Illustration (A) and lateral radiograph (B) of a Lewis and Rorabeck type II periprosthetic femur fracture. (Used with permission of Mayo Foundation for Medical Education and Research. All rights reserved.)

Fracture Classification and Treatment Options

- The ideal classification scheme (1) facilitates communication between clinicians, (2) includes only relevant variables, (3) guides management, (4) has prognostic capabilities, and (5) is simple to use.[2] We thus prefer the following classification schemes for periprosthetic fractures about the knee.

Femur

- Lewis and Rorabeck[3]
  - Accounts for fracture displacement and integrity of the implant
    - Type I: Undisplaced fractures; prosthesis is intact (Figure 70.2A and B)
    - Type II: Displaced fractures; prosthesis is intact (Figure 70.3A and B)
    - Type III: Undisplaced or displaced fractures; prosthesis is loose or failing (Figure 70.4A and B)

Tibia

- Mayo classification[4]
  - Accounts for fracture location, integrity of the implant, and timing of the fracture (Figure 70.5)
    - Type I: Plateau
    - Type II: Adjacent to stem
    - Type III: Distal to stem
    - Type IV: Tibial tubercle

    Subtypes
    - A: Well-fixed prosthesis
    - B: Loose prosthesis
    - C: Intraoperative

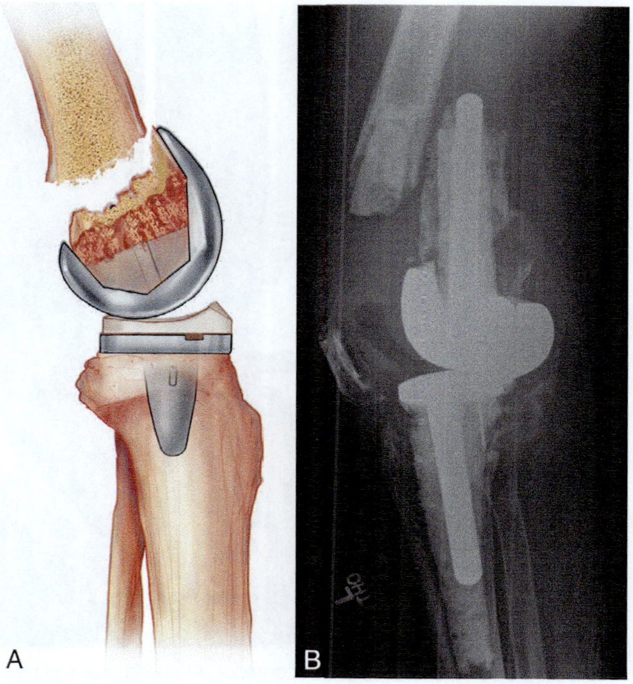

Figure 70.4 | Illustration (A) and lateral radiograph (B) of a Lewis and Rorabeck type III periprosthetic femur fracture. (Used with permission of Mayo Foundation for Medical Education and Research. All rights reserved.)

Operative Planning and Templating

- Every effort should be made to obtain the operative report and implant stickers for the index TKA, with particular focus on the surgical approach and components in place.
- Full-length femur and tibia radiographs are crucial to detect any bony abnormalities (e.g., deformity) or other implants that may affect treatment.
- We provide classification-based treatment considerations for femur and tibia fractures in the following text.

Femur

- Type I: Nondisplaced fractures of the distal femur with a stable prosthesis may be treated nonoperatively or operatively. Nonoperative intervention consists of casting and restricted weight bearing with close radiographic follow-up. Disadvantages of nonoperative management include a fairly high

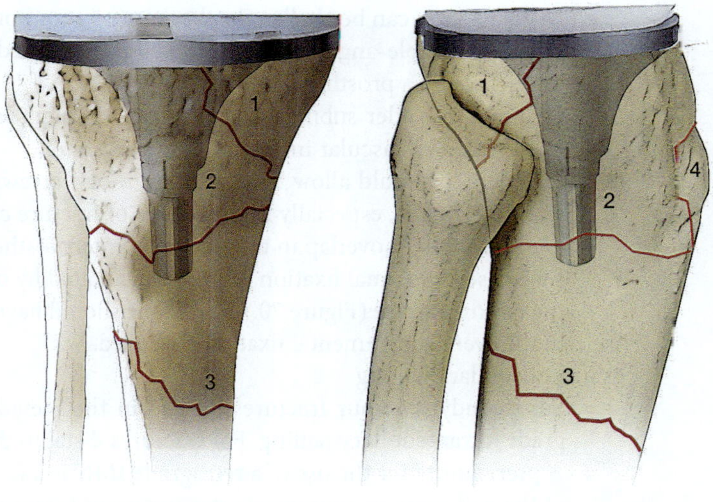

Figure 70.5 | Illustration of the Mayo classification of periprosthetic tibial fractures.

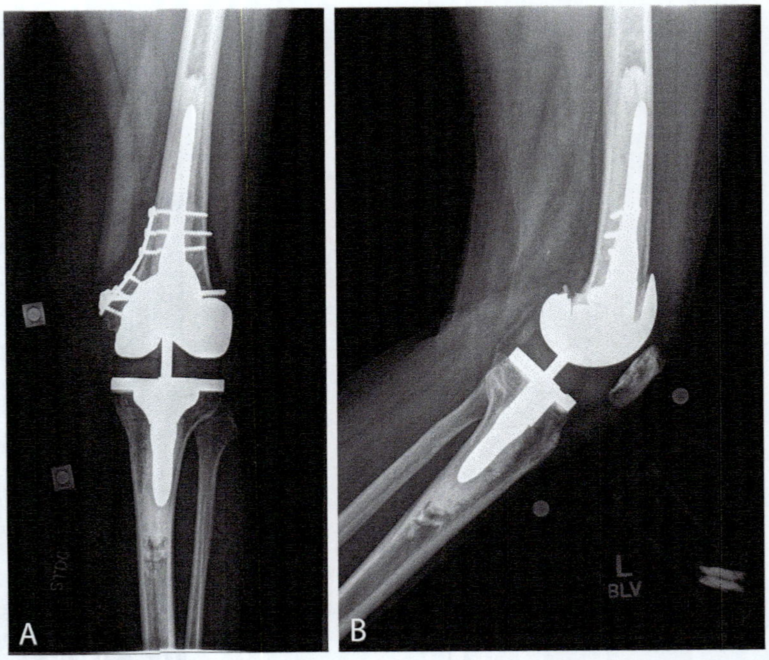

Figure 70.6 | Postoperative anteroposterior (A) and lateral (B) knee radiographs demonstrate a minimally displaced medial femoral condyle fracture that occurred at the time of reimplantation total knee arthroplasty. Lag screw fixation and a buttress plate were utilized in addition to a stemmed femoral component that bypassed the fracture.

risk of malunion, nonunion, and posttreatment functional loss.[5] Operative intervention in the form of plate and screw fixation or a retrograde IMN allows for earlier mobilization and range of motion, but with the inherent risks of surgery.

- Type II: Treatment of displaced distal femur fractures with a stable implant can be approached in several ways. Considerations include fracture pattern, comminution, position and design of the femoral component (cruciate retaining or posterior stabilized), amount of bone attached to the femoral component, quality of host bone, and timing relative to the index procedure. Fractures that occur intraoperatively during the index TKA can usually be managed with use of a stemmed femoral component that bypasses the fracture site with or without supplemental fixation (cerclage cables or wires, plate and screws or lag screws; Figure 70.6A and B).
- For postoperative fractures, goals of surgical stabilization include anatomic reduction, restoration of leg length, fracture union, and early mobilization and range of motion. The following fixation options exist and can be used with or without supplemental bone graft:
  - Periarticular locking plate
    - Distal fixation can be challenging because of poor bone stock and certain femoral component designs. Variable-angle locking plates allow for varied patterns of fixation and are particularly useful around a prosthesis.
    - One may consider submuscular insertion through limited incisions to minimize soft tissue dissection and vascular insult to the fracture site.
    - Plate length should allow for a minimum of 4 screws (8 cortices) proximally. Consider long working lengths, especially in the setting of fracture comminution.
    - Plan for implant overlap in the setting of interprosthetic fracture with hip implants above. In such cases, proximal fixation is greatly facilitated by offset and variable-angle locking holes in the proximal plate (Figure 70.7A-H). One should have cerclage cables or Luque wires available in the event supplemental fixation is needed.
  - Intramedullary nailing
    - Supracondylar femur fractures located in the metadiaphyseal region are amenable to antegrade intramedullary nailing. For fractures distal to this, a retrograde IMN is preferred.
    - A prerequisite for the use of a retrograde IMN is a femoral component that will allow passage of the nail from an appropriate starting point (Figure 70.8A and B). References exist to gauge the compatibility of different TKA models for retrograde IMN fixation.[6]

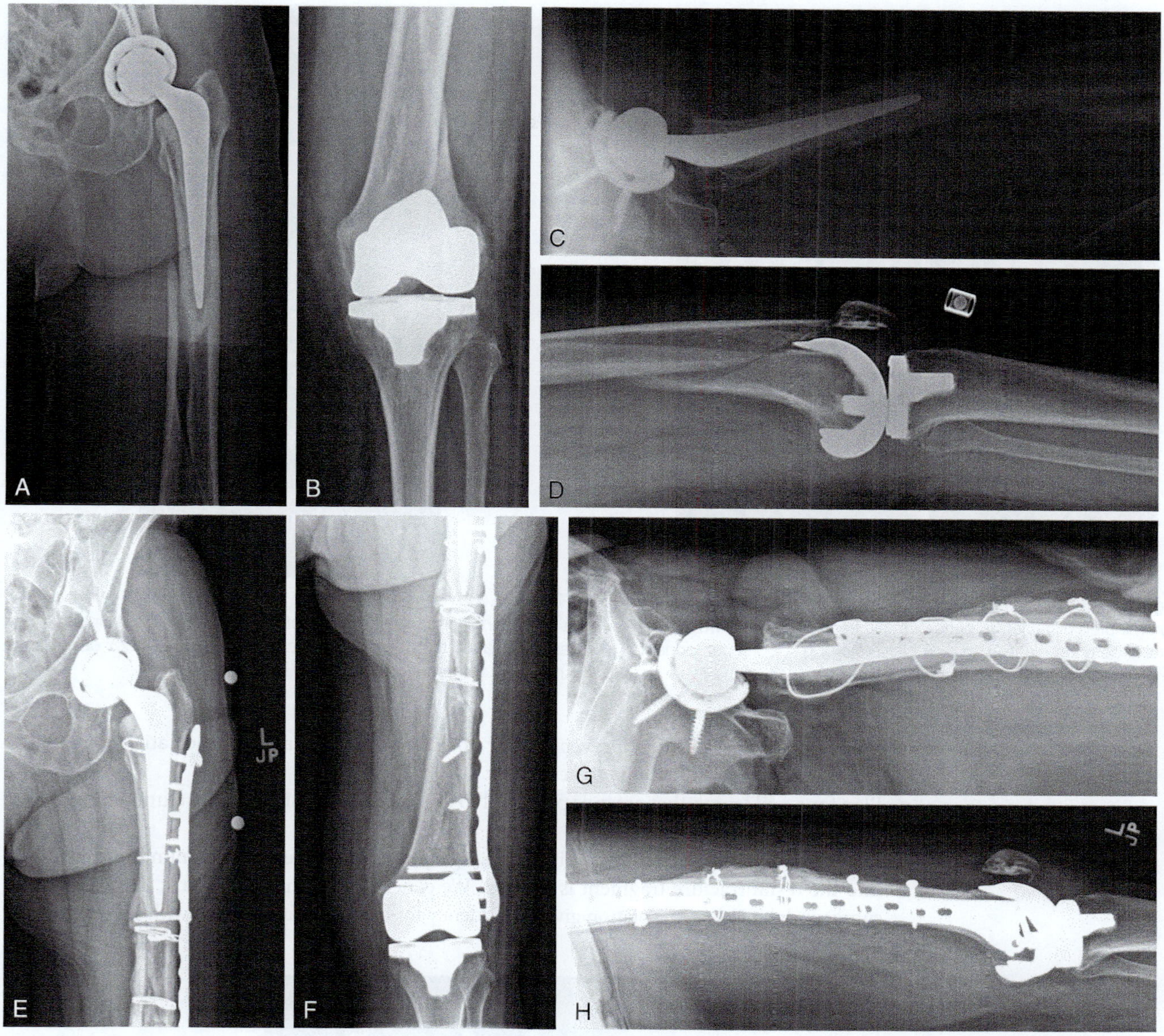

Figure 70.7 | Anteroposterior (A, B) and lateral (C, D) femur injury radiographs of an interprosthetic spiral fracture between well-fixed total hip and total knee replacements. Anteroposterior (E, F) and lateral (G, H) femur radiographs taken 6 months after open reduction and internal fixation using interfragmentary lag screws for compression of the fracture and a lateral-based variable-angle locking plate spanning from the knee to above the lesser trochanter for fracture neutralization and implant overlap. A combination of bicortical nonlocking screws and unicortical locking screws were used about the femoral component of the hip replacement to optimize proximal fixation. Cerclage wires are used sparingly to aid in fracture reduction and to supplement proximal fixation, while taking care to minimize soft tissue stripping.

- Most intramedullary nail systems come in diameters ranging from 10 to 13 mm. Most cruciate-retaining femoral components have a 14-mm window that allows passage of a retrograde IMN 1 to 2 mm smaller.
- We generally recommend using the largest-diameter nail possible given the tendency for these patients to have capacious canals (the intercondylar dimensions of the implant are often the limiting factor, rather than canal size). If needed, a metal-cutting burr can be used to widen a narrow window. The box in posterior-stabilized designs often prevents nail passage, although there are designs that allow it. Surgical techniques have been described for burring a window in closed-box designs[7] (Figure 70.9), although this practice must be weighed against the risk of damaging the prosthesis and retaining metallic debris within the knee.
- It is important to scrutinize femoral component position. Supracondylar fractures fixed with a retrograde IMN are prone to extension deformity, particularly in the setting of a flexed femoral component (Figure 70.10).

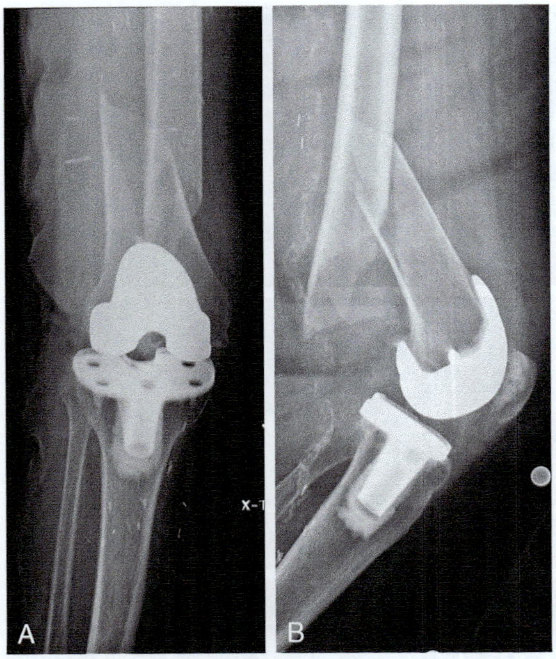

Figure 70.8 | Anteroposterior (A) and lateral (B) radiographs of a comminuted distal femur periprosthetic fracture above a well-fixed total knee arthroplasty with a cruciate-retaining femoral component amenable to passage of a retrograde intramedullary nail.

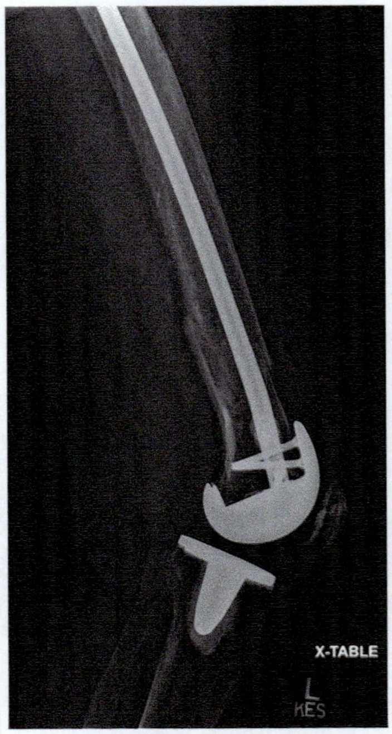

Figure 70.9 | A lateral radiograph of the knee demonstrating fixation of a supracondylar periprosthetic fracture using a retrograde intramedullary nail placed through a window created in a closed-box design total knee replacement.

- Preoperative knee stiffness preventing 40° to 60° of flexion is a contraindication for a retrograde IMN owing to inability to access the start point.
- Plan for a nail length that extends proximal to the lesser trochanter. Avoid an undue stress riser in the intertrochanteric region.
- Retrograde IMNs with multiple distal locking options are preferred; a minimum of 3 screws into the distal fracture fragment is desired. We generally recommend against the use of short supracondylar IMNs in isolation given a tendency for increased failure rates with these implants.

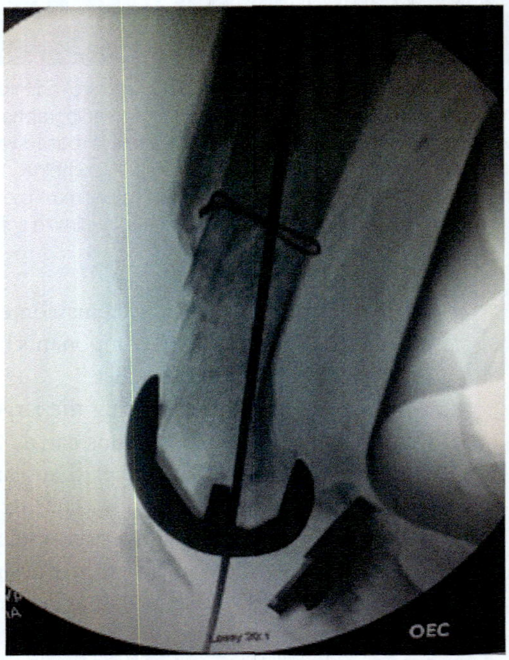

Figure 70.10 | A lateral radiograph of the knee demonstrating how the starting point for a retrograde intramedullary nail can be forced posteriorly by a flexed femoral component, predisposing to extension deformity at the site of a supracondylar periprosthetic fracture. (Image courtesy of Marc A. Zussman, MD.)

        - Although it is possible to pass a retrograde IMN while retaining the polyethylene liner, we recommend having compatible liners available, if possible. Liner removal can facilitate exposure, and replacing the liner at the end of the procedure can help ensure the liner is not damaged and the knee is appropriately stable.
        - Having a backup locking plate available is strongly recommended when the plan is a retrograde IMN. Multiple unforeseen variables, including inadequate distal fixation, can make a retrograde IMN suboptimal and should trigger conversion to the alternative fixation strategy.
    - Fixed-angle plating
        - Two types of fixed-angle plating can be used to stabilize periprosthetic distal femur fractures: a blade plate or a condylar screw plate.
        - These implants are used infrequently with the advent of modern locking plates. Disadvantages include only a single point of distal fixation with a tendency toward varus collapse.
- Type III: A displaced distal femur fracture with a loose femoral component poses a significant challenge.
    - Revision TKA
        - In cases with loose or unstable prosthetic components (or if severe comminution or very distal fracture extension make stable fixation of the fracture fragments unrealistic), revision arthroplasty using stemmed components and metaphyseal cones is an appropriate first-line treatment.
        - This procedure requires the use of cemented stems and may require the use of constrained implants. Structural allograft, augments, and/or augmented metaphyseal fixation (sleeves or cones) may be needed in the presence of bone loss and to protect fixation with the use of constraint.
        - Advantages of revision TKA include the potential for early range of motion and weight bearing if stable fracture fixation is obtained.
        - Preoperative templating of both the femoral and tibial components is essential. In addition to estimating the size of the components, templating is used to gauge bone resection levels and the need for augmentation, as well as the length, position, and size of cemented stems.
        - Selective component retention (e.g., retention of a well-fixed and well-aligned tibial component) should be considered preoperatively based on compatibility with planned revision implants and the degree of constraint anticipated.
        - Surgeons who treat periprosthetic fractures around TKAs must have the expertise and technical support to perform either stemmed revision TKA with metaphyseal fixation or revision to a megaprosthesis, as it is often difficult to determine which reconstructive option is necessary until the fracture is assessed intraoperatively.
    - Distal femoral replacement
        - Revision TKA with a distal femoral replacement can be chosen in the setting of marked comminution, osteopenic bone, and loss of ligamentous support in very elderly patients for whom additional revision surgery is unlikely.
        - In these cases, fracture healing is not required and early range of motion and weight bearing are permissible.

Tibia

- Type IA: Nondisplaced fractures of the tibial plateau with a stable implant can be treated with restricted weight bearing, bracing or casting, and close radiographic follow-up, with consideration of tibial plateau ORIF.
- Type IB: Fractures involving the tibial plateau with a loose implant are an indication for early revision with a stemmed tibial component to bypass the bone defect. The fracture can be addressed with screw fixation, and treatment of accompanying bone defects is based on depth: defects <5 mm deep can be filled in with cement, those 5 to 10 mm can be filled in with cement and screws placed as rebar, and those >10 mm may require metal augments.
- Type IC: Intraoperative fractures of the tibial plateau are often reduced and fixed with a cancellous screw or a plate before insertion of final components (Figure 70.11A-D).
- Type IIA: Periprosthetic fractures that occur in the metadiaphyseal region of the proximal tibia can be treated nonoperatively if the fracture is nondisplaced. For displaced fractures, traditional plating techniques can be used given that rigid fixation can be achieved. If rigid fixation is not possible, long-stem revision bypassing the fracture site is advised. With a well-fixed tibial component, component removal can be challenging and lead to considerable bone loss.

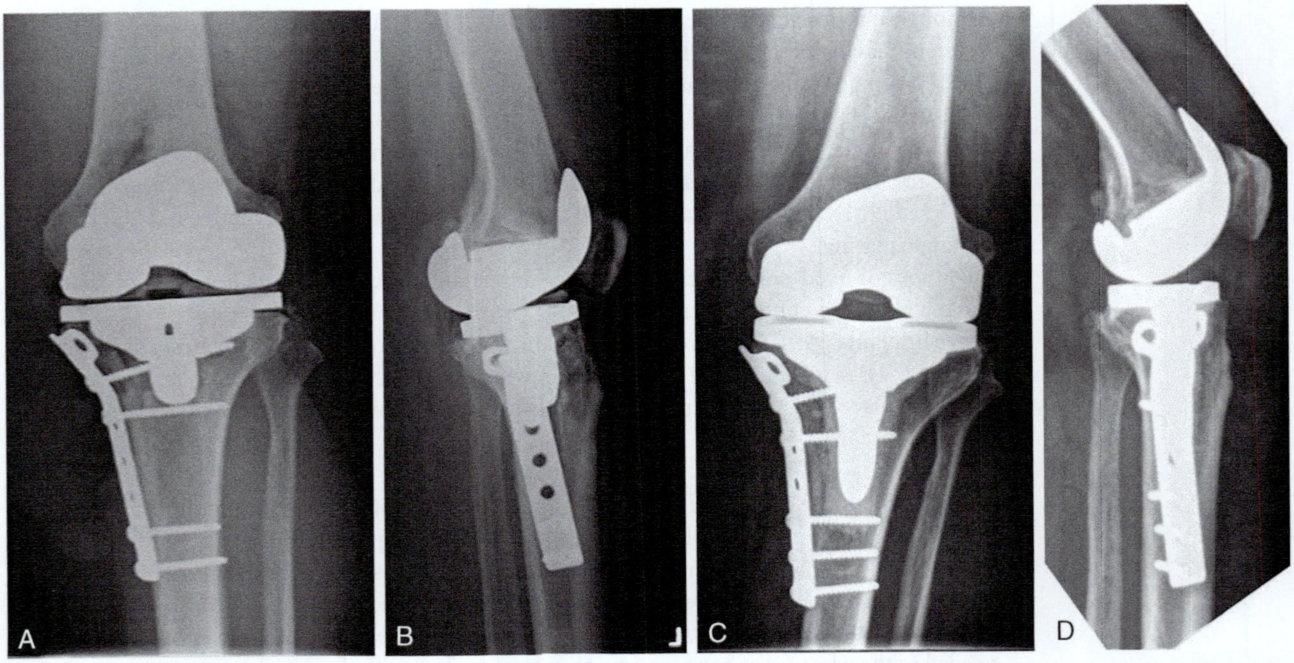

Figure 70.11 | Anteroposterior (A) and lateral (B) intraoperative fluoroscopic images demonstrate a medial tibial plateau fracture that occurred when using the keel punch at the time of primary total knee arthroplasty. Postoperative anteroposterior (C) and (D) lateral radiographs at three months demonstrate uneventful healing after treatment with a stemmed tibial component and medial plating. (Images courtesy of Kevin I. Perry, MD.)

- Type IIB: Fractures that border the tibial stem and are associated with component loosening are best treated with revision to a long-stemmed tibial component. In cases of severe metaphyseal bone loss, impaction bone grafting[8] or metaphyseal sleeves or cones can be utilized.
- Type IIC: Intraoperative fractures next to the stem of the tibial component often occur during removal of a tibial component or preparation and insertion of a stemmed prosthesis. If the fracture is recognized intraoperatively, a longer stem can be used to bypass the fracture. If the fracture is recognized postoperatively, a minimally displaced fracture can be treated with restricted weight bearing for 6 weeks.
- Type III: Fractures distal to the tibial component may result from trauma, limb malalignment, or a complication of tibial tubercle osteotomy. Fractures due to trauma may be treated nonoperatively if minimally displaced with <1 cm of shortening and >50% of contact between fragments. Fractures that fail to meet these criteria should be treated with ORIF. If a malaligned TKA was the cause of fracture secondary to increased stresses, a corrective revision procedure is warranted with a stemmed tibial component to bypass the fracture. Authors have advocated bypassing the fracture by at least one cortical diameter.
- Type IVA: Minimally displaced or nondisplaced tibial tubercle fractures can be treated nonoperatively with immobilization of the knee in extension. If displaced, ORIF with wiring, tendon transfer, or mesh reconstruction is warranted.
- Types IVB and IVC: Tibial tubercle fractures that occur postoperatively or intraoperatively in conjunction with a loose prosthesis require revision of the tibial component and ORIF of the tubercle with screws or wires.

Bone, Implant, and Soft Tissue Techniques

ORIF of the Femur With Periarticular Locking Plate (Lewis and Rorabeck Types I and II Fractures)

- When ORIF is undertaken for a distal femur periprosthetic fracture around a TKA judged to be stable, it is important to scrutinize the fracture pattern to determine whether primary or secondary fracture healing is desirable. This will determine the extent of exposure and fixation construct.
  - Simple fracture patterns (Figure 70.12A-D) are often conducive to rigid fixation with interfragmentary compression to allow for primary fracture healing. In such cases, proximal extension of the lateral approach to the distal femur described earlier is warranted to allow direct exposure and anatomic reduction of the fracture. A locking plate can be placed over the top of the interfragmentary lag screws.

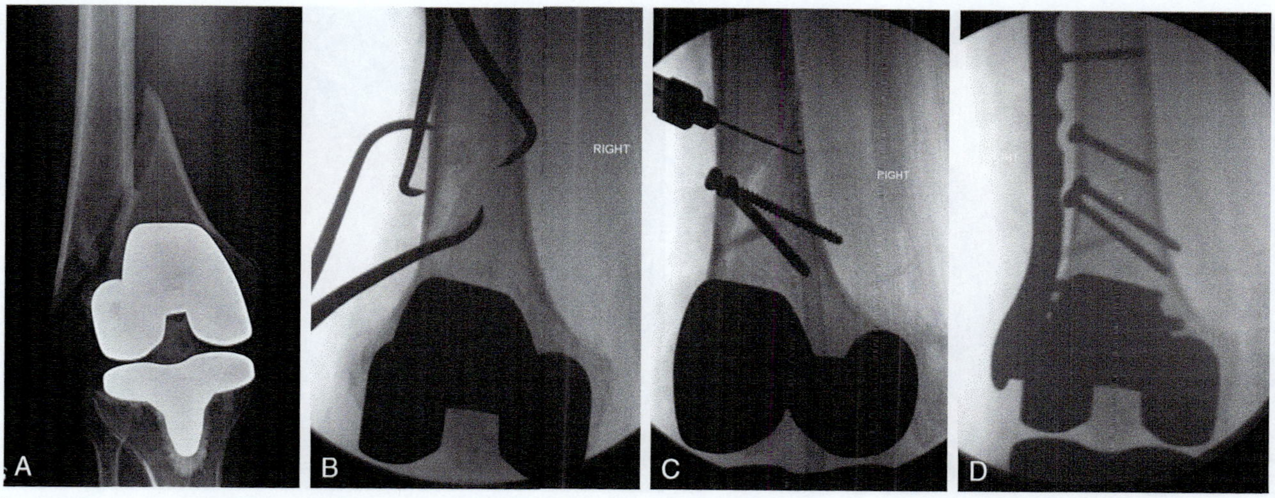

Figure 70.12 | Anteroposterior injury (A) and intraoperative fluoroscopic images of the knee demonstrating anatomic reduction of a spiral periprosthetic femur fracture using serrated reduction clamps (B) and interfragmentary lag screws by technique (C) with a locking plate placed over the lag screws to neutralize the construct (D).

- Comminuted fracture patterns (Figure 70.13A-D) are amenable to secondary fracture healing through relative fracture stability. In such cases, a more limited distal incision can be used to tunnel a lateral-based locking plate in a submuscular fashion, with the proximal screw holes filled percutaneously to form a bridging construct and minimize dissection at the fracture site.
- Indirect reduction aids such as skeletal traction or external fixation can be utilized. An anterior-based knee-spanning external fixator works nicely to maintain provisional reduction while allowing access to the lateral thigh.
- Lateral exposure to the distal femur is completed based on the above-mentioned considerations.
- When satisfactory fracture reduction is achieved, use fluoroscopy to choose a distal femoral locking plate of appropriate length.
  - An understanding of native distal femoral anatomy is important to gauge the adequacy of reduction and proper plate positioning (Figure 70.14A and B).
  - The plate should typically extend above the lesser trochanter and can be contoured to accommodate the vastus ridge.

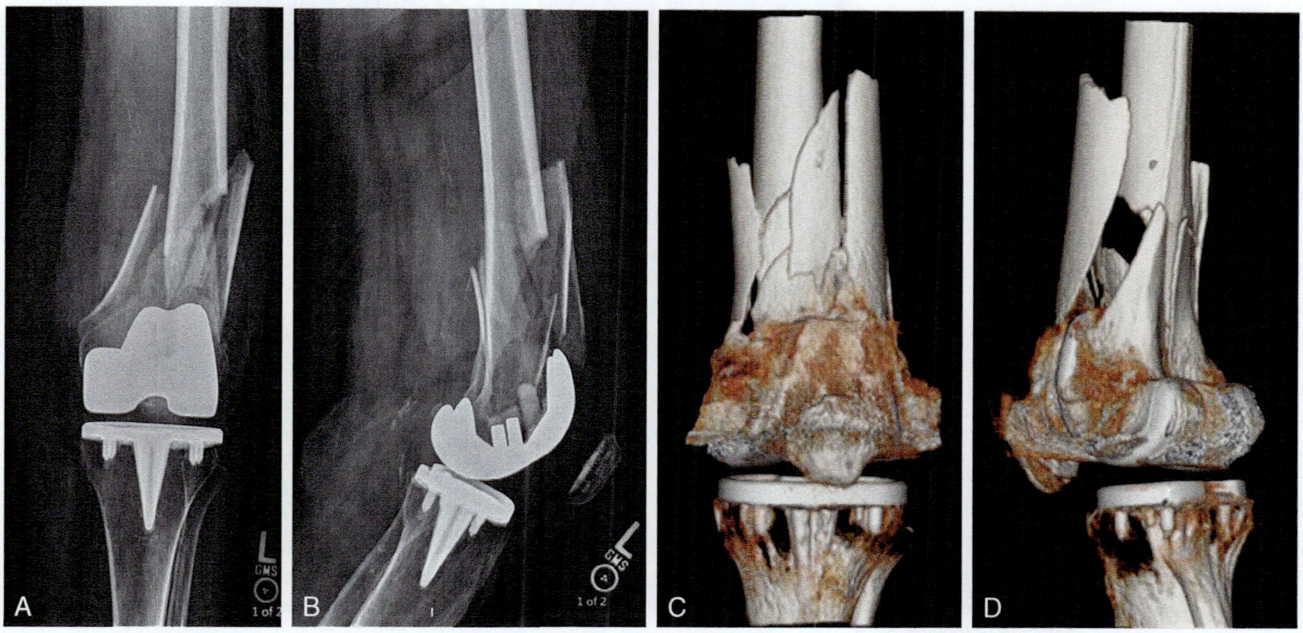

Figure 70.13 | Anteroposterior (A) and lateral (B) radiographs and 3-dimensional reconstruction computed tomography images (C, D) revealing a comminuted Lewis and Rorabeck type II periprosthetic femur fracture amenable to submuscular locked plating.

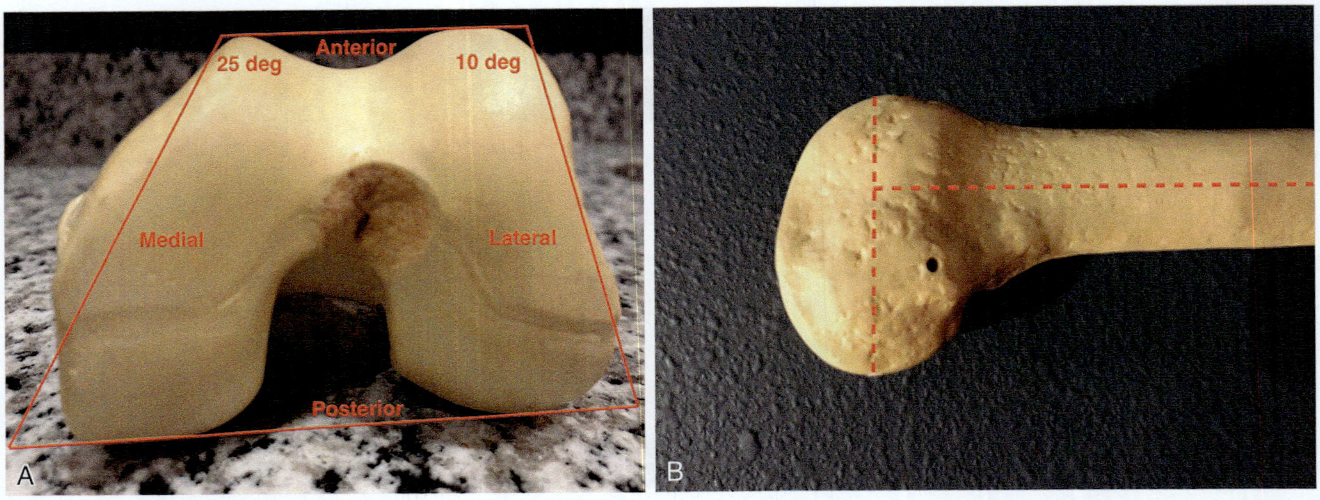

Figure 70.14 | Annotated photo (A) of the distal femur viewed on axis shows its trapezoidal shape, wider posteriorly than anteriorly. The lateral metaphysis of the distal femur is angulated 10° from the sagittal plane, whereas the medial metaphysis is angulated 25° from the sagittal plane. A second photograph (B) of the distal femur viewed from the side shows that the femoral shaft is in line with the anterior half of the distal femoral condyles.

- In a retrograde fashion, use the insertion handle to slide the distal femoral locking plate from the knee to the proximal femur in a submuscular, extraperiosteal manner.
- Use AP and lateral fluoroscopic imaging to verify that the plate is of appropriate length and positioned properly in the coronal and sagittal planes.
    - Avoid posterior placement of the distal plate, which can result in medialization of the condyles (the so-called golf-club deformity; Figure 70.15A and B) secondary to the posterior condylar flare (Figure 70.14A).
- Once satisfied with plate length and position, the plate should be secured to the bone distally using a guidewire in the center hole (Figure 70.16A and B).
    - This guidewire should be parallel to the joint line and provides a pivot point around which the AP positioning of the plate can be manipulated to properly align with the shaft (Figure 70.16C). Of note, fixed-angle plating systems are designed to reestablish the valgus alignment of the distal femur. Placing the distal screws parallel to the joint will help ensure that when the shaft is brought to the plate, the anatomic axis of the femur is restored.

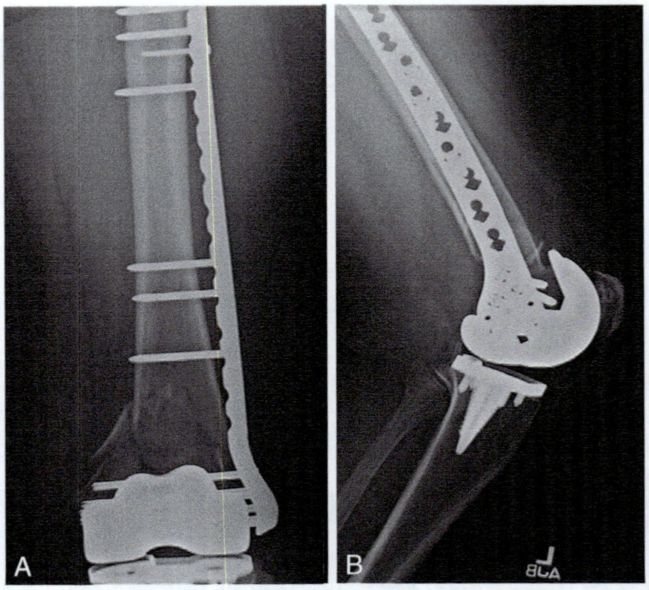

Figure 70.15 | Anteroposterior (A) and lateral (B) radiographs demonstrating medialization of the femoral condyles ("golf-club deformity") after open reduction and internal fixation of a distal femur periprosthetic fracture using a lateral distal femur locking plate.

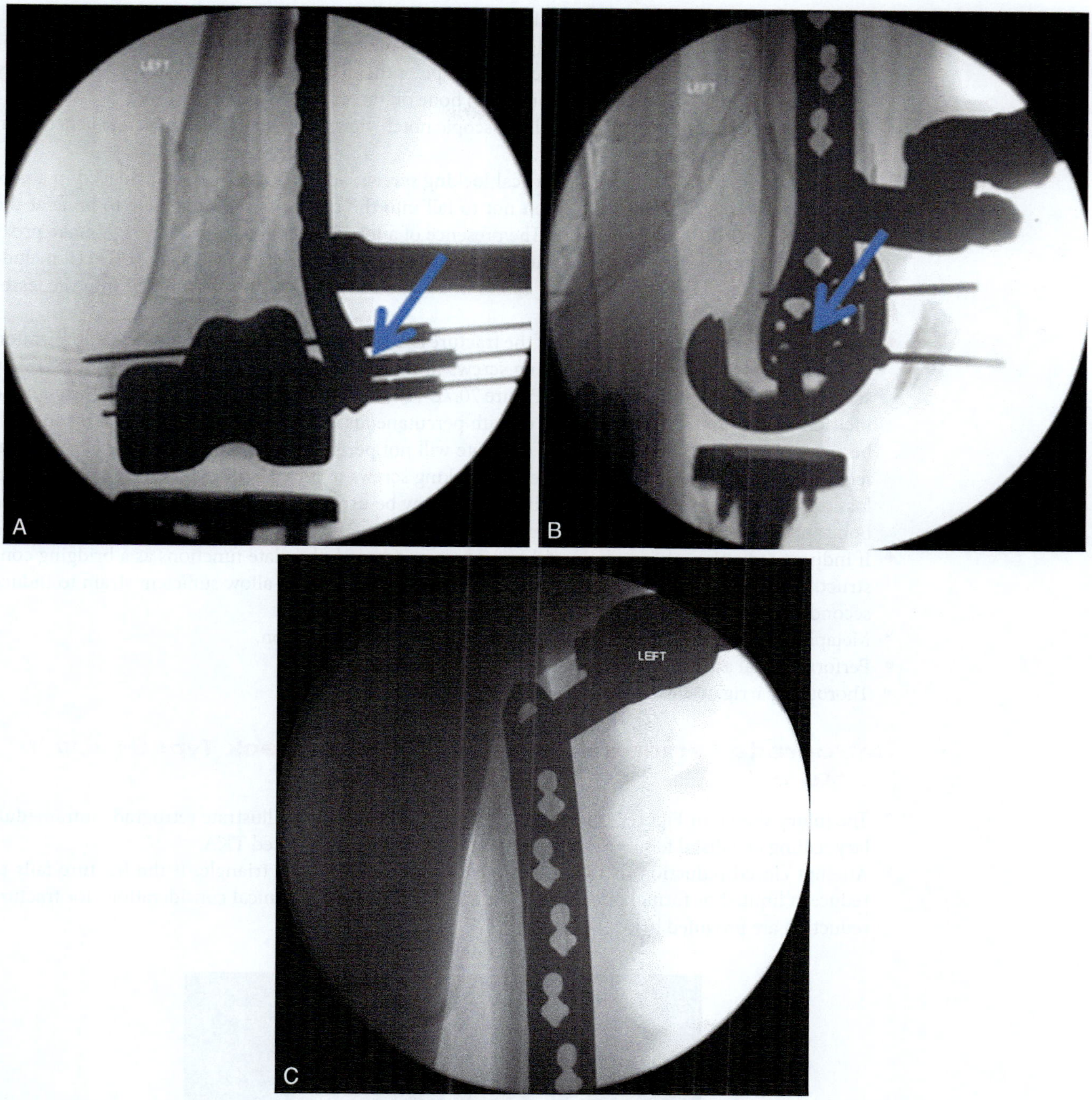

Figure 70.16 | Anteroposterior (A) and lateral (B) intraoperative fluoroscopic images of the periprosthetic distal femur seen in Figure 70.13A-D demonstrating guidewire placement through the central hole of the distal plate (arrows) with a trajectory parallel to the joint line. Proximal plate alignment with the femoral shaft is verified on the lateral view (C).

- The plate should then be secured to the bone proximally with either a K-wire or a "whirlybird" device. This can be done percutaneously.
- Fluoroscopic verification of plate position and fracture reduction is recommended before commencing with screws.
- Place 2 to 3 fully threaded locking screws to secure the plate to the bone distally. A cannulated screw can often be placed over the central guidewire.
- Place at least 1 screw proximally to secure the plate to bone.
    - The first screws should be nonlocking cortical screws. Never place a nonlocking cortical screw after placing a locking cortical screw.

- Place the rest of the locking screws in the distal portion of the plate.
  - An AP fluoroscopic view with the leg in 25° to 30° of internal rotation is needed to verify appropriate screw lengths given the trapezoidal shape of the distal femur (Figure 70.14A). Excessively long distal screws can falsely appear within bone on direct AP view.
  - For cruciate-retaining implants, a fluoroscopic notch view can help to rule out screw penetration posteriorly within the notch.
- The goal for proximal fixation is bicortical locking screws, and this can often be achieved in a percutaneous fashion. Care must be taken not to fall into the trap of pulling the plate to bone at the expense of malreducing the fracture. The presence of a total hip arthroplasty above can make proximal fixation challenging and may warrant alternative fixation strategies (Figure 70.7E-H), including unicortical locking screws and/or cables in addition to a bicortical screw aimed into the lesser trochanter.
- If direct reduction and compression of the fracture is achieved, the plate functions as a neutralization construct. Thus, place 2 to 3 nonlocking screws in the femoral shaft adjacent to the fracture. Every screw hole does not need to be filled (Figure 70.7E-H). These screws can often be placed through the incision used from fracture reduction or with percutaneous techniques. However, the surgeon must be aware that often the precontour of the plate will not perfectly fit the contour of the lateral distal femoral cortex. Thus, the application of nonlocking screws to a well-reduced fracture may result in loss of reduction. In these cases, locking screws may be useful to prevent reducing the plate to the bone and thus malreducing the fracture.
- If indirect reduction of a comminuted fracture is performed, the plate functions as a bridging construct. Thus, adequately space the screws bordering the fracture to allow sufficient strain to induce secondary bone healing (Figure 70.17A and B).
- Metaphyseal bone loss can be bone grafted at the surgeon's discretion.
- Perform a final assessment of knee stability.
- Thoroughly irrigate all wounds and perform a layered closure.

Retrograde Femoral IMN (Lewis and Rorabeck Types I and II Fractures)

- The injury shown in Figure 70.18A-D is used as a case example to illustrate retrograde intramedullary nailing of a distal femur periprosthetic fracture above a well-fixed TKA.
- Attempt closed reduction of the fracture over a knee-positioning triangle. If the fracture fails to reduce, a limited or formal open reduction may be necessary. Technical considerations for fracture reduction are provided below.

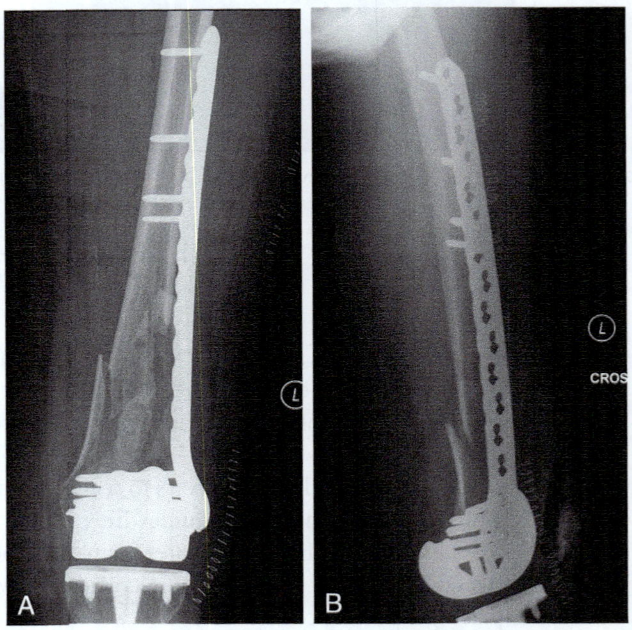

Figure 70.17 | Anteroposterior (A) and lateral (B) radiographs of the femur show the final bridging construct with a lateral locking plate utilized for the comminuted supracondylar periprosthetic fracture seen in Figure 70.13A-D.

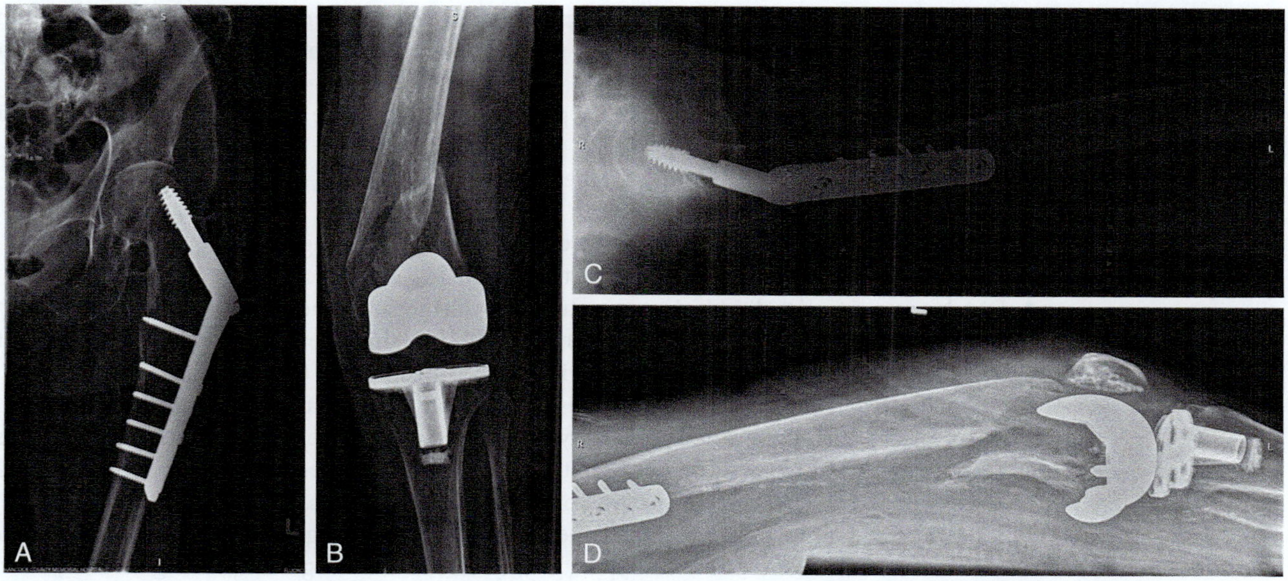

Figure 70.18 | Anteroposterior (A, B) and lateral (C, D) radiographs show a distal femur periprosthetic fracture between a well-fixed, cruciate-retaining total knee arthroplasty and a sliding hip screw from a healed intertrochanteric fracture. A decision was made to utilize retrograde intramedullary nail fixation to facilitate implant overlap while leaving the femoral neck protected.

- Approach the knee through the prior anterior knee incision and a medial parapatellar arthrotomy.
- We generally reserve this technique for femoral components with an open box known to accommodate an IMN. If a decision is made to use a metal cutting burr to facilitate nail passage (either to expand an open box or to create an opening in a closed box), it is imperative to minimize undue damage to the prosthesis and avoid retention of any metal debris.
- With the knee flexed to approximately 40°, utilize fluoroscopy to establish an appropriate starting point within the intercondylar notch (Figure 70.19A and B). Remove the polyethylene insert (if a replacement liner is available) to facilitate access to an acceptable starting point at the apex Blumensaat line on the lateral view and in line with the center of femoral canal in both the coronal and sagittal planes. Advance the starting guidewire in a retrograde fashion on power. When starting to drill, drop one's hand slightly to counteract the tendency for the femoral component to deflect the

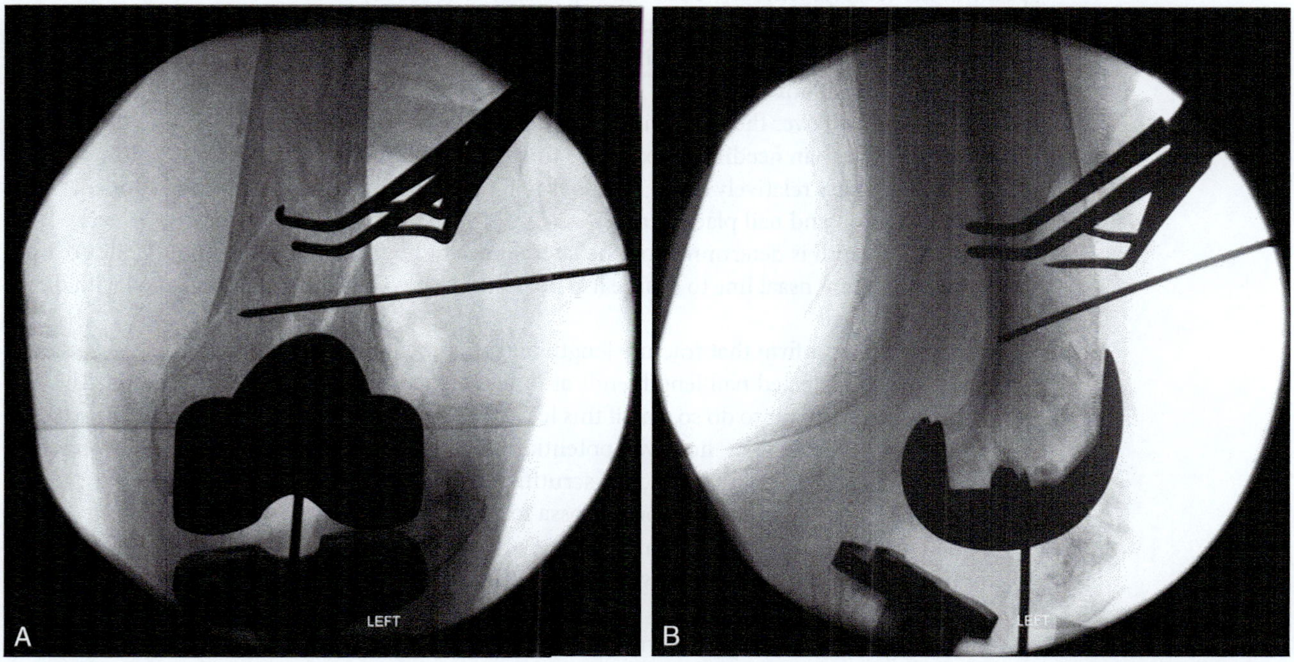

Figure 70.19 | Anteroposterior (A) and lateral (B) intraoperative fluoroscopic images demonstrating the proper start point for retrograde intramedullary nailing of the injury seen in Figure 70.18A-D.

wire posteriorly into the notch. The hand is raised once the wire enters the cortex, so as to be collinear with the femoral shaft. Once the starting guidewire is centered on the AP and lateral images, the wire is passed into the distal femoral shaft.

- Place a soft tissue retractor over the starting guidewire to protect the patellar tendon and prosthetic components.
- Use a cannulated starting reamer to open the distal femur.
- Ensure that the fracture is reduced.
  - Reattempt closed reduction of the fracture over a knee-positioning triangle.
  - Traction is used to restore length; ensure that adequate paralysis is employed.
  - Distal fractures tend to displace in recurvatum through the pull of the gastrocnemius muscle; bumps placed under the knee can relax this deforming force. Blocking screws in distal fractures can create a canal in the metaphyseal region in line with the proximal shaft so that the nail aids in reduction.
  - Alternatively, a femoral distractor can assist with obtaining and maintaining fracture reduction. It can be placed laterally, inserted proximally at the greater trochanter and distally in either the posterior aspect of the femoral condyle or in the proximal tibia. Some surgeons recommend anterior placement to avoid posterior angulation of distal fracture patterns.
  - If the fracture fails to reduce, a limited open reduction is encouraged with a push-pull technique. This can often be done with a ball-spike pusher on the shaft fragment pushing medially and a bone hook on the distal fragment pulling laterally.
  - A formal open reduction is necessary if the above-mentioned methods fail. Laterally based incisions are preferred unless otherwise dictated by an open fracture wound.
  - Restoration of length and correct rotation must be assessed clinically as well as radiographically. In the absence of comminution, the latter can include comparing the thickness of the medial and lateral femoral cortex proximal and distal to the fracture to ensure that they are equal.
- Pass a beaded-tip guidewire from the knee to just below the piriformis fossa. This ensures that reaming will be performed past the level of the lesser trochanter, as the reamers stop at the beaded portion of the guidewire (Figure 70.20A-C).
- Measure the appropriate nail length off of the guidewire. If the measurement is between nail sizes, the shorter nail is selected. Length can be added with an end cap if required.
- Ream the canal with end-cutting cannulated reamers.
  - Typically, begin with an 8- or 9-mm reamer.
  - Fracture reduction must be maintained to avoid reaming eccentrically.
  - Increase in 0.5-mm reamer increments to avoid thermal necrosis.
  - The approximate nail diameter is estimated based on preoperative measurement of the narrowest point of the femoral isthmus. The final nail diameter is ideally selected based on the size of the reamer that provides initial cortical chatter; the canal is then reamed to 1.0 to 1.5 mm over the selected nail diameter. With a TKA in place, nail size may be limited by the inner diameter of the femoral component box rather than canal fit.
- Insert the selected nail over the guidewire (most current systems allow nail passage over the beaded-tip guidewire, rather than needing to exchange this for a smooth-tip guidewire).
  - The nail should pass relatively easily; if it does not, perform careful fluoroscopic assessment of the fracture reduction and nail placement.
  - Nail insertion depth is determined on the lateral knee radiograph. The nail should end proximal to the apex of Blumensaat line to ensure it is not in the knee. This should be confirmed with direct visualization as well.
  - Radiographically confirm that fracture length and alignment remain appropriate.
  - Confirm that the selected nail length ends at or above the level of the lesser trochanter. The nail can be advanced if it fails to do so, and if this leaves the nail countersunk, end caps can be selected to gain nail length. This does, however, potentially limit points of distal fixation with low fracture patterns, emphasizing the importance of scrutinizing the appropriate nail length initially.
  - Take care to remain below the piriformis fossa to prevent proximal nail protrusion.
- Lock the nail distally using the distal interlocking guides.
  - A minimum of 3 interlocking screws engaging the distal fracture fragment is preferred (Figure 70.21A and B).
  - As with ORIF, use fluoroscopy to scrutinize screw lengths given the trapezoidal shape of the distal femur (Figure 70.14A).
  - Consider a locking end cap (which locks the most distal interlocking screw to the nail) in osteoporotic bone.

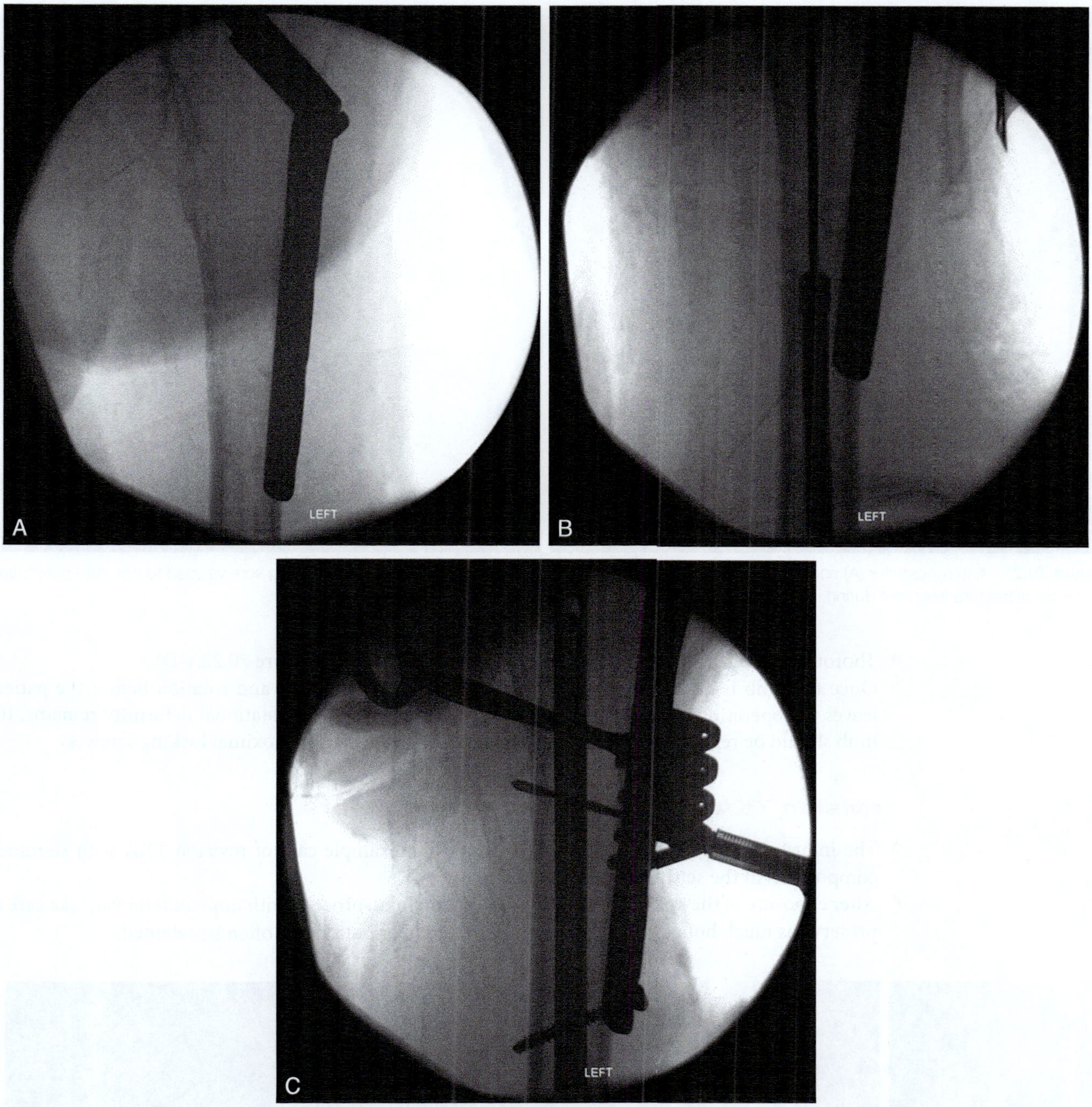

Figure 70.20 | Anteroposterior intraoperative fluoroscopic images from the injury shown in Figure 70.18A-D demonstrate that the shaft screws were removed from the sliding hip screw (A) to facilitate passage of the guidewire, reamers (B), and retrograde nail. Two cortical screws were ultimately replaced through the side plate in a redirected fashion to avoid the nail (C).

- Reassess fracture reduction fluoroscopically after the distal interlocking screws are placed.
  - If shortening has occurred, length can be regained with traction or by back-slapping the nail (exercise caution with this strategy in osteoporotic bone).
- Place anterior-to-posterior, bicortical proximal interlocking screws using the perfect circle technique.
  - Avoid slipping off the femur medially as the femoral artery lies 1 cm medial to the femur at the level of the lesser trochanter.
  - The usual length of proximal interlocking screws is 25 to 35 mm.
- Perform a final assessment of knee stability. If the polyethylene insert was removed to facilitate exposure, it can be trialed and replaced.

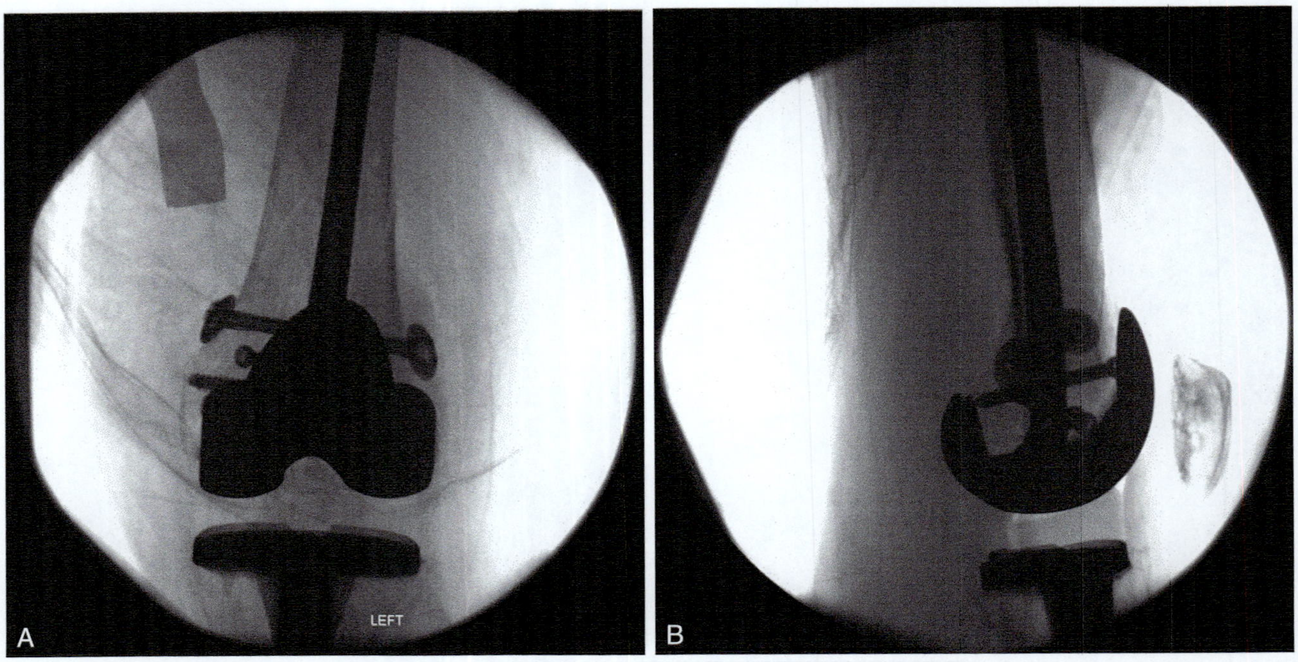

Figure 70.21 | Anteroposterior (A) and lateral (B) intraoperative fluoroscopy images show 4 distal interlocking screws used to optimize purchase of the distal fracture fragment during intramedullary nailing of the injury seen in Figure 70.18A-D.

- Thoroughly irrigate all wounds and perform a layered closure (Figure 70.22A-D).
- Once the limb is undraped, perform a final assessment of length and rotation before the patient leaves the operating theater. If notable leg-length discrepancy or rotational deformity remains, the limb should be reprepared, draped, and corrected by altering the proximal locking screw(s).

Revision TKA With Stemmed Components

- The injury shown in Figure 70.23A-E is used as an example case of revision TKA with stemmed components in the setting of periprosthetic fracture.
- After exposure of the knee using revision TKA principles, proceed with implant removal; take care to preserve as much bone as possible. A well-fixed patellar button can often be retained.

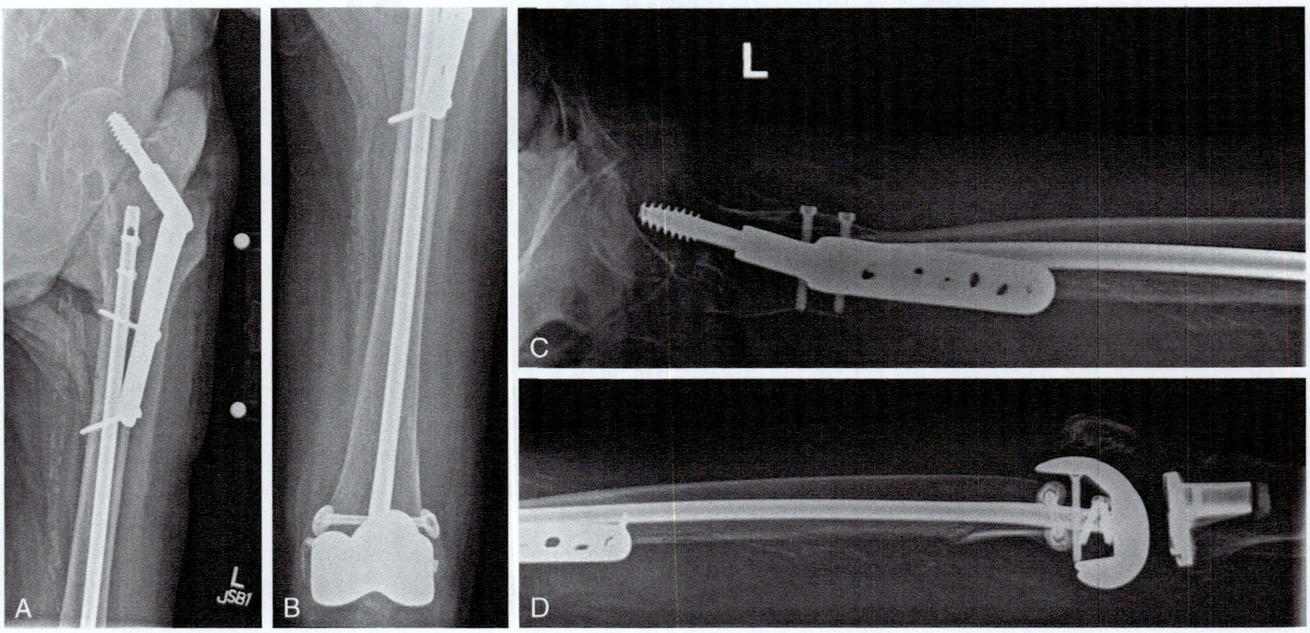

Figure 70.22 | Anteroposterior (A, B) and lateral (C, D) postoperative femur radiographs after intramedullary nailing of the injury seen in Figure 70.18A-D.

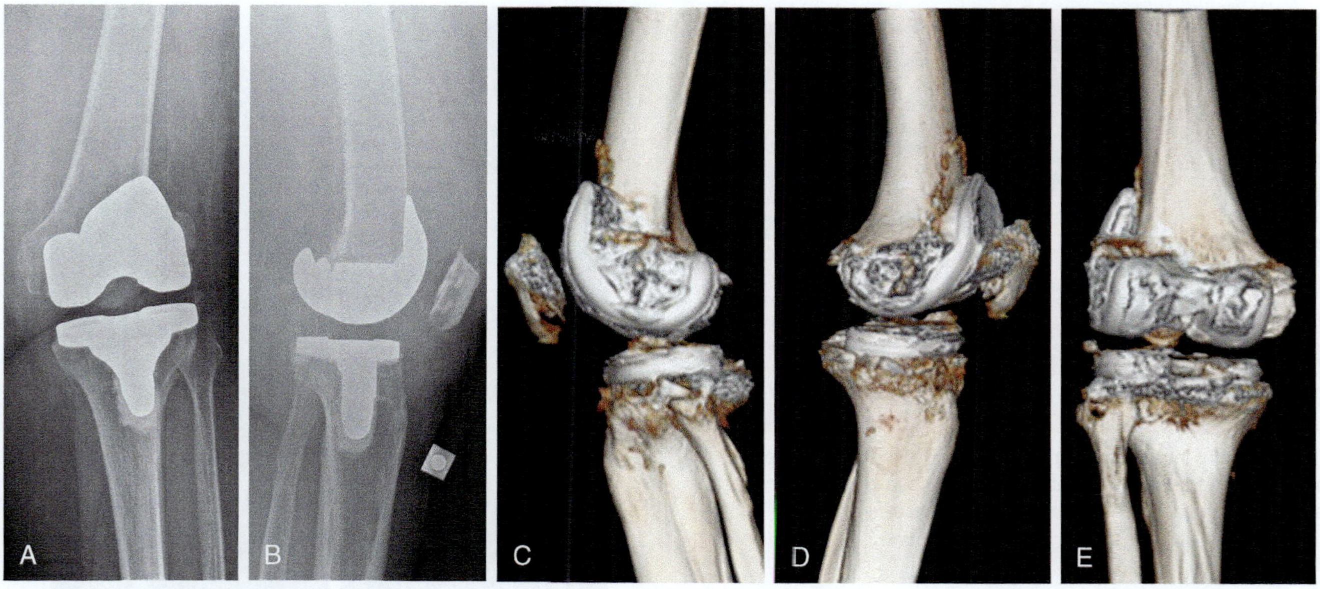

Figure 70.23 | Anteroposterior (A) and lateral (B) radiographs and 3-dimensional reconstruction computed tomography images (C-E) of the knee demonstrating a very low and comminuted distal femur periprosthetic fracture above a total knee arthroplasty that was not amenable to internal fixation.

- Fully debride all cement and fibrous tissue. Assess the extent of bone loss to verify or adjust the anticipated reconstruction plan (Figure 70.24A and B). The following treatment algorithm provides general guidance when it comes to bone loss management in TKA.
  - Contained defects
    - <5 mm: polymethylmethacrylate fill
    - ≥5 mm: porous metal augments
  - Noncontained defects
    - <5 mm: polymethylmethacrylate fill
    - 5 to 15 mm: porous augments, cones, and stems
    - ≥15 mm: megaprostheses versus porous augments, cones, and stems
- Prepare the tibia. The goal is to prepare the tibial canal and create a supportive bony platform on the proximal tibia perpendicular to the mechanical axis.
  - Ream distally
  - Prepare for cone proximally

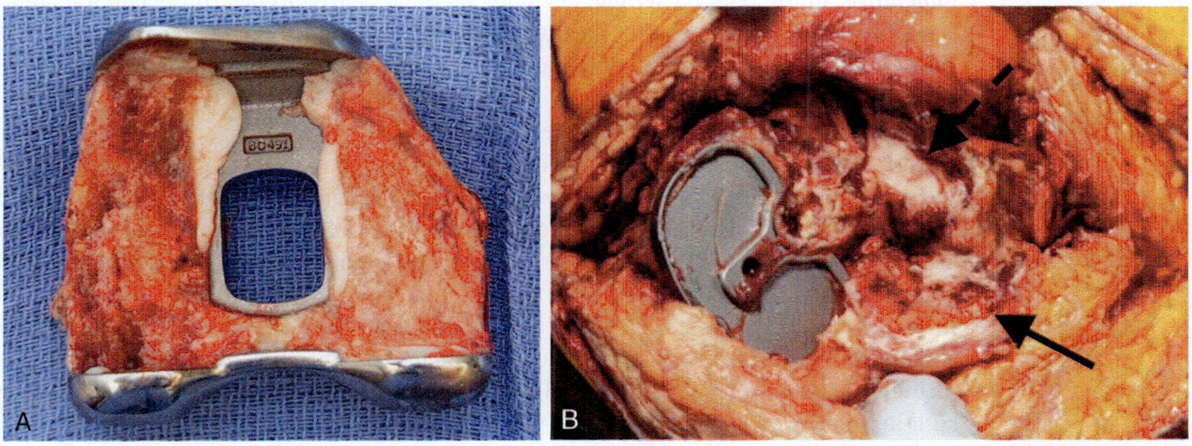

Figure 70.24 | Intraoperative photographs from the case presented in Figure 70.23A-E demonstrate the extracted femoral component (A) and associated uncontained distal femoral bone loss (B), including the vast majority of the lateral femoral condyle (solid arrow) but relatively sparing the medial column (dotted arrow). It was decided that there was sufficient bone for a hinged construct utilizing a femoral cone.

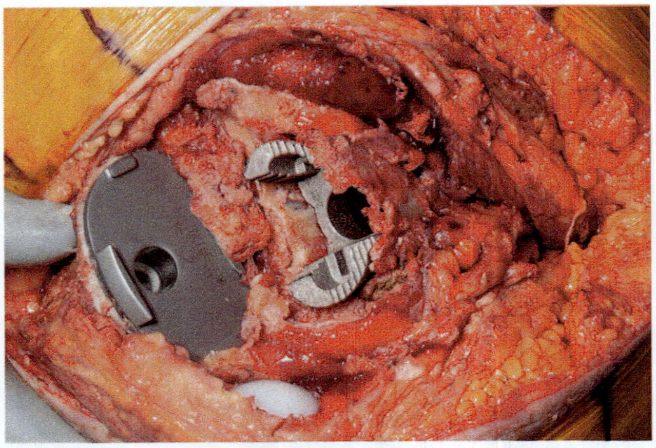

Figure 70.25 | Intraoperative photograph from the case presented in Figure 70.21A-E demonstrating reconstruction of the uncontained femoral defect using a highly porous metaphyseal cone.

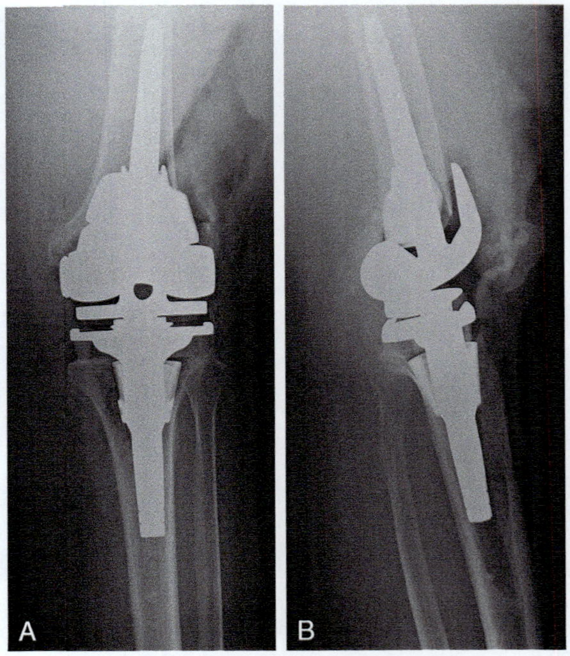

Figure 70.26 | Anteroposterior (A) and lateral (B) intraoperative fluoroscopic images from the case presented in Figure 70.21A-E demonstrating the trial hinged components and highly porous metaphyseal cones in the femur and tibia. Of note, most hinges have excessive valgus built in to the system, so it is our preference to place the femoral component and stem in slight varus to compensate for this.

- Use augments on tibia if polyethylene diameter is estimated to be 20 mm or greater
- The length of the stem required remains controversial but, in the setting of a periprosthetic fracture, should undoubtedly span the fracture after provisional fracture reduction. In general, the more the damage present to metaphyseal bone or the larger the augments needed to reestablish the metaphyseal bone, the longer the stem should be.
- In patients with adequate bone stock, short cemented metaphyseal stems are sufficient. As the bone loss increases, longer stems (>120 mm in length) may be required.
- The above-mentioned stem principles hold true on the tibial and femoral sides.

- Prepare the femur.
  - Progressively ream the femoral canal to the proper size.
  - Size the femoral component based on preoperative templating and intraoperative findings.
  - Determine appropriate femoral component rotation. Rotation of the femoral component is imperative. In the revision setting, key bony landmarks used to determine femoral component rotation are often compromised (the transepicondylar axis, posterior condylar axis, and trochlear groove). In these scenarios, the tibia should be used to establish femoral component rotation and ensure a symmetric flexion gap.
  - Femoral cones may be required (Figure 70.25).
- Perform a trial reduction and radiographic evaluation.
  - When acceptable gap balance is achieved, construct the trial components with the desired stem sizes and augments attached. Distal and posterior femoral augments and tibial augments should be used based on the intraoperative assessment of gap symmetry, bony deficiency, and re-creation of the joint line.
  - Intraoperative radiographs with the trial components in place are advised to ensure appropriate alignment of the extremity, restoration of the joint line, and position of the stems within the intramedullary canals (Figure 70.26A and B). Of note, most hinge components have too much valgus built in, so the goal is slight varus with the femoral component.
- Formal postoperative radiographs are advised (Figure 70.27A and B).

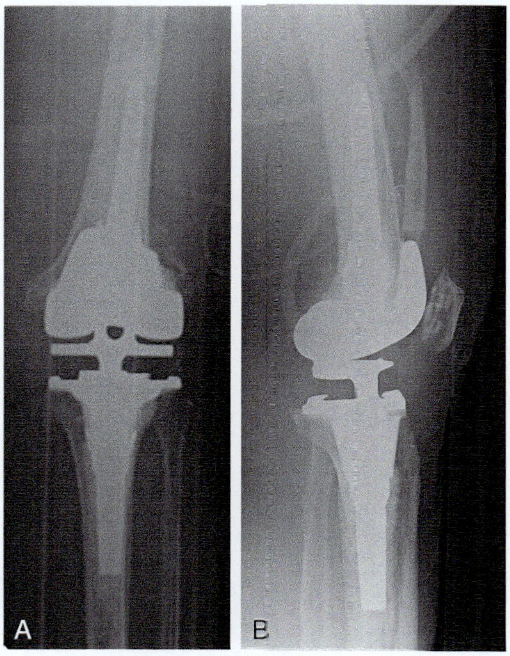

Figure 70.27 | Anteroposterior (A) and lateral (B) postoperative radiographs from the case presented in Figure 70.21A-E demonstrating a modular hinged revision total knee arthroplasty with metaphyseal cones and fully cemented, stemmed tibial and femoral components.

References

1. Garvin KL, Scuderi G, Insall JN. Evolution of the quadriceps snip. *Clin Orthop Relat Res.* 1995;(321):131-137.
2. Rorabeck CH, Taylor JW. Classification of periprosthetic fractures complicating total knee arthroplasty. *Orthop Clin N Am.* 1999;30(2):209-214.
3. Rorabeck CH, Taylor JW. Periprosthetic fractures of the femur complicating total knee arthroplasty. *Orthop Clin N Am.* 1999;30(2):265-277.
4. Felix NA, Stuart MJ, Hanssen AD. Periprosthetic fractures of the tibia associated with total knee arthroplasty. *Clin Orthop Relat Res.* 1997;(345):113-124.
5. Culp RW, Schmidt RG, Hanks G, et al. Supracondylar fracture of the femur following prosthetic knee arthroplasty. *Clin Orthop Relat Res.* 1987;(222):212-222.
6. Thompson SM, Lindisfarne EA, Bradley N, et al. Periprosthetic supracondylar femoral fractures above a total knee replacement: compatibility guide for fixation with a retrograde intramedullary nail. *J Arthroplasty.* 2014;29(8):1639-1641.
7. Maniar RN, Umlas ME, Rodriguez JA, et al. Supracondylar femoral fracture above a PFC posterior cruciate-substituting total knee arthroplasty treated with supracondylar nailing. A unique technical problem. *J Arthroplasty.* 1996;11(5):637-639.
8. Beharrie AW, Nelson CL. Impaction bone-grafting in the treatment of a periprosthetic fracture of the tibia: a case report. *J Bone Joint Surg Am.* 2003;85-A(4):703-707.

Chapter 71
Patellar Instability

TIMOTHY S. BROWN
RAFAEL J. SIERRA

Key Concepts

- Patellar instability is a common cause of anterior knee pain and stiffness following total knee arthroplasty (TKA).
- The most common underlying etiology is malrotation of the femoral, tibial, or both components.
- Revision surgery to address patellar instability should address all malpositioned components and often requires both femoral and tibial revision.

Sterile Instruments and Implants

- Revision TKA instrumentation and implants.

Preoperative Planning

Diagnosis

History

- Prior patellar instability/dislocation
- Prior valgus knee deformity with patellar subluxation
- Difficulty with stairs, getting up from seated position
- Predominantly anterior knee pain, different from preoperative knee pain

Signs/Symptoms

- Anterior knee pain, especially with stair ascent/descent.
- Lateral dislocation of the patella in a flexed position.
- Difficulty actively extending the knee, but reduction of the patella allows active extension.
- Extensor lag, may be present if patella is persistently subluxed or if associated with partial quad rupture.
- Valgus deformity at the knee.
- Excessive external rotation of the lower leg, may indicate internal rotation of the tibial component.

Tests

Examination

- Apprehension with lateral motion of the patella
- Pain with palpation of the patella throughout range of motion
- Patient reduces a patellar dislocation manually as they bring leg into full extension
- Excessively externally rotated foot
- Valgus overall alignment

Radiographs

- Anteroposterior (AP)/lateral of knee
- Long-leg hip-to-ankle radiograph
- Merchant view of bilateral patellae
- Radiographs are reviewed for
  - component fixation (including patellar fixation)
  - polyethylene wear
  - osteolysis
  - component rotation
  - overall limb alignment
  - patellar tracking/tilt
  - patellar subluxation/dislocation
  - patellar thickness and symmetry of bone resection
  - patellar fracture
  - patellar height (baja/alta)
  - extensor mechanism disruption
  - patellar avascular necrosis

Computed Tomography

- Lower-extremity computed tomography (CT) hip through knee is used to better evaluate the rotation of the femoral and tibial components. Careful interpretation of the CT scan is needed so that rotation of the tibial and femoral components is not underestimated or overestimated.

Nonoperative Treatment

Conservative

- Physical therapy may be an option in the patient with mild to moderate anterior knee pain. Patellar bracing is also an option in less severe forms of instability. Frank instability that does not respond to bracing is best treated operatively particularly if an etiology for the instability is elucidated.

Bone, Implant, and Soft Tissue Techniques

Surgical Management

- Surgical management of patellar instability after TKA varies depending on the underlying etiology for the instability.
- Rupture of the medial retinacular/capsular repair (Figure 71.1).
  - In rare instances in which acute patellar instability is the result of failure of the medial parapatellar approach to heal, soft tissue procedures alone may be able to rectify the instability. A palpable defect anteriorly may help diagnose, but occasionally the soft tissue repair stretches out and a defect is not palpable. An ultrasound or magnetic resonance imaging examination might help verify whether the repair has failed.
  - The knee is approached via the previous open medial parapatellar arthrotomy and the patella subluxed with flexion. Verification of tibial and femoral component rotation is always necessary. In addition, the patellar button fixation and symmetry of resection should be reviewed. Tracking of the patella is tested with towel clips or temporary suture fixation holding the arthrotomy together.
  - If the patellar component tracks well, the medial retinaculum is closed and no other intervention is required. If the patella tracks laterally, then lateral retinacular release may be done.
- Malpositioned femoral or tibial components (Figure 71.2).
  - Isolated revision of the patellar component or soft tissue procedures alone are not advised when there is internal rotation of the femoral, tibial, or both components. A total knee arthroplasty revision is performed to specifically position the implants in appropriate rotation and alignment.

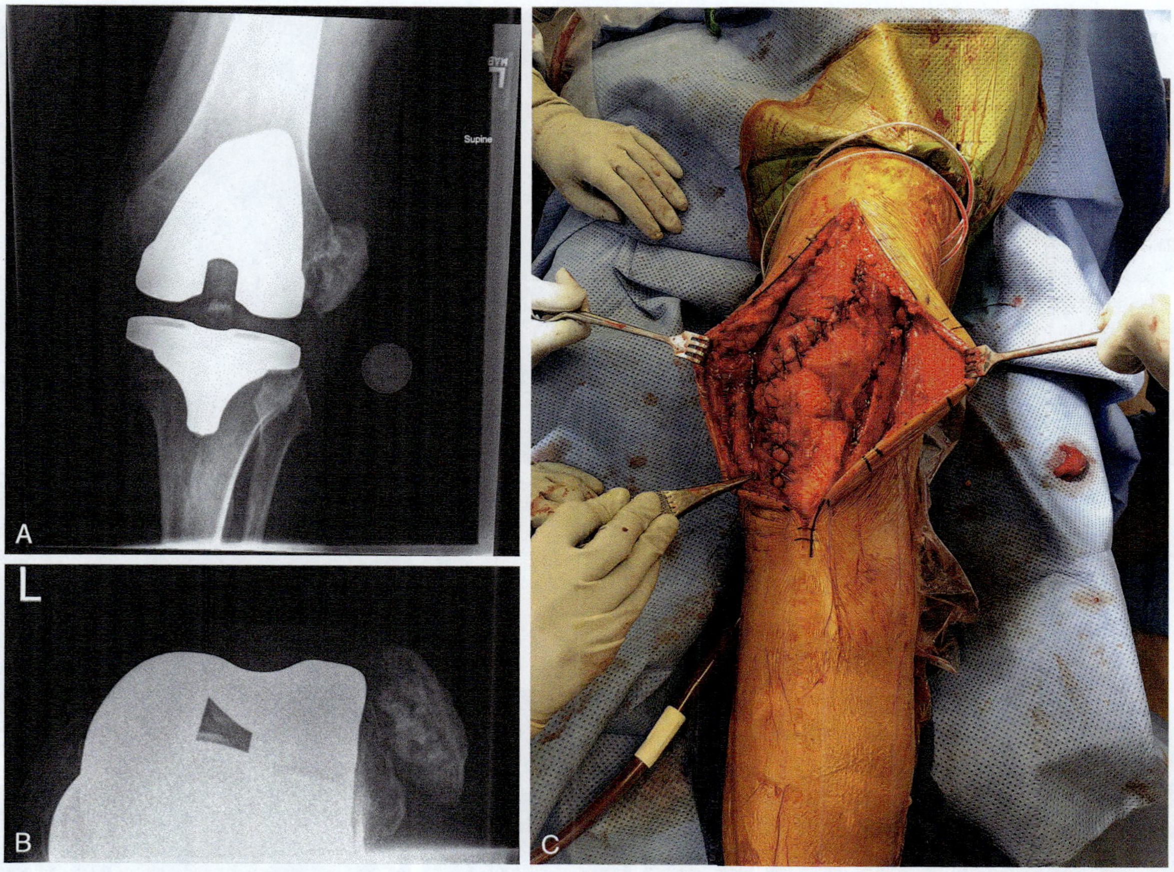

Figure 71.1 | AP (A) and Merchant (B) radiographs of acute lateral patellar instability after a fall 2 weeks following primary TKA. C, Intraoperative image showing primary repair of torn median parapatellar arthrotomy with extensive lateral release.

  - Patellar tracking is tested with implant trials in place. A lateral retinacular release is performed if the lateral retinaculum, iliotibial band, or patellofemoral ligaments are tight and add to maltracking.
  - In cases in which the vastus medialis has stretched out excessively, an extensor realignment and advancement with a pants over vest closure of the extensor mechanism should be performed to tighten the extensor mechanism.
  - If chronic subluxation has led to an incompetent extensor mechanism, the authors' preferred approach is to reinforce the quadriceps extensor mechanism with a Marlex mesh reconstruction (Chapter 73, Revision TKA for Specific: Extensor Mechanism Deficiency)
- Loose or malpositioned patellar component.
  - Isolated revision of the patellar component is attempted in cases in which there is no rotational or angular deformity of the tibiofemoral articulation.
  - The patellar button is removed (see Chapter 61, Revision TKA: Implant Removal).
  - For minimal bone loss, the patellar cut can be revised and the patella prepared for a standard polyethylene resurfacing component.
  - For moderate to severe bone loss, options are a biconvex patella, patellar bone grafting, a trabecular metal patellar button (Zimmer), or rarely resection alone. Patellar component resection is not the best option in patients with patellar subluxation.

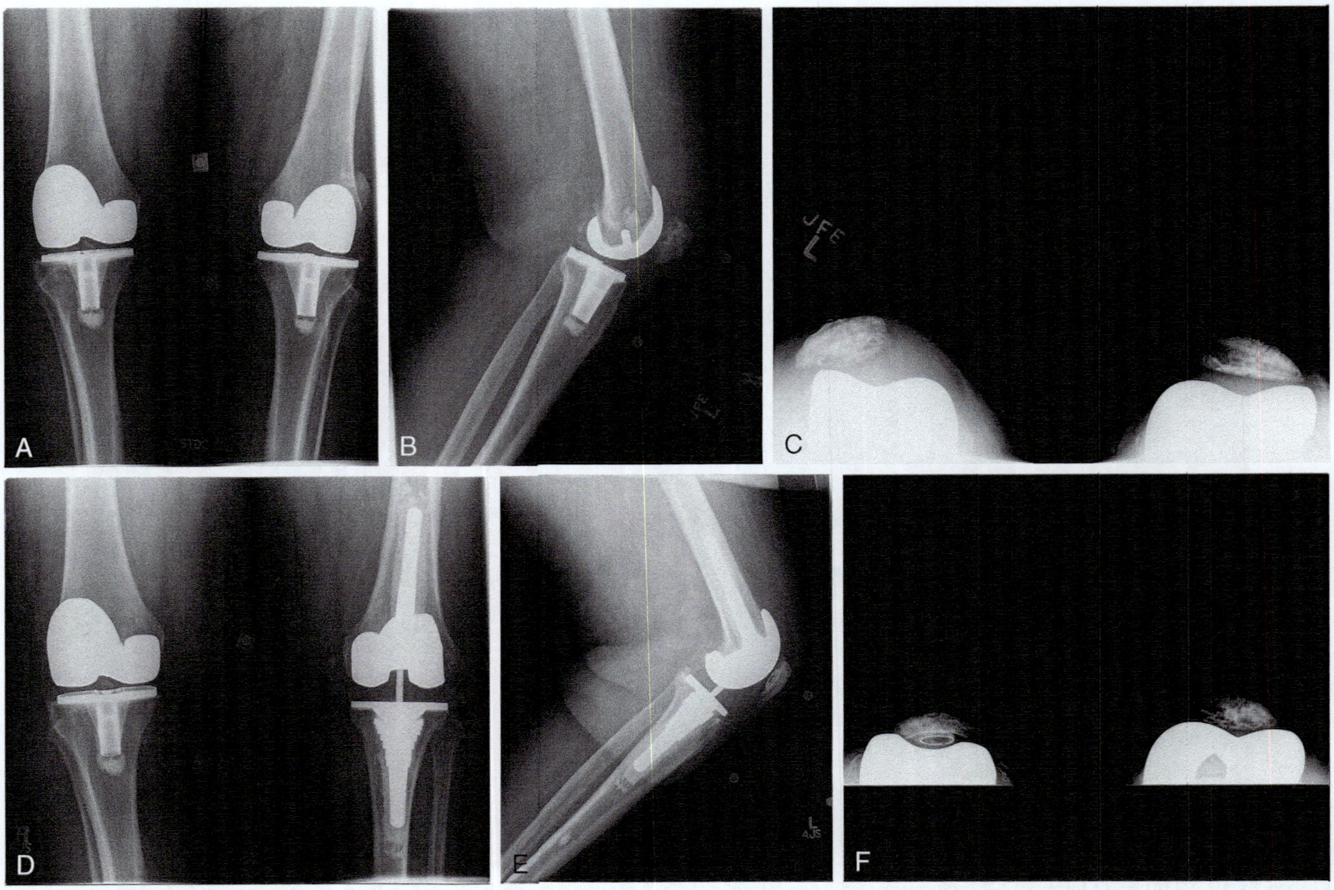

Figure 71.2 | Preoperative AP (A), lateral (B), and Merchant (C) views of a patient with patellar instability and pain with internal rotation of femoral component. Postoperative AP (D), lateral (E), and Merchant (F) views of the same patient following revision TKA and patellar realignment procedure.

Postoperative Care

- Most patients are allowed full weight bearing immediately after surgery.
- Physical therapy to improve active motion is used for the first 6 weeks.
- If extensor mechanism reconstruction or realignment was done, then a 2- to 6-week period of straight leg brace immobilization may be prudent to allow for the soft tissues to heal.

Chapter 72
Patellar Bone Loss

KEVIN I. PERRY
ARLEN D. HANSSEN

Key Concepts

- The majority of patellar revisions are performed with standard or biconvex patellar components. Less than 10% of revision total knee arthroplasty (TKA) are associated with severe patellar bone deficiency requiring one of several alternative reconstructive techniques.
- Severe patellar bone loss, leaving the so-called patellar shell (Figure 72.1), can be managed by simple patellar resection arthroplasty, a gull-wing osteotomy, use of a dedicated porous metal-polyethylene revision construct, or cancellous impaction bone grafting (preferred and described here).
- *Most important concept: None of these patellar reconstructive procedures should be performed as an isolated procedure if the femoral or tibial components are not in proper rotational position.*

Sterile Instruments and Implants

- Typical setup for revision TKA if tibial or femoral revision required
- High-speed burr
- Nonabsorbable #1 sutures

Surgical Approaches

- Standard medial parapatellar arthrotomy

Preoperative Planning

- Determine if only partial femoral or tibial component revision will be required and have proper implants available.

Bone, Implant, and Soft Tissue Techniques

- For severe patellar bone loss, we prefer the patellar bone grafting technique. After performing arthrotomy, leave all peripatellar tissue intact. This includes the thick fibrous rind on the undersurface of quadriceps tendon as this tissue is necessary to create the tissue pouch to contain the cancellous bone graft (Figure 72.2).
- The loose or failed patellar implant is carefully removed to minimize additional bone loss.
- Ensure that tibial and femoral components are rotated properly so that central patellar tracking can be achieved, otherwise patellar reconstruction failure is likely.
- If femoral revision is required, it is often possible to harvest enough cancellous bone in the central portion of the femur during revision of cruciate retaining implants. Additional cancellous bone can also be obtained from the metaphyseal/diaphyseal junction when preparing the femoral canal for a stemmed revision implant.

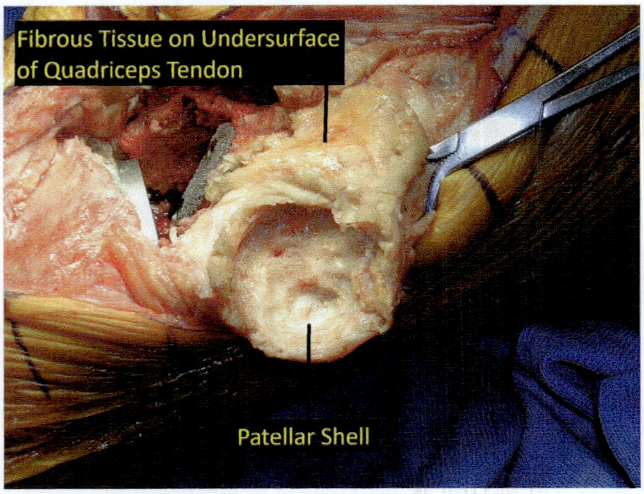

Figure 72.1 | Intraoperative photograph demonstrating a thin patellar shell with fibrous tissue on the undersurface of the patellar tendon.

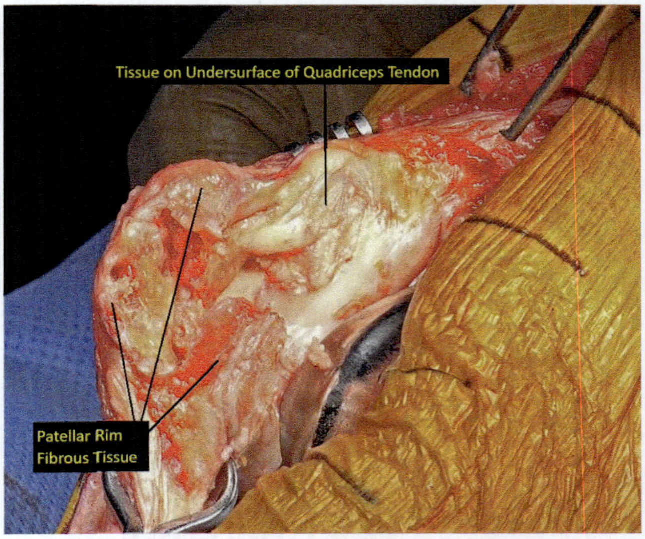

Figure 72.2 | Intraoperative photograph demonstrating fibrous tissue around the patellar rim and on the undersurface of the quadriceps tendon.

- A soft tissue flap is elevated from the undersurface of the quadriceps tendon from proximal to distal being careful to avoid detaching any tissue and creating defects at the superior patellar rim (Figures 72.3 and 72.4).
- If patellar bone stock is less than 10 mm and precludes standard patellar revision techniques, all fibrous material is removed with a high-speed burr (Figure 72.5).
- The tissue flap is then sewn to the fibrous tissue of the patellar rim with multiple interrupted non-absorbable sutures leaving an opening medially to allow introduction of the cancellous bone graft (Figure 72.6).
- If the local available tissue is insufficient, a free flap of tissue from the adjacent fascia lata or fibrous rind in the suprapatellar pouch can be used. If these tissue sources are not satisfactory, commercially prepared tissue products can be used.
- Cancellous bone graft, either harvested autograft or banked cancellous allograft, is then progressively introduced into the medial opening of the so-called pita pocket (Figure 72.7).

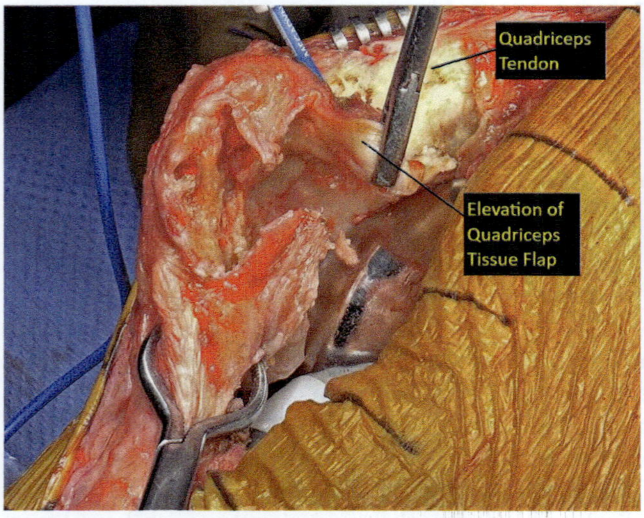

Figure 72.3 | Elevation of the fibrous tissue flap under the quadriceps tendon.

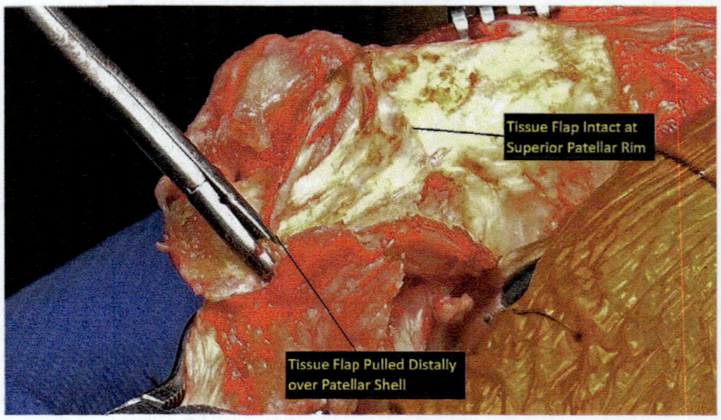

Figure 72.4 | The fibrous tissue flap being pulled distally to cover the remaining shell of the patella.

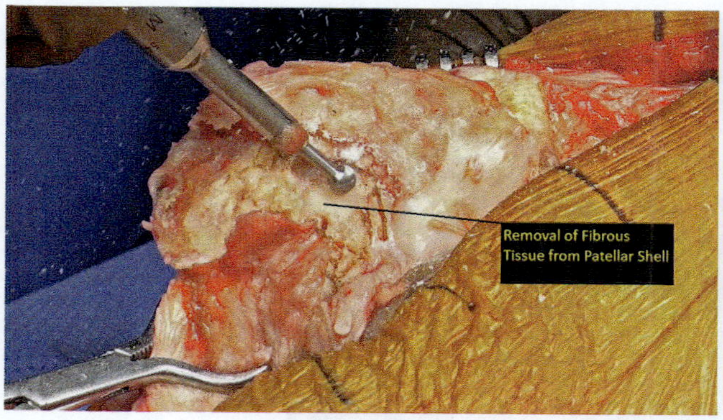

Figure 72.5 | Removal of the fibrous tissue from the patellar shell.

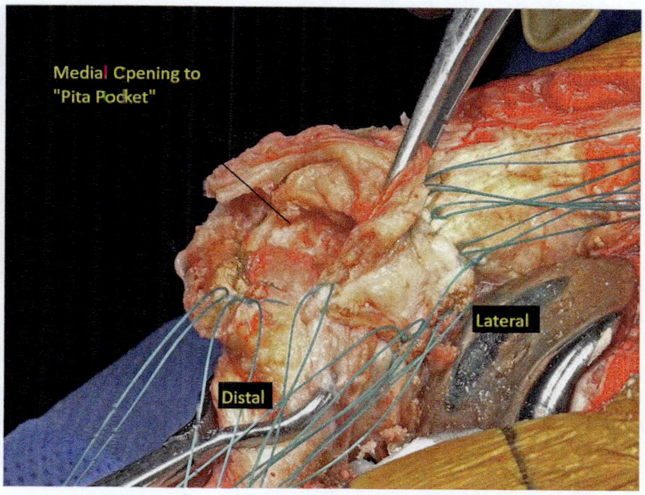

Figure 72.6 | Intraoperative photograph demonstrating the medial opening to the "pita" pocket.

- As small amounts of bone graft are introduced, the graft is tightly impacted into the lateral, superior, and inferior aspects of the pocket with a bone tamp before adding additional bone graft into the pouch.
- Approximately 50 mL of cancellous graft is required to stuff the tissue pouch to a final patellar composite height of greater than 25 mm. Creating this final height is important as the cancellous bone tends to compress about 3 to 5 mm postoperatively as it tracks in the femoral trochlea.
- After impaction grafting, the medial opening is closed with interrupted nonabsorbable sutures (Figure 72.8). The remainder of the patellar rim closure is carefully inspected to ensure a watertight closure.
- Patellar tracking is assessed to ensure central tracking of the patellar construct (Figure 72.9).
- The arthrotomy is then closed over drains with multiple interrupted nonabsorbable sutures.

Postoperative Care

- There are no unique postoperative rehabilitation or weight-bearing restrictions after this patellar bone grafting procedure.

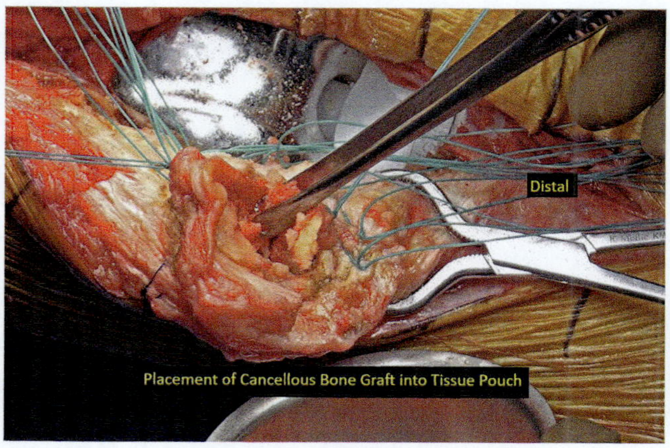

Figure 72.7 | Placement of bone graft into the patellar pouch.

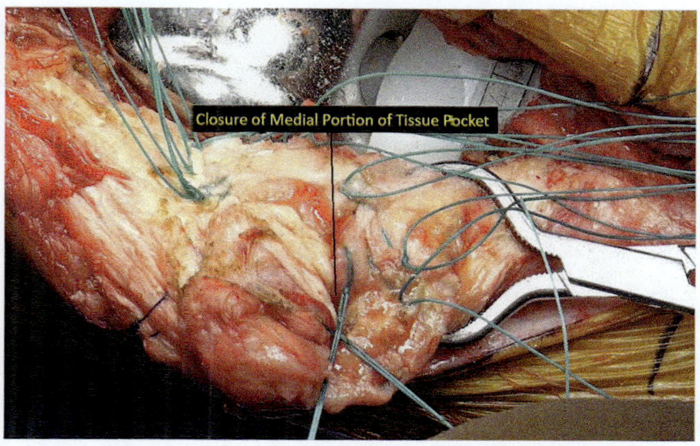

Figure 72.8 | Closure of the medial portion of the patellar pocket.

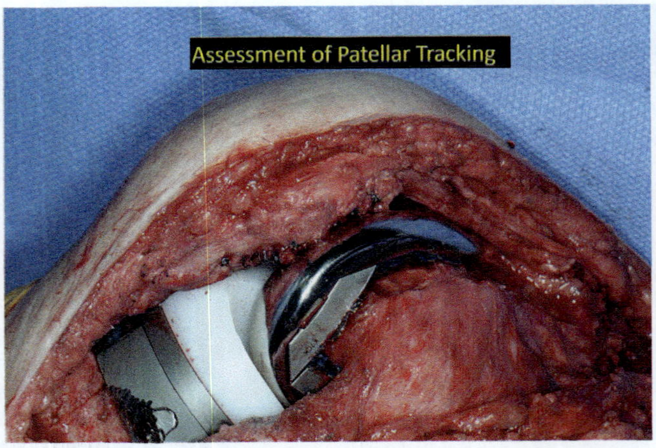

Figure 72.9 | Intraoperative assessment of patellar tracking after closure of the patellar pocket with bone grafting.

Suggested Reading

1. Hanssen AD. Bone-grafting for severe patellar bone loss during revision knee arthroplasty. *J Bone Joint Surg Am*. 2001;83-A(2):171-176.
2. Hanssen AD, Pagnano MW. Revision of failed patellar components. *Instr Course Lect*. 2004;53:201-206.

Chapter 73
Extensor Mechanism Deficiency

MATTHEW P. ABDEL
ARLEN D. HANSSEN

Key Concepts

- Extensor mechanism deficiency following total knee arthroplasty (TKA) can occur owing to disruption of the patellar tendon or the quadriceps tendon or catastrophic patellar fracture. Each situation requires a slightly different anatomic reconstructive approach.
- Principles of the reconstruction depend on whether the extensor discontinuity is acute, subacute, or chronic. If chronic, the quadriceps mechanism retracts proximally and scars to the adjacent soft tissues and femur.
- The rotational position and status of prosthesis fixation should be determined either preoperatively or immediately after surgical exposure as loose or malrotated implants require concomitant revision.
- Some patients with chronic extensor deficiency develop varying degrees of global instability that may be amenable to simple upsizing of tibial insert only.
- If there is concomitant deep periprosthetic infection, a 2-stage approach is recommended. In most cases, owing to the extensor mechanism disruption, a nonarticulating spacer will be required as articulating spacers are prone to tibiofemoral dislocation.
- Extensor mechanism reconstruction has historically been done with whole extensor or Achilles tendon allografts. However, our preferred technique is to use synthetic mesh for reconstruction. The rationale for using mesh is that multiple sutures passed through friable host tissue are stabilized and more secure when those multiple sutures also pass through the synthetic mesh graft.

Sterile Instruments and Implants

- Routine revision TKA instruments and implants
- Specific implants and tibial inserts for partial revision cases
- High-speed burr
- Cancellous bone screws
- 5-0 and #1 nonabsorbable suture
- 10" × 14" sheet of knitted monofilament polypropylene mesh (Marlex mesh; C.R. Bard, Inc., Murray Hill, NJ, USA) (Figure 73.1)
- *Important note: this surgical mesh should be the variety that allows soft-tissue ingrowth and not one of the newer variety meshes that prevent tissue ingrowth.*
- Use of a sterile tourniquet that allows for an extremely proximal skin incision is recommended.

Surgical Approaches

- Utilize the most recent and reasonable skin incision and anticipate considerable proximal extensile exposure to identify and mobilize the quadriceps, particularly in chronic cases.

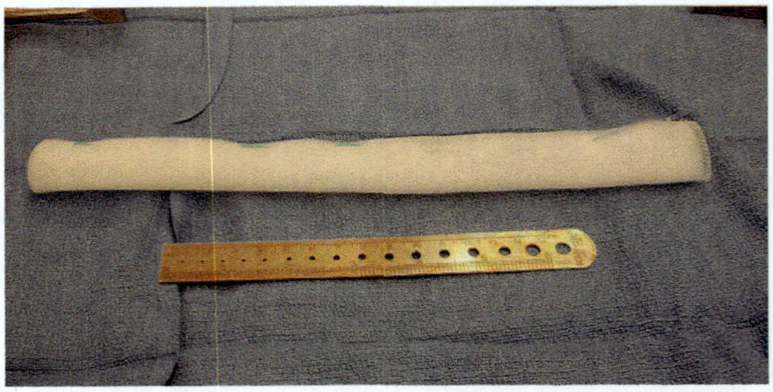

Figure 73.1 | An intraoperative picture of a 10" × 14" sheet of Marlex mesh folded on itself 8 to 10 times and then unitized with a #5 nonabsorbable suture.

Preoperative Planning

- Determine whether existing implants are well fixed and/or well positioned.
- Obtain prosthesis records for indwelling implants and arrange for these specific implants in the event that partial revision might be performed with the extensor mechanism reconstruction.
- If prior reconstructive attempts with allograft have been performed, it is helpful to obtain operative records to review that surgeon's description of technique to facilitate complete removal of allograft tissue.

Bone, Implant, and Soft Tissue Techniques

- Depending on the location of the extensor mechanism disruption, the choice of how to perform the arthrotomy is critical.
- *Patellar tendon disruption.* In these patients, the distal tissue is often thin and redundant. Midline division of this tissue to create equal medial and lateral tissue flaps up to the inferior pole of the patella is important for eventual wound closure and distal coverage of the mesh.
- If the patella is absent, simply extending the arthrotomy in the midline is performed; otherwise, a standard medial parapatellar arthrotomy is performed.
- *Quadriceps tendon disruption.* In these patients the medial and lateral halves of the quadriceps are usually retracted proximally and to their respective sides. The arthrotomy in these circumstances should be performed adjacent to the medial edge of the vastus lateralis to maximize the amount of tissue that remains attached to the vastus medialis muscle. This is very helpful for eventual distal and lateral translation of the vastus medialis at final closure.
- If the patella is present, distal extension of a parapatellar arthrotomy is performed; otherwise, the arthrotomy is carried in the midline down to the tibial tubercle.
- *Important note: Do not resect any redundant native healthy tissue, particularly distally, as often this tissue is required for arthrotomy closure and coverage of the mesh.*
- Determination is made as to whether the tibial and femoral components require revision or whether a tibial liner exchange will confer adequate joint stability.
- The 10" × 14" sheet of mesh is first prepared by folding it to a width of 15 mm that is 8-ply thick (Figure 73.1). Thereafter, it is unitized with a single #5 nonabsorbable suture placed in a running locked fashion along the free margin.
- If the tibial component is retained, the technique for distal stabilization of the mesh is performed by the creation of a proximal tibial window using a high-speed burr (Figure 73.2).
- Wet bone cement is delivered into the tibial trough with a syringe (Figures 73.3A and B, 73.4A and B). It is often helpful to predrip 1 inch of the mesh into the wet cement before placing it in the tibial trough. The mesh is inserted in the tibial trough to a depth of 3 to 5 cm. After the cement has completely hardened, a 4.5-mm (smaller patients) or 6.5-mm (larger patients) cancellous bone screw is placed to transfix tibia, cement, and mesh.
- If the tibial component is revised, the mesh is inserted into the medullary canal simultaneously with implantation of the new tibial component (Figure 73.5).

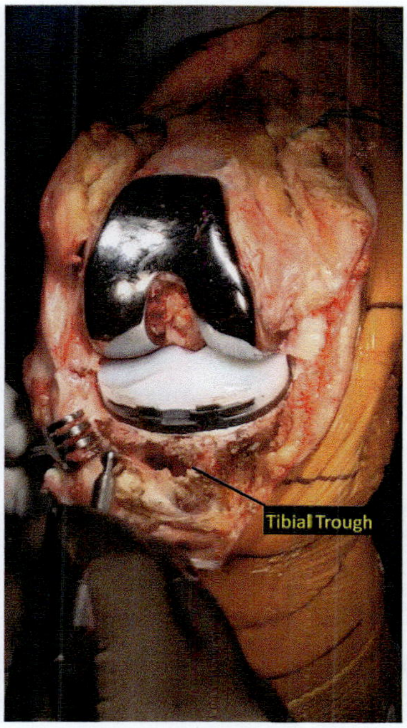

Figure 73.2 | An intraoperative picture of a 1" × 1" × 1" tibia trough created anterior to the tibial keel in a case in which the tibial component is maintained.

- As most cases are chronic, extensile proximal exposure of the quadriceps mechanism is required to release scar on both the ventral and dorsal aspects of the vastus medialis and vastus lateralis (Figure 73.6A and B). Usually the vastus lateralis does not retract as much as the vastus medialis, which can retract surprisingly far proximally.
- The vastus lateralis is then drawn as far distally as possible so that the mesh can be delivered from inside out through a small portal and secured with several nonabsorbable sutures (Figure 73.7).
- The mesh is securely attached to the ventral surface of the vastus lateralis with multiple interrupted sutures, a running Krackow suture, or both (Figure 73.8).

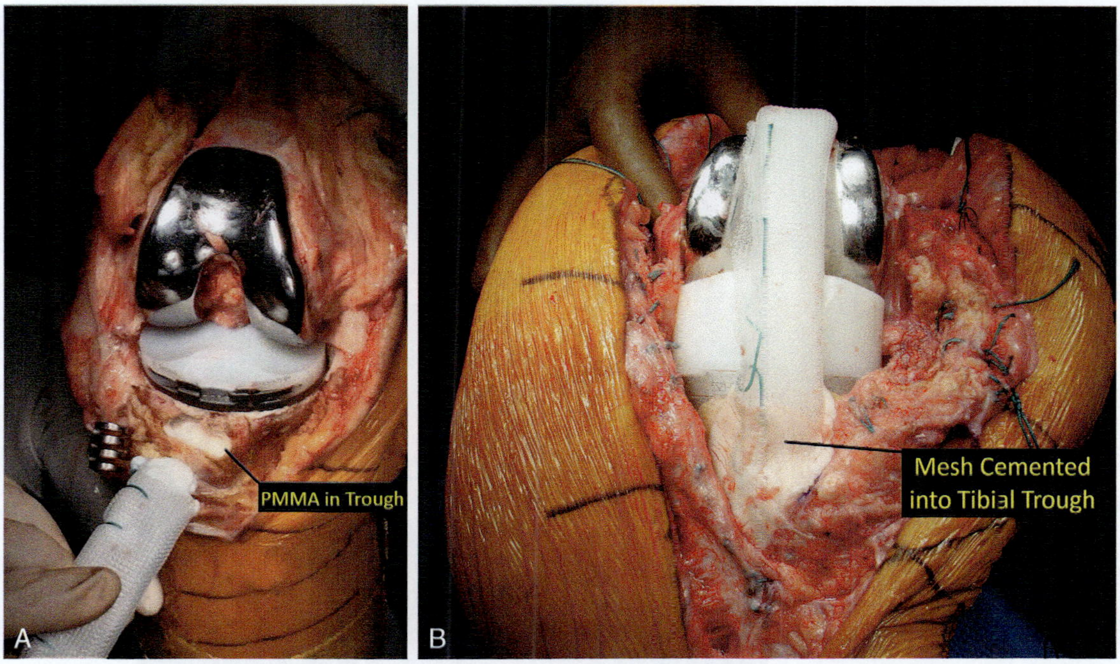

Figure 73.3 | A, Cement is then inserted into the tibial trough through the use of a syringe. The tip of the Marlex mesh is also predipped in the cement before insertion. B, This intraoperative picture depicts the Marlex mesh cemented into the tibial trough. The cement is allowed to cure before moving forward.

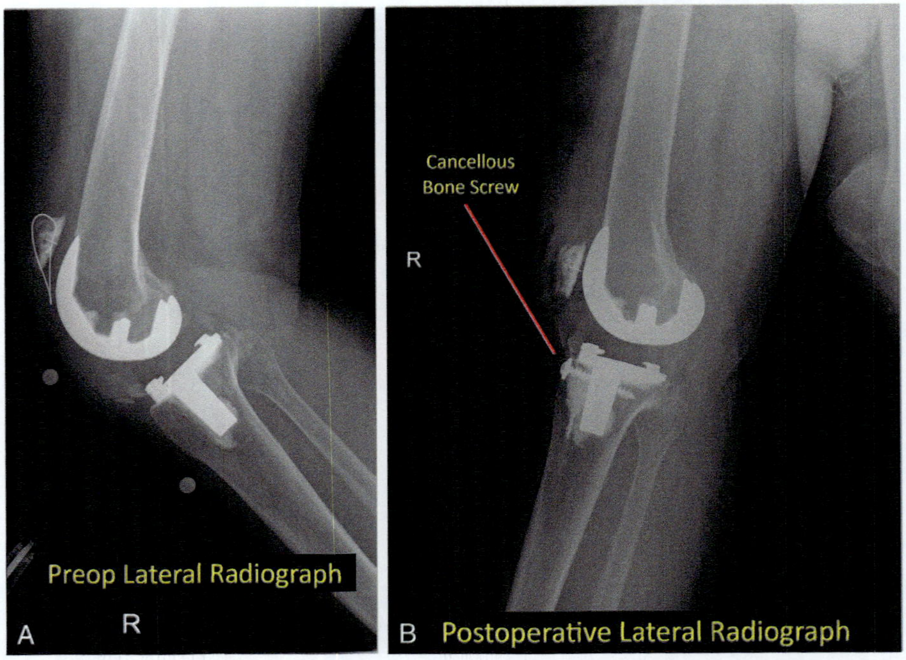

Figure 73.4 | A, Lateral radiograph depicting patella alta, indicative of a patellar tendon disruption after attempted repair at an outside institution. B, Lateral radiograph revealing anatomic placement of the patella after Marlex mesh reconstruction as depicted by the cancellous screw going through the mesh, cured cement, and host bone.

- The vastus medialis is now advanced distally and laterally over the mesh in a pants-over-vest method (Figure 73.9). It is important to make sure the mesh is entirely covered by the vastus medialis so that the mesh does not wick blood and joint fluid into the subcutaneous tissue plane.
- At some point in the distal closure, redundant tissue from the medial or lateral margins should be placed between the mesh and the tibial component so that the mesh is not in direct contact with the prosthesis (Figure 73.10). Occasionally, this is done with a free tissue flap harvested from the fibrous tissue in the suprapatellar region of the knee joint.
- Multiple #5 and #1 nonabsorbable sutures are passed through the vastus medialis and mesh so that every suture incorporates mesh (Figure 73.11).

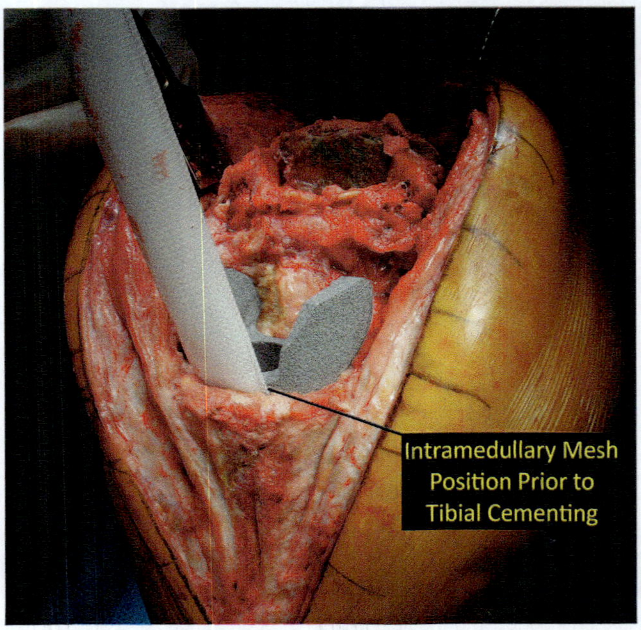

Figure 73.5 | An intraoperative picture depicting a Marlex mesh reconstruction during a procedure where the tibial component is also revised. In these cases, the mesh is placed intramedullary and a tibial trough is not required.

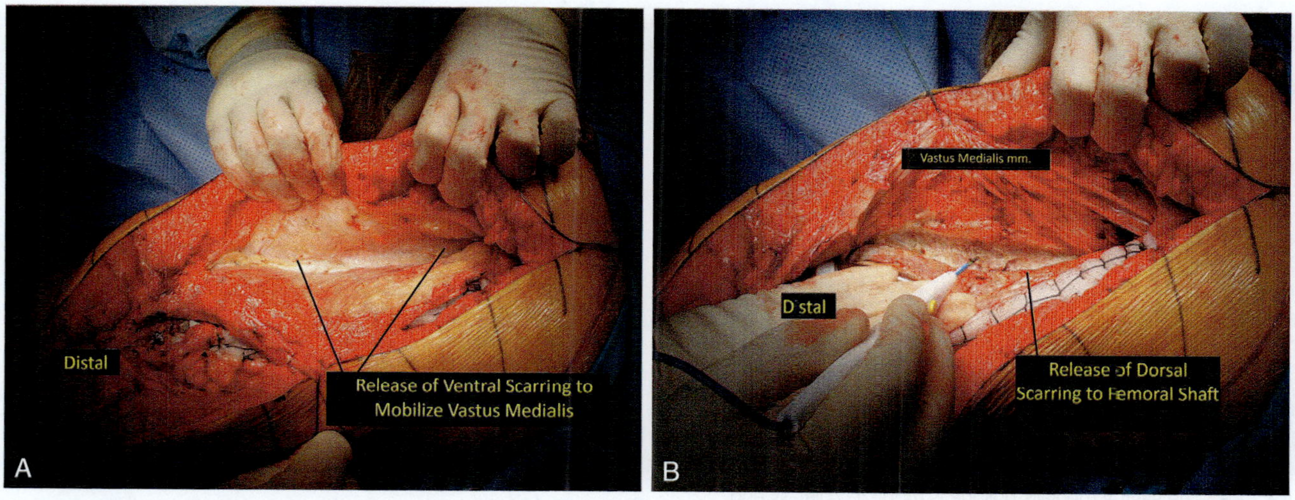

Figure 73.6 I Scar tissue from the vastus medialis oblique must be removed from both the ventral (A) and dorsal (B) aspects of the muscle so that it can be mobilized inferiorly.

- Typically, advancement and closure of the vastus medialis is performed from distal to proximal so that several deep drains can be inserted before final proximal closure. After closure, the knee joint typically has only 30° to 40° of flexion present, although this should not be tested.
- The subcutaneous tissues and skin are closed in the usual fashion, and the limb is placed in a bulky Robert Jones cotton compression dressing with a posterior plaster slab.

Postoperative Care

- At 48 hours, the wound is evaluated and the leg is placed in a long leg cast incorporating the foot with the knee flexed to 5°.
- In extremely obese patients, a custom bivalved thigh-leg-foot orthosis is used, and this can be fit preoperatively.
- The cast is changed and sutures are removed at 2 to 3 weeks. Total casting time is 12 weeks.
- At 3 months, the cast is removed and the limb placed in a hinged knee brace full time for an additional 3 months. The patient is allowed to do only active gravity flexion exercises in the brace, which is adjusted monthly at 45° for first month, 60° for second month, and 90° for third month. The patient is allowed to weight bear during this time with the brace locked at 0°.
- During this time, and after brace removal, it is recommended that the patient use an ambulatory aid such as a cane or walking stick to help prevent a fall that hyperflexes the knee and disrupts the extensor mechanism reconstruction.

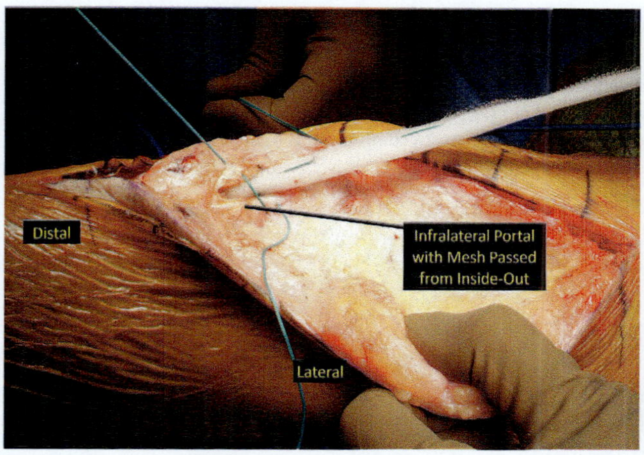

Figure 73.7 I The Marlex mesh is delivered from inside out through a small portal and secured with several nonabsorbable sutures.

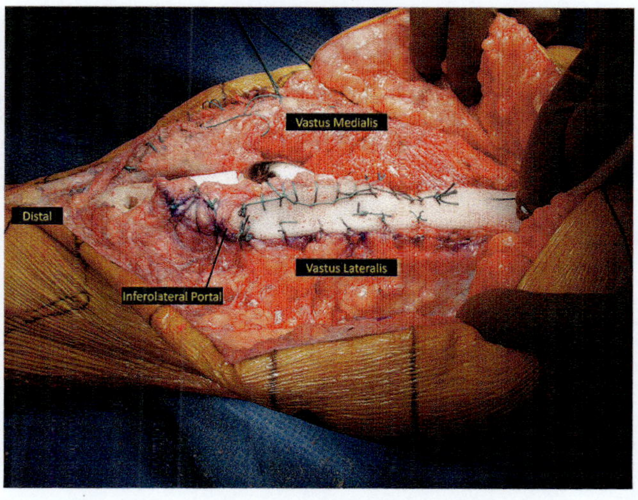

Figure 73.8 I The mesh is secured to the ventral surface of the vastus lateralis with multiple interrupted nonabsorbable sutures.

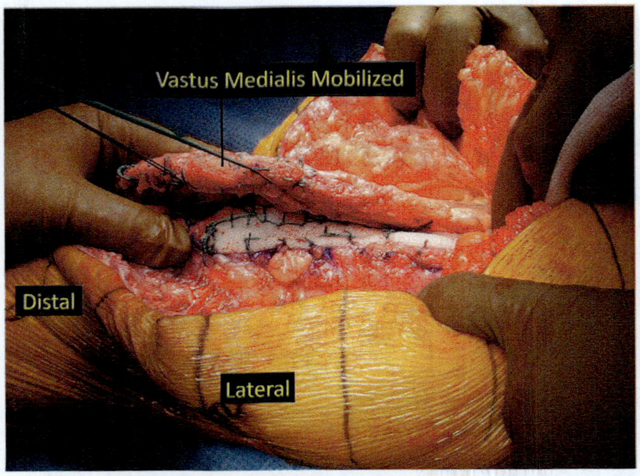

Figure 73.9 | The vastus medialis oblique is mobilized distally and laterally over the Marlex mesh in a pants-over-vest fashion.

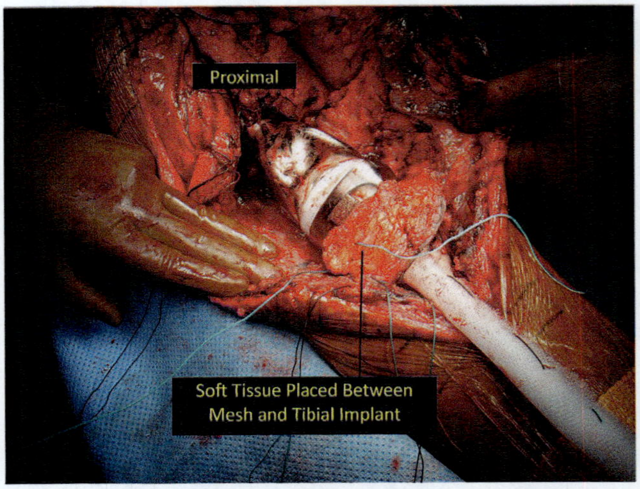

Figure 73.10 | The surgeon should use remaining scar tissue to cover both the ventral and dorsal aspects of the mesh from any portion of the implant and the subcutaneous tissue.

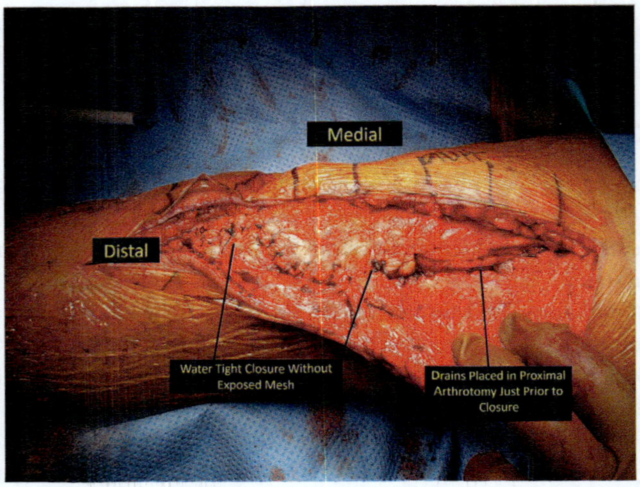

Figure 73.11 | The remaining arthrotomy should be closed with #1 nonabsorbable sutures.

Suggested Reading

1. Browne JA, Hanssen AD. Reconstruction of patellar tendon disruption after total knee arthroplasty: results of a new technique utilizing synthetic mesh. *J Bone Joint Surg Am*. 2011;93(12):1137-1143.
2. Nam D, Abdel MP, Cross MB, et al. The management of extensor mechanism complications in total knee arthroplasty. AAOS exhibit selection. *J Bone Joint Surg Am*. 2014;96(6):e47.

Index

Note: Page numbers followed by "f" indicate figures and "t" indicate tables.

V

W